Basic Concepts of
CLINICAL ELECTROPHYSIOLOGY
in Audiology

Editor-in-Chief for Audiology
Brad A. Stach, PhD

Basic Concepts of CLINICAL ELECTROPHYSIOLOGY in Audiology

John D. Durrant, PhD
Cynthia G. Fowler, PhD
John A. Ferraro, PhD
Suzanne C. Purdy, PhD

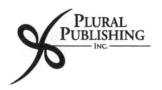

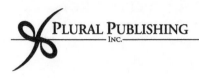

5521 Ruffin Road
San Diego, CA 92123

e-mail: information@pluralpublishing.com
Web site: https://www.pluralpublishing.com

Copyright © 2023 by Plural Publishing, Inc.

Typeset in 10.5/13 ITC Garamond Book by Achorn International
Printed in the United States of America by Integrated Books International

All rights, including that of translation, reserved. No part of this publication may be reproduced, stored in a retrieval system, or transmitted in any form or by any means, electronic, mechanical, recording, or otherwise, including photocopying, recording, taping, Web distribution, or information storage and retrieval systems without the prior written consent of the publisher.

For permission to use material from this text, contact us by
Telephone: (866) 758-7251
Fax: (888) 758-7255
e-mail: permissions@pluralpublishing.com

Every attempt has been made to contact the copyright holders for material originally printed in another source. If any have been inadvertently overlooked, the publisher will gladly make the necessary arrangements at the first opportunity.

Library of Congress Cataloging-in-Publication Data:

Names: Durrant, John D., editor. | Fowler, Cynthia G., editor. |
   Ferraro, John A., editor. | Purdy, Suzanne C. (Suzanne Carolyn), editor.
Title: Basic concepts of clinical electrophysiology in audiology /
   [edited by] John D. Durrant, Cynthia G. Fowler, John A. Ferraro, Suzanne C. Purdy.
Description: San Diego, CA : Plural, [2023] | Includes bibliographical
   references and index.
Identifiers: LCCN 2021017656 (print) | LCCN 2021017657 (ebook) |
   ISBN 9781635501759 (hardcover) | ISBN 163550175X (hardcover) |
   ISBN 9781635501797 (ebook)
Subjects: MESH: Audiometry, Evoked Response | Hearing Disorders—diagnosis |
   Electrophysiological Phenomena
Classification: LCC RF294 (print) | LCC RF294 (ebook) | NLM WV 272 |
   DDC 617.8/075—dc23
LC record available at https://lccn.loc.gov/2021017656
LC ebook record available at https://lccn.loc.gov/2021017657

Contents

Foreword by José Juan Barajas de Prat ... ix
Preface ... xiii
Special Message to Student Readers and Others Aspiring Toward Competent Use of
    Clinical Neurophysiology in Audiology ... xiii
Special Message to Instructors Adopting This Textbook ... xv
Acknowledgments ... xxi
Contributors ... xxiii
Dedication ... xxvii

1 Basic Concepts of Clinical Electrophysiology in Audiology ... 1
Prequel—A Peek at the Auditory Evoked Potentials and Areas of Application ... 1
    John D. Durrant
    Heads Up: Like in Space, It Takes Time to Travel Along the Auditory
        Pathway—So What? ... 2

2 Signals and Systems Essentials ... 7
Signal Generation, Analysis, and Conditioning—Analog Versus Digital Perspectives ... 7
    J. Robert Boston and John D. Durrant
Temporal Versus Spectral Views: The Saga Continues—Impulsive Versus Steady State ... 20
    W. Wiktor Jedrzejczak
    Heads Up: Prequel 2: Why Are Computers So Important in This Area of
        Audiology and Are They Everywhere? ... 29
        Rafael E. Delgado
Signal-Issues Particular to Stimulating the Auditory System and the
    Importance of Being Calibrated ... 34
    Robert F. Burkard
    Heads Up: Wideband Transmission and the Middle Ear Bottleneck ... 43
        M. Patrick Feeney

3 Electrically Connecting to Humans To Access Their Auditory
Neurosensory Systems ... 49
Bioelectric Basics, Interface Dilemmas, and Electrode Montages/Caps—
    One Size Fits All? ... 49
    John D. Durrant, Krzysztof M. Kochanek, and Lech K. Śliwa
Functional Neuroanatomy of "AEP Space" and Underlying Neurophysiological Bases ... 62
    Frank E. Musiek
    Heads Up: Need That Like a Hole in the Head? What About a Nail?
        A Case in Point! ... 77
        Christopher D. Bauch and Wayne O. Olsen

4 Stimulating the Auditory System and the How and Why of an "Evoked" Response — 83

Extracting the Response's Signal From Noise Background — 83
Steven L. Bell

The Good, Bad, and Ugly—Optimizing Response Extraction From Background Noise and How Signal Processing May Become Too Much — 101
Ozcan Ozdamar and John D. Durrant

Heads Up: Interlude—And You Don't Even Have To Raise Your Hand When You Hear the Beep — 115
John D. Durrant, Cynthia G. Fowler, and Suzanne C. Purdy

5 Evoking Responses of the Peripheral Auditory System — 121

First Sign Something's Going On in There: An Acoustic Response of the Inner Ear — 121
Jacek Smurzynski

Heads Up: Otoacoustic Emission Without Turning On Sound? Who Knew? — 134
W. Wiktor Jedrzejczak

CM, SP, and AP: Not Alphabet Soup and First Signs AEPs Are Afoot! — 138
John D. Durrant and John A. Ferraro

Electrocochleography: How Do Electrical Signals Get From Hearing Organs to the "Outside" and What Good Are They? — 147
John A. Ferraro and John D. Durrant

Heads Up: Intriguing ECochG App: Sensing Weakened Wall of Semicircular Canal — 159
John D. Durrant, John A. Ferraro, and José Juan Barajas de Prat

What More Can Electrocochleography Teach, Including About What to Expect Later? — 163
Martin Walger

6 Evoking Responses of the Central Auditory System: Testing the Brainstem — 177

Brainstem Auditory Evoked Potential: General Interpretation—Its Nature and Peripheral Versus Central Systems Aspects — 177
George A. Tavartkiladze

Heads Up: Binaural Interaction in Auditory Brainstem Potentials — 193
Cynthia G. Fowler

Brainstem Responses to Complex Stimuli—Frequency and Envelope Following Responses — 195
David Purcell and Viji Easwar

Heads Up: Speech-Evoked EFR and FFR — 205
Ananthanarayan Krishnan

Auditory Steady-State Response—80-Hz Response — 209
Maria C. Perez-Abalo

Evoked Potential Audiometry Using Auditory Brainstem Response/Auditory Steady-State Response Measurements — 219
Susan A. Small

Differential Diagnostic Applications — 231
Cynthia G. Fowler and Jun Ho Lee

DOUBLE-HEADERs UP
Heads Up: Differential Diagnostic Case Studies and the
  Challenge of Auditory Neuropathy ... 247
  Jun Ho Lee and José Juan Barajas de Prat
Heads Up: Postauricular Muscle Response—Friend/Foe/Why Care? ... 254
  Suzanne C. Purdy

7 Testing Midbrain and Cortical Projection Pathways ... 271
Auditory Middle Latency Response and 40-Hz Auditory Steady-State Response—
  Signals En Route to the Cortex ... 271
  Joaquín T. Valderamma-Valenzuela
Why Evoked Response Audiometry (ERA) Using AMLR or 40-Hz ASSR Measures ... 284
  Cynthia G. Fowler and So E. Park
Differential Diagnostic Applications of AMLR ... 292
  Thierry Morlet and So E. Park
  Heads Up: BIC Update—Whither Beyond Pontine CANS ... 302
    Cynthia G. Fowler and So E. Park

8 Cortical Level Testing ... 313
Call Them Late, But They Were the First AEPs for Practical ERA—LLRs ... 313
  Barbara K. Cone
Why ERA Using Cortical Response Measurement ... 322
  Linda J. Hood, Rafael E. Delgado, and Abreena I. Tlumak
  Heads Up: A Case Spared Operative Treatment Thanks to Testing of Both
    Brainstem and Cortical AEPs ... 332
    John D. Durrant and Martin Walger
Late-Late Shows in AEPdom—Beyond Obligatory Potentials: When Just Turning
  On the Same Stimulus Is Not Enough ... 336
  Mridula Sharma
DOUBLE-HEADERs UP
  Heads Up: Peek at EEG Analyses Via Advanced Signal Processing ... 349
    Ronny K. Ibrahim and Mridula Sharma
  Heads Up: The Change Potential—Sometimes What's Later Tells More ... 352
    Fabrice Bardy

9 Difficult-to-Test Patients—General Methods and Newborn Screening ... 365
Screening Hearing Responses Versus Threshold Estimation and
  Estimating Audiometric Configuration ... 365
  Monica J. Chapchap and Patricia C. Mancini
Bone Conduction Testing—A Special Challenge, Yet Efficacious With Understanding ... 377
  Susan A. Small
Testing Patients Under Natural Sleep or Medically Induced Sedation/Unconsciousness ... 388
  Diane L. Sabo
  Heads Up: Testing Patients Who "Exaggerate" Their Hearing Thresholds ... 395
    John D. Durrant and Cynthia G. Fowler
Testing Patients With Cochlear or Brainstem Implants ... 400
  Andy J. Beynon

10 Testing Potentially Beyond Hearing-Related Yet of Interest in Audiology the Profession — 421

Heads Up: Not Only Electric Fields, Magnetic Fields Too—Confirming Origins — 421
   John D. Durrant, David L. McPherson, and Lionel Collet

Quick Look at Intraoperative Neuromonitoring and Other Evoked Potentials — 428
   Abreena I. Tlumak and John D. Durrant

Heads Up: A Case of Elective Surgery That Could Have Gone Badly Were It Not for IONM — 441
   John D. Durrant and Abreena I. Tlumak

Whose Land Is This? — 444
   Suzanne C. Purdy

Index — 455

Foreword

This book is meant to be a basic introduction for students interested in auditory electrophysiology of the peripheral and central auditory systems, particularly those intending to enter the professional practice of audiology, although certainly not exclusively. This volume provides a guideline and a comprehensive overview of measurement of auditory evoked potentials and other responses of possible interest in this field. It reflects the work of a group of clinicians and scientists who have been working in auditory electrophysiology for years and sharing their research and clinical findings at biennial symposia of the International Evoked Response Audiometry Study Group (IERASG). The group was seeded over a half century ago by its iconic founder, the late Hallowell Davis, easily recognized as the "father" of evoked response audiometry.

The two most key terms of this book are *brain* and *auditory evoked potential (AEP)*. Let's start with *brain*. The only way the brain can grasp reality is through the processing of signals sent up pathways from specialized sensory organs. Evolution has been selecting neurons by trial-error principles. Many of these neurons, gifted with properties that provide them with special physiological characteristics, procure information on sensorial states and that has become a part of our genetic predetermination. From the very moment of our birth, these neuronal circuits are exposed to sensorial experiences that will be stored in our personal memory. Every sensation, being in its own nature secret and abstract, should be regarded as an interpretation and classification of events based on past individual or species-specific experiences. Thus, experience operates on physiological events giving them mental significance. These sensorial experiences become our mental possessions.

Unlike other species that are exoskeleton (crabs), humans are mainly endoskeleton. The bad news is that it is precisely the area where the brain lies that is exoskeleton. In fact, the brain is surrounded by an implacable bony frame and, to make matters worse, the auditory sensorial organ is hidden inside the hardest bone in the human body, the temporal bone, in such a way that our knowledge of brain function cannot be obtained by direct means.

However, the good news is that many years ago we learned that if we attach a pair of electrodes to the surface of the human scalp and connect them to suitable instrumentation, the minute electrical signal recorded could be used to discern brain activity locked in time to a sensory experience. Such signals can even be recorded and processed in a manner that suggests the resulting response reflects cognition—a higher level of the brain's job than mere sound detection. Never before have we had a *toolbox* with such a powerful instrumentation to extract audiological electrophysiological information of the nervous system. Still, it remains the user's responsibility to have the appropriate knowledge base and skill set to properly make use of this important armamentarium and to be mindful in their use in research and clinical strategies alike.

In this text, the reader is led along the temporal sequential process that gives rise to AEPs, a sort of *journey* from the receptor (ear) to the cortex. As expected from conventional audiometry, the stimuli will play a key role in pursuit of the ascending activation of the auditory pathway. The AEPs elicited will take on characteristics in different ways along the way. Tools then will be needed to analyze both stimulus and response. Therefore, before setting off on this journey, our luggage will have to include a substantial *toolbox* by which to reveal important parameters of measurements of their stimulus-response relationships. Another important preliminary concept to bear in mind is that, at all times, we are looking for physiological events that provide only indirect evidence of the phenomenal sense of audition. At the same time, the tools in the box presented will have gotten there only from extensive vetting, which in the clinical sciences is best expressed as *evidence based*. The box contains plenty of technology that has greatly empowered modern advances, including advanced digital-signal processing, but without a truckload of equipment for general-purpose computing.

The tools often will draw on concepts outside of routine audiometry conducted in the course of the basic audiological evaluation. Occasionally something like masking—to help ensure the results have come by way of processing of sound by the ear intended—will be equally of concern in assessing AEPs. Often, and naturally, assessment of these electrophysiological signals will be scrutinized in relation to results of behavioral audiometry. Prior knowledge of that area will help the reader to best understand the intent and information within this book. Such foundation of knowledge then is built on the side of electrophysiological methods, not in isolation nor to its exclusion. Another parallel and important concern from the "culture" of behavioral audiometry is calibration—not only of stimuli and acoustic test environments but also of the AEP test parameters. There will be a goodly number of methodological procedures presented as a part of molding the tools in the box, some of which will be in the vein of audiometry and others will be unique to electrophysiological methodology.

A particular challenge will be to extract signals of interest in less than ideal circumstances. The reader with be challenged to wonder what's real—whether or not the recording of a given AEP and time of measurement actually corresponds to the subject's real biological response. Here too, this concept is not unique to electrophysiology. Again, in behavior, the patient is asked to signal when hearing the stimulus presented. Can the response always be trusted to reliably reflect the patient's true hearing sensitivity? Furthermore, what if during the examination workers next door were preparing a room for, let's say, another/new test booth? If sudden banging on the wall occurred during audiometric assessment, are any responses observed still credible? These or like issues pervade clinical electrophysiology. Some tools will be dedicated to addressing the challenge. Fortunately, the toolbox will prove to be robust in this regard. Some of the "tricks of the trade" in electrophysiology will not be alien but addressable by common approaches (in concept) in behavioral science. For example, in the assessment of a test's reliability, there are similarities between the previous example in judging an individual's response and evaluating success of hearing screening of industrial workers. Were the tests reliable/repeatable or even valid in the first place? Such matters are often approached in good part using statistics. It will be seen that signals can be recorded and treated as sets of data; as such, they too are often treatable statistically (such as with measures of central tendency and tests of correlation).

A clear understanding of the neuroanatomy and neurophysiology of the auditory system will help the clinician to understand the AEP attributes at each level of the auditory system and their interpretation. The editors and writers rightfully do not accept full responsibility to cover such background. Nevertheless, they do endeavor to catalog and present in appropriate depth (for the scope and aims of the book) nuances that most help to account for origins and nature of the AEPs commonly employed in clinical electrophysiology in audiology. Here, it is important to establish at the outset that there is not always a direct relationship between structure and function or that the electrophysiological response does not always reveal the precise locus of a particular dysfunction. Nevertheless, principles will be expressed by which to interpret AEP "findings" for a useful functional level of assessment. Predictably, one of the common final paths between conventional audiological (behavioral) tests and findings of AEP measurement(s) will be the derivation of an estimate of just how sensitive is the patient's auditory system and perhaps other correlations between test modalities. Here the reader is ensured of some interesting "twists" (in effect) along the auditory pathway.

This book gives the opportunity both to beginners and even more advanced students/readers to review the intriguing area of clinical auditory electrophysiology as well as various overviews of areas beyond and/or not necessarily broadly used clinically, yet promising and truly fun facts beyond the primary scope of the text. Within the scope, the text is written in a very practical way and provides comprehensive information of direct application in both clinical settings and for research purposes. The main aim of the book, I submit, has been achieved by trying to answer the questions of what technology to use and when and what is well supported fundamentally—salient principles that are supported substantially by an evidence base. The coverage demonstrates, indeed, that the *toolbox* is bountiful. Now, it soon will be your turn to decide what tools to use for your clinical objectives or perhaps even a research plan. We hope this book can help you make the right choice. Good Luck!

—José Juan Barajas de Prat, MD, PhD

Preface

> **The Producers**
>
> John D. Durrant
> Cynthia G. Fowler
> John A. Ferraro
> Suzanne C. Purdy

i. Special Message to Student Readers and Others Aspiring Toward Competent Use of Clinical Neurophysiology in Audiology

If this page is the first one to which you have jumped, dear reader, please return to the *Foreword*. It will help your mindset for reading this textbook throughout, namely to do so with a sense of curiosity and adventure. Thereafter, let us address the perennial question up front about the content to follow in this preface; it should not "be on the exam", if the *Producers* have any say in this. However, that does not relieve you of the responsibility to read the following, for the best experience and learning with this textbook. The next questions should be, "Who are 'the producers?'" and, "Why are you talking that way?" They (well, we) are the editors of this volume—a document of substantial proportion (OK, it's long) to serve purposes of instruction in a technically demanding, yet clinically important, part of assessment of function of the auditory system. In general, there are numerous academic books produced among the professions intended particularly for students in postgraduate education, often toward a clinical or research accreditation and/or for credentialed workers in the professions trying to keep abreast of the incredibly voluminous literature in the clinical sciences alone. Any authors of such books are expected to speak with authority about what is important to know, where a field is heading, or perhaps about the current or the lack of standards of practice, and so forth. This is a tall order for any singular author to pull off. Here, the production has been envisioned in the context of how the editors hope readers will embrace this book. The production concept of this book is in reference to the likes of projects that give us today's television or cinematic "productions," often in some variant of a series of *episodes* that, with good luck, may be sponsored for multiple seasons of a given show.

The producers of this volume have recruited a considerable number of writers to join them in their production of series that truly are intended to be followed from the first chapter—*season*—and therein sequentially through each series of stories—again, episodes. The sequence comprises the logical building blocks of a foundation of knowledge. Each episode helps to present the topics of the next within a season, and each season leads to the next. While the concept of building a broad foundation of knowledge is the desired outcome, the "build" is not, say, a pyramid or, if a pyramid, then it is being built upside down. This depiction is simply how the auditory nervous system looks. The inner ear is a marvelous and cleverly designed part of this system, but it cannot think. Hence, we need the brain, which physically expands dramatically going up the pathway that is to be followed in our quest to fill the toolbox pondered in the *Foreword*. Special feature stories along the way, entitled *Heads Up* (HU), will entertain you further with still more facts, more advanced concepts, and/or more tools even beyond the scope of the last episode and/or the book. They will not be comprehensive presentations; they are intended more as, well, a heads-up about what else is going on. While perhaps not in routine practice today, they will concern promising methods worthy of at least some awareness. After all, this is a dynamic field.

xiii

The producers are from the rank and file of the profession of audiology, as it has come to be today. They are highly seasoned clinicians and educators as well as having individually contributed to the evidence base of the targeted subspecialty—clinical electrophysiology as applied to enrich audiology. The writers are similarly endowed contributors, the producers have been compelled to contribute as well, and the entire production team has been charged to ensure presentation of practices in this area that are consistent with the ever-evolving stories to be told. The subspecialty presented herein has been more than a half century in the making, through research and technological advances that have led to reasonably stable tools of the trade based on sound principles of understanding of auditory electrophysiology of clinical interest, or at least (again) of considerable promise.

The initial episodes embrace stories that the producers hope are more familiar in subject than not. These topics are not to be belabored in this book; if some readers find any topics beyond their comprehension after thorough reading, they certainly should take a pause to get some tutoring in that area. This textbook is intended for readers with undergraduate or like level of preparation, thus with the expectation that they will have studied hearing science and have some foundation of knowledge in general neuroanatomy and neurophysiology. For readers with such background, perhaps even more, the episodes are intended to serve as overviews. This approach permits the writers to zero in on bits of broader areas that specifically are relevant to readers' understanding and (ultimately) proper interpretation of results of tests of the auditory evoked potentials. As such, it will be advisable to avoid approaching the reading of this book somewhat in parallel to a no-no in reliable research—"cherry-picking" data that best suits the researcher's hypothesis. In that vein and in the present context, you thus are urged not to cherry-pick episodes, namely to read only the one(s) that you perceive as uniquely relevant to your clinical/other interest(s). First, this approach is likely to cause you to miss important lessons about principles; again, these episodes build the foundation for various clinically routine interests. Second, just selectively reading likely will not allow you to become empowered by the knowledge base as intended. The technology is not confined to one part of the brain and/or one clinical application. Therefore, why should users confine the competence of their knowledge? Topics herein are presented to minimize "reinventing wheels," rather starting with some "good wheels" and refining some parameters for the next application and/or level of the auditory system to be evaluated.

The end of each chapter provides a summary of key issues from the episodes and HUs in a brief segment called *Take-Home Messages* (THMs). The previous admonition for avoiding cherry-picking parts of the book to read is naturally followed by the "sin" of only reading abstracts of chapter summaries, journal articles, and so forth. Each THM is intended to be (borrowing jargon from comedic entertainment) somewhat like "one-liners," although often compound sentences taking more than one line of print to make the point. What they are not are "tell-alls," not even collectively. If the main points of the content provided were understood, these quasi-one-liners should be understood immediately. They also can contain some of the many abbreviations introduced in the episodes—an inherent part of vocabulary building—but not being redefined. The TMHs thus are designed to trigger recall, not reteach. They are presented with the conviction that there is no better way to renew memories than to review the relevant part of the chapter when the meaning of the THM is not clearly understood.

Lastly, much effort in production has been invested in producing the figures in a manner to fit the episodes. There are lots of them, but the objectives of this textbook and what all you really need to know (ultimately) to competently practice the methods presented cannot be learned from just looking at the figures and reading the captions. The flip side of that "coin" is not to judge importance of content based on density of figures or tables or, conversely, discounting portions of the text with relatively low numbers of figures. A picture well may be worth 1,000 words, but the narrative is still what frames the picture and expresses the intended relevance to the story in which it is presented. In any event, and by all means, please enjoy.

ii. Special Message to Instructors Adopting This Textbook

To anticipate perhaps a question, dear instructor, neither what the *Producers* have expressed directly to your students in *Preface i* nor what is expressed in the *Foreword* by our distinguished colleague should appear on an exam. However, they do reflect a bit of our motivation and approach to this textbook. The objective here is to address more specifically and thoroughly the authority that this group of editors has endeavored to impart to the book, both regarding the editors' backgrounds and commitments to minimize a couple of problems that sometimes can compromise a multiauthored volume intended primarily to serve as a textbook.

Even single or coauthored books can present difficulties achieving evenness of depth and style of writing throughout, especially given substantial diversity of content across chapters. The senior editor (to discount any self-impression of infallibility on this point) once suffered the sting of a prepublication review of a textbook wherein the reviewer pondered whether the same person had written both halves of the book. Even in books of one to a few authors, illustration materials typically derive from many sources and at times seem somewhat disjointed. Despite these challenges, edited texts often serve well the objective of producing a compendium of works on such topics as state of the science of methods, trends of research in a given area, and so forth. They still make great reference books and intellectual food for more advanced graduate students and postgraduate/professionals who are fully at ease going to the research/comparable literature. Indeed, the authority of such books, by way of skillfully recruited writers, is hard to match by one to few authors, given the relatively high level of technology and voluminous literatures of clinical sciences of today. We contend that for a textbook at the more foundational level, however numerous the contributors, it needs to be inviting and its contents flowing well across the book—the goals to which this volume is dedicated.

The production of this text was developed on the notion of having a group of very knowledgeable writers contribute to a volume wherein each draft would evolve from more detailed organization, interactive editing between editors and writers, and central management of illustration production. These steps in the current textbook were designed to ensure their fit to the main points presented, in synchrony with the table of contents, using novel figures as much as possible, and throughout more or less customizing them to the text's narrative. The picture being worth 1,000 words was not wisdom lost on our producers and writers. When details are expected to be recalled, images supported by adequate/well-correlated narratives can be particularly helpful come exam time. While at the graduate level the students certainly should be prepared to deal with the literature, articles containing voluminous data, and diverse ways of presentation of the data, this process need not be the initial goal all textbooks.

Here then is the product of collective efforts to build a solid foundation of reasonably well-established principles and practices in clinical electrophysiology of audiological interest. Coming full circle back to the written text, writers have been charged to address significant units of foundational knowledge as the editors see them, and therein were "assigned" as highly seasoned and trusted reporters to address various principles to build a substantively essential foundation for clinical work in this area.

The approach taken in this project also reflects the bias of the editors that objective measures today deserve more than a single term of coverage in academic programs, whether in the context of a master's or professional-doctoral curriculum. The mantra here is a priority of building the foundation of knowledge that hopefully will serve well in the growth and development of users of clinical electrophysiology for audiological applications as well as into the next course and beyond during their professional life. In general, the conviction guiding the production of this book is that competency in practice demands competent knowledge bases. For the student/novice reader, it is equally important to present material that will spur on their interests in further foundational building and with a hint that continued education (beyond degrees or certification) will be expected and is indeed essential for anyone intending to continue to practice in the field. We also have aimed to provide exposure and develop in the reader a recognition of various areas that are deemed, at this writing, as not yet ready for "prime-time," routine clinical practice. To this end, instructors also are encouraged to not include content of the *Heads Up* (HU) features (in effect, "short stories") for exam purposes. There is more than ample material for tests of comprehension in the episodes of each chapter to which any given HU is associated. Discuss them in class, nevertheless? Surely. If a term paper is required, they are also fair game for topics (and thus grading). Otherwise, please just let your students read the HUs and "get" what they can from these short stories, perhaps together with your own tutelage to address some of the issues therein and/or enhancing from your own experience. The topics of the HUs often are higher end, yet included to kindle interests for what else is "out there." In some cases, the HUs are used to plant seeds of upcoming episodes, but at that juncture, just a blush. This hopefully will tweak curiosity without "overcharging" their brains with issues not yet essential to the teaching points of the respective current episodes.

The notion of production of a volume dedicated to defining an essential foundation of knowledge for ultimate competency is not novel. In the latter 1980s, the Committee on Audiometric Evaluation, a standing committee of the American Speech-Language-Hearing Association, formed the Working Group on Auditory Evoked Potential Measurement. Academic audiologists recruited were charged to develop a guideline on "Competencies in Auditory Evoked Potential Measurement and Clinical Applications" (1990; *Asha* [Suppl. 2]). In the course of their deliberation, the group decided, in effect, that developing a monograph summarizing information gathered could be useful, subsequently published as "The Short Latency Auditory Evoked Potentials" (1988; *Asha*). This area, after all, was a subspecialty that had led to one of the most pervasive transformations of audiological practices, bringing clinical electrophysiology into routine practice in the hands of clinically certified audiologists. The working group members included editors Fowler and Ferraro. As chair of the working group, the senior editor, with additional help of Dr. Kenneth E. Wolf, subsequently rounded out the coverage to include longer latency potentials, published as a chapter in *Hearing Assessment* (W. F. Rintelmann [Ed.], 1991 [2nd ed.]; Pro-Ed). In the same vein, writers and editor-writers alike were challenged in the current project to present the most salient bases of a given method, application, and so forth but now appraised after over a half century of research and development comprising extensive clinical practice, well-developed evidence bases, and continuing research and development. Thereafter, they were asked to overview promising further advances. To get the writers "creative juices" both flowing and calibrated to the design and intended level of treatment in this textbook, the contributors were advised first to think of the assignment much as that of writing an editorial. From their expertise and scrutiny of the state of the science in their assigned areas respectively, they were asked to express what in their judgment are the most well-established principles and concepts that are truly foundational.

Our editors and several associate reviewers were recruited to help vet the manuscripts—highly seasoned academics in communication science and disorders or allied field who have dedicated substantial portions of their careers to clinical electrophysiology and other objective methods used in audiology today. All have substantially contributed to the evidence base of this book (thus active in research); they also have contributed broadly to higher education, instructional presentations at national/international society meetings, and/or educational publications. Senior editor Durrant was educated in a traditional American program in communication science and disorders (CSD), namely speech-and-hearing therapy in the day. He had a substantial formation in psychology and physiology, leading to a postgraduate education in audiology and physiological acoustics, earning the degree of doctor of philosophy and a postdoctoral fellowship (Northwestern University). He later became clinically certified and ultimately came to direct audiology clinics in the medical schools of Temple University and (more recently) the University of Pittsburgh, with primary and secondary appointments (or vice-versa) in otolaryngology and CSD. He lastly served as the vice-chair of the CSD department and is now a professor emeritus. He also had a 3-year stint of Atlantic-hopping bimonthly to the Université Lyon I (France) as an associated professor of medical physiology. These various posts and sites collectively allowed him over his career to work in nearly all areas covered in this book. A career-long member of the American Speech-Language-Hearing Association (ASHA), ultimately fellow and honoree of the Association, he also contributed to activities of the American Academy of Audiology (AAA). He and his colleague J. H. Lovrinic (professor, Temple University, retired) authored the first foundational book on hearing science for CSD programs by clinical audiologists—*Bases of Hearing Science* (1977, 1984, and 1995 [editions 1–3]; Williams and Wilkins). He continues to be active in the profession nationally and internationally and currently serves as a research scientist for Intelligent Hearing Systems (Miami) in projects supported by the National Institutes of Health. He remains actively involved in the International Society of Audiology, including as a founding associate editor of the *International Journal of Audiology*, and as the former chair of the Council of the International Evoked Response Audiometry Group (IERASG). In addition to his primary responsibility to this project, he managed the final production/reproduction of all figures as they appear herein.

Editor Fowler entered CSD with an undergraduate background in psychology. She soon became interested in auditory electrophysiology, which developed into a career. Upon consummating her clinical and research education (doctor of philosophy, Northwestern University), she served as a clinical and research audiologist at the Long Beach Veterans Hospital and University of California-Irvine, where she taught medical students and residents. At the VA, the audiology group attracted students from around the country and abroad in their clinical fellowship year, including having mentored many who became leaders in the field. She taught auditory electrophysiology at California State University-Los Angeles. She subsequently moved to the University of Wisconsin-Madison, where she continued to mentor students and pursue research in auditory electrophysiology. She subsequently developed and served as the founding director of the doctor-of-audiology program, a joint venture with the University of Wisconsin-Stevens Point. Her research program has been primarily concerned with clinical applications of auditory brainstem responses, yet not exclusively, and overall in pursuit of electrophysiological manifestations of perceptual events and effects of aging. She has been a career-long member of ASHA and elected Fellow of both ASHA and AAA. She has been active in still other professional associations, not the least of which is the IERASG (Council Member). In this project, she bore responsibility to review all contributions with the senior editor and particularly with the charge of copyediting to smooth out writing across the substantial number of contributors, including the other editors with their contributor hats on.

Editor Ferraro came to CSD as a card-carrying biologist (bachelor's and master's degrees with minors in chemistry and psychology). However, he became interested in the auditory system and earned his doctor of philosophy in speech and hearing sciences (University of Denver), followed by postdoctoral work in physiological acoustics (Northwestern University). He started his career at The Ohio State University, but in due course became more broadly recognized for his leadership in the Intercampus Program in Communicative Disorders, between Kansas City (medical center) and Lawrence (main campus), University of Kansas. His decades of chairing of the KU Medical Center Hearing and Speech Department included service as associate dean, associate dean of research, and acting dean of the School of Health Professions. He was particularly active in the Council of Academic Programs in Communication Sciences and Disorders and thereby kept a thumb on the pulse of CSD-education programs, especially through the formative years of the professional doctorate in audiology. He also authored *Laboratory Exercises in Auditory Evoked Potentials* (1997; Plural Publishing, under its former name, Singular Publishing Group)—a step-by-step manual to lead students to successful recordings. A career-long member of ASHA, ultimately fellow and honoree of the Association, and active as well in the AAA, ensured him broad and deep involvement in both didactic teaching and mentoring of students, medical residents, and fellows throughout his career. At the same time he was a dedicated and continuously productive researcher that literally helped to keep electrocochleography "alive" in the profession. He continues to probe evident issues of this technique and to endeavor to keep the method still ripe for current clinical interests.

Editor Purdy is a career audiologist and hearing researcher in New Zealand who has enjoyed extensive collaborations over the years with international colleagues in a number of countries, including Australia, the United Kingdom, China (Hong Kong), and South America. She earned her doctor of philosophy in the United States (University of Iowa) and has been a frequent participant/contributor to professional conventions/scientific meetings there as well as globally abroad. These contributions were recognized by the AAA's 2021 International Hearing Award. She has contributed to the establishment of postgraduate programs in audiology and speech pathology and is currently the head of the School of Psychology, University of Auckland. She succeeded the senior editor as the present Council Chair of the IERASG. Through research, mentoring, and clinical work, she has embraced broadly the measurement of auditory evoked responses and their bases and potential clinical applications. Her work has taken on a range of electrophysiological challenges beyond the conventional, including those aspects that sometimes suffer the waxing and waning of popular interests and/or understanding (as demonstrated in one of her contributed stories).

The three invited reviewers who contributed to the project are also distinguished workers in auditory electrophysiology and related areas. While thus not members of the team contracted by the publisher and indeed purposely valued for their relative independence, they were recruited to help vet the book's content. Reviewer Guy Lightfoot has been a clinically based scientist specializing in auditory electrophysiology and vestibular assessment throughout his career with the English National Health Service, based in Liverpool. He obtained his doctor of philosophy degree working on brainstem-auditory evoked responses and came to run a specialist training course in evoked response audiometry, attracting an international audience for 30 years. He has published results of a number of studies on ERA-related topics and recently contributed the chapter on brainstem-response-based ERA in *Pediatric Audiology—Diagnosis, Technology, and Management* (J. R. Madell et al. [Eds.], 2019 [3rd ed.]; Thieme Publishers). He has coauthored many of the British national guidance documents relating to ERA. Dr. Lightfoot is a long-standing member of the IERASG's Council and a regular contributor to its biennial meetings.

Reviewer Paul Avan is both a physicist and doctor of medicine who has dedicated his career to biophysics, wherein falls the theoretical bases and methods of eliciting and measuring sensory evoked responses. He has developed complementary skills to study objective methods of exploration of the cochlea and auditory pathways, such as otoacoustic emissions (cochlear "echoes"). He validated them on models of mutant mice with precisely defined molecular deficits. These models bridge the gap between two domains that shared very few bits of common knowledge merely a few decades ago, namely audiology and molecular physiology. He today heads the Center for Research and Innovation in Human Audiology at the Institut de l'Audition in Paris, France. He works on the design and validation of electrophysiological equipment with the aim of detecting formerly inaccessible functional parameters. He also has served as an editor of *Les Cahiers de l'Audition*—a professional magazine dedicated to disseminating clinical/research findings, even those of his countrymen who are compelled to publish in English academically and namely to help ensure that the science is also reaching frontline French-speaking workers. This includes physicians and therapists alike, especially in the area of audio-prostheses.

Reviewer David McPherson is a professor of communication disorders and neuroscience at Brigham Young University. He is also a principal investigator in the BYU MRI Research Facility. His current research focuses on the simultaneous recordings of fMRI and evoked potentials. He has also served on the editorial board of several professional organizations and as a consultant to NIH grant reviews. He continues to mentor graduate students and maintain research grants and thus is active in research. He was the first hearing scientist to publish a book dedicated to auditory cortical responses—*Long Latency Auditory Evoked Potentials* (1996; Singular Publishing). He is an elected member of the Society for Sigma Xi at the California Institute of Technology and recipient of the Honors of the Association (ASHA) for his research and contribution to the field of CSD. He is an officer of the IERASG Council. He earned his degree of doctor of philosophy at the University of Washington, followed by postdoctoral studies at the Brain

Research Institute, University of California-Los Angles, in cochlear physiology. He then served on the faculty at the University of California-Irvine and worked extensively with Arnold Starr, currently professor emeritus, University of California and Brigham Young University. Professor Starr was not only his mentor, but a mentor to many others and he is an iconic worker in auditory neurophysiology and pathology and has been a long-time contributor to the IERASG Biennial Symposia.

Finally, frequent mention of the IERASG has been made in these introductory pages reflecting its considerable inspiration and motivation for the production of this textbook, but perhaps eyebrow-raising at the same time. What sort of academic society would persist in calling themselves a "study group." Introspection by the Council and at times in the general assembly of the biennial meetings has been given to the issue of continued use of "Study Group" in the society's name. However, Davis argued at its inception (in effect) as being appropriate apropos its first purpose—practically at the dawn of clinical electrophysiology in audiology as we know it today—to explore what we do not know. Thereto, the content of this book is intended to provide points of departure, neither bottom lines to suggest it as a consummate study of clinical electrophysiology in audiology, nor its reading as a consummate education in this specialty. The producers sincerely hope that this textbook will help instructors to teach their students the fundamentals herein, providing a rich source of illustrations but readily harmonious with other materials and/or manners of presentation per nuances of their respective course/curricular structure. At the same time, these writings hopefully will help to instill in their students the importance of a lifetime commitment to continuing education, as ultimately mandated by the profession and essential in such a dynamic area

Acknowledgments

This textbook was produced ostensibly under the auspices of the International Evoked Response Audiometry Study Group. It is not a formal society in the sense (these days) of a "nonprofit" or an academy. However, the IERAG's Biennial Symposia have been a recognized mainstay in evoked response audiometry and related areas of clinical electrophysiology and hearing science for more than a half-century, founded principally by Hallowell Davis. More recently, the IERASG has become formally affiliated with the International Society of Audiology and has conducted minisymposia within their biennial World Congresses of Audiology. Royalties from the sales of this book are to be donated to help sustain the Biennial Symposia and/or initiatives as these have served to produce high-quality scientific meetings for airing out new approaches and/or continued vetting of even well-established evidence bases, as the scientific method demands. The biennials also have been a forum of complete openness to newer workers/students with and among seasoned workers in the field. These meetings have left the participants with deep and abiding memories for some of the best of times in their careers, have introduced or sustained their participation in the international community, and/or seeded many a new collaboration.

The views expressed herein also should not be taken as opinions or edicts of the IERASG's past or present members, nor of the Council members. The latter are long-time colleagues and career-long workers in the field. For this project, Council members were straightforwardly approached during the development of the proposal to the publisher, namely to hear it out in concept and to thereafter (pending overall support in concept) be invited to join in the actual production of the book. The sitting Council members at the inception and throughout this project and to whom the editors are grateful for their encouragement and confidence were as follows:

Council Chair, Suzanne C. Purdy; Vice-Chair, Andy Beynon; Treasurer, Susan Small; Secretary, Martin Walger; Membership Chairman, David McPherson; Webpage Manager, W. Wiktor Jedrzejczak

Council Members: José Barajas, Steven Bell, Robert Burkard, Monica Chapchap, Barbara Cone, Robert Cowan, Cynthia Fowler, Andrew Dimitrijevic, Ferdinando Grandori, Kimitaka Kaga, Krzysztof Kochanek, Jun Ho Lee, Guy Lightfoot, Ozcan Ozdamar, Maria Perez-Abalo, David Purcell, Mridula Sharma, and George Tavartkiladze.

There are still others too numerous to list who served on the Council and/or were frequent contributors to the Biennial Symposia over the years—scholars for whose exceptional knowledge, contributions to the field, and collegiality the production team and writers readily attribute substantial influence on their own knowledge bases, as often reflected in the reference lists of this textbook.

A special recognition is due to a Council Chair Emeritus for his ever-inspiring influence and leadership—Terence (Terry) W. Picton. A career-long researcher and innovator from the formative years on, he also organized the second Biennial Symposium in the New World—held in Ottawa, Ontario—and authored Human Auditory Evoked Potentials (2011, Plural Publishing) which continues to stand as an outstanding reference in this field.

More detailed information about the IERASG and past biennials may be found online at http://www.ierasg.ifps.org.pl.

The editors would be remiss if not advising that this textbook's contents are not intended to be used as standards (de facto) or reference values in the use of any of the methods described herein, although the writers endeavored to represent characteristic data throughout. Such information is provided uniquely to support stated principles and to make them tangible for the reader.

The final proposal of this textbook was developed by the editors and in cooperation with Plural's Executive Editor Val Johns. We are indebted to her for her devoted commitment from its inception and thereafter the fine work of the Plural team for final production of this textbook, the encouragement of Editor-in-Chief of Audiology Brad Stach, and tireless efforts of our Project Editor, Christina Gunning.

Contributors

José Juan Barajas de Prat, MD, PhD
Medical Director
Clínica Barajas
Santa Cruz de Tenerife, Spain
Foreword, Chapters 5 and 6

Fabrice Bardy, PhD
Honorary Academic
School of Psychology
Faculty of Science
University of Auckland
Auckland, New Zealand
Chapter 8

Christopher D. Bauch, PhD
Emeritus Associate Professor of Audiology
Mayo Clinic College of Medicine and Science
Rochester, Minnesota
Chapter 3

Steven L. Bell, PhD
Associate Professor of Audiology
Institute of Sound and Vibration Research
University of Southampton
Southampton, United Kingdom
Chapter 4

Andy J. Beynon, PhD
Head, Vestibular and Auditory Evoked Potential
    Lab–E.N.T. Department
Assistant Professor
Radboud University & Radboud University
    Medical Center
Faculty Medicine and BioMedical Sciences,
    Faculty Linguistics
Donders Center for Brain, Cognition and
    Behaviour
Medical Neuroscience–Hearing & Implants
Nijmegen, The Netherlands
Chapter 9

J. Robert Boston, PhD
Professor of Electrical Engineering and
    Biomedical Engineering (Retired)
School of Engineering
University of Pittsburgh
Pittsburgh, Pennsylvania
Chapter 2

Robert F. Burkard, PhD, CCC-A
Professor
Department of Rehabilitation Science
University at Buffalo
Buffalo, New York
Chapter 2

Monica J. Chapchap, MS
Electrophysiological Hearing Evaluation
Hospital Sirio-Libanes
Sao Paulo, Brazil
Chapter 9

Lionel Collet, MD, PhD
Conseiller d'Etat
Former Professor of Physiology
Conseil d'Etat
Paris, France
Chapter 10

Barbara K. Cone, PhD, CCC-A
Professor
Speech, Language, and Hearing Sciences
The University of Arizona
Tucson, Arizona
Chapter 8

Rafael E. Delgado, PhD
Director of Research and Software Development
Intelligent Hearing Systems Corporation
Miami, Florida
Chapters 2 and 8

xxiii

Vijayalakshmi (Viji) Easwar, PhD, MSc Audiology
Assistant Professor
Department of Communication Sciences and Disorders and Waisman Center
University of Wisconsin-Madison
Madison, Wisconsin
Chapter 6

M. Patrick Feeney, PhD
VA Portland Health Care System
Director, VA R&D National Center for Rehabilitative Auditory Research
Professor, Oregon Health and Science University
Departments of Otolaryngology, Head and Neck Surgery and Neurology
Portland, Oregon
Chapter 2

Linda J. Hood, PhD
Professor, Department of Hearing and Speech Sciences
Director, Human Auditory Physiology Laboratory
Vanderbilt University Medical Center
Nashville, Tennessee
Chapter 8

Ronny K. Ibrahim, PhD, M.EngSc
Postdoctroral Research Fellow
Faculty of Medicine, Health and Human Sciences
Macquarie University
Sydney, Australia
Chapter 8

W. Wiktor Jedrzejczak, PhD
Professor and Head of the Department
Department of Experimental Audiology
Institute of Physiology and Pathology of Hearing
Warsaw/Kajetany, Poland
Chapters 2 and 5

Krzysztof M. Kochanek, DSc, Eng
Professor and Scientific Director
The Institute of Physiology and Pathology of Hearing
Warsaw, Poland
Professor at Marie-Curie University
Lublin, Poland
Chapter 3

Ananthanarayan (Ravi) Krishnan, PhD, CCC-A
Professor
Department of Speech, Language, and Hearing Sciences
Purdue University
West Lafayette, Indiana
Chapter 6

Jun Ho Lee, MD, PhD
Professor
Department of Otorhinolaryngology-Head and Neck Surgery
Seoul National University College of Medicine
Seoul, Korea
Chapter 6

Patricia C. Mancini, PhD
Associate Professor
Department of Speech-Language Pathology and Audiology
School of Medicine
Federal University of Minas Gerais
Belo Horizonte, Minas Gerais
Brazil
Chapter 9

David L. McPherson, PhD
Professor Emeritus
Department of Communication Disorders
Center for Neuroscience
Research Faculty, MRI Research Facility
Brigham Young University
Provo, Utah
Chapter 10

Thierry Morlet, PhD
Senior Research Scientist
Auditory Physiology and Psychoacoustics Laboratory
Nemours/Alfred I. duPont Hospital for Children
Wilmington, Delaware
Adjunct Professor Communication Sciences and Disorders
University of Delaware
Newark, Delaware
Chapter 7

Frank E. Musiek, PhD, CCC-A
Professor & Director, NeuroAudiology Lab
Department of Speech, Language and Hearing Sciences
University of Arizona
Tucson, Arizona
Chapter 3

Wayne O. Olsen, PhD
Emeritus Professor of Audiology
Mayo Clinic College of Medicine and Science
Rochester, Minnesota
Chapter 3

Ozcan Ozdamar, PhD
Professor of Biomedical Engineering
College of Engineering
Professor of Otolaryngology
Pediatrics and Neuroscience (Grad Prog)
Miller School of Medicine
University of Miami
Coral Gables, Florida
Chapter 4

So E. Park, PhD
Doctoral Student of Audiology
Auditory Electrophysiology and Aging Lab
Department of Communication Sciences and Disorders
University of Wisconsin-Madison
Madison, Wisconsin
Chapter 7

Maria C. Perez-Abalo, MD, PhD
Assistant Professor
Albizu University, Miami Campus
Miami, Florida
Chapter 6

David W. Purcell, PhD
Associate Professor
School of Communication Sciences and Disorders
National Centre for Audiology
Faculty of Health Sciences
Western University
London, Ontario
Canada
Chapter 6

Diane L. Sabo, PhD
Senior Global Product Manager-Hearing Screening and Assessment
Natus Medical Inc.
Beaver, Pennsylvania
Chapter 9

Mridula Sharma, PhD
Associate Professor
Course Director of Clinical Audiology
Department of Linguistics
Faculty of Medicine, Health and Human Sciences
Macquarie University
Sydney, Australia
Chapter 8

Lech K. Śliwa, PhD, Eng
Assistant Professor
Department of Experimental Audiology
Institute of Physiology and Pathology of Hearing
Warsaw, Poland
Chapter 3

Susan A. Small, PhD, RAUD
Associate Professor
Hamber Professor in Clinical Audiology
School of Audiology and Speech Sciences
The University of British Columbia
Vancouver, British Colombia
Canada
Chapters 6 and 9

Jacek Smurzynski, PhD
Professor and AuD Program Coordinator
Department of Audiology and Speech-Language Pathology
East Tennessee State University
Johnson City, Tennessee
Chapter 5

George A. Tavartkiladze, MD, PhD
President
National Research Center for Audiology and Hearing Rehabilitation
Head of the Department for Clinical Audiology
Russian Medical Academy for Continuous Professional Education
Moscow, Russian Federation
Chapter 6

Abreena I. Tlumak, PhD, CCC-A, R. EEG T, CNIM
Formerly, University of Pittsburgh
Department of Communication Sciences and
 Disorders
Pittsburgh, Pennsylvania
Chapters 8 and 10

Joaquín Tomás Valderrama-Valenzuela, PhD
Senior Research Scientist
National Acoustic Laboratories
Sydney, Australia
Chapter 7

Martin Walger, PhD
Professor of Audiology
Audiology and Pedaudiology, Cochlear Implant
 Center of Cologne
Department of Otorhinolaryngology, Head and
 Neck Surgery
University of Cologne, Germany
Chapters 5 and 8

Dedication

This textbook was produced in the spirit of the International Evoked Response Audiometry Study Group and dedicated to the memory of

- *Hallowell Davis, Principal Founder and First Council Chair*
- *Gideon Gestring, Council Secretary*
- *Michael Portmann, Newsletter Editor*
- *Gerhard Salomon, Council Chair*
- *Manfried (Marc) Hoke, Council Treasurer and Newsletter Editor*
- *A. R. Antonelli, Council Chair and Principal Organizer of a Biennial Symposium, Bergamo, Italy*
- *Roger Ruth, past Council Secretary and Principal Organizer of a Biennial Symposium, Charlottesville, Virginia*
- *A. Roger D. Thornton, Council Chair*

. . . and to others too numerous to mention, but not forgotten fellow "peak pickers," who also gave years of service in the development of clinical electrophysiology in audiology and participated in the Biennial Symposia held around the globe.

Basic Concepts of Clinical Electrophysiology in Audiology

The Writers

Episode 1: John D. Durrant
Heads Up: The Producers

■ Episode 1: Prequel—A Peek at the Auditory Evoked Potentials and Areas of Application

The grand tradition of sensory psychology toward the end of the 19th century and the subsequent explosion in both experimental psychology and neurophysiology from early on in the last century was greatly devoted to the exploration of sensory stimulus-response relationships. From the classical psychophysics perspective, this intellectual "game" indeed starts with quantifying nuances of the stimuli employed and subsequently measuring responses to them accordingly.

This textbook is about metrics based on a variety of bodily signals that derive from bodily functions and how they can be intentionally elicited and measured systematically. The primary focus, as bespeaks the title, will be signals of the auditory sensory system (although not exclusively) as it endeavors to process a variety of stimuli, whether environmental or research-based, yet certainly of ultimate clinical use or potential application. However, it is important to address one issue up front, and this hardly will be the last word on this matter. Measurement of the signals surveyed never should be construed literally as measurements of hearing. As this sense is classically defined, it is considered uniquely to be evaluated based upon a subject's voluntary or conditioned behavioral responses. However, this does not preclude measuring these signals to estimate hearing sensitivity, to demonstrate correlation with some behavioral measures of discrimination among different sounds, to corroborate some capabilities of binaural processing, or even to define metrics that reflect some level of cognitive processing of sound.

In general, these signals are substantially accessible by methods of electrophysiology that have come to help researchers and clinicians to better understand certain effects of sound stimuli and/or underlying mechanisms of the brain's response to sound. With understanding, it becomes possible to apply such measures to clinical problems, such as indeed characterizing an individual's hearing capacity or differentiating among certain types of hearing impairments/disorders. The foundation of knowledge that has empowered the presently high level of understanding comes from well over a halfcentury of research and development, instigating one of the most voluminous literatures in hearing science. Consequently, it provides a broad evidence base in clinical applications that has been enticing for robust technological advances and commercialization necessary to put tools of electrophysiology in the hands of researchers and clinicians alike.

To explain, conducting clinical tests using methods described herein are best conceived and approached as N-of-1 experiments. The clinician has some idea that such-and-such may account for a given patient's condition, some test is purported to offer some possible insights, another may confirm a given diagnosis, or otherwise the results may be at least to inform further management of the case. With modern technology, the clinical-electrophysiology "toolbox" is stocked with advanced and powerful tools that are highly efficacious in the hands of competent users. Their particular evidence bases are broadly overviewed herein, demonstrating indeed that these can be useful for teasing apart sophisticated issues of clinical concern and are broadly applicable over the life span.

In fact, the auditory system can be investigated in-depth using current electrophysiological tools, many requiring little of the subject/patient, often even with the individual being inattentive to the stimulus, sleeping naturally or under sedation/anesthesia. Examples include screening infants for possible hearing loss shortly after birth, estimating hearing sensitivity when conventional audiometric results prove unreliable, monitoring auditory function during surgery, differentially diagnosing peripheral versus central auditory lesions, assessing cognitive processing ability, or monitoring clinical treatment. The toolbox, much like a mechanic's tool kit, provides a variety of instruments. What mechanic worth their salt would have a toolbox filled only with box-end wrenches? Different "jobs" require different tools; some require several tools to really do the job.

The overall goal here is to address major types of clinical electrophysiological tools that are prevalent in current audiological practice and overview each one surveyed for their most common applications. Still others will be mentioned at least, if not featured, along the way to hint of potential interests, even if presently the topic is somewhat beyond the primary scope of this foundational textbook and/or not quite ready for "prime-time" (routine) clinical use. Their coverage is to serve as encouragement of continued study beyond "the book." This text is thus intended as a launch pad toward competency in this very intriguing area of clinical practice. Ultimate clinical, hands-on competency starts with a "competent" knowledge base—a comprehensive background upon which to develop and that—together with further study and clinical mentoring—can lead to clinical competency. This foundation must also be such as to support growth (and certainly not to compromise it) in the further pursuit of knowledge, into the future. Any field worth its salt is not stagnant; any competent and seasoned worker will attest to not doing things today entirely the same as when they first became clinically certified and started working in the profession.

Therefore, the focus here is the systematic measurement and use of bioelectrical signals that are elicited (conventionally) at the beginning of the 8th cranial nerve, to elicit in turn activity along the ascending auditory pathway. Final destination—the cortex.

HEADS UP

Like in Space, It Takes Time to Travel Along the Auditory Pathway—So What?

It will be useful to look a bit ahead at the object of affection of the book's writers and editors. Figure 1–1 presents schematically the "big picture of AEPdom"—what collectively are called *auditory evoked potentials (AEPs) or responses*. However, only with a specialized approach can such a panoramic view of these signals be approximated—a singular continuum of *recorded* undulating waves of electrical activity, having been generated all along the auditory pathway from inner ear to cortex. Furthermore and particularly important technically, nor can such a pristine sample of the component AEPs be realized—ever. However, there will be plenty of opportunity to deal with reality reasonably effectively. It will suffice for the moment simply to note that a variety of technical

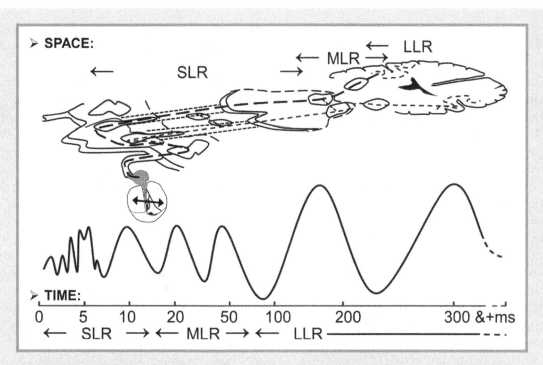

Figure 1–1. Temporal and spatial overviews of auditory evoked potentials and their underlying neuroanatomical origins. Perspective of the examiner is "eyeing" the initiation of the fascinating barrage of neural activity in the time domain (bottom of the figure) while it is traveling "away" toward the considerably larger, and even more elaborate, cortical projections and expansions therein. The three traditionally defined response latency classifications are demarked in time and (in effect) in space, although these divisions are more gray than black-and-white in either domain. Even for a sound like the snap of the fingers, the component waves of AEPs elicited along the way in space add up to hundreds of milliseconds in time, thanks to the multiple "weigh-stations" along the way. Not illustrated but also contributing to this complex wiring and adding time to signal propagation is the relative density of nerve-cell populations along the pathway. *Heavy dashed line*: primary, crossover path; *light dashed line*: secondary/uncrossed-path and/or additional levels of crossover in the brainstem system. (Inspired in part by illustrations of Netter [1962[4]] and Moore [1987[3]] and adaptations by the American Speech-Language-Hearing Association [1988[1]] and Durrant and Feth [2013[2]].)

"tricks" can and will be called upon to allow the examiner to measure reliably a variety of AEPs, as defined practically. This will include efforts to sort out specific influences of stimulus parameters as well as various other factors to which AEPs are sensitive (such as maturation and certain types of pathology). It will be shown that it is possible to target less or more specific levels of the ascending auditory pathway and interpret possible clinical significance of the resulting observations/measurements.

The citizen-wave components in AEPdom are extractions largely from **brainwaves**. It will not ruin the rest of the story to disclose that these waves are searched using fundamentally the tool of **electroencephalography (EEG)**, thus recording the signals of interest most often (but not exclusively) from the surface of the scalp. Furthermore, AEPdom is ultimately about time and space, with time–space coordinates effectively summarized in Figure 1–1. This virtual map reflects the substantial neuroanatomy involved and the signals generated sequentially from events stimulating the *peripheral auditory system*, thus covering more than the *central auditory nervous system (CANS)*. Signals thus can be expected to arise and possibly be recorded whether from the hearing organ, 8th nerve, neural ganglia, and nervelike tracts within the brainstem and midbrain and areas within the expansive cerebral cortex.

One of the major tactical decisions generally dictated by a given AEP test and its purpose is that of the time frame of recording of the particular AEP waves of interest. This is defined routinely by the period of time from the onset of the stimulus to a given peak of the targeted wave component. This measure is called *latency*, so the clock starts indeed in the periphery, upon initiation of the sound stimulus. AEPs are conventionally divided into three broadly defined intervals of latency—those of the *short, middle, and long latency responses (SLR, MLR, LLR)*. The whole issue arises from the simple fact that the neural pathways are not capable of instantaneous transmission of signals from the sensory organ, up the ascending pathway, and to (possibly throughout much of) the cortex. In the backdrop of complexity of the neuroanatomical pathways, the "time–space continuum" gets stretched in ways not entirely intuitive. Overall, the longer the pathway, the longer the total latency to the given wave of activity, at its presumed site of generation. However, the south-to-north trajectory is also not entirely the only possible way for electrophysiological signals to propagate (in effect), and the neuroanatomical architecture is truly three-dimensional. Nevertheless, by the methods considered herein, a number of simplifications will prove to be practical, thus, for instance, focusing only on potentials primarily from a specified level of the system. Making measurements from less or more locations around the head will be dictated by specific clinical interests. Speaking of which, this indeed is where the measurements are recorded routinely for most clinical interests in audiology, generally using methods that are strictly noninvasive and thus causing the patient minimal/no discomfort. The truly remarkable aspect of the AEPs (as illustrated in Figure 1–1) is their mutation, so to speak, along the time–space continuum—a sort of time–space warp occurs. Not only is transmission of signals along the pathway time consuming, the delay effect (again, latency) is progressive in time but in reverse. The signal does not speed up going to the cortex—rather, it slows down! Not only can this activity last for hundreds of milliseconds, this progression is such as to require the time base of the record to be scaled logarithmically (a nonlinear scale) to get essentially all major component waves plotted reasonably on the same page. This is in deference to the ensuing complexities of the ascending pathway wherein the underlying signals travel but also are mutated through space on the way to the cortex and even therein. Also noteworthy is that the peripheral system does not operate like a microphone, transducing sound into electricity nearly instantaneously and directly input to the brainstem, as if it were a public address system. Nevertheless, several component waves (SLR citizens) are witnessed well within an interval of merely 10 ms, and that includes a sequence of signals having traveled already a good bit up the brainstem. Mutation occurs because activation from one level of the system progressively spreads more and more in space, again taking more time, but while also building progressively larger waves, by an order of magnitude or so for some at the cortex—from one-millionth of a volt (1 μV) or less in magnitude (SLR-land) to upward of 10 μV (LLR-land). There then will be quite a variety of approaches in both stimulus generation and response analysis as well as clinical interests that such approaches may serve.

■ Postquel

From this Heads Up overview, the recording of any of the waves of AEPs rightfully can be expected to reveal something about the status of different levels of the brain and/or permit extrapolation from findings of their measurement to predict the likelihood that the auditory system is, firstly, capable of responding to sounds in a given individual. Thereafter, issues of relative sensitivity (re: normal-hearing/neurologically intact patients), if not some aspect predictive of cognitive ability, can be addressed. Various details of underlying neuroanatomy and neurophysiology thus will need to be considered to provide fundamental understanding of what makes the AEPs "tick" and provide rationales for clinical use of their proper measurement. In order to correctly interpret results of AEP tests, it will be important to consider such bases even down to the microanatomical/cellular level at times. The rendering of a decision of abnormal function first relies upon foundational knowledge of normal function and basic aspects of what are or account for nuances of nonpathological findings. Only then can pathological variants be entertained knowingly to deduce what might have gone wrong along Patient X's pathway.

More fundamental matters are essential knowledge before the would-be AEP examiner is ready to escort Patient X into the exam room. These are the various technical aspects involved, such as some of the computer science that is essential for "digging out" relatively small signals in less-than-pristine circumstances. The term "electro" (as in EEG) and "potential" (as in AEP) were used earlier without fanfare. Yet, some basic principles of electricity are essential to understanding both the auditory system and electrophysiological tests thereof, although not too much more than understanding the basic battery-operated flashlight. The term "signals" was thrown around a good bit too, and that implies the need to know some methods of analyzing the bioelectrical activity to be recorded during the electrophysiological examination. There will be some fancy math underlying the signal-processing concepts essential to AEP measurement, yet only conceptually and studied with confidence that the methods themselves can be expected to be implemented broadly in commercially available test systems. These instruments incorporate high-speed computing and hardware both to generate suitable stimuli and to permit detection/other analyses to aid the examiner in rendering their judgment of what the findings mean. Operating today's AEP test systems are much like operating a home computer/laptop and using common software for word processing, electronic-spreadsheet analyses, producing virtual photo albums, and so forth. So, let's go!

■ References

1. American Speech-Language-Hearing Association. (1988). *The short latency auditory evoked potentials: A tutorial paper by the Audiologic Evaluation Working Group on Auditory Evoked Potential Measurements*. Author.
2. Durrant, J., & Feth, L. (2013). *Hearing sciences: A foundational approach*. Pearson Publishers.
3. Moore, J. K. (1987). The human auditory brain stem as a generator of auditory evoked potentials. *Hearing Research, 29*(1), 33–43.
4. Netter, F. H. (1962). *Nervous system* (Vol. 1). CIBA Pharmaceutical Company.

Signals and Systems Essentials

The Writers

Episode 1: J. Robert Boston and John D. Durrant
Episode 2: W. Wiktor Jedrzejczak
Heads Up: Rafael E. Delgado
Episode 3: Robert F. Burkard
Heads Up: M. Patrick Feeney

Episode 1. Signal Generation, Analysis, and Conditioning—Analog Versus Digital Perspectives

As a debut of foundational information underlying concepts of stimulating the auditory system and systematically analyzing signals elicited and recorded from the scalps of humans, this episode is an overview of principles largely from *acoustics* and related areas of *engineering*. Although derived from rigorous physical principles and related mathematics, the presentation here (as throughout this textbook) is largely narrative. This is a story and, hereafter, more stories will follow to provide still more information and insights.

Many of the particulars covered here are common to foundations of conventional audiometry and relevant standards, although further developed toward a knowledge base of their application to clinical electrophysiology in *audiology*.[1,2] For the reader, ideally, much of what is discussed herein will not be news, as such, although perhaps bearing more emphasis and/or some additional concepts that are deemed to be important backdrops of the overall saga of auditory evoked potentials (AEPs), their measurement, and (ultimately) clinical applications.[3] The foundation is laid firstly on signals-and-systems concepts[4] that ultimately empower the clinician to draw from their "toolbox" some truly remarkable "tools of the trade," but of which a variety of foundational concepts are requisite for their knowledgeable use, whatever their use in communication science and disorders.[1,5]

There are classically two views of signals, whether sound stimuli, radio waves, electrophysiological potentials, and so forth. These views are provided respectively by *temporal* and *spectral analyses*, typically by way of graphs of the magnitude of a signal over time or frequency.[4] In other words, the measure of the signal (dependent variable—what happens) is plotted as a function of the value (independent variable—what the user specified), namely scaled in values characteristic of the *domain* of interest—time or frequency. Concepts of *waveform* (overall view) and/or *fine-structure* (instantaneous values) derive from analyses in the time domain. The *frequency makeup* of the signal evidently is a matter for analysis in the frequency domain. Yet in practice, this sometimes seems not to be so "evident," perhaps even at the risk of forgetting/ignoring that the two analyses simply yield different representations of the given signal to be measured. Practice tends to become habit, so there may be simply an "out of sight, out of mind" effect—or worse, a bias to ignore one domain of analysis. The latter might derive from a perception that a certain analysis is "harder" to comprehend, whether due to the underlying math and/or greater demands on the side of instrumentation required.

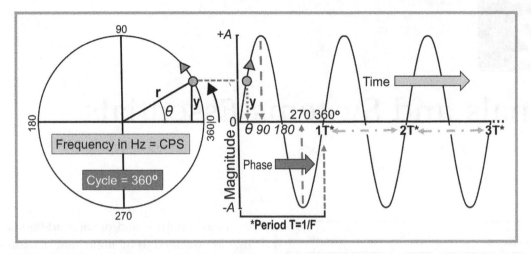

Figure 2–1. Generation of the sinusoid and bases of relations among parameters of amplitude (A), instantaneous magnitude (y), frequency (hertz [Hz] or cycles per second [cps]), period (time [T]), and phase (angle). A phasor at one instance is indicated by radius "r" at angle "θ," a phase here of 30°.

Actually, until the last half-century there was a considerable dichotomy of ease of access to time versus frequency analyses. Yet, the law is the law and never should be out of mind, as a change of parameter(s) in the time domain has consequences in the frequency domain and vice versa—that is inevitable.

Temporal analysis provides the *time history* of the signal analyzed, a convenient way of saying "the instantaneous magnitude of a signal as a function of time." The method is applicable to any signal. A variety of signals, or sounds upon *transduction*, are of interest in hearing science overall, for stimuli serving both audiometric and AEP measurement.[2,3] Easily, the "dearest" and most fundamental signal in audiometry is the *pure tone*, or a reasonable approximation thereof, produced by generating a *sinusoid* (Figure 2–1). Having mentioned transduction of a signal brings up the important point that *analysis* and *generation* or *synthesis* are actually two sides of fundamentally the "same coin." The outcome of analysis is, again, the time history of a given signal; generation is "playing the record" of that history. The initial definition focused for simplicity on instantaneous magnitude versus time. Similarly for simplicity, this may be the only information conveyed about the time history of a given signal/sound. The graph in Figure 2–1 tells the complete story. The graph shows a point moving counterclockwise around the circumference of a circle at a constant speed, indicated by the arrow. The distance of the projection of this point on the *x*-axis from the origin describes a sine wave, as shown to the right. Any time point on the sine wave can be related to the corresponding angle theta (shown in the figure). This angle is called the *phase* of the sine wave at that time point, and phase is also an essential parameter for complete specification of a sinusoid. This figure summarizes various aspects of the generation—also apropos analysis—of the sinusoid conceptually and the common parameters of measurement, which also serve as measurement of other functions.

A variety of functions of practical value, in both the clinical and research laboratories, are illustrated in Figure 2–2, including those underlying real-world/environmental sounds. They are equally useful for generating acoustic stimuli and methods of measurement of AEPs. Their analysis and synthesis have become efficacious thanks to modern electronics and computing. The variety is exemplified, ranging from simple to complex in several ways. Panels A and B permit comparisons among signals of similar and different *periods*, the reciprocal of frequency: T = 1/F (see Figure 2–1). Figure 2–2 also demonstrates a variety of waveforms—*sinusoidal* versus

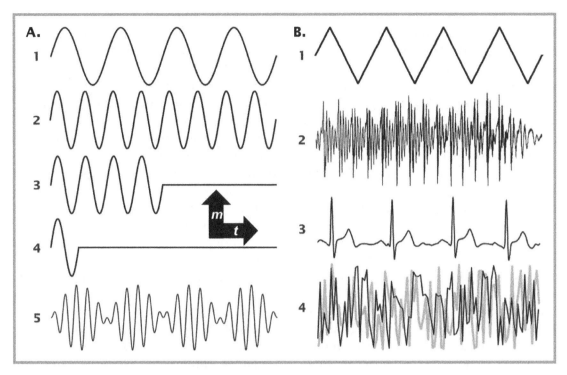

Figure 2–2. Sample signals representative of a wide variety of functions of didactic and practical interests in both analysis and synthesis (see text). **A.** Variations on the theme of the sine function. **B.** More complex functions, periodic and beyond. Time domain analyses: magnitude (m) versus time (t).

more **complex**. Functions A.1, 2, and 5 represent signals that are effectively **steady state**, thus infinitely long in principle. Functions A.3 and 4 show **transient** signals resulting from the application of **gating** (*a.k.a. windowing*) of an underlying **carrier** (A.2 in this example). These are variants of brief "bursts" of the underlying function (perceived as tones when acoustically presented)—***sinusoidal pulses*** (a.k.a., ***tone bursts***)—and are fundamentally one of the most common transients used in both conventional audiometry and tests of AEPs. Examples A.3 and 4 imply that any number of cycles can be included in such tone bursts. Example A.5 presents a more complicated ***modulation*** than simply turning the carrier on and off and at the same time can be generated as a steady-state signal. In this example, a higher frequency carrier than A.2 is modulated (varied) in magnitude by another sinusoid of a different period (in effect, that of A.1 in this example). Both ways of modulating the magnitude of a carrier signal are of common interest in practice in eliciting/measuring AEPs and neither results in functions (A.3–5) that would produce pure tones upon transduction to sounds. (More on this story to come.)

Still other complexities are exemplified in Figure 2–2B that are of practical interest, though not necessarily for generating sound stimuli. Function B.1 is not even perfectly reproducible as a sound, although it can be transduced to make a sound of some quality (like a pleasant, or not so, "buzz"). This signal often is used in technical applications, such as testing test instruments themselves. It is every bit as periodic as the sinusoid. Example B.2 characterizes some of the complexity and novelty of speech, in this case a vowel phoneme (/e/, as in "sake"), which is both periodic and quasi-steady state. In contrast, consonants in running speech tend to be aperiodic and transient.

The functions and methods overviewed in this episode apply equally to signal generation (starting with synthesis) and analysis. Several examples also will be shown later to more or less characterize kinds of interference that can give the AEP examiner headaches. Signal B.3 (interestingly enough, so stay tuned) is a bodily signal that is quite special—a matter of life or death (to be melodramatic)—the *electrocardiogram (ECG)*. Though evidently made up of recurrent transients, normal biological function depends on its periodicity and steady state as well as the waveform of the elemental signal. Function B.4 is an example of a signal of *random* magnitude and period, and, in a sense, it is the antithesis of the continuous sinusoid/tone. It is commonly characterized as noise and indeed can appear as a form of interference for other signals of interest. In the illustration, to further express its randomness, the plot in black line—deriving from a brief window of analysis to demonstrate the detailed ups and downs of its erratic waveform—is overlaid on a sort of shadow of itself (in gray line) from an instant earlier, and none of which is repeatable point by point other than by chance. Although not all these examples, when used to generate sounds (for instance, noises for masking in audiometry), represent environmental sounds directly. Nevertheless, several are more or less representative and all are of practical interest.

The simplest way to understand analyses of signals is first to consider the basic consequences of the complexity of signals beyond the simple/singular sinusoid and by way of synthesis,[1] starting with combining just two sinusoids but of different frequencies. In general, changing the magnitude of one component of a two-component signal will change the resultant waveform, unless both components are changed the same way. The simplest example would be changing the magnitude of one component to zero, but the "same way" also means same phases. Illustrated in Figure 2–3A, function 1 is the result of combining two harmonically related sinusoids (functions 2 and 3). The resultant (1) continues to show the influence of the fundamental (lower-frequency) function (2), but its waveform has changed substantially from that of a pure sinusoid. In the condition of function 1, the two *frequency components* also are seen to have a common starting phase. The condition for the resultant/function 4 is that of giving a 90° phase lag to function 3. Virtually demonstrated by Figure 2–1 was the fact that instantaneous magnitude at a given time is like a vector in trigonometry—a *phasor*—a quantity with both magnitude and phase (an angle in trigonometry). Combining two sinusoids, unless of identical phase, is not friendly to mere arithmetic addition and is further complicated given multiple frequencies. Indeed, the waveform is changed upon manipulating relative phases (function 4 versus 1). It can be deduced from this basic demonstration that (in effect) by applying phasor addition of still more frequency components, it is possible to build a signal of any complexity. Conversely, it is possible mathematically to analyze the frequency makeup of signals of any complexity.

An overall measure of magnitude is often required in practice, and, in particular, some way to equate effectively the relative intensity of sounds among the variety of sounds overviewed thus far, including from Figure 2–2A, function 1 versus 4. A common objective is to do so such that upon transduction to sound, the same sound level would be equal. In audiometry for example, this is the challenge of relating effectiveness of speech versus pure tones to stimulate/test hearing. The example set by complex tones #1 and #2 demonstrates the same challenge, given differences in *peak magnitudes* or *amplitudes* (A_{o-p}) The law of conservation of energy demands an outcome of equivalence in overall intensity, since the frequency makeup has not changed between the two resultants, as in the adage about getting something for nothing. While seeing is supposed to be believing, here appearances prove misleading. However, hearing in this scenario prevails in defense of the law; the two resultant sounds will have the same perceived magnitude or *loudness*. So, what gives?

Even for the simple sinusoid or pure tone, how best to measure magnitude (acoustically, electrically, or otherwise) is a challenge and a "depends" situation. Taking on the latter first, it depends on what is of particular interest or is required. In conventional audiometry, it is that of calibration of the test instrument's output, for instance (a topic coming soon), testing frequency by frequency. While instantaneous magnitude varies throughout the cycle, sinusoids and more complex functions alike will present positive and negative maxima. Another possible metric of magnitude is measurment of the difference *peak-to-peak amplitude* (A_{p-p}), which also is valid for a variety of interests and sometimes

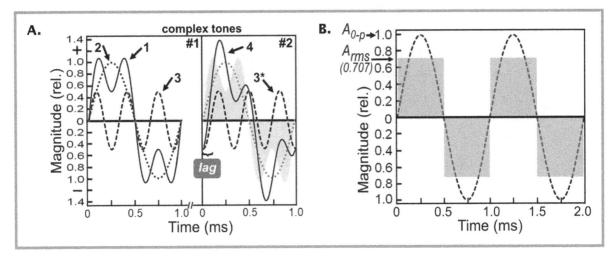

Figure 2–3. A. Addition of two sinusoids, represented by functions 2 and 3 (for instance 1000 Hz and 3000 Hz), are used here to synthesize a new signal, function 1. If prolonged and transduced by an earphone, #1 would be perceived as a complex (not pure) tone. For complex tone #1 (and thus function 1), both frequency components are initiated at a relative phase of 0°. For complex tone #2, the higher frequency sinusoid (3*) has been given a phase lag, namely a starting phase of –90°. The resultant, function 4, reflects a substantial change in peak amplitude and waveform. **B.** The values of a sinusoid deviate equally above and below the zero axis. Computing the root mean square (RMS) value, $A_{RMS} = 0.707\ A_{0-p}$. The gray-highlighted areas represent equal areas under the curves, upon which mathematically this metric is based. Magnitudes relative (rel.).

even the chosen parameter. Yet, neither A_{0-p} nor A_{p-p} resolves the quandary presented by signals 1 and 4, and the first impression is that function 4 looks bigger and so (transduced) ought to sound louder! A measure that does provide resolution and that is readily available via modern electronic instruments and/or computing is the ***root-mean-square (RMS) amplitude***. As illustrated in Figure 2–3B, A_{RMS} is computed across all instantaneous magnitudes. Its equation effectively looks at areas under the curves; the equivalent rectangular areas are shown in gray. A_{RMS} is well known in statistics as the standard deviation. For the sinusoid, the relationship to the peak amplitude is simple: $A_{RMS} = 0.701 A_{0-p}$ or roughly one-third of A_{p-p}. More complex signals are not so simple, but they too are measureable with the help of appropriate electronic/computing algorithms to compute A_{RMS}.

If time and frequency measures are simply two views of a signal, then the logical expectation is after the signal is generated and passed through transducers, the acoustic signals should sound like the time analysis "looks." What more analysis is needed? Well, the problem is that time analysis overlaps the frequency components making up complex sounds, so the detailed makeup often is not so obvious. Some knowledge from speech science might lead to an informed guess of the makeup of the signal back in Figure 2–2B (function 2, a vowel sound), but hardly a definitive deduction. Distinguishing among various types of signals/sounds is difficult without analyzing their spectra. The compelling contribution of the spectral view is indeed that of frequency makeup and, if comprehensively analyzed, includes both magnitude and phase spectra. It would be exceedingly tedious to arrive at such information by trying to match the target signal via synthesis, as in Figure 2–3A.

Thankfully, the great mathematician Fourier worked out the analysis two centuries ago—in modern times called the Fourier transform. Modern computing provides the means practically and efficiently (approaching "real time") to do so—via the ***Fast-Fourier Transform (FFT)***.[6] Figure 2–4 illustrates FFTs/spectra for functions that, upon transduction, would be perceived as simple (panel A) versus complex tones (panels B and C). In panel A, the spectrum demonstrates the "purity" of a single sinusoid

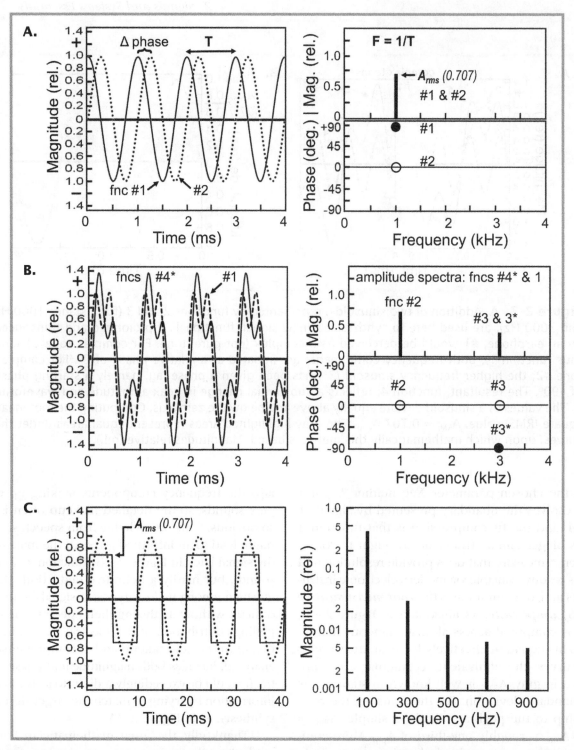

Figure 2–4. Sample signals of a fundamental frequency (F) of 1000 Hz, that is a period (T) of 1 millisecond; temporal analyses are on the left and spectral analyses on the right for signals as follows: **A.** Sinusoid of two different starting phases (fnc #1, +90° and fnc #2, 0°), where these signals are representative of an input versus output signal of some system. This would represent a 90° phase shift/change (Δ) occurring in the signal as it passed through that system. **B.** Sum of two sinusoids (from Figure 2–3: fnc #1 = fnc 1 of complex tone #1; fnc #4 = fnc 4 of complex tone #2; component sinusoids as before). **C.** Square wave overlaid on a sinusoid, matching its effective (RMS) amplitude. Magnitudes relative (rel.).

(amplitude spectrum), while the phase spectrum readily permits computing precisely the phase difference (function #1 versus #2). This is possible via the time history, but is tedious for more than the simplest *phase shifts*. The functions for panel B are from Figure 2–3A—the resultants of synthesis of the two-tone complexes #1 and #4 (functions 1 and 4, respectively). Turning the table, suppose the purpose had been the analysis of an unknown signal like this, having been measured from the output of a microphone. Its "decomposition" via the FFT readily reveals its frequency makeup. Precise phase information also is provided by the FFT and would reveal a phase difference (for frequency component/function #3) as indeed the basis of the difference between the two "versions" of this two-tone complex.

The example in panel C is a bit special and as intriguing as the triangle wave featured in Figure 2–2B, function 1. This is a square wave; it also is virtually impossible to transduce it perfectly according to its time history, although also sounding like a buzz if played through an earphone. This is another example of a signal useful for testing electronic systems, for instance, as a marker for magnitude and/or time, given a precisely calibrated source. It is interesting theoretically because it is clearly periodic, seems simple enough (in detail, more so than the sinusoid), but with an impressively rich spectrum. The specific progression of summed components (only partially represented in Figure 2–4C) extends along the frequency axis to infinity, given a pure square wave.

Spectral analysis and the resulting frequency-domain view often provide complimentary/comprehensive information about the nuances of a signal. Outstanding examples are time histories and spectral analyses of signals like speech. Figure 2–5A shows analyses of another vowel, /ɛ/, in its overall time-domain analysis. The spectrum provides further insights, including how the *spectral envelope* (pattern of frequency distributions of the magnitudes of the spectral components) reveals the concentrations of energy in the *formants* that so characterize vowel sounds.[7] Spectral analysis reveals similar (not shown) frequency-wise energy concentrations of consonants, known as *hubs*. Again, consonants are remarkably different from vowels, particularly for their "noise"-like qualities, such as /s/, or the naturally impulsive plosives like, /t/.

The common feature characterizing all the signals illustrated between Figure 2–4 and Figure 2–5A, regardless of simple or complex waveforms, demonstrates the concentration of energy at discrete frequencies. Such *discrete spectra* are "expressed" ideally as a series of lines graphically, hence the alternative moniker of *line spectra*. These spectra are in sharp contrast to those of random noises and many environmental sounds. Noises come in many spectral "flavors"; *Gaussian* and other *white noises* (Figure 2–5B, left panel) have broad interest in acoustics, psychoacoustics, and AEP measurement. The time histories of random noises change from instant to instant in real-time analyses or from test to retest samples, varying randomly in magnitude and phase. A white noise (connoting white light) has at least a relatively broad and flat-topped frequency band (Figure 2–5B, right panel) when its spectrum is averaged over a relatively long time and with no lines/discrete foci of energy. Energy is spread continuously over the bandwidth of the noise, hence characterized by the term *continuous spectrum*. "Gaussian" refers to the underlying function (the normal probability function, familiar from statistics). Gaussian noise is "white," but not all white noises are Gaussian; the "pure" version has an infinite bandwidth that (when long-time averaged) is perfectly flat over frequency, to infinity if truly Gaussian.

Incidentally, the measurement of random noises/signals is another application that is served well by the RMS value (as demonstrated in Figure 2–5B). It, in turn, enables many applications wherein reasonably fair comparisons of overall power among diverse signals can be made. This is not only to characterize the similarity or differences among signals like tones, speech, noises, and other sounds. It is especially valuable to have a metric for such contrasts, such as in the case of a single-frequency component in a background of noise—the *signal-to-noise ratio (SNR)*. This can be applied to production of certain sound stimuli, like speech in noise with SNR as the independent variable of some study. An example might be that of characterizing and exploring the discrimination ability of speech in noise in normal-hearing versus hearing-impaired

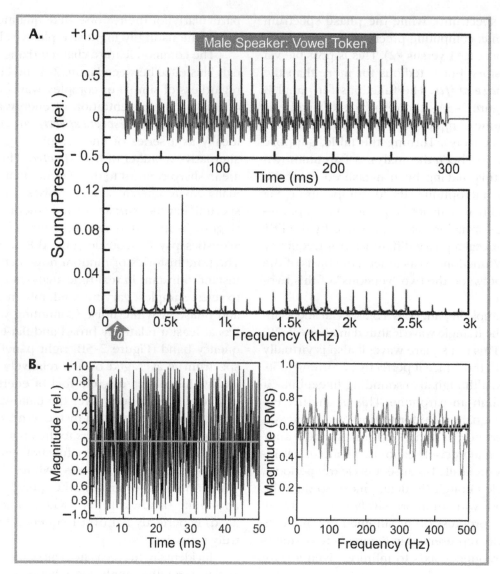

Figure 2–5. A. Another sample time history of a speech token, the vowel /ɛ/ as in "bet" (*top panel*) and spectral analysis below. The spectral envelope strongly reflects characteristic vowel formants excited by the fundamental frequency (f_0) of the male speaker's voice (on average, 108 Hz). (Courtesy of Dr. D. Purcell.) **B.** Another sample of random noise, time history, and spectrum (over the first 500 Hz), contrasting a relatively short-term (*darker gray line*) and substantially longer-term average spectrum (*black line*), versus the idealistic flat spectrum (*light-gray line*) of true Gaussian noise.

subjects wearing a new model of hearing aid. A higher or lower SNR of this signal would cause more or less difficulty in conditions respectively of lower versus higher SNRs of the speech tokens. But would it be any more so for users of the new hearing aid? Or by what SNR difference, if so? The same logic may be applied in signal analysis, as in the measurement of AEPs, as noise is pervasive. A higher or lower SNR of the targeted potential would tend to suggest more or less reliability of the measurement, respectively.

The value of temporal and spectral analyses in revealing insights into the inherent complexity of speech and noise can be taken to portend similar

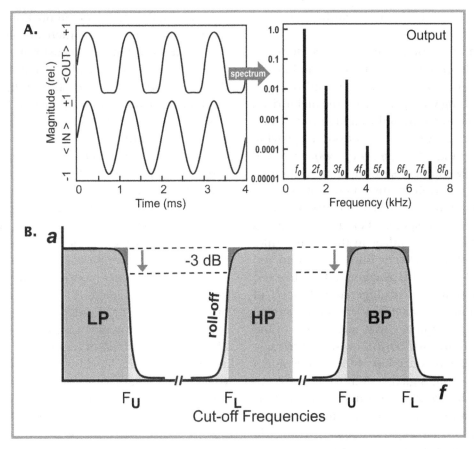

Figure 2-6. A. Effects of an asymmetrical amplitude nonlinearity in the reproduction of a sinusoidal signal (IN). The fundamental of the output signal (OUT), f_0, equals the frequency of the input signal, but the output includes numerous distortion products—$2f_0$, $3f_0$, and so forth, although harmonically related (reminiscent of the square wave). **B.** Frequency responses (*black-line plots*) of low-pass (LP), high-pass (HP), and band-pass (BP) filters. Cutoff frequencies (F), at the half-power or three-decibel-down points (–3 dB), are indicated; subscripts U and L indicate upper- and lower-frequency cutoffs, respectively.

value in understanding workings of the auditory system and applications for measuring and understanding AEPs. Some effects on signals are inherently "diagnostic." For instance, compare the output signal of a system that has been fed a sinusoid, as in Figure 2–6A. Having nearly converted the input sinewave to a square wave certainly is an eyebrow-raising alteration or ***distortion*** of the input signal's time history. In this case, the distortion is manifested as a ***nonlinearity*** of amplitude at the output of the system (in general). Another nuance—subtle at a glance, but hardly trivial—is an ***asymmetry*** in the output signal. The spectrum shows just how seriously the system is distorting the input signal at its output. If the system is now excited by two or more frequencies at once, such distortion becomes even more interesting. It proves to be the sort of system that generates ***difference tones***.[1]

Difference tones have been observed in hearing for centuries, but only in the latter half of the 1900s could they be demonstrated readily by electrophysiological and related responses of the auditory system, which is even useful for purposes of clinical tests (as will be demonstrated in a subsequent episode). Particularly intriguing, such effects of auditory processing are not readily evident to a listener, nor is nonlinearity in the auditory system necessarily a bad thing.

Distortion of the output signal of a system—in the broadest definition as changes effected at the output—is not necessarily nonlinear and/or diagnostic of something wrong. True, if some high-priced audiovisual system connected to a high-priced digital television cannot be counted upon to provide an impressive range of *frequency response*, the owner rightfully can be disgruntled. Nevertheless, there are various applications wherein it is desirable (even for that high-end ATV system) to manipulate the frequency response. Perhaps as received (for whatever reasons) and/or in the setting (like room acoustics), the listener finds the sound too "boomy" (low frequencies exaggerated) and/or too "bright" (high frequencies exaggerated). Indeed, in many applications in laboratories or clinics, it can be useful to apply a frequency-wise attenuation of the amplified signal. *Amplification* or *attenuation*—increases or decreases of *gain* of the output signal relative to the input signal—often can be accomplished essentially linearly over considerable dynamic ranges. Attenuation selectively of some frequency ranges also can be accomplished linearly using *filters*. Basic examples of three broad types of filters are illustrated in Figure 2–6B: *high-* or *low-pass* filters primarily pass energy above or below certain cutoff frequencies and in combination to effect a *band-pass filter*.

Depending on stages of implementation in the instrumentation, the type of filter (electrical versus acoustical) and the applications as well as the shape of the filter function (per the frequency response) can be varied. Variations occur in terms of not only *cutoff frequencies*, but also shape and rate of the rejection rate or *roll-off* (slope) of the response over frequency (generally expressed in decibels per octave). However, as the roll-off will not likely be instantaneous above and below a given cutoff frequency in practice, it is often specified at some starting point along the frequency axis where the signal amplitude has "fallen" below the plateau of the frequency response of the filter. A common example is the level of half-power or –3 decibels. Areas in Figure 2–6B shaded in midgray tone thus represent the idealistic response and bandwidth intended, while the lighter and darker gray bits represent under- and over-attenuation (respectively), often demonstrated by practical filters, including those often used in AEP measurement. In general, when it comes to considerations related to production/control of sound stimuli, filtering can be implemented with more precision, flexibility, and cost-effectiveness electronically than acoustically. Indeed, the more "exotic" filter functions are more easily designed and implemented electronically—if not computationally, digitally, using logic/logic-controlled circuitry or computers.

Nevertheless, acoustic filtering happens, intended or not. Various acoustic effects can and often do impose frequency-dependent changes in the audio system's output (in reference to the intended/input signal). High-fidelity sound enthusiasts are well familiar with the adage that the sound (output) is only as good as the loudspeakers. There also are some positive, impressive, and even enjoyable examples of acoustical filters (in effect): stringed, wind, and percussion musical instruments as well as the voice. These all demonstrate more or less the same underlying principle. The same acoustics are pertinent to the outer ear and baffle (the head) in which it is "mounted." This is the phenomenon of *standing waves*, which introduces a resonance-like effect (increased gain around some frequency) that can add significantly to nuances of the spectrum of any sound presented to the ear.[2] The underlying principles are summarized in Figure 2–7, well understood from the classical examples of vibrating strings (panel A) and tubes (panel B, like that of a pipe organ). Enhancement occurs at specific multiples of the fundamental frequency of vibration or sound, respectively.

The ear canal being terminated by the eardrum indeed looks acoustically like a pipe, one end open and the other closed, hence "playing" by the rule in panel B. Standing waves form at odd-numbered multiples of the fundamental mode (lowest frequency at which they occur). Consequently, a sound pressure at the input (open end of the ear-canal pipe) will receive a "boost" (gain) at the eardrum at the "right" frequencies. As the motion of the air particles encounters some frictional resistance or absorption along the skin-lined tube, this means some gain too on either side of the optimal frequency, around 3.4 kHz. Thereafter, there will be

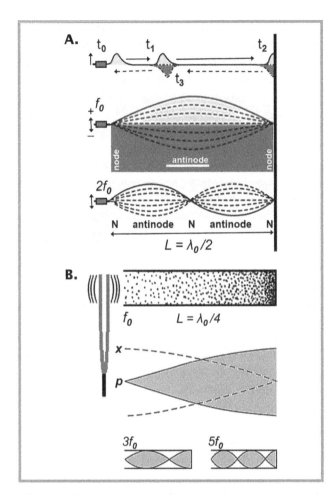

Figure 2–7. A. Generating standing waves on a string. The string is imagined as a jumping rope wherein the handle is cut off at one end, tied to a rigid wall, but also as being elastic (more like bungie cord than regular rope). An upward jerk at the other end at t_0 starts a wave toward the wall, progressing over time. "Snapshots" at different instances of the round-trip of propagation at t_1 and so forth indicate the initial wave (1) to have been reflected ultimately (3) at the fixed end of the rope (2). At the right frequency (f_0) of up–down motion (instead of just a jerk), per length of a string (*L*), a standing wave is formed of largest displacement but also at integer multiples. **B.** Acoustic standing waves similarly can be excited in a pipe with one end closed, such as by the sound from a vibrating tuning fork. Insets: higher modes (resonances, in effect) occur only at odd-numbered multiples. Displacement (***x***) of air particles in the tube are readily displaced at the opening but not at the closed end. However, this builds up sound pressure (***p***) and subsequently reinforces sound pressure at the orifice.

a diminution until approaching the third mode of the ear-canal pipe ($3f_0$) and so on, but with an overall roll-off in gain. This system, though, is connected naturally to another, with far more acoustical consequences—the middle ear. Suffice it to say for the moment, the overall frequency response of the combined outer and middle portions of the ear impart considerable filtering of the sound energy reaching the cochlea for the outside world, indeed accounting for the shape of the minimum audibility curve (plot of sensitivity versus frequency) and frequency limits of hearing.

Technology was considerably restrained by dependence largely upon analog devices for centuries, starting with mechanical/acoustical systems in endeavoring to "control" the sound environment of the listener. Electronic/digital signal generators, signal processing circuits, and high-speed computing algorithms progressively have exploded in the high-tech age of personal computers, media recorders and players, and telecommunication devices. Still, perhaps despite "illusions" of compact disc players, cell phones, full surround sound, and so forth, neither the digitally analyzed nor synthesized signal is without some level of distortion—perceived or not. Understanding of the issue here starts with understanding that analog-to-digital conversion and "going digital" literally distorts the truth.

It is well beyond the intended scope of this text to provide comprehensive discussion of methods of digital signal analysis or generation, but key points are readily discussed and will suffice for purposes here.[3] Electrophysiological signals to be recorded or audio-frequency signals to generate sounds are ***analog***; they are continuous in amplitude and time. Yet, they must be represented in the computer as binary numbers. A signal, whether "coming or going," will be represented in the computer and ancillary digital circuitry as fundamentally binary pieces or ***bytes*** ("words" of bits, a number-based sequence of 0s and 1s). This implies that the incoming/outgoing signals—relative to the actual/desired signals—are "sliced and diced" in both magnitude and time. Consequently, the ***analog signal*** must be converted: ***analog to digital (A–D)*** or ***digital to analog (D–A)***, respectively, and it must be sampled in a timely manner. These processes are not instantaneous, although they may seem so at times and timing of sampling certainly must be precise. The "pace" will be set by an internal high-frequency controlled oscillator—the **clock** of the computing device employed.

Shown by Figure 2–8B–D are steps of the digitization process in reference to panel A (graph of the desired signal). The original signal only can be represented by a series of steps or dots (one per each conversion), no matter how high-speed the A–D and D–A conversions are. **Digital sampling** is like a picture in a children's coloring book—it is necessary to connect the dots. Limitations of the quality of the "picture" are determined by the effective **magnitude resolution** and **sampling rate** (per temporal resolution). The sampling rate also limits the maximum frequency that can be appropriately represented. The **sampling theorem** states that a given sampling rate can represent frequencies in a signal accurately only up to one-half the sampling rate; this is called the **Nyquist frequency**.

Fortunately, modern AEP test systems benefit greatly from high-quality, sophisticated technology that only rarely "runs into" practical limits imposed by pushing the limits of the sampling theorem and/or yielding appreciable distortions of the digital "picture" of the desired signal. Hence, most modern evoked response test systems likely will not degrade substantially response analysis or stimulus quality. Still, it remains important to have the basics in mind to ensure against being misled and/or having unrealistic expectations. Here (looking again at Figure 2–8), the first obstacle is a large enough digital "word" used in the A–D/D–A conversion to make the binary numerical steps in amplitude very small, such as that of a 12-bit conversion. Resolution of a signal's amplitude is $1/2^{12} = 1/4096 \simeq 0.02\%$ of the voltage range of the converter. This is not just about a "pretty" picture of the signal. When the signal is transduced to sound, it is indistinguishable from the analog version by hearing. On the analysis side, there is also the matter of being good enough to resolve a desired signal from a background of noise, thus limiting the ultimate SNR. This perhaps begs the question of why not just use huge binary-word conversions? They take time, and there are "no free lunches," especially when cost containment is a consideration for the manufacturing of economical test instruments and costs passed on to the consumer.

The conversion also must be very fast to avoid the problem of inadequate sampling rate. This consideration also is not only to improve the illusion of an ever more perfect "analog like" signal; rather, it is to avert creation of false signals—an effect called **aliasing**. In television shows/movies in which the scene is a moving car or wagon, rotation of the wheels rarely appears to be at a reasonable rate, at times not even in the right direction. The apparent rate/direction in such cases is an "alias," as the frames/second of the movie or (digital) video camera were too slow to keep up with the actual angular velocity. The effects of a high enough sampling rate (left graph) versus not high enough sampling rate (right graph) of a familiar signal are illustrated in Figure 2–9. Both graphs show results obtained with a sampling rate of 1000 Hz, thus a Nyquist frequency of 500 Hz. A 100 Hz signal is well below the Nyquist frequency, while 900 Hz is equally well above. The two sets of samples yielded are identical; hence, the inverse transformation yields the same function for both data sets. The 900 Hz signal (right panel) is misrepresented by aliasing as a 100 Hz signal!

There is a mathematical procedure (an inverse transform) that can be used to **interpolate** the sampled signal values to obtain a set of values approximating the original signal (see Figure 2–8, panel D, left, gray line). However, the interpolation is accurate only if the sampled signal contains no energy above the Nyquist frequency; yet, any real signal may/often does contain energy above the Nyquist frequency. That energy can distort interpolation by the aliasing process referred to previously, in which high frequency energy is represented at frequencies below the Nyquist frequency and will create a false interpolation (see Figure 2–9).

Practically speaking, relatively low sampling rates for a given frequency of a signal tested may be adequate; this is another "depends" situations. The user must consider what upper limit of frequency of input/output signal will provide adequate **time resolution** (for a given rate) and toward what objective? As a general rule of thumb, 8 points/cycle allows pretty good representation of the waveform of a signal like the sinusoid. Even using only 4 points readily shows it to be (at least) an alternating signal, but it would not permit distinction among sine, triangular, and square waves. At the

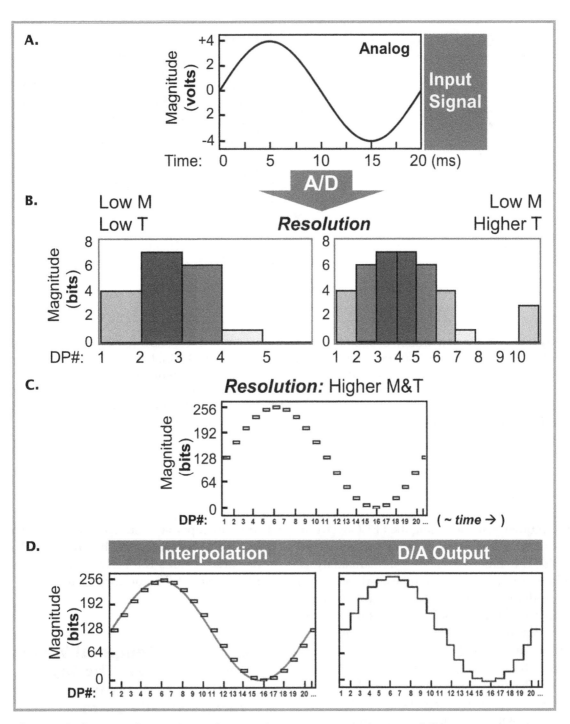

Figure 2-8. Digital sampling of an analog (input) signal (**A**) at different resolutions in magnitude—4-bit (**B**, both) versus 8-bit (**C**)—and in both magnitude and time (**B**, right graph versus **C**). Panel **D**, left (*gray line*): Interpolation applied to the digital version of the signal to better approximate the analog input signal. Panel **D**, right: "Playing" a digitized sine function via a D/A converter's output.

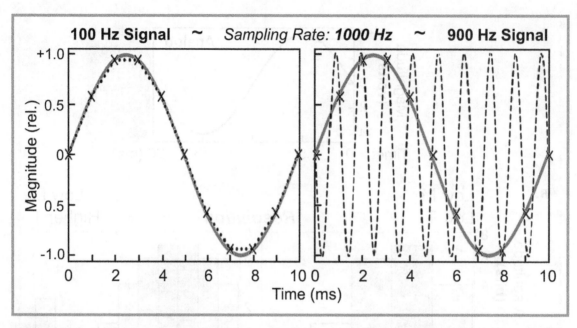

Figure 2–9. Demonstration of sampling-rate effects. Both panels show results obtained using a Nyquist frequency of 500 Hz (sampling rate/frequency = 1000/2). Left: x's demark the sampled values for the 100 Hz signal being measured. The overall representation of the analog signal sampled provides a reasonable approximation to the actual function when the x's are connected by point-to-point interpolation (*dotted line segments*). Right: values for a 900 Hz signal under test. However, the actual signal's time history is as shown by the dashed line. Both sets of data were also interpolated by a computer algorithm (*solid gray line*). Although in both a "prettier" approximation to a sine function, the interpolation on the right clearly is false, due to aliasing.

Nyquist frequency, if computing the FFT (spectrum) of the signal, the frequency could be measured, but this is also the limit of frequency domain analysis.

Whether in analysis or synthesis, these issues bear consideration. Generally, an analog low-pass, **anti-aliasing filter** is used as part of data acquisition or outputting to other devices to minimize the amount of energy (both in the signal of interest and in the background noise) above the Nyquist frequency. Because filters are never ideal, oversampling is a good practice whenever possible. Nevertheless, even with considerable oversampling, the digital version shows its true nature; it is still not analog (see Figure 2–8D, right).

The various observations made of time and frequency domain in this episode must now be taken a few more steps forward, substantial steps aimed at additional concepts especially important to several aspects of testing auditory evoked responses. These concepts are foundations of the stimulus-response-test paradigms that have evolved and today are methods routinely used in clinical neurophysiology of the auditory system.

■ Episode 2: Temporal Versus Spectral Views: The Saga Continues—Impulsive Versus Steady State

The first episode was dedicated to basic aspects of signals in both time and frequency domains. There also was some dabbling into systems of relevance on several sides of those and/or underlying concepts that will be embraced subsequently in the progressive development and expanding scope of methods of auditory evoked response measurement as well as their ultimate clinical applications. As diverse were the signals exemplified, there remain other details of particular importance in this area of clinical audiology that require attention, as a lack of knowledge and understanding of them can undermine competent tests and interpretation of their results. The saga of signals and systems thus continues.

The simplest signal in terms of its time domain is a mere *direct-current (DC) pulse*, as illustrated in the left panels of Figure 2–10. When acoustically transformed (by earphone or loudspeaker), DC pulses make a clicking sound, much like the snap of the fingers. This simplest of pulses can provide a balance of temporal brevity and broad-frequency spread of energy that inherently has commanded much attention in the measurement of AEPs,[1,3] the particular example of which will be considered substantially in the upcoming episode. Meanwhile, back to basics. For its utter simplicity in the time domain, the spectra of such pulses are impressively complex and are other examples of *continuous spectra* (right panels of Figure 2–10). As seen by their spectra, there occur *spectral nulls* in relation to the *duration (D)* of the pulse. Like frequency and period, the frequency of the first spectral null—where magnitude falls to zero—and duration of the

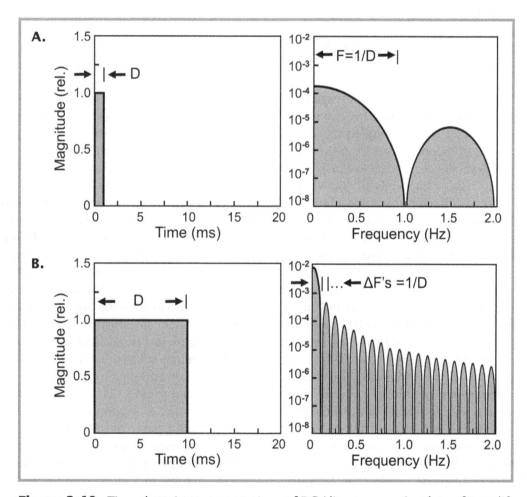

Figure 2–10. Time-domain representations of DC (direct-current) pulses of two different durations (D) (*left panel* **A/B**) and their respective spectra (*right panel* **A/B**). *Gray fill*: energy distribution in the time and frequency domains, respectively. Frequency intervals (ΔF) between spectral nulls is equal to 1/D.

pulse are reciprocally related. In the example of panel A, given a duration of 1 ms, $F = 1/10^{-3} = 1000$ Hz for the first null/zero. In between the nulls (which, in principle, continue to an infinite frequency with only initial ones graphed for simplicity) are spectral *lobes* (the "hills" between the zeroes). Lengthening the pulse's duration (by 10-fold in panel B), the spectrum appears more elaborate, but that is merely an artifact of imposing the same frequency range on both. Although neither of these durations of pulses (1 ms and 10 ms) represent DC pluses typically used to produce sound stimuli in hearing science (including AEP tests), their spectra are very important for understanding other signals that are commonly used. This is because the spectrum of the simple/DC pulse, regardless of duration, demonstrates what to expect; its spectrum is entirely predictable!

As a stimulus, the spectrum of a DC pulse connotes more of a "splat" than anything remotely tonal, relative specifically to test stimuli of pure-tone audiometry. What if *frequency specificity* is also a priority, even if such brevity should be required? It might be tempting to try simply to use the briefest "beep" possible, rather than "beeeeeeeeeeeeeeeeeeeee . . . p" (as in conventional audiometry, lasting hundreds of milliseconds). Intuitively, there will have to be some number of periods of a given test frequency to "focus" energy around the desired frequency. Figure 2–11A shows the spectrum of a *sinusoidal pulse*. Its *carrier*, a sinusoid of a given frequency, is *gated* (*windowed*) for a particular duration; in this example, to turn 1000 Hz on and off for 10 ms and as quickly as possible. The choice of a duration (D) of 10 ms is to permit a direct comparison of its spectrum to that of the 10-ms DC pulse in Figure 2–10B. The resulting spectrum of a gated sinusoid is seen to have a prominent lobe of energy centered at the carrier's desired frequency (good news). Still, there is a good amount of *splatter* of the rest of the energy about the main lobe (less good to bad news, pending needs of the application). The window applied here is rectangular, just like the DC pulse, and the consequences in the frequency domain are much the same. Just as the simple pulse demonstrates a continuous, rather than line, spectrum, so the spectrum of the sinusoidal pulse is also continuous, although becoming riddled with spectral nulls. In other words, in between the nulls, the spread of energy under the spectral envelope is still continuous.

The concept of envelope is useful at times, as hinted earlier and as in this example, to characterize overall aspects or salient features of the spectrum, applicable as well in the time domain (see again Figure 2–11, left panels)—the *temporal envelope*. It thus "contains" the fine structure of the signal. Both fine structure and envelope (shaped by gating of the signal in the time domain) are seen to contribute spectral nuances. The enlightening effects of these examples perhaps seem to "muddy the waters" of frequency specificity for any stimuli of interest, if assuming at least some interest to preserve a tonal quality of the resulting stimulus. Demonstrated by the example in Figure 2–11B, a longer window duration is helpful but does not eliminate the splatter problem. Furthermore, such a duration, although appropriate for testing some AEPs, exceeds the duration of the response itself for others, a possible conflict for the intended application. Consequently, there is inevitably a compromise between windowing aimed at controlling/containing spectral splatter versus the desired duration of the sinusoidal pulse. This is one of several "no free lunch" messages that will be learned as a part of how evoked responses of the auditory system are stimulated and measured effectively. There also will be differences in the significance of this trade-off, from application to application. If indeed needing a stimulus clearly perceived as a tone rather than a transient—like the click which is the most popular variant—the duration inevitably must be on the longer side, by tens or more milliseconds, depending on just how "clear" a tonality is desired and how much splatter is tolerable. The latter can add to the perception of a click added to the "burst" of tone. What to do?

A possible "work around" is found in the fact that the "gating game" is one of trading off sideband splatter of energy versus that distributed within the main lobe of the spectrum. In other words, how the spectrum rolls-off (attenuates) above and below the carrier frequency relative to the bandwidth of spread immediately around the carrier frequency. Such trade-off is well illustrated by Figure 2–12, comparing spectra of a classical *tone burst* in panel A—with its *rectilinear window* (straight-

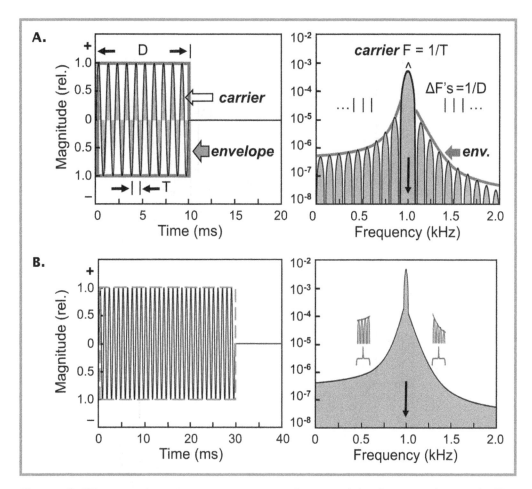

Figure 2–11. Time-domain representations of sinusoidal pulses gated on and off to yield rectangular windows of two different durations (D) and their respective spectra. Interval ΔF is again equal to 1/D, whereas period T determines the frequency of the carrier and, in turn, the peak of the main lobe, given a sinusoidal carrier. Temporal and spectral envelopes are highlighted. **A.** Sinusoidal pulse corresponding in duration to the DC pulse in Figure 2–10B, with similar spectral lobes and the same spectral nulls, but now both above and below F. **B.** Extending duration (3-fold in this example) generates more lobes and nulls (shown by insets) but overall similar spectral envelope. However, given more time devoted to the carrier frequency, its main lobe is both narrower and reaches a higher magnitude.

line-demarked envelope)—to that of a more sophisticated gating—like the **Blackman window** in panel B.[8] The former (panel A) is a bit of improvement over the rectangular windows of the earlier examples, exhibiting a pretty tight center lobe for an overall duration about half that of the example in Figure 2–11A, but still having relatively high levels of sideband splatter of energy. The Blackman window (panel B) offers excellent reduction of side-band splatter around the main lobe of the spectrum, although at some cost (per the no free lunch admonition)—a somewhat broader main lobe. It also is important to bear in mind the cost of reducing overall the **effective duration** of the window—loss of energy.

Effective duration is about the area of the temporal envelope.[9] At first glance, signals A and B in Figure 2–12 appear to have the same durations,

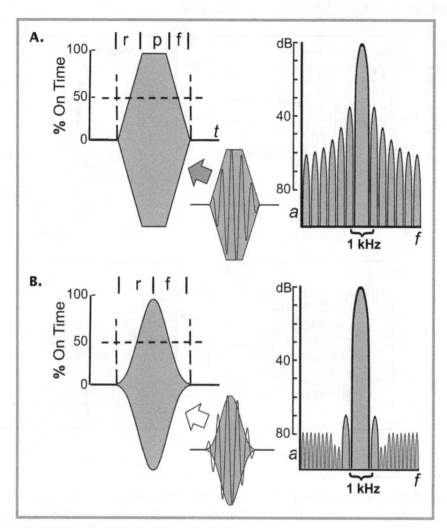

Figure 2–12. Spectra for two different windows (panel A versus B) for sinusoidal carriers of the same frequency. Temporal envelops are for rectilinear (**A**) and Blackman (**B**) gating functions. The insets show that the sinusoidal function contained in the rectilinear envelope does not quite fit in that of the Blackman function, despite the same overall durations. The issues of effective rise/fall (r/f) and plateau (p) durations as well as shape of the envelope substantially impact their respective spectra. Note: here the magnitude axis is scaled in decibels—dB—in deference to its advantages in such analyses and as a preview to the upcoming episode.

in reference to the times at which their respective temporal envelopes "take off" from the baseline (magnitude = 0) and "return" to zero. Nevertheless, these signals do not have quite the same effective duration. Only for the signal in Figure 2–12A is the computation of effective duration simple. The window is formed of a combination of right-triangular **rise-fall times** and a rectangular **plateau** portion (see inset, panel A). For r = f, overall D = 2/3 r+p. For the likes of the Blackman window (panel B), it is necessary to call upon calculus to evaluate overall energy. A popular approach is simply to measure duration from the points of 50% on- and off-times. The idea is that the energy above and below the 50% level add up to that of the equivalent rectangular window. Outlining the "first 50%"

of signal A and overlaying it on B readily shows that the two signals presented still cannot have precisely the same areas without some adjustment apropos the actual areas within these envelopes. Furthermore, adjustment of the areas between the two windows still would not give them the same spectrum. Longer on-/off- windows and still other windows (like the extended cosine) also are of interest in some areas of AEP measurement, including gating of more complex stimuli, like speech. Therein, rise, fall, and plateau durations or equivalent envelop parameters also must be considered. Lastly, in signal analysis (rather than synthesis as emphasized thus far), the effects and issues overviewed apply for the same reasons. Consequently, in sampling a signal, like that of an AEP, similar considerations must be given, lest the signal "capture" window significantly distorts its true time history and spectrum.

Compromises of effects seem to be everywhere. However, choices of parameters of the temporal envelope (per the underlying mathematical function of the window) are generally dictated by practical considerations as well. The broad popularity of the Blackman window is its hard-to-beat sideband-splatter suppression. If the slight broadening of the main lobe of its spectrum does not exceed about one-third octave, that advantage will likely outweigh its disadvantage. This is because one-third octave is the nominal bandwidth commonly attributed to the cochlear-based critical bands of frequency processing (as demonstrated by psychoacoustic measurements). It thereby is considered to be "frequency-specific enough," even with overall durations less than 10 ms and at least in comparison to results of pure-tone audiometry.

The inevitable "bottom line" is that there is always a trade-off between frequency and time resolution of the signal, whether in synthesis or analysis. This is a consequence of the Heisenberg ***uncertainty principle***, which refers to the limits of precision that can be determined for some pairs of properties.[10] The inherent challenge is that of localizations (thinking graphically) in the time and frequency domains. To demonstrate further this principle, consider a frequency-by-time (F-T) "space," as presented in Figure 2–13 (lower panel); the backdrop is rendered in black, as if looking out into the dark void of deep space at night. The time-history

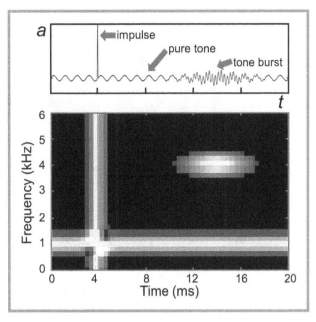

Figure 2–13. Demonstration of the uncertainty principle for the curious mix of signals seen in the time history (*top graph*)—essentially pure tone, impulse, and tone burst (see text). Magnitude is represented by brightness of the images, for simplicity, represented by steps of gray tone from black to white.

graph at the top portrays the following: (1) a relatively long sinusoidal pulse approximating a pure tone; (2) an impulse (extremely brief DC pulse); and (3) a brief tone burst. All three have three dimensions—time, frequency, and magnitude. Magnitude, though commonly measured as sound pressure in hearing science, is an expression of the energy in these sounds. A glimmer of light has the same meaning out in space, suggesting the presence of energy. The long tone burst is seen to be localized fairly well along its frequency axis, lighting up F–T space, any splatter faithfully following on either side, yet indefinitely on this time scale. The energy of the impulse appears perpendicular to this (nominally) pure tone, concentrated fairly well in time, yet indefinite in frequency. Then there is the brief tone burst, designed to meet the aim of localization in both frequency and time. Nevertheless, it looks more like a galaxy far, far away, puzzling the observer as to how far it reaches beyond its "bright" center in either dimension.

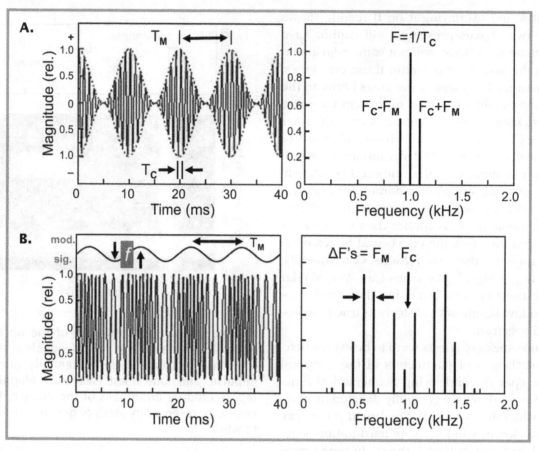

Figure 2–14. Time-domain representations of (**A**) amplitude—AM—and (**B**) frequency modulated—FM—sinusoidal carriers of frequency F_C and their respective spectra. T_M and F_M: parameters of period versus frequency of modulation (wherein $F_M = 1/T_M$).

In classical pure-tone audiometry, the carrier is presented as a "long-enough" tone, namely equal to or greater than the limit of duration at which further prolongation would not yield a lower threshold of response.[11] Although technically still "tone bursts" (sinusoidal pulses), these signals yield nearly steady-tone qualities for audiological applications. However, there are other ways to approach the aim of frequency specificity. A virtually endless tonal carrier can be generated and modulated in other ways, such that the modulation itself is an "event" capable of eliciting an AEP (for instance). Two modulations of broad interest are shown in Figure 2–14, *amplitude* (*AM*, panel A) and *frequency modulation* (*FM*, panel B). The most basic AM is the sort of tone bursts illustrated earlier but simply repeated in a "train" for steady-state stimulation (if that is the objective). The example of AM in panel A is that of changing the amplitude of the carrier—rather than simply abruptly turning it on and off—according to the sine function (as mentioned briefly in the first episode). In the case of FM, it is the period of the carrier that is being so modulated. Energy again is concentrated around the carrier frequency, although it no longer is a "pure" tone. Yet, as illustrated, these too have discrete (line) spectra.

In sum, the major contrast among the foregoing signals considered (including those of the previous episode) is that some are essentially ***impulses or transients*** while others are ***steady-state*** signals. This distinction is not that of, for example, a DC pulse versus and AM signal. As hinted previously but reconsidering the point at the most basic level, repeated DC pulses within an observation/measurement window also will be steady state. It is worth repeating by illustration (see Figure 2–15A) that, treated effectively as a singular event, the DC pulse will behave indeed as an impulse, and its spectrum will be purely continuous. However, as illustrated in Figure 2–15B, a train of DC pulses lasting effectively indefinitely will yield a discrete spectrum. The spectral lines will occur at intervals of $f = 1/T$ where T is the period of the *repetition rate* or frequency. Meanwhile, the spectral envelope, including spectral nulls, will be the same of the single pulse's spectrum.

Being able in some applications to use steady-state signals for stimuli will prove to provide certain advantages for analyses applicable to the response elicited. While both time- and frequency-domain measures will always be applicable in principle, practical considerations will play a role in such a way to favor one domain over the other; for example, the time domain for exploring impulsive responses and the frequency domain for steady-state responses. Regardless, the laws of physics prevail, and both T and F domains always must be kept in mind. Some advances of research and development in clinical electrophysiology in audiology only have occurred by being so minded. For

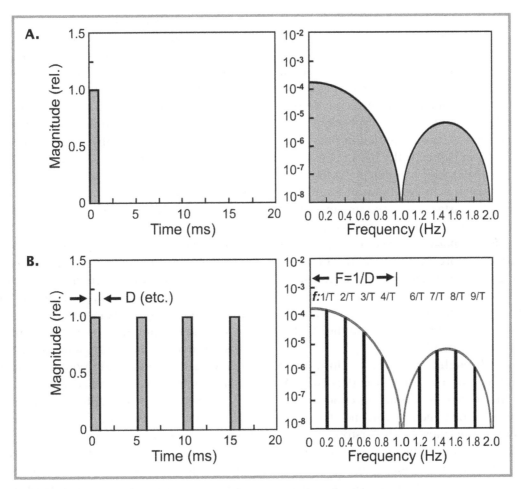

Figure 2–15. Time-domain representations of a DC pulse treated as a single transient event (**A**) versus in a train of DC pulses (continuous repetitions), thus steady state (**B**). Panel A, for convenience of direct comparison, is simply a replot of Figure 2–10A. Although the resulting spectrum in the latter case (panel B) is discrete (a line spectrum), the spectral envelope has the same lobes and spectral nulls as in panel A (a continuous spectrum). The spectrum of the pulse train also continues on along the frequency axis indefinitely. T is the period of repetition at the rate (frequency), *f*.

instance, in an upcoming episode, the innovators of the specialized stimulus paradigm discussed had to think beyond the status quo and more about a type of transient signal that is well appreciated by chirping birds—a pulse which is based on FM.

From this and the first episode, the ways of evaluating signals and the underlying methods of synthesis or analysis provide various useful prospects to specify all sorts of sounds used in AEP assessment and to analyze the recorded responses themselves. All this applies regardless of temporal or spectral complexity of either stimulus or response. For example, easily some of the most "demanding" paradigms are those involving speech. Recalling Figure 2–5, some parts of speech naturally look like a burst of a complex tone, most notably the vowels. They can be treated (for some purposes) as steady state by "tricks" of synthesis and/or analysis or naturally via singing. Alternatively, windowing can be applied to make speech tokens relatively more brief (impulsive) signals than in natural speech. A given speech token then is readily limited in time when its natural duration is practically too long for measuring the particular AEP of interest. At the same time, natural speech is in good part of interest for its complexity, for instance, consonant-vowel transitions. Consonant-vowel tokens, like "ba" and "da," with appropriate windowing make for signals still abrupt in attack (short on-time) and brief enough to suit testing of some AEPs, across time and space of AEPdom. Both natural and synthesized speech have applications and inherently practical uses in hearing science overall and clinical auditory electrophysiology, in particular.

Noise was brought up right away in the first episode, and for good reason—it is pervasive. As mentioned, noise also is of interest/concern as a quasi-steady-state phenomenon. This and other uses/ definitions of "noise" must be understood as oversimplifications, relative to the variety of real-world noise. Examples given are often particular to the application, such as masking noises used in conventional audiometry. In signal analysis, coincidental presence of noise on the particular signal of interest potentially puts optimal analysis of the targeted signal at risk. The most common example in AEPdom proves to be brainwaves themselves, including those targeted in classical electroencephalography (EEG).

On the side of signal synthesis, coincidental noise effectively adds a sort of distortion of the desired signal; this also possibly indicates a problem with the instrumentation generating the signal/sound.

Noises are not all bad. They can be synthesized deliberately for use as sound stimuli. They can be modulated for certain effects, starting with a simple burst of noise used as a stimulus as well as for a masker. Not all noises of interest are as statistically predictable as Gaussian noise, which has the same underlying math as the Gaussian distribution broadly employed in statistics. Yet for practical purposes, recall that white noise (simply by way of its long-term constant RMS over a certain bandwidth) is an ally, readily molded by filtering into defined bands of noise. Therefore, when masking is required in evoked response testing, maskers can be applied as needed, starting with comparable situations and rationales as in behavioral audiometry. Speech presented in background noise (as in various behavioral clinical tests) have applications in clinical electrophysiology too. Lastly, such "noise" (for instance) can be more naturally/environmentally relevant if synthesized in the form of "speaker babble."

Throughout the history of efforts to measure auditory evoked responses (AEPs and more, as soon to be explored), all the types of signals surveyed here have found some viable or at least potential application for both research and clinical applications. As a stimulus-response "game," AEPs and other evoked responses more or less mimic or are more or less influenced by stimuli. This also dictates the need of a variety of analysis techniques. Therefore, both time- and frequency-domain analyses and both transient and steady-state paradigms are encountered with different advantages/disadvantages, at least within practical means/limits respectively. Types of signals and analyses in clinical practice have emerged dramatically over the past several decades. Yet, their evolution is naturally conservative, inherent to the nature of scientifically developed methods and mandates for evidence-based clinical practice for routine use. This follows the considerable precedence set by research and development in conventional behavioral audiometry and related methods, including a mandate for a standard of stimulus calibration.

HEADS UP

Prequel 2: Why Are Computers So Important in This Area of Audiology and Are They Everywhere?

Writers of both episodes of this chapter have freely discussed various signals of interest for their analysis or synthesis, all presented graphically and made accessible to a broad range of users (not only mathematicians, engineers, etc.) thanks to computing. Computing places the necessary functions at users' fingertips via the keyboard or other devices. Is this and related technology, indeed, pervasively found in audiology today?

As will be seen in subsequent episodes, there is no question that computing is pervasive in clinical electrophysiology in audiology. A good part of AEP measurement, conveying at least preliminarily the results "on the fly," post-test processing, reporting of results involving graphical analyses, and quite a bit more makes computing an inseparable part of such testing. This includes generation and control of the signal to be used to drive the transducer (including D/A conversion) and controlling devices (including A/D conversion) to render the signal picked up in the form upon which computations can be made—digital. Certain limits of what can, versus cannot, be expected reasonably—as the user sets out to have the computer do their bidding—were also noted. However, limitations have become progressively less and less, while computing "power" has become progressively more economical. Last but not least, is the evolution of software that allows test instruments to be user-friendly in clinical applications for maximizing test efficiency while minimizing start-up training on use of the instrument itself. Today, the clinical user need not be a "computer whiz" as such software has become increasingly more intuitive to use and since such intuition is fostered by users' familiarity with general-purpose tools such as electronic spreadsheets, word processors, and other applications. This, in turn, is a far cry from the early days of clinical electrophysiology, yet thereafter benefitting progress realized thanks to the several (in effect) quantum leaps of the technology highlighted in this Heads Up and indeed robust bases by which computing is truly pervasive in audiological test instrumentation.

That modern computing is the product of leaps and bounds of the digital electronics era, the outcomes are more than meets the eye—in fact, making some of the most complex processes common place. This is also an era in which computational devices need not be *general-purpose computers*—like the desktop or even a compact laptop—rather, programmable computational *integrated circuits* to produce even turnkey electronic instrumentation. The familiar clinical-diagnostic audiometer is virtually unrecognizable as a "computer"; but is it? Modern test instruments indeed are crammed full of similar/same circuits in computers, thanks to numerous advantages of both production and utility of "packages" of variable mixes of *hard-, firm-, and software*. The results are a range of instrumentation from (indeed) turnkey to dedicated processors linked to a general-purpose computer. This feature's title begs two provocative questions per what is state of the art—perhaps more to the point, state of the science and technology—and, in effect, why and how has computing become so pervasive in audiology and allied fields and implicitly, in particular, in clinical electrophysiology in audiology?

Innovation is critical for the advancement of all fields and audiology is no exception.[12] Over the past half-century, computers in the field of audiology have enhanced the clinician's ability to conduct measurements and analyze data on levels that previously were not possible.

However, innovation bears substantial risks and costs to manufacturers and users alike. The selection of the proper technology for a given

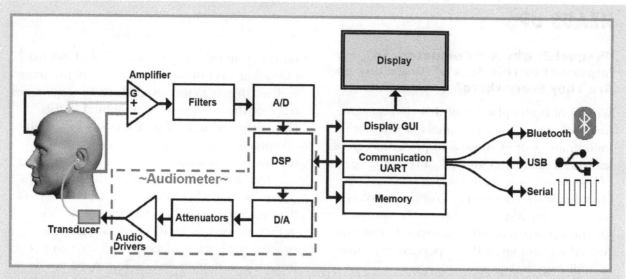

Figure 2–16. General block diagram of an acquisition system for measuring auditory evoked responses (see text).

application is critical in order to accomplish the required task in an efficient and cost-effective manner without increasing complexity unnecessarily. The wrong technology can cause excessive cost and personnel training with no benefit for practical/clinical use. Some of the earlier computer-linked test instruments suffered, for example, from being rather slow and/or inflexible. Clinicians were often hesitant to move into the "new age" when their "trusty" and largely analog test system (despite its limits) permitted greater efficiency per test. This is still true to some extent with software updates and other computer improvements. The clinician, by nature, needs instruments that are easy to use and reliable in order to meet the ever-increasing demand for services.

The overall goal of implementation is new/increased capabilities at effective costs. There has been a huge proliferation over recent decades wherein computing is the central tool for many applications. ***Digital signal processors (DSP)*** based on integrated circuits is one of the primary advances empowering the emergence thereof. DSP, in turn, has evolved rapidly by way of ***large-scale integration*** of ***logic circuits*** on printed circuit boards or "chips" with phenomenal miniaturization. Meanwhile, the types of electronic circuits and materials has greatly improved processing speed and memory capacities. These advances are not unique to computers but are also seen in ancillary circuits that ***interface*** the computer (whether internal or external) and development and advances of dedicated sophisticated circuits to enhance ***peripheral devices***. This includes the likes of high-resolution color monitors and high-speed hard-copy printers.

Shown in Figure 2–16 is a typical implementation of a DSP-based AEP acquisition system. Electrodes to detect these electrical potentials are connected to a bioelectrical amplifier and interfaced to both condition the signal recorded and provide the patient isolation from the rest of the system's electronics. Further signal conditioning includes filtering to help suppress unwanted components from either physiological or external activity/noise. An A/D converter digitizes recorded signals at a predetermined sampling rate. The digital signals are processed and analyzed by the DSP to carry out computations to extract the targeted AEP from background EEG/other electrical activity. The DSP also generates the digital stimulus signal which is converted to an analog signal by the D/A converter. A digitally controlled attenuator is used to adjust the output signal to the desired level, including reference values stored in memory. The audio drivers provide the required power to drive the transducers to produce the sound stimulus. The DSP is also connected to various components in order to provide memory storage and/or communication with other peripheral devices. The ***universal asynchronous receiver/transmitter (UART)*** can provide communication with other computers, printers, and other devices using (high-speed) serial transmission, a ***universal serial bus (USB)***, and/or wireless Bluetooth connectivity. The ***graphical user interface (GUI)*** provides display capabilities which can be integrated with touchscreen technology, including directly on the system as particularly important for handheld devices. Consequently, the design can be used for a general-purpose device with audio stimulation and electrophysiological recording capabilities controlled by a personal computer (PC) using a USB connection or a dedicated handheld device with built-in display and Bluetooth communication. In general, the basic building blocks are the same: stimulation, recording, processing, and communication components. As outlined lastly in Figure 2–16, a portion of the AEP test system is seen to be inherently an audiometer. With additional programming, the same system can be operated much as a conventional audiometer, including manual tone presentation and plotting thresholds on an audiogram for subsequent printout. The audio drivers generally can handle both air- and bone-conduction transducers, as also used in evoked response audiometry.

To exemplify the benefit of such advances, consider the history of the printer—not the entire history to make the point but just a couple of "leaps" more recently. For some time in development, communication with relatively economical printers, whether next to the computer or over some distance (perhaps via telephone lines), was made essentially by modestly elaborating the "twisted" pair of conventional telephone lines. The data transfer was strictly a serially transmitted code and inherently at a very slow transmission rate. However, at least for a nearby printer, a practical and much faster approach was to use more lines in parallel (one per bit of the binary word [like eight-bit words]). This was a quantum leap in speed for both printouts of text and graphics. The downside was that it was not practical to run very long cables without risk of degradation of the signals involved. Fortunately, another leap soon ensued, ironically a reconsideration and further development of serial communication. Enter the USB, prevalent and with subsequent improvements and ongoing refinement to this day. Still other developments followed, such as wireless transmission, and developments in computing itself, such that large documents can be sent to the computer and the user can move on with routine use of the computer itself, rather than having to wait for the printout to be completed. Or just forget a printout; email it or load it into a centralized record-keeping system, per advances in electronic record keeping that can be accessed from anywhere in the world, virtually instantaneously.

DSPs and other modern microcontrollers are the ***central processing unit (CPU) or "brains"*** for many clinical devices that allow the implementation of various online (often virtually in real time) signal analysis/generation techniques. Advanced DSPs provide powerful integration of signal processing capabilities of spectral analysis, filtering, memory, and communications to peripherals, reducing the overall number of components required for any design and (therefore) reducing the overall size of circuit boards and instruments.[13] All these advances contribute to processing efficiency and the ability to provide users with additional and more complex automated response analysis features. Conversely, their limits partially define the overall computer efficiency of the device. Speaking of which, the advances in the speed and size for these "brains" has enjoyed leaps in development that seem to be unthinkable, yet today, they are being developed in an environment of presumption that the next generation will have the speed required by the innovators. More than a half-century ago, it was postulated that the number of transistors that can be integrated into a given area would double every 2 years.[14] The time frame today is actually 18 months. This has resulted in tremendous processing speed and miniaturization of integrated circuits.

Under the "hood" of applications is math-based **algorithms** to any given problem, such as spectral analysis or even the most modest tools like a virtual pocket calculator. DSPs such as the TI320D6746 are capable of performing 2100 million floating point operations per second (MFLOPS) and performing FFTs in a few microseconds.[13] This provides sufficient processing power to perform essentially real-time speech processing, that is with minimal delay.[15] Again, analyses modules incorporating familiar electronic spreadsheets formats are now found in AEP and other audiological test instruments. The digital code on which the computational modules function is programmed via firmware (usually unchangeable by the user) or software (programmed by the manufacturer but in principle changeable, for instance via updates). Flexibility has long been a major challenge to technological advances and thus another major goal of innovation. The combination of firm- and software provides expediency to place in the instrumentation marketplace a product that meets current needs but also flexibility for some time to come to fix and/or upgrade system performance. This is, as well, to offer the user more options, either to accommodate forthcoming utilities and/or others than might have been needed or afforded with the initial acquisition.

In general, there is little utility in developing computer-based systems that are not adaptable to changing needs and/or difficult to use. User interfaces must meet several objectives/qualities. First, they must be able to connect to a variety of inputs and outputs of the instrument. Portability is particularly key in the modern age—a constant nuisance early on in the history of evoked response test instruments. Portability empowers usage in/at cramped spaces, patient's bedside, operating rooms, newborn nurseries, and even outpatient clinics, where "enough" space is likely more a luxury than a given. Space demands include or are influenced by needs to service more clients and accommodate still other test equipment, as clinical science overall has become extensively instrumentation dependent. Open architectures, allowing CPU-based designs to be interfaced with a broad range of input and output components sharing a common data transfer method, can accommodate a variety of uses/formats and at the same time promote both portability and cost reduction. These designs can be repurposed by adding different hardware/firmware components or uploading different software modules.

The need for technological development/innovation, in any event, will remain constant. Above all, continued development of user-friendly interfaces is essential—ideally the more intuitive the better—and implementation in systems that are ever-more flexible and portable. The emergent systems must at the same time enhance both utility and performance. AEP test instruments were developed before broadly implemented **operating systems** like Windows. Consequently, over the past couple of decades, developers have added to their challenges that of working in an operating system's environment not of their own design, namely that might better "fit" their instrumentation package (for example, to optimize efficiency of their own programs). Fortunately, this at least has made interfacing specialized tests to postprocessing and/or output utilities more universally based, like converting data files to one readable by Excel. For each utility there is a variety of subroutines that are essential to aid the examiner toward optimal evaluation of the measured responses and any posttest processing that might help in interpretation of the results as well as in efficient report writing.

As technology and new ideas continue to evolve, the clinician can expect to see emergence of all sorts of new systems and/or specific advances to have computers assist them by doing what computers do best—high-speed controlling of signal acquisition and subsequent computational processing. Processing examples in AEP acquisition include automated peak labeling and deconvolution of responses acquired at very fast stimulation rates toward expediting tests and/or other objectives.[16,17] Meanwhile, the clinician will be better able to do what they do best—think—contemplating the information needed to evaluate the patient's problem and adapt efficiently to changing needs to follow whatever clue with the right test (rather than a rigid protocol). The clinician can have sophisticated test protocols readily at their fingertips and analytical tools thereafter, with less time invested in routine stages of the testing—again, for more time contemplating what the clinician wants/needs to know for as fully competent and comprehensive evaluation possible. There are indeed a variety of machine/automated processes that can be handled well by computers (some to be mentioned soon), including to level the "playing field" of examiner expertise (in effect) and/or make even clinical electrophysiology conducive to teleaudiology.

In routine tests presented in upcoming episodes, as a first step in AEP evaluations, the examiner may be perceived to have to do most of the work, first starting with entering personal and relevant clinical information about the client. The test system thus will already be running, but not necessarily just patiently awaiting the examiner's keystrokes. Then, some routine system checks will be in order, just as in conventional audiometry. If any issue, some troubleshooting tools and/or protocols will be available, as needed. The clinician certainly will have some chores of preparation of the patient. In any event, the system will not sit there for long, including while the examiner is connecting it to the patient. It will be put to work before the evaluation itself has been initiated, as the system will provide a running display of the time history of the ongoing EEG/other background activity. It then will (or on-command will) execute a quantitative check of the connections to the patient. It will have or then will be "commanded" to set essential instrumentation parameters as well as loading a specific test utility desired and/or a test protocol stored in memory (for instance, a sequence of commands for a series of test conditions). All of which having replaced, in the "days of yore," the tedious and often error-prone setting/turning of mechanical switches and dials. Welcome to the modern age of clinical electrophysiology and—with an assurance by history—that of continued refinements of tools for the clinician's toolbox!

Postquel 2

This feature was a humble tribute to innovators, researchers, developers, and instrumentation manufactures who have so enthusiastically taken on the challenge to engage and invest in research and development to bring, over decades of effort, these tools to researchers and clinicians alike. For the reader, it effectively extends the first episode of the book, Prequel 1, to now have considerably overviewed the object of these workers' affection—the ever-fascinating evoked responses of the auditory system—and the genre of instrumentation that empowers workers who endeavor to better understand them and to use evoked response tests as effectively and conveniently as possible on the frontline of clinical service. However, these initial "stories" are but the tip of the proverbial iceberg—in this case, base of knowledge. Moving forward, the collective details overviewed will begin to be picked apart, numerous further details revealed, and concepts further defined or refined toward the big picture. Enjoy the show!

Episode 3: Signal-Issues Particular to Stimulating the Auditory System and the Importance of Being Calibrated

Auditory perception cannot be measured directly, as perception reflects an individual's state of mind and cannot be detected by others. To investigate auditory perception, it is important to manipulate parameters of the acoustic stimulus and document the response of an individual, a group of individuals, or a population. Imagine a study of some auditory effect. When the response to a given stimulus is behavioral (for example, raising a hand or pushing a button), the experiment might be called psychoacoustics or perhaps speech perception. If the response is an AEP, the study might be neurophysiological. Most importantly, either way, if the *acoustic stimulus* is not known with appropriate accuracy, then the responses assessed are truly meaningless.

The most fundamental step in measuring the acoustic stimulus is *transduction*. *Sound* is a vibration that travels through a medium. That vibration can be produced by numerous mechanical systems: the vibrating vocal folds, the biosonar pulse of a dolphin, a tuning fork, or the earphones used to watch a movie on a plane. For a mechanically generated sound, such as from a tuning fork, it is only possible to change the frequency by manipulating the mass and/or stiffness of the tuning fork. The level of sound from a tuning fork only can be manipulated by the strength of the strike used to set the tuning fork in motion or moving the listener closer or farther away from the tuning fork. Thus, mechanical manipulations of an acoustic signal are challenging and ultimately limit the types of sounds that can be delivered to a subject or patient. With the development of modern electronics, it became possible to create almost any electrical stimulus desired. By changing the modality of this stimulus from electrical to acoustical, it is possible to use the power (and ease of use) of electronics to control the acoustic stimulus. A transducer is a device that converts the modality of energy. The field of *electroacoustics* thus concerns the conversion of an electrical stimulus to an acoustic stimulus—by use, for instance, of an *earphone*—and the conversion of an acoustical signal to an electrical signal by a *microphone*, for example. The pure-tone audiometer has become a highly accurate device for determining the threshold of hearing. This device would not have been possible without the great strides in the fields of electronics and electroacoustics during the 20th century.

As discussed in the first two episodes, the time and frequency domains are two different ways of representing acoustic or other signals. For each time-domain signal, there is a unique frequency-domain representation. In AEP testing, it is quite common to create an acoustic transient—such as the *acoustic click*—by exciting an earphone with a brief-duration rectangular electrical pulse. Figure 2–17 shows the frequency-domain representation (the amplitude spectrum) of two DC pulses: one with a duration of 1000 μs (= 1 ms) essentially replotted but rescaled from Figure 2–15 and the other with a duration of only 100 μs. The time-domain view of these two pulses would appear quite similar. However, as demonstrated in the last episode, the spectrum changes quite dramatically across different pulse durations, with regard to width of spectral lobes and consequently intervals between spectral nulls. It is the 100-μs pulse that is of special interest here. To recap—with D = 100 μs, spectrum does not plunge to zero amplitude until 10,000 Hz ($F = 1/D = 1/10^{-4}$ Hz). There will also be higher frequency lobes and nulls (as was illustrated in Figure 2–10). For 100 μs duration, this will occur at 20,000 Hz and above, but for simplicity, they are not shown in Figure 2–17. The frequency region below the first spectral zero—the main lobe—is where most of the energy of a 100 μs click stimulus is concentrated and is pronounced especially for transducers used conventionally in audiology. Thus, by manipulating the duration of the click stimulus, the bandwidth can be manipulated specifically to control the upper cutoff frequency of the click stimulus or (more specifically) the frequency of the first spectral zero.

Every transducer shapes the spectrum of the acoustic output relative to the spectrum of the electrical signal input to the device. The resulting filter function is known as a *transfer function*, which affects both the level and the timing (or phase) of the response. The focus for the moment will be on the amplitude spectrum, rather than the phase spectrum. As emphasized earlier, this neither means that

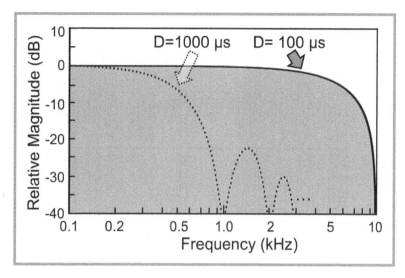

Figure 2–17. Frequency domain representations of 100 and 1000 μs DC-pulses, which when transduced, produce "click" stimuli. The 100 μs DC-pulse is employed to produce acoustic clicks used conventionally in AEP testing. The 1000 μs plot will be familiar from the last episode (see Figure 2–15A) but note the use here, in effect, of log-log coordinates—decibels by log frequency. Both scale values in equal-ratio intervals, for example 0.1 to 0.2 kHz and 1.0 to 2.0 kHz (re. octaves).

phase changes are not there nor will not need to be considered for some applications. Figure 2–18 shows the time domain representations of some familiar electrical signals (left panel) and their acoustical counterparts (right panel) following transduction. There are a number of changes to the input signal possible following transduction. One is that there is overshoot in the amplitude of the stimulus over the initial cycles. Once the stimulus is turned off, the acoustic signal still responds. These effects are called ***ringing***. While it is possible that ringing is due to the transfer function of the transducer used (earphone, for instance), it may also be due to the reflections in the recording environment, whether this be a small acoustic volume (such as a coupler, as discussed below, or ear canal) or a room. After all, acoustic couplers and rooms have their own filter functions—again, transfer functions. There also is a delay introduced by the transduction process, of ~1 ms in this example. This delay also could be due in part to the transduction process itself or to the physical distance between the earphone/loudspeaker and the microphone. As sound travels at ~340 m/s in air at sea level and at room temperature, the 1 ms delay might mean that the microphone is 0.34 meters from the earphone's vibrating diaphragm.

An ***acoustic coupler*** is defined by standard ANSI S3.6-2018, as a "cavity of specified shape and volume used for the calibration of an earphone or microphone in conjunction with a calibrated microphone adapted to measure the sound pressure level developed within the cavity of the coupler."[18] The transfer functions of the transducer, the coupler, and even the recording microphone can lead to distortions of the stimulus, in addition to those revealed by Figure 2–18. One example is ***harmonic distortion***, where there is energy not only at 1000 Hz (the frequency of the electrical stimulus driving the transducer) but also at its integer multiples known as harmonics—2000 Hz, 3000 Hz, 4000 Hz, 5000 Hz, etc. There are other types of distortion, such as ***intermodulation distortion***, which occur when presenting an electrical signal at two or more frequencies. An example is the result of delivering two electrical sine waves at 2000 Hz (f_1) and 2400 Hz (f_2) to an earphone. In the acoustic signal, there is not only energy at these two frequencies but also at

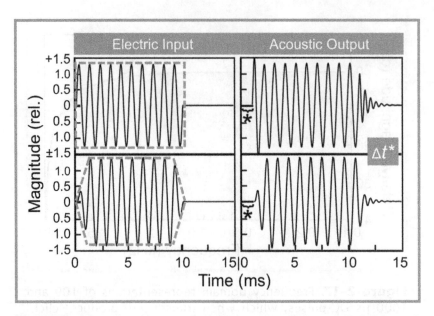

Figure 2–18. Time domain representations of electrical (*left panel*) and acoustical (*right panel*) waveforms of 10 ms duration—a 1000-Hz tone burst (sinusoidal pulse). Temporal envelopes are outlined, top panel for a simple on–off gating of the carrier and bottom panel for a rectilinear temporal envelope including 1-ms rise–fall times (recall Figure 2–12A). On the right, deviations from the intended input function are evident for both windows. "Ringing" perhaps seems clearest in these examples at the offset of the stimulus (as a spurious oscillation), yet the effect is also manifest, equally importantly, at the onset (as overshoots). Also noted* is some delay (Δt) in real time in the actual onset of the acoustic output.

summation and difference frequencies, like those equal to f_2-f_1, f_1+f_2, etc. There is an important intermodulation frequency at $2f_1-f_2$, called the cubic difference tone, particularly important to the analysis of one of the first evoked auditory responses to be discussed in later episodes of this book.

While perhaps not often paying particular attention to phase spectrum, there is an important phaselike stimulus parameter—***polarity***. Figure 2–19 shows a positive-voltage electrical pulse (panel, top) and the acoustical output when the pulse is passed through a transducer, such as earphones which are commonly used in conventional audiometry and AEP testing. The acoustical output represented by a positive-polarity initial response is condensation (C) in this figure. In panel A (bottom), a negative electrical voltage pulse is shown along with an initially negative output of the earphone—rarefaction (R). Condensation represents an acoustic overpressure (an increase in pressure above atmospheric pressure), while rarefaction represents an acoustic underpressure (a decrease in pressure from atmospheric pressure). Looking at this figure, a few things are apparent. First, when the polarity of the electrical pulse is inverted, so is the acoustic pressure waveform. Second, there are clear differences in the time-domain electrical and acoustical waveforms. The electrical pulses are unipolar and of a finite duration (100 μs), but the acoustical responses contain both polarities. In other words, both rarefaction and condensation phases are in the acoustic response, regardless of electrical pulse polarity. Also, the acoustic-response duration is substantially longer than the electric-pulse duration. These latter effects are because the earphones (and possibly the coupler used to mate the earphone and microphone or the external ear in the case of "real-ear" measures) act as filters of the electrical signal—they also have a transfer function. Acoustically then, there appear clear consequences of manipulations of stimulus polarity. However, the more important question is whether such stimulus characteristics are manifested in AEPs in some manner and, if so, the extent to which they are helpful, are a nuisance, or simply can be ignored. Suffice it to say for the moment, stay tuned.

The acoustic consequences of the earphone/coupler transfer functions are often seen more readily in the frequency domain, as shown in Figure 2–19B. This panel shows the electrical and acoustical spectra of a 100 μs pulse stimulus ("click"). The main lobe of the electrical pulse has its first spectral zero at 10 kHz (replotted from Figure 2–17). While there is clear evidence that the acoustic spectrum follows some aspects of the electrical spectrum, there equally are departures of the acoustical spectrum from the electrical spectrum. The click plot is simplified (for illustration purposes), yet there appears to be an acoustic resonance in the 1 to 4 kHz range (more possibly pending real-ear and earphone nuances), and the acoustical spectrum drops off at a lower frequency than does the electrical spectrum (~5 kHz rather than 10 kHz). In any event, these differences in the acoustic spectrum are the cumulative result of the earphone and acoustic coupler transfer functions.

As stated in the introduction of this episode, a percept cannot be measured directly in any sensory modality, including hearing. Consequently, a subject's perception must be measured in reference to the physical characteristics of the signal that elicits it. The field of psychoacoustics relates the nature of the acoustic signal to response thresholds or some suprathreshold aspect of perception, like loudness, pitch, or timbre. In the physiological domain, there are several dependent variables of AEPs, including response detection limit, timing (latencies), and amplitudes of the various AEP peaks (recall Figure 1–1) that may be related to various stimulus parameters. If the physical properties of the acoustic stimulus are not precisely known, then the response is difficult or impossible to interpret, again whether that response be perceptual or physiological.

Therefore, "applying" sounds to evaluate sensory responses requires some method of ***calibration*** of the stimulus. Calibration is defined in broadest terms as verification that certain desired parameters of a stimulus are within defined tolerances. The importance of calibration can be readily appreciated by an example. Suppose someone is exposed to a very loud sound from a blast while vacationing in Odense, Denmark and had a hearing test there; they had a retest upon returning home in Buffalo, New York. The determination of whether the patient's hearing threshold changed from the time it was measured in Odense versus upon return to Buffalo is based on the assumption that the audiometers used for both tests were

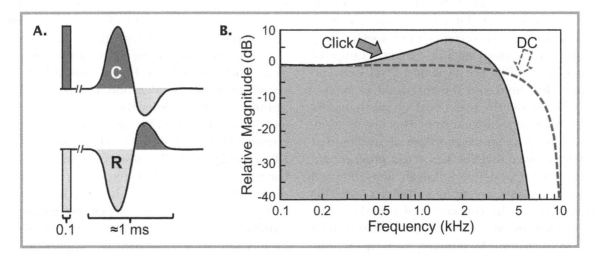

Figure 2–19. A. Electrical input and acoustical output signals of condensation (C) and rarefaction (R) click stimuli. **B.** Their common amplitude spectrum with that of the DC-pulse input for comparison. The click output is modeled here in general trends; actual acoustic data would reveal details according to the nuances of the transducer, coupler, and microphone used.

measuring—within acceptable tolerances—exactly the same thing. The manner in which the acoustic output of the audiometer is measured in practice is dictated by a **national** or **international standard** and becomes critical in such a scenario. If the acoustic output of the audiometers in Odense and Buffalo indeed are calibrated to identical values (again, within acceptable tolerances), then both audiologist and patient can feel confident that any differences in the Odense and Buffalo audiograms relate to the patient's hearing—whether the same or having changed—and not to differences in the acoustic output of the two audiometers—false similarities or differences. Some aspects of acoustic calibration that are important include the following:

Reference sound pressure

Transducer and coupler used

Stimulus envelope

Transducer distortion

Ambient noise level in the test room

A discussion of acoustic calibration starts with the **decibel (dB)**, which often is used, sometimes not fully understood, and thus possibly "abused." Hence a review never hurts, starting with the definition of the decibel. It is a tenth of a Bel. A Bel is the base-ten logarithm of the ratio of two sound powers or of two sound intensities, where **acoustic intensity (I)** = power/area: Bel = $\log(I_1/I_2)$.

Early work studying the dynamic range of hearing—the difference in sound level between absolute threshold and the threshold of pain—revealed it to extend across more than twelve orders of magnitude of sound intensity. This observation, and results of some psychophysical studies that followed, showed that listeners detect proportional change rather than simple arithmetic steps in sound parameters, namely according to **Weber's law**. This discovery led to the conversion of sound intensities on a logarithmic scale using the base ten or common logarithm. In normally hearing people, in their most sensitive frequency range (1–2 kHz), threshold was ~ 10^{-16} watts/m^2, which became the reference intensity for measures of sound **intensity level (IL)**. However, it is easier to measure **sound pressure** than sound power or intensity (sound pressure requires just a single microphone), and it was determined that 10^{-16} watts/m^2 in sound intensity was roughly equivalent to 0.00002 newtons/m^2. As 1 N/m^2 is also known as a pascal (Pa), then the approximation to best threshold in normally hearing humans is often referred to as 20 µPa. Herein, this value will be referred to as the **reference sound pressure** for making **sound pressure level (SPL)** measurements in air. In contrast, the reference sound pressure for underwater measurements is different—it is 1 µPa.

Back to the dB, as it is a tenth of a Bel, thus dB = 10 $\log(I_1/I_2)$. From **Ohm's (acoustic) law**, sound intensity is proportional to the square of sound pressure, so dB = 10 $\log(P_1^2/P_2^2)$. When a number is squared, the logarithm is doubled, hence the following equation is derived: dB = 20 $\log(P_1/P_2)$. Finally, applying the reference sound pressure of 20 µPa produces a standardized dB unit known as **sound pressure level (SPL)**: dB SPL = 20 $\log(P_1/20 \text{ µPa})$. For determining the level of a long duration sound, such as a tone (a sinusoid) from a pure-tone audiometer, either the "fast" or "slow" exponentially **time-weighted scales** of the measurement instrument—the **sound level meter (SLM)**—may be used. The "fast" function has a time constant of 125 ms, while the "slow" function has a time constant of 1000 ms. As it takes 3 to 4 time constants for these functions to approximate their asymptotic value, even the "fast" function would substantially underestimate the true SPL of the transient stimuli often employed in AEP testing.

Determination of the SPL of an acoustic transient (such as clicks and brief sinusoidal signals) requires special consideration. Two methods are in popular use to measure the SPL of acoustic transients frequently used for AEP testing. One method requires a special feature of a SLM to measure **peak SPL (pSPL)**, while the other uses an oscilloscope (or equivalent digital system) that can instantaneously trace and display the time history of the analog output of the SLM, namely to measure **peak equivalent SPL (peSPL)**. Note that pSPL also can be measured using the methods applied to determine peSPL.

On some SLMs, in addition to allowing the measurement of SPL using the "fast" or "slow" exponential time-weighting, there is also the option to measure pSPL. Using the "peak-hold" feature, the SLM captures the highest instantaneous SPL during a measurement interval, which can be reset manually. Note that this is not an RMS measurement, which "averages" the measurement over a time interval, rather it just measures and holds the largest instantaneous SPL. If measuring the SPL of a tone in the "fast" (or "slow") meter mode and comparing that to the measurement in the "peak hold" mode (pSPL), the latter would be 3 dB greater. The reason is the *crest factor*—the ratio of peak to RMS of a sine wave—which is 3 dB (namely, a ratio of 1.414 = the square root of 2). Simply put, pSPL = 20 log(P_p/20 μPa), where P_p is peak pressure.

The peSPL method is a two-step process. In the first step, the stimulus of interest is routed through the SLM to the oscilloscope/comparable analyzer, such as running an audio-analysis software program on a computer. The intrepid calibrator notes the voltage on the oscillographic display (Figure 2–20), either the maximum baseline to peak voltage (bpV) or the maximum peak-to-peak voltage (ppV). The upper waveform simulates a click stimulus that has been routed through the SLM to the analyzer. Considering again Figure 2–19, there is commonly an asymmetry between the R and C phases of the acoustic output, for a given input pulse's polarity. In Figure 2–20, the (nominally) rarefaction click is featured, thus the R phase is quite a bit larger than the C phase. A choice here is whether to quantify the signal by measuring the peak or the peak-to-peak pressure. (Note that the actual value here is not sound pressure, rather simply voltage of the SLM's output signal, but voltage is the electrical analog of sound pressure.) Now it is time for the second step, requiring a sine wave to be presented through the earphone. The level of the tone is adjusted until matching the voltage—either in reference to baseline-to-peak voltage (bpV) or peak-to-peak voltage ppV. Then the operator reads the SPL on the SLM and that is taken as the peSPL of the click stimulus (or other acoustic transient).

Should this measurement be for the bpV or the ppV? That issue is discussed later in the context of *calibration standards*. For now, it is enlightening to measure both and see how the two measurements differ. Figure 2–20 shows the voltage of the sine wave adjusted to the click bpV versus that to be equal to the ppV of the click. Two observations

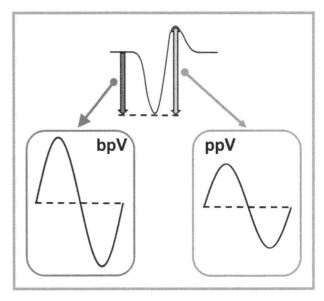

Figure 2–20. Schematization of measurements to determine peSPL (bpV—base-line-to peak voltage; ppV—peak-to-peak voltage; matching sinusoids, respectively; see text).

here are important. The two approaches will often yield different numerical values of peSPL! The second important observation is that the peSPL using the ppV approach can NEVER be larger than the peSPL observed with the bpV approach. If the maximal amplitudes of the rarefaction and condensation phase are exactly equal, then the two approaches will provide identical peSPL values. If a transient is critically damped and thus only producing a condensation or rarefaction phase (a challenging feature to create with a real earphone), then the 2 measures can differ by 6 dB (with the peak-to-peak approach producing the lower value).

To sum up, the question is what is the numerical relationship between pSPL and peSPL? Using the bpV approach for peSPL, the pSPL is 3 dB greater than the peSPL, as the two are related to the crest factor of a sine wave, again 3 dB. The peSPL assessed using the ppV approach is anywhere from 3 dB to 9 dB less than the pSPL, so the differences are not trivial.

Performing the peSPL match of the click to the reference signal is represented by Figure 2–21A. Here, the reference is 2000 Hz for demonstration purposes. The value 1000 Hz is popular in practice—or in the case of brief tone bursts, the frequency

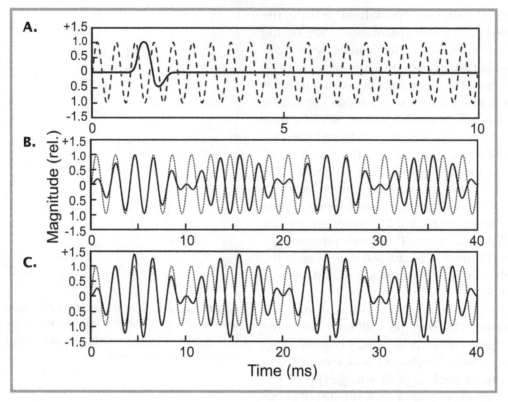

Figure 2–21. Peak-equivalent matching to an audiometric tone for an acoustic click, here using the condensation phase (**A**) and an amplitude modulated carrier (**B/C**). Comparison of sound pressures attained upon matching the AM to the reference signal according to peak-equivalent (**B**) versus A_{RMS} (**C**). In the latter scenario, the peak SPL will be 3 dB higher than that of the reference.

of the given carrier, generally an audiometric frequency. However, a bit of "unsettled law"—that is not explicitly represented in the standards available—is what to do with steady-state sounds, like a sinusoidal AM tone. In principle, it should not be a problem to just do the same match, as illustrated in panel B. FM also would not make any difference; the level of the modulated and unmodulated driving signals are the same. Actually, the FM stimulus could be calibrated simply using the protocol and calibration table for pure-tone audiometry. To explain, when the audiometer is calibrated, it is set to produce a continuous signal, readily measured using the SLM directly. (No oscilloscope/other equipment needed.) This then is simply matching (in effect) the A_{RMS} to that of a pure tone. This also could be done with the sinusoidal AM stimulus. However, as the carrier is being turned on and off essentially, the matching RMS to the standard for a given dB HL requires a driving signal to the transducer that is 3 dB higher in pSPL, as seen in panel C. This could be of some concern.

The highest test level used routinely with clicks and presumed to be safe—to avoid auditory fatigue or worse consequences of possible overstimulation—is 90 dB nHL. The pSPL then approaches/reaches 130 dB.[19] Not much higher than this, the examiner risks crossing into a region of the dynamic range of hearing that can cause discomfort and potentially permanent damage to the ear. In the steady-state area of AEP testing, there seems to be an assumption of safety to use levels up to 110 dB HL because this is a level that can be produced by audiometers for most test frequencies. Still, neither this nor the level itself—magnitude—are the sole issues for risk of injurious sound exposure. The other dimension of an exposure is duration—time. This is because it is the energy of the overall exposure, in essence magnitude × time, with potential tradeoffs between the two parameters for what can be considered a "safe" exposure. Unlike transient stimuli, including the standard tone burst used in audiometry (~500 ms or less), steady-state stimuli in AEP-measurement applications are turned on continuously for minutes at a time for each stimulus presentation; presentations, in turn, will recur with little recovery time throughout the test session (lasting perhaps a half hour or more). On the magnitude side of the exposure, calibration by way of peak equivalence is clearly more conservative and potentially less risk prone, more so if adhering also to a 90 dB nHL limit. Certainly, any other approach should be taken cautiously and with due consideration of the factors summarized.

To accurately measure SPL in general, the first thing needed is a microphone, but specifically one for which the ***frequency response*** and overall ***sensitivity*** are known. Failing that, a way is needed to determine sensitivity. Frequency response is the sensitivity across the frequency range over which measurements are to be made. Sensitivity of a microphone is the relationship between the sound pressures at the microphone diaphragm to the voltage at the microphone output—for instance, 50 mV/Pa. A power supply may be needed to provide a bias voltage depending on the type of microphone (for example, many non-prepolarized condenser microphones require a 200 V bias voltage). Thereafter, an amplifier and some type of voltage detector is used; a digital oscilloscope works particularly well. Some filtering capabilities are also useful—dBA and dBC weighting scales, and/or octave band filters, or perhaps even third-octave band-pass filters. For some purposes, the ability to "average" the voltage over time to simulate the "fast" and "slow" time-weighted averages is useful. Fortunately, SLMs can be purchased that have these features built-in. Still, not all SLMs have the same capacities and, in turn, are typed according to standards. Type I is the most capable. As noted previously, the SLM also must have the "peak-hold" feature in order to measure pSPL. Otherwise, pSPL (and peSPL) can be determined with an oscilloscope and SLM (or equivalent system), as described previously.

Figure 2–22 is a collage of photographs of hardware that is useful for calibrating an earphone used for audiometric purposes, including the measurement of acoustic transients. An SLM is shown in panel A. It is shown with a 1" condenser microphone, which can mate directly to standard 6-cc and 2-cc couplers commonly used in audiometer calibration. Panel B shows the digital readout of this SLM. Various couplers are shown in panels A and C. These couplers include those that are used with supra-aural earphones (like the TDH-39 and -49 earphone), often called 6-cc couplers. Other couplers are used for insert earphones (such as the ER3A tubal-insert earphones), often referred to as 2-cc couplers. A pair of supra-aural earphones are shown on the upper right portion of panel C, while an insert earphone is shown on the right side of panel A. It is helpful to have acoustic calibrators, which produce a known SPL at one or more frequencies. Two such calibrators are shown in panel A, upper right side. Again, acoustic transients can be measured by routing the AC output of the SLM to (for example) a digital oscilloscope, as shown during calibration of an acoustic click in panel D.

Standards are essential not only for calibrating the acoustic output of audiometers, but also AEP test equipment, again in order to ensure that everyone is measuring the acoustic output in the same way. In many cases, the standards select certain measurement parameters that are either arbitrary or the result of compromises made during the development of a standard. At the same time, it is fair to say that standards often ensure that everyone is measuring the acoustic stimuli in exactly the same wrong way. Yet, there is far more gained than lost with this approach. There are both national and international standards related to audiometric equipment, and there are several international standards related to the measurement of acoustic transients. Table 2–1 shows a brief list of national and international standards with which the reader should be familiar. In this table, the national standards included are those from the United States, developed by the American National Standards Institute (ANSI). The international standards are developed by either the International Electrotechnical Commission (IEC) or the International Organization of Standards (ISO). The ANSI standards include two very important standards for calibration of audiometric equipment. ANSI S3.6 is a detailed standard on how to calibrate the audiometer. Many of the calibration measurement procedures (and tolerances) specified by

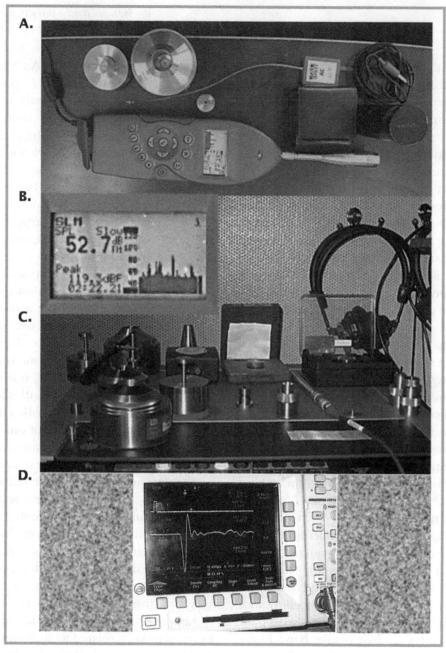

Figure 2–22. A–D. Photo collage of instrumentation used for acoustic calibration, including the calibration of transients (see text).

Table 2–1. Some Standards Relevant to Audiometric Testing and the Measurement of Acoustic Transients

▪ ANSI S3.1-1999 (R2018): Maximum Permissible Ambient Noise for Audiometric Test Rooms
▪ ANSI S3.6 (2018): Specification for Audiometers
▪ IEC 60645-3 (2020). Electroacoustics–Audiometric Equipment–Part 3: Test Signals of Short Duration
▪ ISO 389-6 (2007). Acoustics–Reference Zero for the Calibration of Audiometric Equipment–Part 6: Reference Threshold of Hearing for Test Signals of Short Duration

ANSI S3.6 can be used when calibrating AEP test equipment. ANSI S3.1 includes specifications regarding acceptable octave and third-octave band ambient-noise measurements in the test room when assessing hearing threshold, so that ambient noise does not substantially elevate hearing thresholds. Whether these ambient noise levels are those that should be applied when using AEP measurements to estimate hearing thresholds is subject to debate and bear further scrutiny.

Standard IEC 60645-3 specifies how to measure the level of acoustic transients, specifically requiring the use of the peak-to-peak peSPL approach. ISO 389-6 contains reference equivalent threshold sound pressure levels (RETSPLs), average hearing levels of normal hearing subjects (0 dB; commonly expressed as "normal hearing level", nHL), using the peak-to-peak peSPL method, for several couplers and earphones. These RETSPLs can be used for either clinical or research purposes, just as the dB HL values are used for the pure-tone audiogram.

In summary, the versatility of modern electronics along with the availability of high-quality transducers allow the generation of almost limitless acoustic stimuli. Thorough analyses and specifications benefit from both time- and frequency-domain analyses. Electroacoustic transducers (and couplers) have their own transfer functions and under many real-world conditions, the acoustic stimulus is not an exact replica of the electrical stimulus. It is critical that acoustic calibrations be performed on a regular basis so that the stimuli used for clinical or research purposes are the desired stimuli, within acceptable tolerances. National and international standards specify exactly how the stimuli should be manipulated and measured, and they provide the tolerances that are deemed acceptable.

PS: Further Readings

A few readers will find themselves wanting (or needing) some background material for further reading. Many sources of information are available about acoustics, sound measurement, and acoustical standards. Those listed in the following texts are a convenient subset of the many sources available in the AEP or audiology literature. There are, no doubt, newer editions of some, perhaps many, of these references. The book by Hunt (1992) provides a rather detailed history of acoustics.[20] Harris (1998) is an outstanding textbook about many aspects of sound measurement and control[21] and should be on the shelf of anyone serious about sound measurement. A good overview of sound measurement for audiologists[2,22] can be found in Yost and Nielsen and in Durrant and Feth. The calibration of acoustic transients[3,23] is covered by Durrant and Boston and Burkard and Don. Standardization and acoustic calibration[24,25,26] are covered in some detail in monographs edited by Burkard as well as Wilber and Burkard. Bon appétit!

HEADS UP

Wideband Transmission and the Middle Ear Bottleneck

Not all sound energy is efficiently transmitted via the outer and middle ear to the cochlea. Due to the effective area ratio between the tympanic membrane and the cochlear oval window, combined with the lever action of the ossicular chain of the middle ear, the most efficient transfer of sound energy between the ear canal and cochlea occurs in the frequency region of 800 Hz to 4000 Hz. Pop quiz: What sounds important to humans have significant frequency content in that region?

Conventional tympanometry informs the clinician about the status of the middle ear by examining its function at a frequency of 226 Hz, for which it is not efficiently passing sound to the cochlea in the first place. This frequency is used because it is convenient for calibration and because most middle ear disorders affect low frequencies (due frequently to the stiffness component of the middle ear transfer function).

What if the interest is evaluating the auditory system at higher frequencies? Is the middle ear affecting the measurements? Is the middle ear a bottleneck? Even answering such questions escapes measurements via routine tympanometry or only barely acquires measurements via other conventional immittance tests.

This Heads Up is about how well **wideband acoustic immittance (WAI)** can be estimated over the full auditory range.[27,28,29]

WAI permits assessment of how the middle ear "bottleneck" is affecting transmission of higher frequencies that could directly affect both pure-tone audiometric thresholds and threshold estimation and other applications of tests of auditory-evoked responses. WAI involves a variety of measurements made using a wideband stimulus, for example the click (recall Figure 2–17). WAI measurement takes advantage of signal processing methods common to those used to obtain AEPs, described in chapters to follow. However, WAI measurements can be made using a train of as few as a dozen clicks (presented at high repetition rates), sufficient to obtain a robust response in a fraction of the time typical of typical AEP tests. Hence, adding little time to what may be an already substantial test session for a given patient, the WAI test is not a burden.

How and what then is measured? The signal processing applied can extract the sound power (in effect) from an incident waveform (the click) using a ***probe microphone***. Therefore, the microphone is directly in the ear canal as part of an overall probe system including connection to a transducer to deliver the sound stimulus. The objective is to determine the amount of sound power that was reflected by the middle ear. The ratio of the reflected sound power to the incident sound power is taken as metric of **energy reflectance (ER)**. That is often transformed to **absorbance** as **1-ER**. As a power-based quantity, the absorbance at the tympanic membrane is essentially the same as the absorbance at the probe in the opening of the ear canal; therefore, there is no worry about subtracting out the ear canal volume, as done in conventional tympanometry. If all the sound is absorbed by the middle ear at a given frequency, the absorbance is 1.0, but if all the sound is reflected by the middle ear, the absorbance is 0.0.

Many of the early WAI studies were dedicated to examining absorbance at ambient pressure, similar to most auditory measurements (that is, other than tympanometry). However, these days there are commercial systems that permit the measurement of absorbance as the ear canal pressure is varied, similar to conventional tympanometry. This may be helpful in obtaining meaningful measures of auditory function in cases where the patient has negative middle ear pressure, namely by (in effect) correcting for the tympanometric-peak pressure. As pathological pressure in the middle ear only makes the "bottle neck" worse, this test condition permits "seeing" the absorbance of the rest of the conductive apparatus, to a certain extent. Wideband acoustic immittance (WAI) thus provides an assessment of how the middle ear bottleneck is affecting transmission of higher frequencies that, again, could directly affect pure-tone threshold, AEP, or other evoked responses.

Figure 2–23 shows a normal adult absorbance pattern (gray line).[29] Note that the middle ear absorbs less sound power at frequencies below 1000 Hz and above 4000 Hz. Even less power may be absorbed and available to the cochlea when the middle ear is not normal, indeed in cases presenting with clinically significant negative middle ear pressure, such as occurs even with the common cold. The ear with negative middle ear pressure (panel A, black line) has lower absorbance below about 4000 Hz and higher absorbance above 4000 Hz. Results of an investigation of effects of changes in ear canal pressure comparable to negative middle ear pressure showed elevated pure-tone thresholds and thus less sound power absorbed by the cochlea.[30] Hence, the objective WAI results were confirmed by the common and presumptive gold standard of conventional (behavioral) audiometry.

Changes in middle ear stiffness induced by the acoustic (stapedius) reflex are detectable with wideband absorbance measures and have

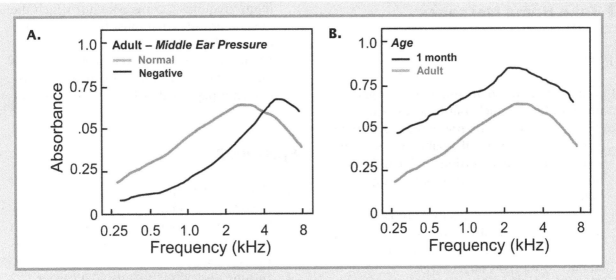

Figure 2–23. A. Effects of ear-canal static pressure on middle ear absorbance (1-ER; see text)—normal/ambient and (effectively) negative pressures in an adult. Modeled functions based on data from Feeney and Keefe (2001; upper curve)[31] and Feeney et al. (2014; lower curve).[30] **B.** Effects of maturation; absorbance in a 1-month-old infant versus the adult. Modeled functions based on data from Sanford and Feeney (2008)[33].

been shown to result in a sensitive measure of the acoustic reflex threshold.[31] Increased compliance (the inverse of stiffness) occurs with ossicular disarticulation and results in a high, narrow peak in absorbance. This eventually may come to be used as a clinical signature of that disorder.[32] These and other such clinical findings show WAI to yield the sort of information provided (within their respective technical limits) in both conventional tympanometry/immittance tests and bone-conduction audiometry.

Particularly enlightening, thanks to advancements in the research and development of WAI, are observations in young infants. An immediate technical advantage beyond those noted previously is not causing the child alarm by applying pressure changes to the ear canal. Absorbance measurement may be obtained readily at ambient pressure in infants and children. WAI has been instrumental in detecting and/or explaining developmental changes of the conductive apparatus.[33] As shown in Figure 2–23B, absorbance in a 1-month-old (black line) is higher than that of an adult ear across frequencies from 0.25 kHz to 8.0 kHz. Does this mean that a 1-month old can hear better than an adult because more sound is absorbed? Probably not, nor would that be consistent with conventional wisdom. Low frequency absorbance in this population is very likely different because sound from the probe is absorbed by the inherently more compliant (developing) ear canal of the infant, compared to that of the adult. Consequently, low-frequency maturation of auditory function overall is probably due in part to increased ear-canal ossification over the first 6 months of life.

At this writing, WAI has yet to be adopted clinically for routine use. Nevertheless, it is a powerful tool by which to enhance comprehensiveness of assessment of auditory function and, at the same time, adding to potential efficacy of routine real-ear objective assessment of the initial stages of sound "processing" by the auditory system, including real-ear calibration of stimuli used in all hearing tests. Herein is a method that actually goes beyond conventional calibration (estimation of SPL at the eardrum) by estimating what is getting through to the cochlea. Many advances have come forth via research and development of WAI; its future is bright.

Take Home Messages

Episode 1

1. It takes time to do anything, but not just a matter of how much, but how it goes.
2. Oscillatory signals do not entirely dominate hearing interests, yet they abound, but still account for only a portion of signals/sounds in the environment and/or of hearing interests.
3. Signals overviewed reflect two broad types—more or less "impulsive" versus essentially steady state, even if modulated (other than simply turning on/off).
4. Fundamentally understanding signal generation is understanding analysis.
5. Time and frequency are inseparable quantities but can provide different views—the time history versus the spectrum.
6. Speech is attractive as both environmentally relevant and neurologically intriguing, yet not always the most straightforward for all tests of interest.
7. Noises can be a consequence (such as a bad connection of a microphone) or generated purposefully (like masking sounds used in audiometry).
8. Even a handful of signals and their spectra demonstrate two types—discrete (line) or continuous.
9. Distortion of signals can be a consequence and can be troubling, as in the case of nonlinearity of amplitude (generally the primary symptom of a bad sounding intercom system).
10. Shaping signals in time and/or frequency also can be a consequence or caused purposefully, as in the use of filtering to limit frequency range.
11. Effecting T/F changes in signals is generally done electronically, but acoustical consequences also can affect the overall output of a system (like incidental formation of standing waves).
12. Analyzing/generating digitally real-world signals—such as AEPs or sounds eliciting them—requires a conversion for which there are certain rules that must be observed for best results.
13. Digital processing/signal generation "rocks" but not without its limits/nuances; as crime does not pay, an alias is not a good thing.

Episode 2

1. Time versus frequency domain analyses teach the admonition of "no free lunches"; the energy of brief pulses is splattered over broad frequency ranges, although with ups and downs.
2. Turning on and off a sinusoidal carrier (a form of amplitude modulation) splatters energy similarly, although the carrier frequency still dominates its spectral/central lobe.
3. Shape of the temporal envelope also affects spectral lobes and envelope, and the spectrum is continuous despite numerous dips/zeroes along the F axis.
4. Signals that are both very brief and highly frequency specific are not easy to come by, reflecting the challenge posed by the uncertainty principle.
5. An attractive alternative to transients are stimuli almost following pure-tone audiometry—the use of virtually steady tones/pulse trains, all having discrete (if complex) spectra.
6. The signal types and analyses overviewed have all "found their way" into use in stimulus-response analyses and measurement of AEPs (stay tuned).

Heads Up

7. Computers are pervasive in modern instrumentation, and are especially important to AEP testing; the overall goal is implementation of new/increased capabilities at effective costs.
8. There is little utility in developing computer-based systems that are hard to use.

Episode 3

1. Manipulating the acoustic signal is done mostly pretransduction.
2. The temporal envelope matters; furthermore, transduction from the electrical to the acoustic domain can change the stimulus.
3. Electrical polarity of the input signal also matters.
4. The need/rationale for calibration is critical; the decibel for the measurement/expression of sound pressure also must be understood for what it is in principle and how it is computed.
5. The measurement of SPL of acoustic transients differs from that of long-duration stimuli, and how it is measured also matters.
6. Standards prescribe how to calibrate sounds within certain tolerances.

Heads Up

7. The middle ear is neither transparent nor treats all sound frequencies equally.
8. Wideband absorbance immittance (WAI) is not just another "flavor" of tympanometry; it is much more comprehensive, essentially a calibration of the middle-ear transfer function.
9. Not yet fully deployed in routine clinical practice, WAI is an excellent research tool with great promise clinically.

References

1. Durrant, J. D., & Feth, L. L. (2013). *Hearing sciences: A foundational approach*. Pearson Education.
2. Durrant, J. D., & Feth, L. L. (2014). Physics of sound and electroacoustics. *Seminars in Hearing, 35*, 278–294.
3. Durrant, J. D., & Boston, J. R. (2006). Stimuli for auditory evoked potential assessment. In R. F. Burkard, M. Don, & J. J. Eggermont (Eds.), *Auditory evoked potentials: Basic principles and clinical application* (pp. 42–72). Lippincott-Williams & Wilkins.
4. Rosen, S., & Howell, P. (1991). *Signals and systems for speech and hearing*. Academic Press.
5. Speaks, C. E. (2018). *Introduction to sound: Acoustics for the hearing and speech sciences* (4th ed.). Plural Publishing.
6. Heideman, M. T., Johnson, D. H., & Burrus, C. S. (1984). Gauss and the history of the fast Fourier transform. *IEEE ASSP Magazine, 1*(4), 14–21.
7. Rabiner, L. R., & Schafer, R. W. (1978). *Digital processing of speech signals*. Prentice-Hall.
8. Blackman, R. B., & Tukey, J. W. (1958). *The measurement of power spectra*. Dover Publications.
9. Dallos, P. J., & Olsen, W. O. (1964). Integration of energy at threshold with gradual rise-fall tone pips. *Journal of the Acoustical Society of America, 36*(4), 743–751.
10. Gabor, D. (1947). Acoustical quanta and the theory of hearing. *Nature, 159*, 591–594.
11. Hirsch, I. J. (1975). Temporal aspects of hearing. In E. L. Eagles (Ed.), *The nervous system: Human communication and its disorders* (Vol. 3, pp. 57–162). Raven Press.
12. Delgado, R. E., & Miskiel, E. (1991). Innovative computer software and hardware design solutions and applications in the field of speech and hearing. *Journal for Computer Users in Speech and Hearing, 7*, 88–93.
13. Texas Instruments. (2017). TMS320C6746 fixed- and floating-point DSP. https://www.ti.com/lit/ds/symlink/tms320c6746.pdf?&ts=1589739871256
14. Moore, G. E. (1965). Cramming more components onto integrated circuits. *Electronics, 38*(8), 114–117.
15. Davies, P., & Delgado, R. E. (2018). SignalMaster—An open hardware and software system for speech and signal processing. *The Journal of the Acoustical Society of America, 143*(3), 1736–1736.
16. Delgado, R. E., & Özdamar, Ö. (1994). Automated auditory brainstem response interpretation. *IEEE Engineering in Medicine and Biology, 13*(2), 227–237.
17. Delgado, R. E., & Özdamar, Ö. (2004). Deconvolution of evoked responses obtained at high stimulus rates. *The Journal of the Acoustical Society of America, 115*(3), 1242–1251.
18. ANSI/ASA S3.6-2018. *American National Standard specification for audiometers*. Melville, NY: Acoustical Society of America. Melville NY.
19. Hall, J. W. (1992). *Handbook of auditory evoked responses* (p. 267). Allyn Bacon.
20. Hunt, F. V. (1992). *Origins in acoustics*. Acoustical Society of America.
21. Harris, C. (1998). *Handbook of acoustical measurements and noise control* (3rd ed.). Acoustical Society of America.

22. Yost, W., & Nielsen, D. (1985). *Fundamentals of hearing. An introduction* (2nd ed.). Holt, Rinehart and Winston.
23. Burkard, R., & Don, M. (2015). Introduction to auditory evoked potentials. In J. Katz, M. Chasin, K. English, L. Hood, & K. Tillery (Eds.), *Handbook of clinical audiology* (7th ed., pp. 187–206). Lippincott Williams & Wilkins
24. Burkard, R. (2014). Standards and calibration. Part 1: Standards process, physical principles, pure tone and speech audiometry. *Seminars in Hearing, 35*(4), 267–360.
25. Burkard, R. (2015). Standardization and calibration. Part 2: Brief stimuli, immittance, amplification, and vestibular assessment. *Seminars in Hearing, 36*(1), 1–74.
26. Wilber, L., & Burkard, R. (2015). Calibration. In J. Katz, M. Chasin, K. English, L. Hood, & K. Tillery (Eds.), *Handbook of clinical audiology* (7th ed., pp. 9–28). Lippincott Williams & Wilkins.
27. Keefe, D. H., & Simmons, J. L. (2003). Energy transmittance predicts conductive hearing loss in older children and adults. *The Journal of the Acoustical Society of America, 114*(6), 3217–3238.
28. Allen, J., Jeng, P., & Levitt, H. (2005). Evaluation of human middle ear function via an acoustic power assessment. *Journal of Rehabilitation Research & Development, 42,* 63–78.
29. Feeney, M. P., Hunter, L. L., Kei, J., Lilly, D. J., Margolis, R. H., Nakajima, H. H., . . . Voss, S. E. (2013). Consensus statement: Eriksholm workshop on wideband absorbance measures of the middle ear. *Ear and Hearing, 34*(7 Suppl. 1),78s–79s.
30. Feeney, M. P., Sanford, C. A., & Putterman, D. B. (2014). Effects of ear-canal static pressure on pure-tone thresholds and wideband acoustic immittance. *Journal of the American Academy of Audiology, 25*(5), 462–470.
31. Feeney, M. P., & Keefe, D. H. (2001). Estimating the acoustic reflex threshold from wideband measures of reflectance, admittance and power. *Ear and Hearing, 22*(4), 316–332.
32. Feeney, M. P., Grant, I. L., & Mills, D. M. (2009). Wideband energy reflectance measurements of ossicular chain discontinuity and repair in human temporal bone. *Ear and Hearing, 30*(4), 391–400.
33. Sanford, C. A., & Feeney, M. P. (2008). Effects of maturation on tympanometric wideband acoustic transfer functions in human infants. *Journal of the Acoustical Society of America, 124*(4), 2106–2122.

Electrically Connecting to Humans to Access Their Auditory Neurosensory Systems

The Writers

Episode 1: John D. Durrant, Krzysztof M. Kochanek, and Lech K. Śliwa
Episode 2: Frank E. Musiek
Heads Up: Christopher D. Bauch and Wayne O. Olsen

■ Episode 1: Bioelectric Basics, Interface Dilemmas, and Electrode Montages/Caps— One Size Fits All?

Electricity is the hallmark of the modern world. This form of energy is also essential to biological systems. Living creatures are dynamos—generators of electricity—not that they should be viewed as one huge battery. Humans and animals alike are fabricated from innumerable cells that are about as many equivalent tiny batteries and other electrical-circuit components, and this is only their brains! At the molecular-biological level are paths of communication that make cells work, so communication truly is the "name of the game" of living organisms. Cells come together to form organs of the body; these parts often have to communicate with each other at that level as well, lest—for example—one hand indeed does not know what the other is doing. Broadly in neurophysiology there are two systems of communication within the body—chemical by way of hormones and *bio-electrical*. Both are involved in vertebrates. The latter derives from electrical events initiated within neurons—the "wiring" of the nervous system. The former involves a system also at the cellular level and expressed broadly in the nervous system by *synaptic transmission*, specifically chemical synapses that release a chemical substance/neurotransmitter to act on the next neuron (for example). This is in contrast to the more archaic *direct electrical synapses* or *ephaptic coupling* via cell-to-cell contact, like the shorting of uninsulated electrical wires that have inadvertently come into direct contact. Still, electricity is conducted and propagated effectively to some body parts (like legs) over considerable distances (from the spinal cord), such as to alert the brain (central system processor) of a stubbed toe (activated pain sensor) and warn of risk of an imminent fall. Electrical systems' signals can be sampled certainly from tapping into cells directly but also by way of strictly noninvasive pickup. Conversely, electricity can be passed to the body to activate some organs. The electrical paths to/from the outside world are often bidirectional, implying the possibility to detect electrical signs at the body's surfaces generated from within. At the same time, this is not necessarily readily so, despite the impression of how easy it is to be victimized by an electrostatic shock. The underlying principles are essential to a comprehensive understanding and competent application of clinical electrophysiology.

Familiar samplings of bodily electrical activity are the *electrocardiogram (ECG)* (recall Figure 2–2B, function 3) and "*brain waves*" via the *electroencephalogram (EEG)*. Electricity is not always well understood by users in practice, but common experience teaches several relevant concepts needed here—starting with the common flashlight.[1] Electrical components such as the flashlight's battery, light bulb, and on-off switch are connected to form a circuit for the current from the battery to circulate. The light bulb is a form of resistor; a resistor's job is to oppose/control the flow of electrical current (like a water faucet's valve). Without *resistance*, as without friction in mechanical systems, this simple circuit would be in a runaway condition that would quickly discharge the battery, or worse. The worst-case scenario (parts melting/burning) happens due to the inevitability of some resistance in the wires and contacts among them. The light-bulb resistor effects a controlled burn, generating light from the heated element (filament). However, it cannot do so indefinitely and will ultimately "burn out," even if the battery was not to have fully discharged. Both the flow of the *electrical current* supplied and pushed by the electrical force of the battery—*voltage*—can be measured. The same is true in bioelectrical systems, as in measurement of the *auditory evoked potentials (AEPs)* sampled in brain waves. With little exception, the parameter of interest will be voltage, as implied by the "P" in AEP (voltage and potential difference being synonymous).

The flashlight circuit largely exemplifies well enough the basic principle of a living cell, such as the skin cell. Dead cells forming the uppermost skin's surface are essentially dead batteries, and not rechargeable ones! In the hearing organ/other systems, both sensory and nerve cells at rest look like charged batteries, although their resting membrane potentials are barely one-half-tenth that of a common flashlight battery. Motor, cardiovascular, sensory, and neural cells have an additional ability: they are irritable. *Irritability* is not an emotion here; it is the ability to discharge and subsequently recharge. In sensory and neural cells, activities are transient changes in voltages that may be tapped via clinical electrophysiology; they give rise then to the sorts of sensory evoked potentials soon to be explored extensively for their clinical utility in audiology.[2]

That is because voltage discharges are the upshots of activation of these cells—from the sensory cell as a *transducer* and the nerve cell as a conveyor of the *event*, hence event-related potentials, as are AEPs. To do so knowledgeably, it is necessary to be familiar with some "realities" of connecting to the clinical subject/patient effectively and especially safely.

Cells work by common principles of physical laws, the most basic being **Ohm's electrical law**.[1] The voltage of the flashlight battery and a cell's resting membrane potential derive from a polarization due to separation of plus and minus charges chemically/biochemically by the processes therein. Batteries source *direct current (DC)*—a unidirectional flow. The battery of an automobile is fundamentally the same, yet current tapped to recharge car batteries and to power devices in homes and industry today are supplied in the form of *alternating current (AC)*, wherein the polarity flip-flops at ~50/60 Hz. Other examples of AC potentials, as noted earlier, include that of the sinusoid fed to an earphone to generate a pure tone; the vast majority of component potentials of AEPs also are AC. The bottom line for purposes here is that both DC and AC concepts apply to their nature, their origins, and the methods involved in their measurement, sooner or later. Nevertheless, it is often desirable when possible to simplify concepts by treating a given effect that may be truly AC-like by way of a DC analogy. Furthermore, the "law" of Ohms applies broadly, although with some twists, as will be clarified along the way.

For all the parallels of bio- and physical electricity, current flow in the two environments is different. In the outside/physical world, current flows by movement of free electrons in the conductor (typically metal/wires); in the body, currents are mediated by movement of *ions* (charged atoms/molecules). Enter the *electrode* and methods of their application to the body to span this "gap" for effective connection between the physical test instrument and the patient being examined. Truly sensitive and stable measurement or *recording* of bioelectric signals is more challenging than might be supposed from television or the movies or even direct experience of having had an ECG. The pickup devices—electrodes—"slapped" onto areas of the chest and/or back provide quick and stable measurements of this critical signal. In reality, the

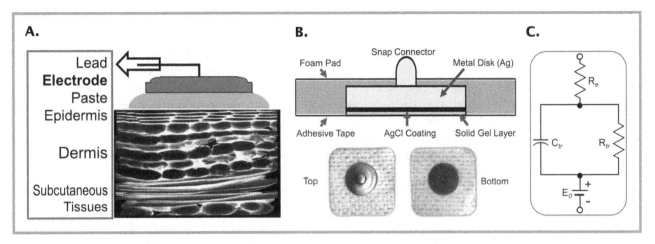

Figure 3–1. A. Metal electrode on skin of which the diversity of cell structure is schematically represented in a simulated magnified-x-ray view of cross section; the electrode "rides" on electrolyte paste, cream, or gel of sufficient amount to avoid direct metal-to-skin contact. **B.** Disposable silver-silver chloride (Ag/AgCl) electrode: schematic cross section (*top*) and actual example (*bottom; top/bottom* views of electrode). **C.** Simplified equivalent electrical circuit of electrode and electrode-skin contact: E_0—half-cell potential (resulting from ion concentration gradient near the electrode interface); R_e—electrode resistance; and R_{tr} and C_{tr}—"transition" resistance and capacitance, making up the electrode impedance (inspired by Neuman[3]).

examiner was not merely touching the skin with a bare wire or equivalent conductor, and there are still other considerations and preparations that can prove to be somewhat grossly inadequate, if done improperly, as follows: (1) inappropriate materials and/or mechanically unstable interfacing (again, not merely touching wire/metal to skin); (2) the skin itself has nuances that demand appropriate preparation, and this must be done methodically; (3) there is often more to the effective electrode than meets the eye and/or the need of more specialized electrodes for certain applications; (4) the potentials of interest for assessing auditory functionality are, at their greatest magnitudes, typically orders of magnitude less than the ECG (in turn, still much smaller than the flashlight battery's voltage); and (5) multiple electrodes are always involved. The ECG analogy fits particularly well apropos the last point—namely, several electrodes minimally that are placed purposefully for optimal sampling of potentials desired to be measured.

Spanning the electron-ion gap ought to be simple enough given the body being made up extensively of water, much of it like seawater. A material like silver can be electroplated with salt (NaCl) to form a coating of ***silver-silver-chloride (Ag-AgCl)*** for an excellent current flow, even at frequencies down to DC (in principle). In signal-ese, "DC" also is nominally defined as zero frequency or arguably an AC of infinitesimally small frequency. This property of Ag-AgCl then serves very well the purpose of recording of any signal from AEP-dom. This point would end this discussion nicely were it not for the largest organ of the body—back to the skin! Skin is made up of multiple layers, schematically illustrated in Figure 3–1A. As the outermost layer is dead skin, it is no good as a battery and not much better as a conductor. Worse is that it is also more or less oily, or still worse, it has additives like skin and/or hair lotions and so forth that the patient may have applied to their skin. A good connection thus requires both appropriate electrode design and adequate preparation of the skin to improve ***conductivity*** through the skin to the electrode. Electrodes like those used routinely for testing AEPs are illustrated in Figure 3–1A and B. All are fundamentally a metal plate, even if very small and/or not readily evident by the eye (as in panel B). The metal part is connected to a wire lead, to be connected in turn to the test instrument. As hinted previously and illustrated, direct metal-to-skin contact is to be avoided; this is to minimize mechanical instability of conductivity of the physical contact. This is ensured by having a "cushion" of ***electrolyte paste***—a salt-impregnated substance that in practice may be a paste, cream, or gel. The electrolyte paste (like seawater) is electrically conductive; in pastier forms, it can help to keep the electrode in place. This otherwise can be accomplished using a piece of gauze pad over the top of the electrode, making physical contact between it and the underlying skin beyond the perimeter of the electrode itself (panel A). Tape is another useful option, especially on bare skin, and a generally useful material to have on hand. A double-sticky tape is inherent to the electrode design of disposable electrodes (panel B) and will be further illustrated shortly. First, there is still more to the "preparation story," indeed critically important for the best results. Here, the proverbial admonition that "haste makes waste" could not be truer.

Therefore, integral to the application of the electrode for adequate conductivity is the proper preparation of the skin itself. The surface of the skin immediately under the intended site of the electrode placement must be clean to reduce oil, makeup, and/or skin/hair treatment that could compromise conductivity. The adhesive support of the electrode will also be more effective. Alcohol "wipes" or saturated gauze pads are commonly used for both preparation and posttest cleanup. Although life cannot be "breathed" back into the dead skin cells, conductivity can be improved—a second purpose of the electrode paste. Absorption of the electrolyte itself is the aim, which can be facilitated using a Q-tip or small piece of gauze pad to massage it into the skin. Working in hair-born areas is an additional challenge for securing the electrode and cleanup subsequently, but it is manageable generally with pushing aside the hair and using one of the pastier electrolyte pastes (versus creams or gels) and a piece of gauze pad over the top (as noted previously). Securing the electrode leads diligently is worth emphasizing too, including anticipating nature's "call" or other emergencies that can/do happen midexamination. The leads can then be disconnected from the test instrument, rolled up, and secured to the patient's clothing, allowing efficient reconnection upon continuation of examination.

Excellent electrodes, in addition to Ag-AgCl, are gold/gold-plated and silver/silver-plated types. Recording of near DC (very low-frequency AC signals), typical of cortically generated AEPs (long-latency responses; recall Figure 1–1), demands especially good application techniques and often the Ag-AgCl type electrode. The electrical circuit formed from the combined skin and electrode proves to be more complex than that of the flashlight with its DC battery, lightbulb, and metal-to-metal contacts among parts, even within the on-off switch. The flashlight is an example of a purely resistive circuit. Resistors fundamentally control current flow in AC circuits without regard for frequency. The good news is that AC signals can be expressed over gaps between conductors, literally. The alternating-polarity charge building up on one side of the would-be contact can induce alternating-charge buildup on the other side—in this case, from the skin to the electrode. This is due to ***capacitance***, the most basic form of which is two conductors separated by an insulator or dielectric. Only the continuously changing force field provides a continuous flow of current from one side to the other—so not DC. For a given material (some plastics, for instance), the thinner and thus closer the spacing, the better the AC conductivity. This factor might seem to be eliminated by proper preparation of the skin, especially by way of the electrolyte, but the material of the skin and its layers are both more or less conductive and less or more insulative. Capacitance is distributed in this circuit along with resistance, as schematically represented in the equivalent "lumped" circuit in Figure 3–1C.[3] This is why true DC recordings are difficult to achieve, short of connecting into the bloodstream. Nevertheless, there is a DC element in the circuit, batterylike, but for one electrode, sort of a half battery called the "half-cell" potential. This effect can exacerbate the general problem of any movement of an electrode; so mechanical stability is paramount. "Where's the good news?" The answer is working with relatively higher-frequency waves of AEPs, as typically generated in the auditory nerve, brainstem, and beyond. Especially for the shorter latency (thus higher-frequency) AEPs that are frequently the focus of tests used in audiology, Ag-AgCl electrodes do not hurt. However, they are far less critical for reliable recordings, if accomplished using good metal electrodes and assuming good preparation of the electrode sites in the first place. Much of the clinical work also is done with some kind of high-pass filtering, particularly at the front end of the system, which helps further

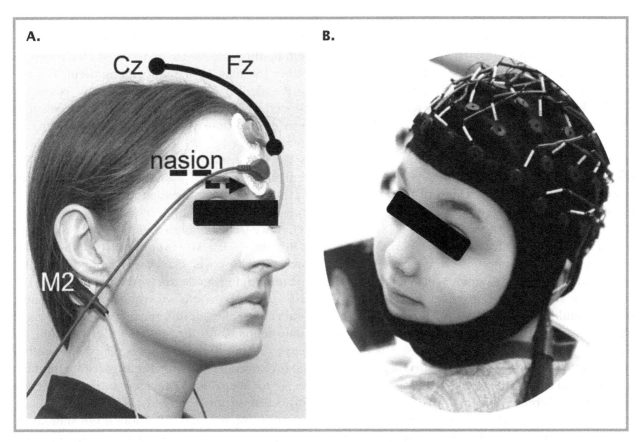

Figure 3–2. A. Clinically popular, basic electrode montage (for single recording channel), comprising electrodes at midhairline (approximately between F_z and F_{pz},), M2, and nasion. C_z and midhairline are some of the most common placement sites used for clinical electrophysiology in audiology. **B.** Electrode cap used for high-density recordings of auditory evoked potentials across the scalp's entire surface.

to stabilize the recording (that is, rejecting low-frequency noise/interference, whatever its origin).

Measurement of goodness of conductivity is very important for reliable response recordings, and this is the first measurement made in a competently performed AEP test. The less good news is that this cannot be measured with a basic and relatively inexpensive volt-ohm meter. However, the form of opposition that this element imposes in the circuit is like elastic elements of the middle ear and other vibro-mechanical systems, namely with components of stiffness and mass (in addition to friction). How they behave is frequency dependent because these elements do not siphon off energy from the system into heat of frictional resistance, rather affecting timing by the property of ***reactance***. Combining resistance and reactance, the net opposition to current flow is ***impedance***.[1] Consequently, this must be tested at some frequency, often like 15 Hz to 30 Hz or higher.[4] The electrode impedance (Z) is tested between electrode pairs or one electrode referenced to the average of others. For AEP work, it generally is desirable to have less than 2,000 to 5,000 ohms with a good balance among electrodes. This is a troubleshooting tool as well, when the recording tends to be of poor quality, as an electrode might have somehow lifted from the skin.

Electrodes are connected to an AEP test system at the stage of the (pre-) amplifier, just ahead of the analog-to-digital converter of the test system (recall preview and figure of the Heads Up of Episode 2.2; also to be discussed in greater detail in the next chapter). Depending on application, a number of electrodes will be placed on the scalp, with a minimum of three (see Figure 3–2A). For fully mapping activity of the brain with high spatial resolution across the scalp's surface, some 20 to 100 electrodes may be needed and secured using an electrode cap (panel B). The minimum configuration (for a single-channel recording) comprises two electrodes that are nominally "active" (like the + and – leads of a battery tester) or wherein one is intended to measure a signal relative to a reference that presumably is neutral. In either case, the measurement is that of a potential difference between the two, in order to sample the desired signal/response. The third is not a part of this measurement, yet no less important; it serves as a connection to the electrical ground and thus is important for safety. As clinical electrophysiology necessarily involves electrical connections to the patient—and even inadvertently the examiner—it is important to emphasize safety first! Consequently, only equipment should be used that has been certified to be electrically safe. The ground connection is protective only if the test equipment is used with the standard three-pronged plug (per current national/international standards), while avoiding extension cords or multiplug adaptors that might defeat proper grounding. All of which—including the EP test system itself, metal desk, cart for system transportation, and a metal-shielded test booth—should be evaluated by electrical safety personnel for proper grounding. This is a life and death matter! Such precaution also is prudent for minimizing electrical-system interference and stimulus artifact, if not as well as for the effective shielding of the subject from becoming a virtual antenna for extraneous electrical noise. These issues will come up recurrently and for good reason—they are not to be "poo-pooed." The focus for now is more on where and why connections are typically made from an anatomical point of view.

Very often in routine clinical testing the hookup illustrated in Figure 3–2A (plus or minus some variations of placement, per the specific AEP test) will suffice for one or two channels of recording. Still more electrodes could be added, even with this one-at-a-time electrode placement. For substantially higher numbers of electrodes, an electrode cap (again, see Figure 3–2B) is far more practical. For consistency of results of AEP tests across examiners/clinics, the actual sites of electrode placement need to be chosen according to or at least referenced to a standard of electrode sites for EEG evaluation, such as the International 10-20 system illustrated in Figure 3–3.[5,6] The name of this system neither means use of 10 or 20 electrodes, but rather the relative spacing among them. The base of the skull from the EEG perspective is taken to be defined by the line subtended between reference points demarked by the nasion (front) and inion (back of skull). The other important referent is the very top of the skull—the vertex (C_z). The remaining standard points are referenced according to percent of distance among them, 20% or 10% of the hemi-circumference from C_z to the base reference (from head side view, at the preauricular point of the ear). The overall matrix of these placements are to cover classically defined regions of the underlying cerebrum (see Table 3–1). The relative scaling is to ensure comparable mapping of brains regardless of differences of head size, as the brain tends to fill the space of a given skull. The letter naming the site follows the major anatomical divisions of the brain; the subscripted numbers or "z" for "zero" indicate sites to the right (even), left (odd), or midline (zero). The earlobe (A) and mastoid (often called "M," though not standard) is widely used. A/M are frequently used electrode sites for AEP work along with C_z, F_z, P_z and other sites pursued in the context of individual AEPs of interest. Such details will be divulged along the auditory pathway, in effect, and thus throughout the rest of the book.

Electrode placement is important, if not critical, to sample optimally the desired signal and/or minimize untoward pickup of unwanted signals—like muscle potentials from swallowing and eyeblink—and/or spurious physical-electrical noise—like from a machine running nearby, even the computer of the test instrument. Nevertheless, nonstandard placements may be used for alternative strategies but at least should be explained in the clinical notes and ideally in reference to the standard. However, placement of an electrode approximately at "midhairline" (as is the case is in Figure 3–2A) is broadly popular for routine testing of short latency responses (SLRs) from the brainstem. Even if well accepted in practice, it is not helpful to mislabel this site by just picking the (perceived) next closest "standard" site. Although hairline is variable/variably judged among individuals, it generally falls neither at F_z nor at F_{pz},

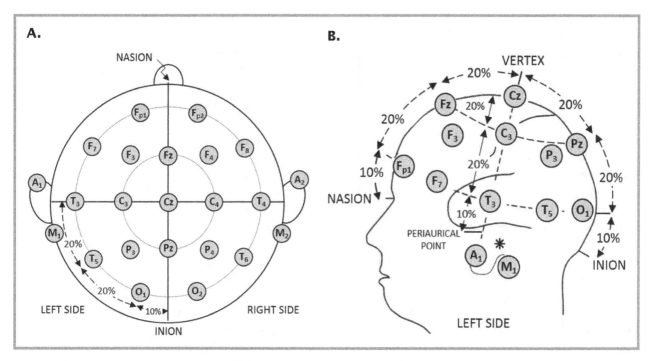

Figure 3-3. Basics of the International 10-20 system[5] for systematically positioning/referencing placement of electrodes for recording brain waves—top (**A**) and lateral (**B**) views. Percentages designate distances among sites relative to the hemi-circumference of the head. Capital letters are defined as follows: F—frontal, C—central, P—parietal, O—occipital, T—temporal, A—auricular. Subscript "Z" (for zero) denotes midline positions; even numbers designate right-side placements and odd numbers designate left-side placements. ✶ = reference point for measuring laterally the hemi-circumference of the head to the vertex, the top of the skull. In practice, the mastoid (M) is often used as an electrode site, rather than the earlobe (A). (See Table 3-1 for more detailed definitions.)

Table 3-1. Definitions of 10-20 System and Relation to Areas of the Cerebrum

Electrode Placement Site		Prefrontal (Fp)	Frontal (F)	Temporal (T)	Parietal (P)	Occipital (O)	Central (C)	Auricular (A) Mastoid (M)	Midline sagittal plane (z)
Underlying Region of Cerebrum		Prefrontal cortex	Frontal lobe	Temporal lobe	Parietal lobe	Occipital lobe			Corpus callosum
Electrode Symbols	Left	Fp1	F3, F7	T3, T5	P3	O1	C3	A1, M1	Fpz, Fz, Cz, Oz
	Right	Fp2	F4, F8	T4, T7	P4	O2	C4	A2, M2	

as illustrated. It falls (at least on average in young males) midway between the two. This begs the question of why not just use F_z or F_{pz}? The "hairline" strategy is to minimize working in hairy areas–like C_z in most patients. Certainly the examiner may need to do so for practical reasons, such as in testing infants (simply for expediency) and newborns (again, per utmost efficiency and avoiding the baby's "soft spot" on the cranium). Yet, this is moving the electrode potentially away from a better site(s) and/or risking compromising the quality of the recordings (by virtually optimizing pick of extraneous potentials). In any event, working with hair may be unavoidable. An example is desiring to see potentials that are optimally recorded from C_Z and/or when desiring to sample possible right-left hemispheric differences by recording simultaneously from C_3 and C_4. Returning to the notion of going as far down the scalp as F_{PZ}, this has another risk but that which will be more evident with a few more "doses" of theory. Whatever configuration of electrode placements—***electrode montage***—deemed useful by the examiner, the use of the 10-20 system in sensory-EP testing is not intended to dictate from where to record. It is to encourage choosing sites systematically and to precisely reference the electrode placements used. Where to record for a given AEP or other EPs (like visual evoked potentials) in a given application must be learned from the literature, which grew out of the extensive research and development of this technology.

How different electrode montages "see" the bioelectric activity on the scalp is a challenging topic. A compelling approach is that of dipole-source modeling,[7,8] which has been enlightening but also is based on "heavy-duty" math applied to large arrays of data from numerous channels of recording from electrode caps. Nevertheless, more general/basic notions are intuitively accessible and will suffice for more basic concepts here, but also can provide useful insights to guide clinical practice.

The AEP generator in this "story" is taken to behave like a sort of dipole antenna, radiating from somewhere in the volume of the brain, like a radio signal. As such, it has an orientation characterized as having plus and minus poles, like the simple battery. As current flows between the + and – poles locally, voltage created in the surrounds become progressively weaker with distance, yet it is still picked up at considerable distances. The upshot of such dynamics is demonstrated by example by one of the long-latency responses (LLRs) arising from cortex, reflecting dramatically the changing "view" possible by location of the electrode (like an antenna). A virtual demonstration of the effect is in order; here is the setup. Recordings are at sites moving down the hemi-circumference of the skull from the top of the head to the skull base and below; below the skull's surface, this "trek" will pass over the superior temporal gyrus. The montage supposed is close to that yielding the data used to model waveforms which were results from an actual and now-classical experiment.[9] For this demonstration (versus more conventional/clinically oriented work), a sort of monopolar antenna is referenced to an essentially neutral site. A truly electrically neutral (zero-potential) site anywhere on the scalp actually proves difficult to come by and/or not entirely pleasant for the subject, like the tip of the nose. This can be thought of (continuing the radio analogy) as holding a walkie-talkie with a small vertical antenna, first held starting at an elevation of about 45°, then rotating it clockwise toward 0°, and then further clockwise.

Therefore, starting the simulation with the "active" electrode at C_Z (the most popular clinical test site for LLR tests), this sequence demonstrates diminishing magnitudes of the waves that ultimately "flip over," as illustrated in Figure 3–4A. The flip-over proves to occur in the vicinity of the superior plane of the superior temporal gyrus, site of the auditory cortex, and the general area of the source of the N_1-P_2 complex. In practice, a more beneficial montage for the examiner is simply recording between C_Z and M_1 (tracing CT* in Figure 3–4A), thereby virtually doubling the N_1-P_2 peak-to-peak amplitude. This is not quite as good as C_Z-N (last tracing, panel A), but moving down the neck may offset the advantage by increasing electromyographic (EMG) interference from neck muscles, soon to be considered with other realities of the challenges of real-world AEP recordings. Meanwhile, "lowering" one electrode down from top and along the side of the head clearly will diminish the amplitude of the recorded potential. Might this be ill advised? Yes, if unintended; for example, if having intended to record indeed from C_Z but placement of the electrode was inaccurate. This could happen upon a mismeasurement of the ear-to-ear distance over the top of the head or miscalculation of the midpoint. The "z" sites fall precisely in the midsagittal plane. Intentionally selecting sites on each side of the head, below C_Z, nevertheless can be interesting, namely to compare right- versus left-hemispheric responses. Clinically this could yield results of diagnostic significance and, in general, is enlightening about the

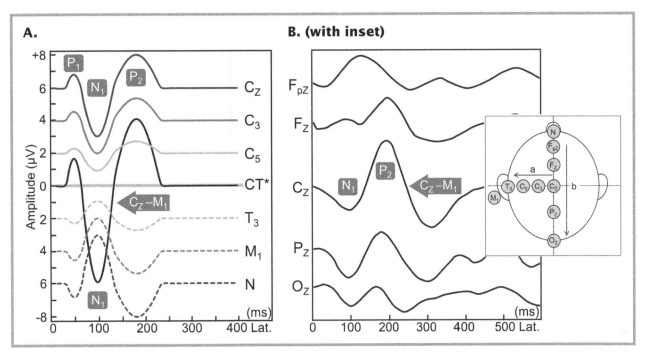

Figure 3–4. A. Simplified computer model of the P_1-N_1-P_2 complex, following trends of peak latencies of the average long-latency response (LLR) in young normal-hearing adults; amplitudes and overall polarity of response adjusted to approximate trends of recordings of the classical demonstration by Vaughan and Ritter (1970)[9] (see text)—effects of measurements repeated as if tracked over sites descending laterally from vertex (C_z) to below the mastoid (N), referenced to tip of the nose. **B.** Actual recording of a comparable response at C_z, tracked from nasion to O_z. Responses as illustrated by panels **A** and **B** are typical of suprathreshold LLRs elicited using tone-burst stimuli in the middynamic range of hearing—clinically, around the center of the conventional audiogram (per dimensions of hearing level by frequency).

distribution of a given AEP over the entire scalp. Modern, clinical test systems often support at least four or more channels of recording, so "looking" at multiple sites at the same time does not mean added test time. Lastly, locations anteriorly or posteriorly (not just more or less laterally) also make a difference, as illustrated in panel B. Such locations become less favorable for the most robust recordings of AEPs and are overlooking other systems' cranial "turf," such as that over O_z favoring visual-evoked potentials.

In general, AEP measurements more often are less about proximity of electrodes to generators literally and more about orientation of recording montage, in reference to location and orientation of the generators of a given AEP. The spread of electrical currents in a uniform conductive medium (like salt water) is analogous to a signal radiating from a broadcast station—in all directions and uniformly. In such a medium, a radiating dipole source develops voltage (force) fields, as illustrated in Figure 3–5A, from current flowing locally between the poles. The spread progressively widens with distance, with loss of signal strength. Nevertheless, even at a distance, the relative location and orientation of the source and polarity of the field would be discernible. The human head is far from such a pristine medium, composed of multiple materials stratified in multiple layers (like skin of the scalp, membranes like the dura matter, and bone) with their own influences on the net spread of the signal. Meanwhile, the generator of a given potential may have a certain angle of orientation in reference to the scalp's surface. The nature of such a situation at the two extremes for its "view" is illustrated in panel B—broadside versus on end. Presumably, the results simulated in Figure 3–4A reflect the scenario on the left in panel B.

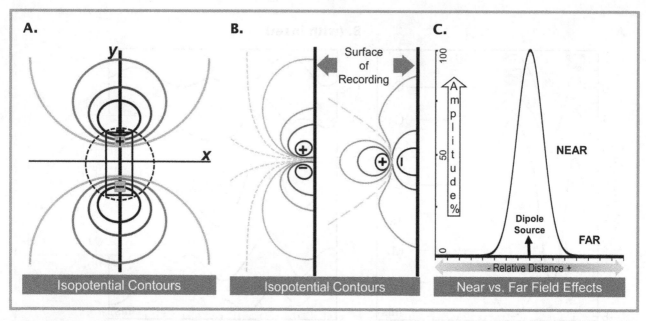

Figure 3–5. Illustrations of cross sections of (in reality) three-dimensional voltage/force fields. **A.** Isoelectric fields expanding from a dipole source in a homogeneous conductive medium (like salt water), at one instant, likened to a battery (*dashed line* symbolizing current flow between the poles locally); relative strength represented in gray scale (lighter = weaker; reflecting approximately halving the potential with each expansion illustrated). **B.** Effects when the source is near a surface (like brain tissue under the skull); relative to contours in **A**, strength is divided by approximately 4 with each expansion of spread from the source. **C.** Concept of near- versus far-field effects on strength of potentials overall recorded as a function of relative distance from the source. (Panels **A** and **B**: based on theoretical concepts and data of Kooi [1978];[10] panel **C**: inspired by Wood and Allison [1981].[11])

The view from the surface of generators within the cranium cannot be expected to reflect all that is going on within, certainly not from any one montage's "view."[10] Nevertheless, the generators of multiple LLRs readily can be recorded from the top of the central auditory pathway, shown well by the demonstration earlier, but with the twist that the N_1-P_2 signal to be sampled most robustly is "straddling" the auditory cortex, suggesting an orientation of the force fields (as in Figure 3–5B, left). Still, the generators of the cortical AEPs are relatively close to the location of the electrodes, especially in reference to side of the recording in reference to the ear stimulated. As illustrated in panel C, the relative influence of mere distance from the generator is determined by the issue of whether the electrode is recording effectively in the ***near*** versus ***far field*** of a given generator.[11] SLRs that are of keen clinical interest have generators in the brainstem, so inevitably and unequivocally they are recorded from the far field. Those AEPs are considerably weaker than LLRs (from the cortex), yet not uniquely by virtue of distance from the generators. Practically, this is not a problem, as long as there is still enough signal strength for detection—and there is!

This is not to say that such "distant" recordings do not pose some challenges for reliable recordings or at least some nuances that must be considered. One is that of sampling activity specific to the side of generation relative to ear of stimulation. Hemispheric differences in cortically generated AEPs have more of a "chance" to be found, given the size of the cerebrum and wide separation of the right and left auditory cortices. However, along the brainstem portion of the auditory pathway, the generators on the two sides are far less separated, down to a few centimeters just above the pontine part that generates major component potentials of the brainstem SLR of clinical interest—the auditory brainstem response (ABR). Should it be possible to observe an effect of side of head used to record the ABR with monaural stimulation? For that matter, how much difference should recording montage make at all for the ABR/any far-field potential?

This certainly is a relevant question for clinical purposes, but there remains much more background information to cover before jumping into the clinical arena. Still, the issue fundamentally can be approached from signals-and-systems concepts already covered, namely to arrive at reasonable deductions and expectations. Thereafter, only time (and further reading) will tell. The star of this "show-and-tell" will be phase! There is a classical time-domain technique that, developed well before digital circuits and computers, permitted fairly precise measures of phase or phase differences using an oscilloscope (again, a device or like program on a computer system) capable of instantly plotting the time histories of signals on the screen (recall Figure 2–22D). Generally, its use is dedicated to measurement of instantaneous magnitude of a signal (like voltage from a microphone) and for which the horizontal axis is under control of a time-base oscillator (user controlled but signal defined internally). Such devices also support feeding the horizontal input with another external signal (user defined). For instance, one sinusoid can be plotted against another. If both signals—nominally vertical and horizontal inputs—are of the same amplitude, frequency, and phase, a straight diagonal line of 45° inclination will be observed. If a phase delay is applied to the vertical input signal, this pattern—called a Lissajous—will begin to open up into an ellipse as the phase shift between the two signals increases. It then becomes a full circle by a 90° shift and so ongoing through 360° (back to 0°, in effect, as longer shifts are ambiguous to measure with this method). With a far more elaborate effort by way of 3-D (three-dimensional) analyses of ABRs, researchers have applied sophisticated Lissajous analyses to tracking the sequence of its waves, thus as the signal evolves in AEP time and space. These are ***three-channel Lissajous trajectories*** (3CLTs).[12] The 3CLT results provided considerable understanding of the complexities of the multiple components generated in the lower auditory pathway (8th nerve and pontine brainstem), especially the combined time-space distribution of the force fields for each of the major wave components. However, such instrumentation is not necessary to place the issue under scrutiny, simply using results essentially from a clinical test system.

Time for another demonstration: Voltage fields of generators of interest in routine clinical tests are substantially "concentrated" in planar segments that fortunately, for purposes of demonstration, fall close to the coronal plane (that is, cutting through the head ear to ear). Serendipitously, commonly performed tests are essentially in 2-D, and this also will be good enough for purposes to make a decision on the question at hand. In other words, should it matter upon testing one ear whether the recording montage effectively provides a view from one side of the head or the other? Figure 3–6A illustrates a montage not quite typical for clinical tests of the ABR in particular, although it has enjoyed both research and clinical interests in the LLRs—"tying" the earlobe/mastoid electrodes together electrically. The "trick" here is to somewhat attenuate activity along the horizontal (H) axis, while focusing particularly on that of the vertical axis (V).[13]

Why the V axis for this demonstration? This is to the essence of the query. This amounts to the issue of recording from the surface of a sizable head something going on very deep in that complicated volume conductor. Figure 3–6B is an approximation to the "vertical" recording of the ABR, as a reference. Why? Because if this is all there is to the response, game over! The view from in deep far-field space must be essentially identical from both sides then (whether stimulated from the right or left ear). Two-dimensional-Lissajous analysis can be applied to actual conventional recordings (montage in panel C) for each side with right-ear-only stimulation. Plotting the contralateral ($C_Z - M_1$) versus the ipsilateral signal ($C_Z - M_2$) should reveal effects of sidedness of the recording, if they are measureable. Even though tying/sharing the vertex electrode between the two channels, the plane of views between the two sides are different by approximately +45° on each side of the sagittal plane. As seen in panel B mid-figure), the first (left most) of the three wave components scrutinized shows little phase difference (2CLT collapsed

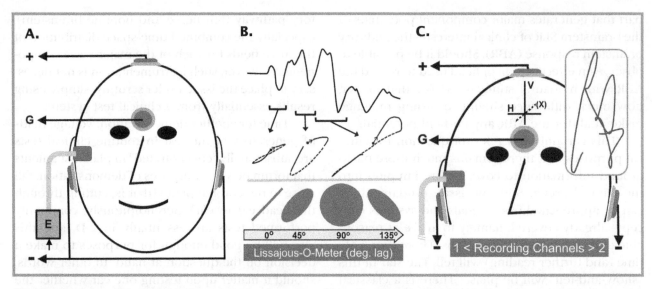

Figure 3–6. **A.** Simplified montage and approach to approximate recording of a purely vertical component (V) of a brainstem potential, versus a horizontal (H) component (see text). Plus and minus connections to the recording amplifier, including the ground (G; recall Figure 2–16). The exaggerated/giant electrodes are reminders of electrode fundamentals; the connection is actually by metal + electrolyte. **B.** Tracing, *top*: modeled response based on actual recordings as posited initially to be seen essentially the same, whether stimulated versus recorded from one side or the other. *Middle* figures: 2D Lissajous tracings (which are keenly phase-sensitive); segments from an actual 2-channel recording for the montage illustrated in panel **C**. Bottom images: for reference, simulated 2-channel recording wherein the response is modeled by a sinusoid of equal amplitude and period, but upon changing phase-shifts between channels per indicated phase differences). Conclusion: In fact, the ipsilateral and contralateral "views" of the brainstem potentials can be different, especially for full-blown suprathreshold responses in the mature adult subject, as illustrated here. **C.** Cartoon illustrating a common montage for a two-channel recording of AEPs. Insets: A "tattoo" on the forehead indicating perpendicular axes in 3D analyses, as approximated in the actual montage used for analyses of 3CLTs. A vignette showing the looping patterns of a characteristic, flat (2D) "projection" of a plot of a real subject's 3D results, portraying their evolution over time (roughly, *bottom to top*). (Based on data from Durrant and coworkers [1994].[14])

nearly to just a diagonal line, for reasons that will surface later but are not surprising when given all the facts). The next one shown pertains to the input level of the auditory brainstem pathways and demonstrates a clear shift between ipsilateral and contralateral viewpoints (resembling the reference Lissajous pattern at the bottom of panel B for a 45° phase shift). The last one is more complex as it pertains essentially to a two-wave complex. Again, some phase difference per view, at least for the component peaks; in any event, not a perfect straight line that would suggest no/0° phase shift.

Profits of 3CLT work have shown small but significant deviations of the true axes of wave-component generators of the brainstem potentials from orthogonal (perpendicular) planes/axes of the brain in 3D. This outcome is illustrated by results from 3CLT analysis for the normal-ear-side potentials based on results from an actual clinical subject.[14] Shown in the inset of Figure 3–6C are the Lissajous segments corresponding to the two-wave complex, with an overall lean to one side of the V axis. The "mysterious X" axis is that running through the skull base from front to back. For the total picture of 3-D voltage space of the brainstem generators, it is not negligible, but additional activity contributed along this axis to the normal response is relatively small. An important insight from 3CLT analyses are segments for the two-wave component, tending to lean anteriorly away from the coronal plane and thus "pointing" more toward F_Z. The practical upshot is that placement of an electrode neither at C_Z nor midhairline are necessarily optimal for the ABR, yet in practice have been found to provide comparably reliable results.[15] Moving further down the forehead toward F_{PZ} also is workable, but predictably at risk of a lower signal strength and/or must be evaluated as well for whether there is relatively more or less possible interference by extraneous signals (such as EMG from the underlying frontalis muscle).

The full 3CLT display (again inset, Figure 3–6C) together with the sequential nature of activation of auditory pathway reminds once more that the AEPs extend in both time and space. The signals among different generators will interact or be combined by both phasor (in time) and vector addition (in space). The signal initially excited in the peripheral auditory system is transmitted to the central system, where there is more "traveling" in space; this takes time yet accrues more activity along the way. The battery model used liberally here is certainly an oversimplification but will be embraced one more time for just one more thing. The reality of the AEP recording is that the potential observed in real-time is an AC signal. A way to think of this is that the battery (as a DC device) is rotating, essentially as in the diagram of the generation of the sinusoid (recall Figure 2–1), although not producing as "well behaved" signal as a quasi-sinusoid, as illustrated in Figure 3–7A. Imagined here is that the test subject is simply a sort of basketball made of something like pigskin (at the risk of mixed metaphors between sports), but not dry skin. Rather than inflated with air, it is filled with seawater for a uniform conductive medium. A battery is rotated relative to the time history of some AEP-component potential, and electrodes on the surface will see a wave ensue. In panel B is a schematic human with several generators per early waves arising along the space continuum in

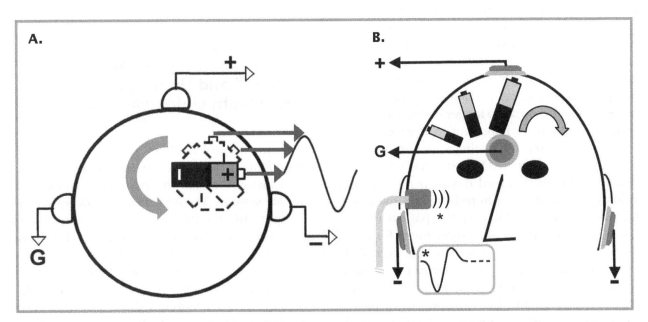

Figure 3–7. A. Rotating battery symbolizing generation of alternating-current auditory evoked potentials. **B.** The response is taken to be initiated with the acoustic click; after acoustic and other delays (stay tuned), the neural response is initiated, using the ground (G) lead as the starting line. The curved arrow in both panels denotes the rotation of the battery-ish dipole, in effect. *Note:* If these batteries are analogous to AAAA, AAA, and AA types respectively (from distally to proximally along the auditory pathway), perhaps an excess of artistic freedom has been taken, since these batteries supply the same voltage; for peace of mind of the seasoned battery user, please consider the analogy to be with regard to their respective amp–hr rating (not merely voltage) or simply that it is only a cartoon.

time. Here the batteries' positive poles (demarking angles of inclination) suggest different starting times (thus phase differences) among them with 9 o'clock demarking initiation of the stimulus—an acoustic click delivered by earphone. The component generators thus are portrayed to have inherent latency differences. It is also notable that perhaps the battery size also progresses along the way. The analogy thereby has been taken effectively into substantial and significant realities of the auditory pathway as a signal generator. How reasonable are these various expectations considered will be scrutinized in due course, beginning with looking for the fundamental bases of their generation. This requires delving into neuroanatomy and neurophysiology of the auditory system (next up!).

However, after all the theoretical and technological discussion, there are concrete issues in AEP measurements, learned as much in clinical as in research laboratories—in the "schools of hard knocks." Whatever strategic decisions that might be defended by theoretical discussions or even guidelines of practice, few things trump the importance of good electrode preparation—the point of departure of all clinical electrophysiology. The wires from the electrodes form another kind of antenna themselves, more literally akin to radio antennas and/or simply a possible means by which the electrode (contact part) may be moved—or worse—be lifted, so as no longer making good/any contact. It is always important to keep electrode wires relatively short to minimize pickup of electrical interference (pursued later in detail). The leads certainly should be taped down to the patient's skin or nearby clothing to reduce movement artifact as well as possibility of the patient (again) having to leave the examination room for a bit. The electrode leads also should be kept away from leads from the stimulus generator to the acoustic transducer (earphone or bone vibrator) to which the cable may have to lay on/against some part of the patient's body. It is arguable that all electrode leads individually or together (as a bundle) should have a metal shield. Similarly debated is braiding the leads from the electrode connector box to as close to the electrode as practical.[16] The right kind of braiding itself acts somewhat like a shield as one of the leads will be connected to ground. Braiding also reduces unsightly/troublesome entanglement of the leads, often five or more. The specific application is also a determinant as to the extreme the examiner should pursue to minimize risk of poor/unreliable recordings. Lastly, it generally is useful to have a "harness" of electrode leads of different colors to not only minimize confusion of contacts but also to attempt to have a routine electrode placement by color. Far safer is connection by purpose—which electrode at what location of the head needs to be connected to what jack on the electrode box. In any event, the examiner should double-check before leaving the patient at the start of the test, including status of course of the stimulus source. As in conventional audiometry, the clinical day for the "electrophysiology lab" should have begun with a systems check!

The "tools of the trade" and underlying theory/concepts both bespeak the need for a systematic approach in every case, regardless of experience. Meticulous attention to various preparatory steps to interfacing the AEP measurement system to the patient truly are essential for competent work.

■ Episode 2: Functional Neuroanatomy of "AEP Space" and Underlying Neurophysiological Bases

The generation of auditory evoked potentials is dependent on fundamental structural and functional factors in both the peripheral and central auditory systems. The *peripheral auditory system* is responsible for the collection of sound waves that represent a listener's acoustic environment. The sound waves are channeled to the middle ear which further transforms them, efficiently passing their energy along to the inner ear. Therein, the hearing organ *transduces* them into *bioelectrical signals*. These signals thus effectively encode sounds into forms of signals by which they ultimately can be utilized by the *cortex*, informing the listener about their sound environment.[17,18] These transformational processes work similarly to those of other *sensory nervous systems*, wherein analogous stimuli are encoded also to enlighten the listener about odors, pressure, light, and so forth, as they navigate the real, multidimensional world. The real world also requires of a listener locomotion to explore the environment beyond the immediate surroundings, so sensory signals ultimately must be interfaced to the motor nervous system and at the same time may not be isolated from other signals within the nervous system (like the cardiovascular and gastrointestinal systems). Consequently, that the listener may encounter music deemed "sickening" may not be just a metaphor. The listener's environment consequently must be rendered effectively into a form of electrical signals representative of the features of sensory stimuli of primary importance to normal function of the nervous system. For hearing naturally, those nuances are the temporal and spectral characteristics of sounds in the environment, considered in the last chapter.

These *transformative* transduction processes of the auditory nervous system[18] create electrical signals that indeed can be recorded and displayed via *clinical neurophysiology* as what are called *evoked potentials* (recall Figure 1–1). These potentials for clinical purposes are taken to be (in some way) as being faithful "byproducts" of a change from ostensibly mechanical signals into electrical representations. On the other hand, the AEPs with rare exception do not approximate direct analogs of the stimulus and, as demonstrated more extensively in later chapters, are often quite unlike the stimulus. The previous episode begged questions, in effect, of what does the sound "look like" via conventional methods of measurement, akin to asking what are the effects of the coupler to the microphone when comparing its measured spectrum to that of the electrical input/driving signal fed to the transducer. In testing AEPs, the eardrum replaces the microphone and the ear itself is the coupler, then begging the question of what the sound will "look like" (in analytical terms, per Episodes 2.1 and 2) once its energy is fed through the peripheral auditory system. Getting the sound energy to the *organ of Corti* is just for openers in the generation of the AEPs, hence the overall importance of a review of structures of the auditory system. Naturally, there is an expansive amount of detailed anatomy and neurophysiology to present the topic comprehensively. First, eliciting and measuring AEPs is not just about the ear, as implied by the "opening remarks." Second, as implied by Figure 1–1, the *central auditory pathways* command a considerable amount of neuroanatomical turf that only expands going up in the central nervous system (CNS). Volumes of research articles and books have been produced over the past centuries and reflect the work of innumerable scholars in a variety of fields, making a "brief" overview seemingly laughable. More comprehensive sources are provided for readers wanting to dig deeper into the topic.[19,20] Yet, what is practical is an overview of information on aspects of both the peripheral and the *central auditory nervous system (CANS)* that substantially influence the generation and/or "behavior" of AEPs relative to stimuli of common interest in their measurement and clinical application. In turn, this information supports the bases of clinical interpretation of AEP findings. Thus, onward; back to basics!

In the auditory system, the periphery[20,21] is located mostly in the *temporal bone* and is represented by three anatomical categories, summarized pictorially in Figure 3–8A. The first (situated most laterally) is the *external/outer ear* that includes the prominent *pinna (or auricle)* and the *external auditory meatus*, in turn terminated by the *tympanic membrane* (eardrum). The tympanic membrane divides the outer from the *middle ear cavity* (second category) which encompasses the *ossicular chain*, comprising the *malleus, incus*, and *stapes*—often referred to as the "conductive apparatus." The stapes conducts sound into the next major part—the *inner ear*—and, specifically of interest, the *cochlea*. This coiled structure comprises 2½ to 2¾ turns in humans. It has a bony spiral skeleton that is broad at its *base* and narrow at its *apex*. Peering into the cochlea by way of a cross-sectional view (panel B), the cochlea has a membranous ultrastructure which forms three distinct canals or scalae—the *scala tympani, media*, and *vestibuli*. The scala tympani and vestibuli are filled with *perilymph*—essentially *cerebral spinal fluid (CSF)*. In contrast, the scala media contains *endolymph*, produced in the endolymphatic sac. Perilymph has relatively high sodium (Na) and low potassium (K) concentrations, whereas endolymph is characterized by high K and low Na. *Reissner's membrane* is a barrier to separate the respective contents of scala vestibuli from that of scala media, while the *basilar membrane*

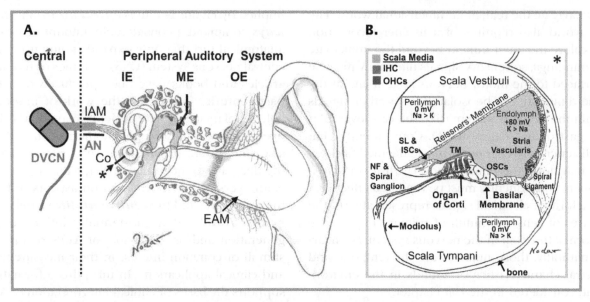

Figure 3–8. Sketches of the peripheral auditory system. **A.** Major divisions—outer, middle, and inner ear (OE, ME, and IE), moving laterally to medially, respectively, and indicating connection to the dorsal-ventral cochlear nucleus (DVCN) in the pontine brainstem, centrally (acoustic/8th nerve, AN; internal auditory meatus, IAM). **B.** Cross section, looking basal-ward at the indicated plane * through the first coil of the cochlea (Co) in panel **A**. The "bone" indicated in the drawing points to the dense bone of the cochlear shell and this, in turn, is embedded in bone like of the rest of the skull. Various functionally important contents of the cochlea are directly indicated as well as the following: inner and outer hair cell(s) (IHC and OHCs); the spiral limbus (SL); inner supporting cells (ISCs); tectorial membrane (TM); and outer supporting cells (OSCs). The relative concentrations of sodium (Na) versus potassium (K) and nominal resting-direct-current voltages observed in the perilymph- versus endolymph-filled spaces (scalae vestibuli and tympani versus scala media) are also indicated, respectively. (Adapted from *The Auditory System: Anatomy, Physiology, and Clinical Correlates, Second Edition* [**A:** p. 1; **B:** p. 97], by F. E. Musiek and J. A. Baran, 2020, Plural Publishing. Copyright 2020 by Plural Publishing. All rights reserved.)

(BM) partitions scala tympani from scala media. This membrane has an important feature for to the hydro-mechanical response to incoming sound energy, that of progressively widening from base to apex with a concomitant inverse change in stiffness, namely decreasing from ***base*** to ***apex***. This parameter is fundamental to the ***traveling wave*** phenomenon, the overall- or macro-mechanical contributor to cochlear signal processing in the frequency domain (considered in more detail in a subsequent episode).

Located on the BM is the organ of Corti. On the distal/radial wall—relative to the core of the cochlea, the ***modiolus***—are the ***stria vascularis*** and ***spiral ligament***. Progressing in a proximal direction are the ***supporting cells***: Claudius', Hensen's, Dieters', and outer and inner pillar cells, more evident in the more close-up view of Figure 3–9A. They support the auditory sensory cells—***outer hair cells (OHCs)*** and ***inner hair cells (IHCs)***. The outer and inner pillar cells also form the ***tunnel of Corti***, significant both for its architectural form (triangular; light but strong) and biochemical contents—***cortilymph***. Like perilymph, it too is much like CSF. Cortilymph thus bathes the exterior of the hair cells in a Na-rich solution (rather than high K like endolymph, as required for their general well-being). This is equally a truism for nerve fibers that must course through this fluid to innervate the hair cells.

Also illustrated is innervation of the hair cells. Connecting to one IHC actually are a number of ***type I auditory nerve fibers***, whereas there are a number of OHCs that connect to one ***type II*** *auditory nerve fiber.*[22] Both are ***afferents***, that is, members of the ***ascending pathway***. However, only about 5% of afferents innervate OHCs. Consequently, roughly a half-dozen OHCs must share one afferent fiber, which implies that their input ultimately to the CANS is perhaps summed for enhanced sensitivity of the system and/or of another signal-processing importance. Additional details of innervation will be considered shortly. For the moment, it is the overall picture that is of interest and has been the basis of a one-time, and for a longtime, mystery. All those OHCs and so few nerve fibers—what gives? There is also a small (yet significant) population of ***efferent/descending*** nerve fibers—but not shown (for simplicity)—with one subgroup ending near the bases of IHCs and the other terminating on afferents or directly on the bases of OHCs. The latter further support the suspicion of an "alternative reality" of importance of the OHCs.[23] Upon movement of the BM, the hair cells and auditory nerve fibers are the elements that are key players in the electromechanical transduction process. Effective stimulation of these cells leads to the generation of gross/compound electrical responses of the cochlea—***cochlear microphonic, summating potential***, and ***whole-nerve nerve action potential*** (to be explored extensively in a subsequent chapter).[24]

The electromechanical process in the cochlea[17,21] starts with the rarefaction and condensation phases of the motion of the stapes, exciting traveling waves along the BM; as commonly illustrated, upward (toward scala vestibuli, Figure 3–9B) and downward (toward scala tympani) movements result, respectively. The upward BM movements (per directions/phases of displacements and/or velocities, thus

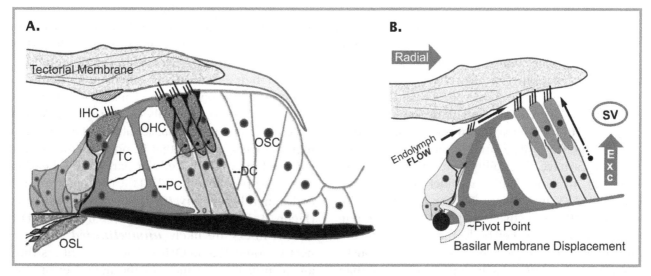

Figure 3–9. A. Simplified drawing of a magnified cross section of the organ of Corti. Moving toward the modiolus: OSC—an outer supporting cell (a Hensen cell in this case); DC—a Deiters' cell; PC—a pillar cell; TC—tunnel of Corti; OSL—osseous spiral lamina. *Note*: The tectorial membrane is illustrated both as approximately how it would be in the living organ, extending out over the OSCs, versus typical histological specimens wherein it generally is seen to be shriveled up considerably. **B.** Partial view (from panel **A**) with focus on macro- and micromechanical events at the instant of maximal excitatory displacement (Exc., nominally "upward" meaning toward SV—scala vestibuli—during the rarefaction phase of sound input). This effects a radially directed shearing displacement of the stereocilia, either by way of their contact directly with the tectorial membrane (outers only) or fluid flow (both). The partially dashed arrow denotes the motile (motoric) effect of the excitatory phase of stimulation, a shortening of the OHCs, to be discussed in more detail in a subsequent episode. (Adapted from *The Auditory System: Anatomy, Physiology, and Clinical Correlates, Second Edition* [**A**: p. 104; **B**: p. 13], by F. E. Musiek and J. A. Baran, 2020, Plural Publishing. Copyright 2020 by Plural Publishing. All rights reserved.)

toward scala vestibuli) result in the opening of pores on the *stereocilia* (hairs) by *tip links*. This action regulates the electrochemical process that leads to either depolarization ("up") or hyperpolarization ("down") of the hair cells, respectively. The detailed, resulting displacement of the stereocilia is peculiar to their relationship with the overlying *tectorial membrane*. The upward movement of the BM results in a shearing displacement relative to the surface of the hearing organ, pushing radially away from the *spiral limbus* (refer again to Figure 3–8 as well as Figure 3–9B). A downward movement of the BM reverses this action, with ultimately a sort of inhibition effect. The ionic exchange over the hair-bearing end of the hair cells drives down (depolarizes) or up (hyperpolarizes) the resting membrane potentials of the hair cells' interiors. Consequently, SV-ward movement is excitatory, driving up the discharge rates of the afferent neurons, whereas the opposite direction of movement causes reduction of the discharge rate.

The point of maximum stimulation along the BM reflects the optimal stimulation apropos the principle of *place coding of frequency*, although timing of excitation—apropos phase or other synchronization—is also conveyed efficiently over a broad range of frequencies. The degree of deflection of the BM at the maximum point of stimulation reflects the intensity of the stimulus. Both IHCs and OHCs have the ability to transduce stimuli efficiently from mechanical to bioelectrical, but the OHCs bodies also can expand and contract (see Figure 3–9B)—effectively lengthening/shortening along the axis of the cell body and so doing at very high rates (high frequencies). As hinted previously, the role of the OHCs is substantially different than that of the IHCs, and the difference in pattern of innervation—convergent versus divergent, respectively—proves to be "another story." The *motility* of the OHCs works as a biological, electromechanical amplifier by enhancing the magnitude of BM movement and also sharpening its peak displacement per distance along its base-apex continuum. This amplifier operates for low intensity stimuli, gradually decreasing gain as the stimulus becomes more intense. As such, one of the physical-world-like roles of the OHCs—as in audio-/radio electronic systems, including hearing aids—is a sort of *automatic gain control*. The result of what is truly a unique biological mechanism in sensory systems is the provision of exquisite sensitivity, yet avoiding excessive rate of growth of loudness of the stimulus.[17] This function is particularly important considering the extraordinary dynamic range of hearing (recall Episode 2.3) while dealing with listening tasks such as speech recognition at both low- and high-sound levels and often in competing noise.

That the hair cells generate potentials (for purposes of this book) is the most important point at this stage of discussion, namely to elicit release of a *neurotransmitter* substance stored in vesicles at the bases of the HCs and thereby exciting the innervating afferent neurons.[25] As noted at the outset of this episode (generally speaking), the hearing organ in mammals thus employs a chemical transmission system of *synapses* to interface between the bases of the HCs and the dendrites of nerve cells, in turn between subsequent neurons along the auditory pathway. As portrayed in Figure 3–10, there are multiple distinctions between type I and II auditory neurons. Their cell bodies form the *spiral ganglia* within the bony modiolus, and their axons progress medially through the *internal auditory meatus*. The auditory neurons are connected to hair cells by *synaptic ribbons* which are known to be susceptible to damage from high intensity sounds (that is, not only the stereocilia and internal, subcellular parts of the hearing organ). Approximately 90% of the neurons are type I and generally are *myelinated bipolar neurons* (Figure 3–10) connecting to about 3,000 IHCs. The type II fibers are likely *unmyelinated* and connect to some 12,000 OHCs. The type I fibers thus are responsible for most of the neural excitation along the auditory pathways, including generation of AEPs. Type II fibers appear unlikely to have significant impact on excitation of either peripheral or central components/potentials of AEPs, although this has not been completely ruled out.

The critical action of synaptic transmission has several key players. Again, located at the end of the base of a hair cell, or end buttons of an axon, are the vesicles that store the neurotransmitter—for hair cells, *glutamate*. The neurotransmitter is released into the *synaptic cleft* and picked up by receptors in the *dendrites* of a nerve cell. Therefore, *post-*

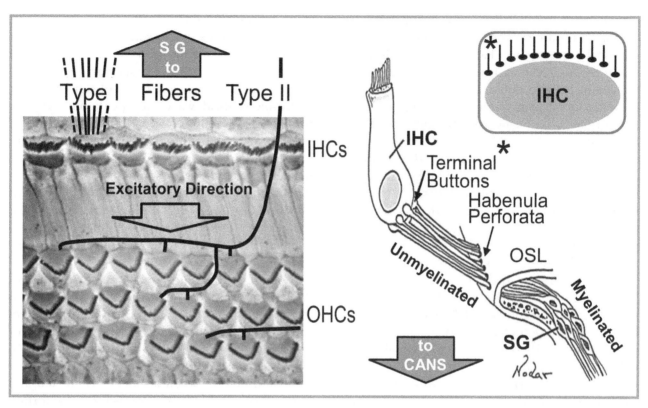

Figure 3–10. Left: Quasischematic representation applied to an electron-scanning micrograph of the surface of the organ of Corti, here presented in photo-negative to appear as if illuminated from below and revealing examples of innervation patterns of underlying neurons (drawn). The iconic mosaic of this surface is particularly noteworthy for differences of patterns of stereocilia of OHCs versus IHCs. **Right**: Both types of neurons have cell bodies forming the spiral ganglia (SG), but here the Type I is more distinctive as a bipolar neuron which, past the openings in the osseous spiral lamina (OSL), become myelinated. Inset: Representation of the numerous terminal buttons appearing at the base of an IHC. (Adapted from *The Auditory System: Anatomy, Physiology, and Clinical Correlates, Second Edition* (**Left**: pp. 9 & 17; **Right**: p. 180), by F. E. Musiek and J. A. Baran, 2020, Plural Publishing. Copyright 2020 by Plural Publishing. All rights reserved.)

synaptic (graded) and ***neuronal (spike-action) potentials*** are generated as part of this connectivity. Recapping the sequence of having elicited vibration of the BM: a nominally upward motion results in a shearing displacement of the stereocilia leading subsequently to increased excitation of the afferent fibers of the spiral ganglion cells; downward motion reverses this action, acting like an inhibitor. The latter is due to ionic exchange over the hair-bearing surface of the hair cells that actually drives up the resting membrane potentials of their interiors, and this subsequently reduces the resting (in-quiet) or ***spontaneous rate*** of nerve-fiber firing.

Many spike-action potentials are generated by the auditory nerve fibers, and (as implied previously) many of them are spontaneously active, even in absolute silence. Such "hyperactivity" bespeaks the exquisite sensitivity of the peripheral auditory system. Workers in animal research have sophisticated methods, including the use of extremely fine electrodes to pick up discharges of a single neuron—the ***single-unit***. For that matter, recordings via similar methods have been made of the receptor potentials of single hair cells. Individual action potentials have different ***latencies*** depending on several factors, including intensity and frequency of the stimulus and whether or not the fiber is myelinated. Again from the front end of the auditory pathway on, auditory neurons tend to manifest spontaneous discharges without external stimulation (from the environment). Indeed, spontaneous rates are one of the parameters by which neuronal responses are characterized—for instance, relatively high versus low rates. This and other behaviors help to define their apparent roles in the auditory nervous system's encoding and subsequent processing of the acoustic stimulus. Hence, the excitation of auditory neurons should not be conceived as akin to turning on/off a light, but rather more like modulating the pattern of a blinking light. The other upshot is that the nervous system is inherently noisy electrically, not quiet even when the listener is in an anechoic, sound-isolation chamber.

The single-unit recording, however, is an invasive method and in sharp contrast to methods by which AEPs are recorded, even for wave components attributable to the 8th nerve. A multitude of spike-action potentials can be excited across a nerve bundle and contribute to the overall potential that is recordable from the nerve's surface and beyond; these are **compound action potentials**, as illustrated in Figure 3–11A. The greater the number of fibers that are stimulated, the greater the number of "spikes" from any number of neurons, so the larger the compound action potential will be as the stimulus's intensity is increased. This "action" is predicated on the relative synchronicity of the spike discharges, and the peak compound potential reflects the highest probability of discharge. There nevertheless is always some delay between the onset of the stimulus and earliest stimulus-related spike potential, then "biased" by degree to which the individual spikes are synchronized. Measuring the onset of the compound action potential is one way to measure **latency** of such potentials, but the more practical/most popular approach in clinical neurophysiology is to measure from stimulus onset to the peak of the compound action potential. The latency of the 8th nerve response is dependent on the effective site of recording, traveling wave velocities to places along the hearing organ predominantly contributing to excitation, **synaptic delays**, and **nerve conduction velocity**.

By the length of the hearing organ, traveling wave velocities have a substantial influence that affects the frequency-dependence of latencies of the 8th nerve action potential, as will be demonstrated in later episodes. For the moment, the point is that frequencies of the sound stimulus are not encoded exactly at the same time. Since higher frequencies stimulate the basal part of the basilar membrane, it takes less travel time for their hydro-mechanical waves to "peak out." Higher frequencies literally elicit a quicker response of the neurons innervating the base than those more toward the apex, stimulated at lower frequencies. Related to this mode of stimulation of the nerve, there also is a relative broadening of the pattern of vibration along the hearing organ from base to apex, so the higher-frequency fibers inherently yield a more synchronous response than lower-frequencies fibers.

Nerve conduction velocity is greatly dependent on the amount of **myelin** on the axon of the nerve fiber. Highly myelinated nerve fibers can have a velocity nearly 90 m/s, while that of unmyelinated fibers are often less than 5 m/s. The basis of this difference is demonstrated by a simulated race between a model myelinated and unmyelinated fiber in Figure 3–11B. The former demonstrates **saltatory conduction**. The insulative myelin has gaps along the axon—**nodes of Ranvier**. This forces electrical discharges of the cell membrane to "leapfrog" from gap to gap.

It is noteworthy that all AEPs are some form of compound potential, although they are not built uniquely of action potentials. The most pristine way to clock neural transmission along a portion of the auditory pathway is by using electrodes placed directly on the nerve or a wire/needle electrode penetrating the brain near a neural tract, but this is evidently invasive for the subject. Using again the predominantly noninvasive approaches of clinical neurophysiology, net conduction velocities fortunately are demonstrable by latency differences among some wave components of AEPs, especially those generated primarily along the peripheral nerve or a nervelike tract in the CANS (to be detailed shortly). Examples are the latency differences between the distal and proximal portions of the 8th nerve—normally around 2 ms—or between the inferior and superior extent of a nerve tract running through the pontine portion of the brainstem—about the same or slightly less. However, noninvasive methods of recording electrical activity of the brain do not permit disambiguating

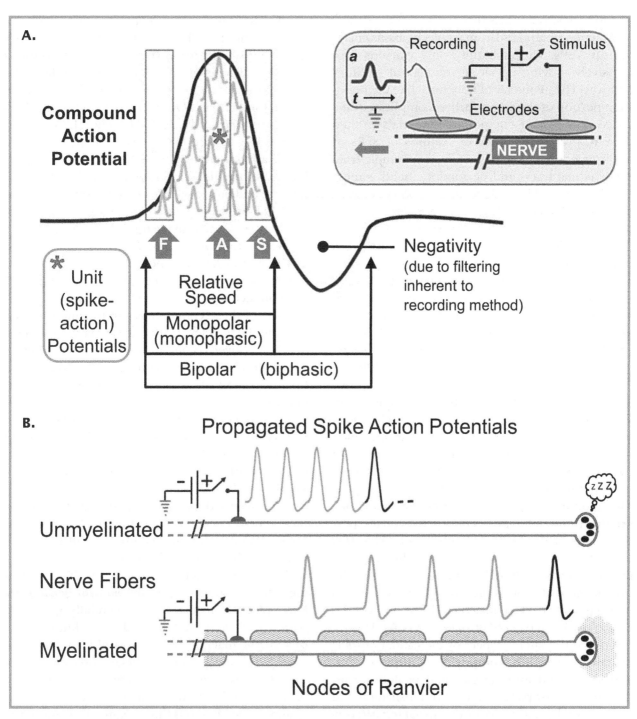

Figure 3–11. A. Synthesis (in concept) of a compound nerve action potential like that of the 8th nerve versus single-unit potentials when recorded per the inset diagram. (Courtesy of Dr. D. L. McPherson.) **B.** Illustration of how propagation velocities of neural discharges along an axon are facilitated by the peculiar insulation of myelinated nerve fibers—breaks or the nodes of Ranvier—which force discharges to jump along the way and thereby cover more "turf" with each action potential.

dendritic field potentials (from arbors of dendrites) from action potentials (from trunks of axons) making up AEPs. The ambiguity only worsens progressively moving up/along the central auditory pathway. The geometry of structures like the brainstem portion of the CANS further complicate time-space relations of compound potentials excited therein. Precise relations of features of SLRs of AEPs generated in the brainstem, for example from some axonal tracts and/or dendritic fields, simply may be oriented in such a way as to defy the generation of detectable "waves" using electrodes on the skull's surface. With this caveat, nevertheless, likely contributors to the brainstem components of the most broadly used SLR clinically have been reasonably mapped per likely generators.[26]

Exploring the neuroanatomy of the central auditory pathways has been an ever-ongoing challenge to researchers and never a "light read" for the scholar. Still, the salient features strongly suspected or known to "support" the production of AEPs can be overviewed in an informative manner and prove useful in practice, starting with a schematic representation as in Figure 3–12A and cross-referenced to a photograph of an actual human specimen (panel B). This pathway—auditory nerve through medial geniculate—first will be discussed anatomically, followed by its pertinent neurophysiology.[27] The auditory nerve exits the **internal auditory meatus** through the **porus acousticus** on the posterior side of the **petrous portion (or pyramid)** of the temporal bone. The 8th nerve then projects into the **cerebellopontine angle** and enters the brainstem at the **pons-medulla junction** for its neurons' axons to terminate via a bifurcation (splitting in two) in the **cochlear nucleus (CN)**. The CN located in the lateral aspect of the caudal **pons** is actually a complex (comprising multiple nuclei) and segmented into anterior and posterior **ventral** and **dorsal** parts. It gives both ipsilateral and contralateral projections to the **superior olivary complex (SOC)** and **lateral lemniscus (LL)**. The anterior segment of the CN connects via the ventral **stria** primarily to the SOC and the **inferior colliculus (IC)**. The posterior ventral CN and dorsal CN project via the intermediate and dorsal stria to the contralateral SOC and LL. Ipsilateral projections of the CN are much less numerous and connect to the SOC with some fibers going directly to the IC. The SOC, located deep in the pons, includes a lateral and medial segment, the **trapezoid body (TB)**, and several **peri-olivary nuclei** (thus too, a complex). The fibers coursing contralaterally to the SOC terminate there or continue on directly to the IC via the LL. The SOC also has some projections to the **nuclei of the LL** (NLL). The LL (as hinted earlier) looks much like a nerve in concept—but is called a **tract** within the CNS—and indeed seems like a "super highway" functionally between the inferior and superior sides of the pons. However, the NLL is often bypassed. Again, the contralateral pathway seems to provide the more robust "wiring" of the pontine brainstem. Yet, the NLL is located in the rostral lateral aspect of the pons and has dorsal and ventral segments. The left and right NLL are connected by the **commissure of Probst**— the first of these commissures in the auditory system and the next level (after the TB, etc.) to support some crossover communication between sides of the bilateral ascending pathways. The NLL output thus is to the IC by both ipsilateral and contralateral routes!

The next major structure in the auditory pathway is the IC, which is somewhat like a pearl in appearance and is located in the posterior aspect of the **midbrain** (see Figure 3–12B, structure #3). The IC can be viewed as having three divisions—central (major), dorsal, and lateral. Like the NLL, the IC has a commissure connecting the left and right nuclei. Almost all auditory fibers from the lower nuclei in the auditory brainstem have synapses with the next-order neurons at the IC. Interestingly, the IC projections to the **medial geniculate body (MGB)** bilaterally are essentially ipsilateral paths. Each is a well-defined tract, known as a **brachium**, that courses in a rostral-lateral manner. The MGB is located in the dorsal- and caudal-most aspect of the **thalamus**, essentially acting like a "grand central station" for many sensory and other systems. The MGB has three segments: ventral (the key auditory part), medial, and dorsal. The MGB fibers project ipsilaterally via the **internal capsule** to the **primary auditory cortex (PAC)**, to be discussed later. For now, the spotlight will be directed to neurophysiology of the subcortical ascending pathway.

A key factor in discussing the auditory neural pathway is the concept of **neural arborization**,

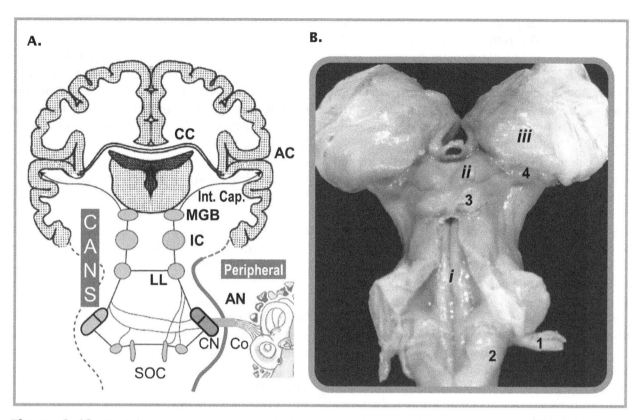

Figure 3–12. A. Schematic representation of major neural wiring along the neural pathways of the central auditory nervous system (CANS). CN—(dorsal-ventral) cochlear nucleus; SOC—superior olivary complex; LL—lateral lemniscus and its nucleus; IC—inferior colliculus; MGB—medial geniculate body; Int. Cap.—internal capsule; AC—auditory cortex; CC—corpus callosum. **B.** Posterior view of an actual human brainstem. Although viewed exteriorly, there are notable prominences bespeaking several key, underlying pathway components: Remnants of the incoming 8th nerve (1); CN, dorsal portion (2); IC (3); and MGB (4). A few additionally notable landmarks are the following: fourth ventricle (i); superior colliculi (which serve the visual system, ii); and thalamus (pulvinar, iii). (Adapted from *The Auditory System: Anatomy, Physiology, and Clinical Correlates, Second Edition* [**A**: p. 1; **B**: p. 206], by F. E. Musiek and J. A. Baran, 2020, Plural Publishing. Copyright 2020 by Plural Publishing. All rights reserved.)

as implied by the foregoing overview. Proceeding from caudal to more rostral structures, for example at the level of the thalamus,[28] the neural subpopulations just described become progressively larger as well as more diverse morphologically. For example, in the human there are approximately 30,000 fibers in the 8th nerve, yet hundreds of thousands in the IC and perhaps millions in the PAC. Germane to arborization is that a neuron at one level connects to many neurons at a higher level, hence the extensive branching. Neural arborization along the ascending auditory pathway relates to a number of relevant concepts of evoked potentials. The upshot is that the evoked potential generated by the 8th nerve is inevitably smaller in amplitude than most brainstem potentials and both are smaller than those from the auditory cortex. Neural arborization can also be related predominantly to sequential processing. That is, at each level of the auditory pathway there is more capability related to more available neurons to do increasingly more complex processing along the pathway of various nuclei. Yet, it must be borne in mind that there are still more complications to the wiring of the brainstem CANS, including possible interactions of ascending and descending paths.

Here, a pause in the "tour" of the CANS is in order to ponder one of the recurrent questions of auditory neural processing throughout hearing-science history. This is the extent to which the auditory system expresses throughout its organization and to which frequency-dependent auditory functions depend on **tonotopical organization** or **tonotopicity**. It is a natural question because the front-end "wiring" of the auditory system essentially looks (on the input side of the 8th nerve) very much like the makings of a point-to-point wiring scheme. Classically, this is called a labeled line system, as the primary nerve fibers course from synapses with the hair cells in a very orderly fashion. This implies functional significance and thus worthy of preservation centrally, in this case as an underlying mechanism for frequency discrimination and pitch—the place code. Historically, the evidence thereto has waxed and waned, most notably apropos organization at the cortex. Consequently, any tour of the CANS begs attention to this issue.

From the auditory nerve through the CANS, there certainly exists a tonotopical organization.[29,30] The practical issue is how to reveal it. Illustrated in the upper-left inset of Figure 3–13A is the cross-section of the 8th nerve, auditory branch coursing through the internal meatus, along with the vestibular branches and the facial nerve. The auditory branch looks a bit like a twisted cable of electrical wires but does reflect substantial frequency-wise groupings. Nature's intent then appears to be to maintain orderly frequency-dependent connections of the 8th nerve fibers to the second-order neurons in the CN. Indeed, tonotopicity proves to be pervasive along the ascending pathway, having been demonstrated in all major nuclei.[28,31] The "trick" to demonstrating it is the use of single-unit recordings and finding an axis of exploration along which the electrode picks up spike-discharges according to a frequency-by-place progression (panel A). However, in endeavoring to explain comprehensively how the auditory system processes frequency, tonotopicity is not necessarily rigorously manifested in the "wiring" of the entire system nor necessarily of functional importance, at risk of exclusion of other neuroanatomical/neurophysiological mechanisms. In other words, tonotopicity neither excludes possible detection of AEP-relevant "signals" attributable to other mechanisms nor maintains that such signals can be revealed uniquely by a singular stimulus-response paradigm and/or looking in only one domain—time versus frequency (recall Episode 2.2). Another strength of the brainstem CANS suggested by Figure 3–13B is that another key characteristic is its parallel processing of multiple "channels" of information sent up the central pathway.[32] This starts with bifurcation of the 8th nerve upon entering the brainstem, to be further "multiplied" by second-order (DCVN) and higher-order neurons forming the complex wiring of the ipsilateral and contralateral paths (see Figure 3–12A). Such a complex and dynamic processor at this level of the CANS is important to various auditory functions and their respective efficiencies as well expected from processing (for instance) speech. This not only requires both temporal and frequency cues but also deals with the substantially nonlinear encoding of intensity in the peripheral system, lest frequency resolution come to suffer even at conversational levels of speech.[33,34]

Frequency indeed is only one of multiple parameters of real-world sounds that are far more often complex rather than simple, such as speech and music. These and even simple tones (especially at low frequencies) involve encoding dependent upon temporal cues as well. Among populations of the neurons sampled in the brainstem, a variety of temporal patterns of discharges actually are observed during testing with tone bursts, as illustrated in Figure 3–13B. The relevant neuroanatomical aspect includes greater diversity of the cell type/morphology of neurons, centrally versus peripherally. The neurophysiological aspect includes electrophysiological manifestations of activity, as demonstrated by single-unit recordings from neurons at multiple sites within a given nucleus. Only one of the five patterns of spike discharges in panel B essentially replicates that of the primary neuron, as will be scrutinized further.

The more fundamental parameter of a stimulus is its intensity.[35] In general, intensity coding along the auditory nerve and brainstem pathway is related to rates and density of neural discharges. Therefore, the density of discharges reflects a combination of the basic relation (for example) of increased rates of spike action potentials with increasing intensity and the increase of numbers of nerve fibers activated as the stimulus intensity increases. However, spike rates are not limitless;

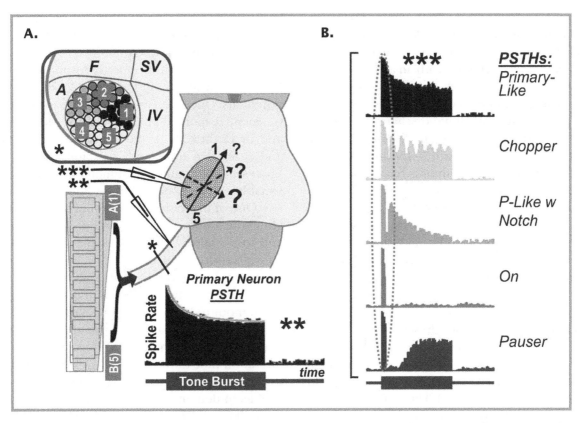

Figure 3–13. A. Illustration of concept of sampling tonotopicity of response of neurons in the 8th nerve or a given nucleus of the brainstem, using the single-unit recording method with micropipette electrodes. The cochlea is portrayed here functionally as a bank of narrow band-pass filters to process frequency by being placed along the basilar membrane from base/high frequencies (B5) to the apex low frequencies (A1). (*Gray shaded overlay* is to remind the reader of its underlying change in width.) Upper Inset: Cross-sectional view of all the nerves occupying and traversing the internal auditory meatus to the brainstem: A, auditory; SV and IV, superior and inferior vestibular; F, facial nerve. Varying gray-scale highlighting nerve fibers represents (grossly) groupings by frequency per place of origin of primary auditory neurons along the hearing organ. (Inspired by figure, courtesy of Dr. M. Don.) Main figure: Drawing primarily of the pontine brainstem (anterior view) with a generalized nucleus therein, to be explored and results compared among time and frequency characteristics of primary-/first-order neurons of the nerve versus second- or higher-order neurons of the pons and beyond. One objective would be to determine any trajectory of the electrode that might show systematic changes of characteristic frequency, "echoing" cochlear place of origin of excitation. Lower Inset: Results from a model of those typical of the rate of spike action potentials during tone-burst stimulation, seen to vary quasirandomly in time, yet defining a distinctive envelope (highlighted by the gray curve). **B.** Other simulated results illustrative of the variety of the poststimulus time histograms (PSTHs) of second- and high-order neurons, with nicknames per pattern. (Based in part on data of Pfeiffer [1966][36] and inspired in part by Kiang [1975][32].)

rather, they are limited by **refractory periods** of neurons. Fortunately for the auditory system, refractory periods of both neurons of the 8th nerve and brainstem can be quite short, for some neurons as low as 1 ms; thereby, a given density of discharges can be maintained at relatively high stimulation rates. This is in contrast to responses of cortical neurons (taking a peek ahead).

Returning now to further examining details of the sort of data portrayed in Figure 3–13B, an important neurophysiological index (available from single-unit recordings) is demonstrated: measuring the spike-discharge rates of axons before, during, and after exciting it with an acoustic stimulus.[32,36] This has proven to be a key indicator of differences among neurons of different orders along the auditory pathway. Spike-discharge activity is tallied and represented by ***post-stimulus-time histograms (PSTHs)***. Figure 3–13 thus illustrates characteristic patterns of stimulus-related increases in spike rate versus spontaneous rates. Yet, the most salient feature in the face of such diversity is the high prevalence of an ***on-effect***, as is also true of the pattern of PSTHs seen in results from the 8th nerve (lower inset, panel A). The firing rate pattern was for a time thought to be related to the particular type of nerve cell (morphologically defined), but the more recent view is that the firing rate is related to the particular circuits formed, whatever the morphology. In Figure 3–13B, the functions shown are modeled after PSTHs obtained from recordings from the CN but can be seen in other/"higher" nuclei as well. The PSTH in panel A thus provides a "reference" pattern per its stark simplicity of the primary auditory neuronal response, which in turn is uniform across the 8th nerve. At the CN level and beyond, this pattern is also seen commonly—hence called "primary-like," so it is not uniquely characteristic of primary (first-order) neurons of the auditory system. Still, this pattern is important, showing how well the CN (and nuclei beyond) retains and passes along the response pattern of the 8th nerve. On the other hand, the neural population is virtually exploding via arborization. Therefore, other/different patterns are expected. There indeed are other patterns, and they are the more exotic plots in panel B (pulsar, etc.).

The diversity of patterns portrayed by high-order neurons is taken to indicate an enhanced processing capacity of the features of sound. However, there remains a strikingly pervasive commonality of the initial time segment of these PSTHs; the on-effect remains very strong (see dotted-line ellipse in Figure 3–13B). This effect unequivocally can contribute to the generation of AEPs and guide ideas of efficient ways to measure/test them. Those potentials typically generated early on and arising toward the beginning of the AEP space-time continuum, the SLRs (for instance), are elicited well by very brief stimuli with little to no advantage of durations beyond some milliseconds! Still, the on-effect may not account necessarily for all types of AEPs and/or variations within types of responses—longer latency transient responses and/or steady-state potentials. Once effectively getting past the robust transient response "empowered" by the on-effect and/or farther along the space-time continuum, and at least in some test paradigms, more timely processing of nuances of stimuli (as encoded) reasonably can be expected to be evident in the AEP.

One of the more complex functions "serviced" along the auditory pathway is sound lateralization and localization.[37,38] Listeners have incredible binaural sensitivity, discrimination, and localization ability, supported by a robust brainstem and higher organization of the CANS, which thus is dedicated throughout to binaural processing of sound. Classical behavioral measures are subjects' abilities to detect interaural intensity differences (IID) and interaural time differences (ITD). These have been explored in animals via single-unit recordings as well as in demonstrating for example ITDs of less than 100 μs.[17] The SOC's two main structures, the lateral and medial nuclei, have very specific frequency representation. The LSO's "mapping" of frequency progresses from low to high in a lateral-to-medial direction, while the MSO exhibits a frequency range from dorsal (low) to ventral (high). At the IC (central nucleus), the progression of characteristic frequencies is in a dorsolateral (low) to ventromedial (high) direction. In the ventral nucleus of the MGB, low-frequency neurons are located more laterally, thus with higher frequencies represented more medially in this structure.[37]

At the SOC, there thus exists bilateral representation of monaural inputs. The SOC again has neurons that are highly sensitive to IIDs and ITDs. The former facilitates localizing a sound source to the side at which sound is more intense, whereas the latter enables localization of a source to the side at which sound waves first arrive (apropos distance between ears). The SOC neurons are very sensitive to time differences, namely on the order of tens of microseconds and thus providing a basis of precise localization based on ITDs. The ITD is the primary cue for localization of low to mid frequency sounds (for which IIDs are reduced/negligible due to sound-wave diffraction around the head). The SOC neurons' keen IID sensitivity is crucial to localization of higher-frequency sounds. In the SOC there are complex interactions between inhibitory and excitatory neurons that constitute a critical part of this underlying mechanism of localization. A simple example is that sound waves from the contralateral acoustic field garner (in effect) a greater excitatory response than from the ipsilateral side. This action provides a greater differential of activity at the SOC. The brainstem auditory pathway thereafter plays an important role in binaural processing by preserving and refining that of the SOC. Consequently, compromise(s) of nuclei anywhere along the brainstem pathway are expected as well demonstrated in both basic and clinical research to decrease localization/lateralization accuracy.

Moving on in space and with some more neuroanatomical details, the MGB projects neurons to the *internal capsule* that will eventually reach the PAC (again see Figure 3–12). This pathway carries activity practically from all auditory fibers arising from the brainstem structures.[39] The PAC receives input mostly from the ventral portion of the MGB. This neural tract has been termed the *thalamocortical pathway*. For purposes here, the interest will be primarily on *Heschl's gyrus*, but it is important to know that other cortical structures—such as *planum temporale*, *insula*, and *peri-Sylvian area*—play key roles in higher auditory processing. Heschl's gyrus is located about 2/3 of the way along the Sylvian fissure, on the *superior temporal gyrus* (Figure 3–14A and B). There can be one, two, or three Heschl's gyri in the normal human brain. In general, the left Heschl's gyrus is larger than the right. This gyrus is bordered anteriorly by the *planum polare* and posteriorly by planum temporale. The auditory cortex has been viewed as a dense neural area known as the core (central area in Heschl's gyrus), surrounded by a belt, in turn surrounded by a parabelt. The core is considered the center of activity with belt and parabelt regions as extensions. There are many cortical outputs from Heschl's gyrus, some known and some unknown. Two main output pathways are the *superior longitudinal fasciculus* (intrahemispheric) and *corpus callosum* (interhemispheric)[40] (see panel B). The former projects primarily to the frontal lobe, and the latter projects to auditory areas in the opposite hemisphere.

The interpretation of tonotopical organization at the cortical level of the CANS has long intrigued and challenged researchers,[41] starting with that of Heschl's gyrus. The consensus (again) has wavered, but there has been increased clarity of understanding, especially more recently thanks to functional-imaging studies. Results of these studies indicate a rather complex arrangement of nerve fibers of low-to-high characteristic frequencies in the PAC. The findings together show the tonotopical map of high frequencies to be situated at the anterior and posterior edges of this gyrus and to form a sort of "V." The mid-frequencies fall inside the tonotopical region of high frequencies and form (in turn) a smaller "V" with the low frequencies, thus represented inside the map of midfrequencies.[42]

Intensity representation at the auditory cortex, as in other areas, is related to neural firing rates and number of neurons activated (density). However, the firing rate of cortical neurons for increases in intensity may show at least nonlinear functions and/or nonmonotonic increases, if not rather abrupt decreases slightly above response threshold. FM and AM signals as stimuli provide a much stronger response from cortical neurons, compared to steady unmodulated signals. The alterations in frequency and intensity (respectively) serve to stimulate more neurons than continuous tones. Research interests in cortical responses to modulated carriers has increased recently due to popularity and expanding clinical use of the *auditory steady-state responses*. High modulation rates (>60 Hz) evoke responses predominately from the brainstem, whereas lower modulation rates (≤40 Hz) arise arguably from as far up the auditory pathway as the PAC.

The wiring of the brainstem was shown (previously) to manifest a "majority" of successive orders of neurons forming the ascending pathway and having crossed over in reference to the side of stimulation of the peripheral system. This organization is substantially expressed in the cortex, but upon increasing expansion of innervation toward further processing of the stimulus "code" and ultimately conveyance of information to other parts of the brain. Therefore, the auditory cortex also plays a critical role in accurate localization/lateralization of sound sources and other binaural processing.[43,44] At the cortical level, IIDs and ITDs remain robust

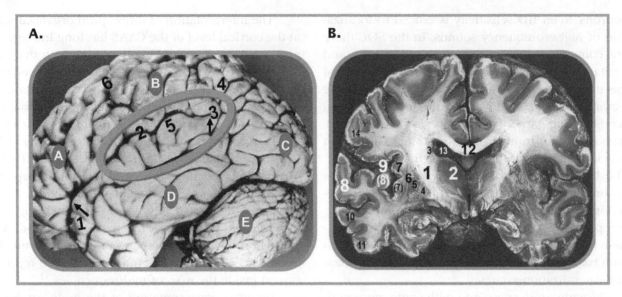

Figure 3–14. A. Photographs of the convoluted surface of the human cerebrum. Lateral view showing major areas of the brain and auditory areas expressed at the brain's surface (area within the ellipse). Frontal lobe (A); parietal lobe (B); occipital lobe (C); temporal lobe (D), temporal pole of the temporal lobe (1), Sylvian fissure (2), with the beginning and end of this fissure demarked by arrows; supramarginal gyrus (3); angular gyrus (4), superior temporal gyrus (5); central sulcus (6). Also included (for general reference) is the cerebellum (E). **B.** Photograph of a frontal section (midcoronal) of the whole cerebrum, vividly representing white versus gray matter of the brain. Highlighted are some of the main anatomical features of interest here of the otherwise seemingly innumerable structures in its detailed neuroanatomy. Those labeled represent minimal "turf" of direct relevance to an understanding of origins of cortical AEPs and knowledgeable use of them clinically in audiology and/or auxiliary areas (such as intraoperative monitoring). Internal capsule (1); thalamus (2); caudate (3); globus pallidus (4); putamen (5); external capsule with claustrum (6); insula (7); superior temporal gyrus (8); Sylvian fissure (9); middle temporal gyrus (10); inferior temporal gyrus (11); corpus callosum (12); lateral ventricle (13); inferior parietal lobe (14). (Adapted from *The Auditory System: Anatomy, Physiology, and Clinical Correlates, Second Edition* [**A**: p. 26; **B**: p. 276], by F. E. Musiek and J. A. Baran, 2020, Plural Publishing. Copyright 2020 Plural Publishing. All rights reserved.)

cues for locating sound sources. In addition, complex interactions between excitatory and inhibitory cortical neurons (akin to those seen in the brainstem) play a role. It well has been documented that greater cortical activity occurs for sounds emanating from the contralateral, compared to the ipsilateral, sides. Results have shown, for example, poor localization abilities in the sound field opposite the hemisphere in which the auditory cortex has been damaged. It also is at the cortical level that much integration across sensory and other systems must occur, including the localization of sound sources in the 3D-space in which the listener (again in the real world) must navigate and while maintaining accurate sound localization, for example while moving the head in one direction and walking in another. Cortical processing also builds upon and/or refines mechanisms of selective attention, processing sounds of interest in diverse backgrounds of complex sounds/noise, as well as memory and learning.

This episode has presented admittedly a whirlwind tour of the auditory pathways and is certainly far short of neuroanatomical/neurophysiological bases to explain all that a listener needs "between the ears" to process fully the acoustic environment. Yet, this "short story" hopefully has been an easy read while having been a substantial charge/recharge of memory cells. The facts will come up from time to time in the episodes that follow, but they may not necessarily be pointed out literally. Rather, the writers of these episodes will tell their stories with the expectation that these memory cells are in good working order. Should the numerous terms doled out in this episode have been a bit soporific, tune right in on the next Heads Up feature—a real eye-opener that "this stuff" is important!

HEADS UP

Need That Like a Hole in the Head? What About a Nail? A Case in Point!

The introductory chapter of this text suggested a sort of "road map" by which some auditory-specific brainwaves can be generated, evolving along the way from underlying neuroanatomical structures and neurophysiological processes, which are summarized in this episode. It would be misleading to suggest that the resulting electrical responses always reveal precisely the locus and nature of any dysfunction that might occur. The sheer population of neurons, their many synapses, and complexed branching make pinpointing the locus of dysfunction along the pathway a considerable challenge. Injuries, space-occupying tumors, other pathology, and diseases (like multiple sclerosis) thus can have less-than-finely defined impacts. Functional consequences also simply can be variable, especially over time. The keyword here is "functional." Tests of the AEPs can produce results at times that are correlated well with those of radiographic imaging, yet they are not of the same genre of tests, nor that of histopathology.

Nevertheless, an injury directly involving the auditory pathway can be expected to have a significant impact on auditory function. One or more of the tests from the audiologist's toolbox, however, may yield results strongly suggesting site of lesion. A dramatic case in point is that of a victim of a nail gun accident on the job.[45] Extraordinarily, the accident was disabling but not fatal. The nail gun discharge derived from the victim's fall from a ladder that initially rendered him unconscious. The nail had entered via the posterior fossa and penetrated both the cerebellum and pons. He subsequently suffered some motor, speech-motor, and balance impairments and complained of some difficulty of hearing.

Thankfully, he did not suffer major auditory dysfunction by conventional audiometric assessment. Hearing sensitivity remained within normal limits bilaterally. Acoustic (stapedial) reflexes were intact. Still, the word recognition score for one ear was reduced. Naturally, this level of information processing is more demanding of the system than mere detection of a sound.

As illustrated in Figure 3–15, the nail had traversed the pons of the brainstem on a bit of a vertical incline. The locus is prime turf for auditory brainstem/short-latency responses (like the ABR). However, dramatic and straightforward adverse effects of the sharply penetrating projectile are readily evident in the responses that were elicited via either ear. The highly prominent fifth wave of the normal ABR is missing on both sides.

Data from another case study, that of a unilaterally necrotized—thus missing—inferior colliculus (secondary to surgical radiological treatment of the cerebellum),[14] permitted an estimation uniquely of wave-V component computationally. An approximate model is added to Figure 3–15 to further illustrate the most specific functional impact of this nail gun accident, as manifested in this particular bioelectric response.

This case is not to imply that AEP tests can be expected to be sensitive only to lesions that effectively blow holes in the auditory pathway. There is much more to response measurement and interpretation than simply judging presence or absence of a certain wave, although any such absence is certainly important. Stay tuned!

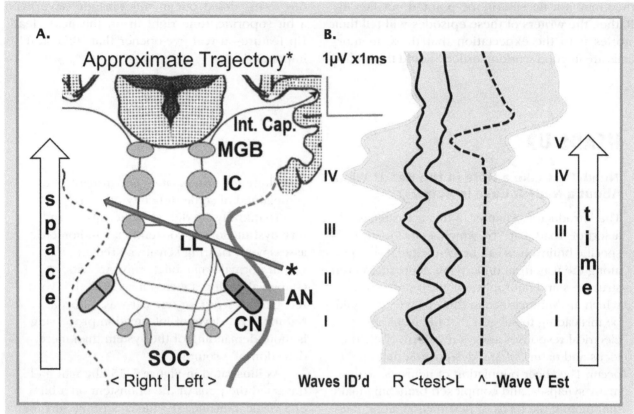

Figure 3–15. Partial copy of Figure 3–12A to illustrate (approximately) the trajectory of a nail that had passed through the brainstem of a victim of an accidental firing of a nail gun. To parallel the space dimension in this incredible clinical case and survivor, the patient's brainstem responses for right and left ears are plotted (based on data of Bauch and associates [1999][45]) both vertically on the page and in proximity to facilitate noting any substantive right/left-response differences. In turn, they are readily evaluated in the virtual "shadow" cast by a model response characteristic of otoneurologically intact adult subjects, tested at stimulus level characteristic of conversational speech. If arguably affected otherwise (beyond normal variability), the wave called "V" is unequivocally absent bilaterally; this is demonstrated further by comparison with a model of this wave component alone (Wave V Est; based on computation of Durrant and coworkers [1994][14] using data from an equally exotic case—see text).

Take Home Messages

Episode 1

1. Electrical energy is well used in both physical and biological realms, but not quite in the same ways, nor readily interfaced.
2. Electrodes are designed to provide reliable contact and stability, when properly applied, and goodness of contact is readily measurable and always should be verified.
3. Careful attention to principles and adequate time invested for good preparation of the subject is the essential first step toward a successful recording of evoked potentials.
4. If AEPs reflect activity in space within the head, the electrode montage aids the examiner to properly view them from "outer space."

5. Although not having to be perfectly followed (if justifiably so) and given other "maps," a long-standing and useful specification for electrode placements on the scalp is the 10-20 system.
6. AEPs arise from and/or are recorded clinically largely far away from their sources, yet still require various considerations of electrode placement per the putative generator site.
7. Despite layers of skin and underlying bone, surface recordings reveal events below, although pinpointing them is another matter (stay tuned).
8. Although a structure like the pons in the brainstem is small and far from the scalp's surface, AEPs can be recorded and to some extent show ipsilateral/contralateral differences.
9. As a sort of dipole modeling of brainstem AEPs, a rotating battery at each "weigh station" in space is imagined, with progressively longer phase lags (latencies in time) yet larger waves.

Episode 2

1. Anatomy of the temporal bone is largely that of the peripheral auditory system.
2. The sound transduction system (organ of Corti) is an electromechanical system of elaborate bioelectric wiring and function.
3. Signals from the brain bearing auditory information derive from barrages of compound potentials fed to the brainstem to excite both axonal and dendritic field potentials in the CANS.
4. The central auditory pathway is wired elaborately/redundantly (via arborization), favoring growing compound potentials along the ascending pathway in magnitude and breadth (in time).
5. The on-effect and other neurophysiological nuances combine to provide robustly recordable responses, thus certainly at but to some extent beyond the onset of the stimulus.
6. Upward cortical-ward projections and cortical pathways continue with great expansion, thus further complexities of brain waves, and further growth and complexities of responses.

Heads Up

7. Extraordinary cases can facilitate understanding principles of clinical electrophysiology of the auditory system; this case was dramatic, yet not melodramatic.
8. Damage to a relatively focal region of neuroanatomical space can manifest at a more or less specific time (latency) of an AEP wave, but many lesions are not so localized.

References

1. Silver, H. W. (2018). *The ARRL handbook for radio communications, volume 1: Introduction and fundamental theory*. ARRL.
2. Freeman, A. R. (1975). Properties of excitable tissues. In E. E. Selkurt (Ed.), *Basic physiology for the health sciences* (pp. 31–53). Little, Brown & Co.
3. Neuman, M. R. (2020). Biopotential electrodes. In J. G. Webster & A. J. Nimunkar (Eds.), *Medical instrumentation. Application and design* (5th ed., pp. 267–332). John Wiley & Sons.
4. Durrant, J. D., & Philips, C. M. (1979). An AC ohmmeter for electrode impedance measurements. *Journal of the Acoustical Society of America, 65*(4), 1065–1066.
5. Jasper, H. H. (1958). Report of the committee on methods of clinical examination in electroencephalography. *Electroencephalography and Clinical Neurophysiology, 10*, 370–375.
6. Jurcak, V., Tsuzuki, D., & Dan, I. (2006). 10/20, 10/10, and 10/5 systems revisited: Their validity as relative head-surface-based positioning systems. *Neuroimage, 34*(4), 1600–1611.
7. Ponton, C., Eggermont, J. J., Khosla, D., Kwong, B., & Don, M. (2002). Maturation of human central auditory system activity: Separating auditory evoked potentials by dipole source modeling. *Clinical Neurophysiology, 113*(3), 407–420.
8. Dimitrijevic, A., Michalewski, H. J., Zeng, F. G., Pratt, H., & Starr, A. (2008). Frequency changes in a continuous tone: Auditory cortical potentials. *Clinical Neurophysiology, 119*(9), 2111–2124.

9. Vaughan, H. G., Jr., & Ritter W., (1970). The sources of auditory evoked responses recorded from the human scalp. *Electroencephalography & Clinical Neurophysiology, 28*(4), 360–367.
10. Kooi, K. A. (1978). *Fundamentals of electroencephalography* (2nd ed.). Harper & Row.
11. Wood, C. C., & Allison, T. (1981). Interpretation of evoked potentials: A neurophysiological perspective. *Canadian Journal of Psychology, 35*(2), 113–135.
12. Pratt, H., Bleich, N., & Martin, W. H. (1985). Three channel Lissajous' trajectory of humans' auditory brain-stem evoked potentials: I. Normative measures. *Electroencephalography & Clinical Neurophysiology, 61*(6), 530–538.
13. Terkildsen, K., & Osterhammel P. (1981). The influence of reference electrode position on recordings of the auditory brainstem responses. *Ear and Hearing, 2*(1), 9–14.
14. Durrant, J. D., Martin, W. H., Hirsch, B., & Schwegler, J. (1994). 3CLT ABR analyses in a human subject with unilateral extirpation of the inferior colliculus. *Hearing Research, 72*(1–2), 99–107.
15. van Olphen, A. F., Rodenburg, M., & Verwey, C. (1978). Distribution of brain stem responses to acoustic stimuli over the human scalp. *Audiology, 17*(6), 511–518.
16. Hall, J. W. (1992). *Handbook of auditory evoked responses*. Allyn Bacon.
17. Durrant, J., & Feth, L. (2013). *Hearing sciences: A foundational approach*. Pearson Publishers.
18. Picton, T. (2011). *Human auditory evoked potentials*. Plural Publishers.
19. Phillips, D. P. (1988). Introduction to anatomy and physiology of the central nervous system. In A. F. Jahn & J. Santos-Sacchi (Eds.), *Physiology of the ear* (pp. 407–429). Raven Press.
20. Moller, A. (2013). *Hearing: Anatomy, physiology and disorders of the auditory system* (pp. 1–3, 49–69, 115–191). Plural Publishers.
21. Harrison, R. (2012). Anatomy and physiology of the cochlea. In K. Tremblay & R. Burkard (Eds.), *Translational perspectives in auditory neuroscience* (pp. 3–7, 65–89). Plural Publishers.
22. Spoendlin, H. (1981). Neuroanatomy of the cochlea. In H. A. Beagley (Ed.), *Audiology and audiological medicine* (Vol. 1, pp. 72–102). Oxford University Press.
23. Dallos, P. (1992). The active cochlea. *Journal of Neuroscience, 12*(12), 4575–4585.
24. Dallos, P. (1973). *The auditory periphery: Biophysics and physiology*. Academic Press.
25. Spoendlin, H., & Schrott, A. (1989). Analysis of the auditory nerve. *Hearing Research, 43*(1), 25–38.
26. Moore, J. K. (1987). The human auditory brain stem as a generator of auditory evoked potentials. *Hearing Research, 29*(1), 33–43.
27. Musiek, F., & Baran, J. (2020). *The auditory system: Anatomy, physiology and clinical correlates* (pp. 11–18). Plural Publishers.
28. McMullen, N. T., Velenovsky, D. S., & Holmes, M. G. (2005). Auditory thalamic organization: Cellular slabs, dendritic arbors and tectothalamic axons underlying the frequency map. *Neuroscience, 136*(3), 927–943.
29. Woolsey, C. N. (1971). Tonotopic organization of the auditory cortex. In M. B. Sachs (Ed.), *Physiology of the auditory system: A workshop* (pp. 271–282). National Educational Consultants, Inc.
30. Romani, G. L., Williamson, S. J., & Kaufman, L. (1982). Tonotopic organization of the human auditory cortex. *Science, 216*(4552), 1339–1340.
31. Brugge, J. F., & Geisler, C. D. (1978). Auditory mechanisms of the lower brainstem. *Annual Review of Neuroscience, 1*(1), 363–394.
32. Kiang, N. Y. S. (1975). Stimulus representation in the discharge patterns of auditory neurons. In E. L. Eagles (Ed.), *The nervous system: Human communication and its disorders* (Vol. 3, pp. 81–96). Raven Press.
33. Sachs, M. B., & Young, E. D. (1979). Encoding of steady state vowels in the auditory nerve: Representation in terms of discharge rate. *The Journal of the Acoustical Society of America, 66*(2), 470–479.
34. Young, E. D., & Sachs, M. B. (1979). Representation of steady state vowels in the temporal aspects of the discharge patterns of populations of auditory nerve fibers. *The Journal of the Acoustical Society of America, 66*(5), 1381–1403.
35. Pfingst, B. E. (1986). Encoding of frequency and level information in the auditory nerve. *Seminars in Hearing, 7*(1), 45–63.
36. Pfeiffer, R. R. (1966). Classification of response patterns of spike discharges for units in the cochlear nucleus: Tone burst stimulation. *Experimental Brain Research, 1*(3), 220–235.
37. Casseday, J. H., & Covey, E. (1987). Central auditory pathways in directional hearing. In W. A. Yost & G. Gourevitch (Eds.), *Directional hearing* (pp. 109–145). Springer-Verlag.
38. Joris, P. X. (1996). Envelope coding in the lateral superior olive. II. Characteristic delays and comparison. *Journal of Neurophysiology, 76*(4), 2137–2156.
39. Brugge, J. (2012). Auditory cortex: Anatomy and physiology. In K. Tremblay & R. Burkard (Eds.), *Translational perspectives in auditory neuroscience* (pp. 15–19, 239–282). Plural Publishers.

40. Bamiou, D. E., Sisodiya, S., Musiek, F. E., & Luxon, L. M. (2007). The role of the interhemispheric pathway in hearing. *Brain Research Reviews, 56*(1), 170–182.
41. Walzl, E. M. (1947). Representation of the cochlea in the cerebral cortex. *Laryngoscope, 57*(12), 778–787.
42. Saenz, M., & Langers, D. (2014). Tonotopic mapping of the human auditory cortex. *Hearing Research, 307*, 42–52.
43. Neff, W. D., & Casseday, J. H. (1977). Effects of unilateral ablation of auditory cortex on monaural cat's ability to localize sound. *Journal of Neurophysiology, 40*(1), 44–52.
44. Beitel, R. E., & Kaas, J. H. (1993). Effects of bilateral and unilateral ablation of auditory cortex in cats on the unconditioned head orienting response to acoustic stimuli. *Journal of Neurophysiology, 70*(1), 351–369.
45. Bauch, C. D., Olsen, W. O., Lynn, S. G., Reading, C. C., & Dale, A. J. (1999). Penetrating injury to the brainstem after a nail gun accident: A case study. *American Journal of Audiology, 8*, 57–64.

4

Stimulating the Auditory System and the How and Why of an "Evoked" Response

The Writers

Episode 1: Steven L. Bell
Episode 2: Ozcan Ozdamar and John D. Durrant
Heads Up: John D. Durrant, Cynthia G. Fowler, and Suzanne C. Purdy

■ Episode 1: Extracting the Response's Signal From Noise Background

This episode introduces a major challenge for recording auditory evoked responses: the task of extracting very small signals embedded in lots of interference/noise. It discusses the methods that are typically used to reduce measurement noise. Finally, the episode shows how, after noise reduction, clinicians are able to identify evoked responses in the residual background noise.

When recording *auditory evoked potentials (AEPs)*, the examiner is generally recording very small signals. The *auditory brainstem response (ABR)* (one of the short latency responses) represents one of the smallest potentials. The peak amplitudes of ABRs are often less than one-millionth of a volt (1 µV). Corresponding *auditory steady-state responses (ASSRs)* are typically less than 0.1 µV in amplitude. In contrast, *long latency responses* (from the cortex) are relatively large, upward of tens of µV. If the problem was only that the signals targeted are very small, then it might not be much of an issue—simply amplify them a few thousand times. However, when the signals are measured from the head, the electrodes pick up other signals/voltages from the body and other equipment than the ones of interest. These are referred to as "noise." Worse, they can be and often are much larger than the targeted AEP. Examples of these extraneous signals include the *electroencephalogram (EEG;* resting activity of the brain), corneo-retinal potentials of the eyes, and voltages generated by muscle activity such as the heart beating, eyeblinks, muscles of the head and neck contracting, and activity of other muscles of the body. Muscle activity is particularly a problem if the subject becomes restless and starts fidgeting during acquisition of the AEP.

The EEG signal is typically around 10 µV peak to peak or more. Figure 4–1 shows an example typical of EEG data (panel A) and a typical ABR (panel B) shown on the same scale. The key point again is that the resting brain activity and other noise (relative to the AEP) is much larger than the signal of interest. The signals picked up from electrodes on the head are added together. What is seen appears to be only the EEG and other interference because the tiny signal of the ABR is buried in this noise. Note: In general engineering terms, unwanted signals are commonly referred to as "noise." In clinical electrophysiology, "noise" generally refers to electrical interference and not to acoustic noise (sound).

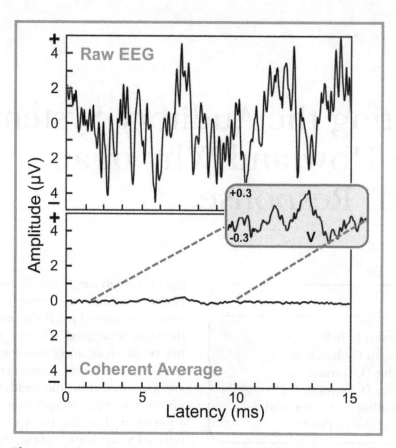

Figure 4–1. Typical magnitudes of the EEG (electroencephalogram or resting brain activity—Raw (not computer processed/averaged) and the Coherent Average* of the auditory brainstem response, plotted on the same scale (*to be discussed in more detail shortly). Inset: Projecting the window of the response itself (the actual stimulus-elicited portion the epoch analyzed) and on its typical amplitude scale; the wave called "V" is featured again on the virtual "big screen."

In addition to *physiological noise* that is generated by the body, there is also *nonphysiological noise*. The latter comes from the environment. Attaching electrodes to a subject, the leads can act as an aerial and pick up electromagnetic signals. These include fields given off by wires powering equipment or electronics therein. Power line (mains) interference can come from elsewhere in the building. Other sources might include mobile phones, computers, elevators (lifts), and other medical equipment in neighboring areas. Nonphysiological signals can also be picked up by the recording equipment and hence contribute noise to the recording.

The challenge is how to extract the AEP of interest from the much larger noise background. As a preview, one of the main utilities of AEPs is their application in estimation of hearing levels of patients by presenting a sound to the ear and trying to measure the tiny responses of the brain to that sound. The sound is made quieter until the subject no longer hears it and so it should not elicit a response from the brain. However, the magnitude of the target-signals at low sound levels becomes progressively smaller—fractions of a millionth of a volt (for the ABR)—as the hearing threshold is approached. If there is any interference, it becomes especially difficult to determine if the signal is present, and this potentially leads to an erroneous conclusion that the patient has a hearing loss, when in fact they do not. It has been demonstrated that variations in ABR waveforms can even affect the interpretations made by experienced clinicians. In a study, given recordings of ABRs made at different stimulus levels, clinicians varied by up to 60 dB in estimates of hearing thresholds of the patients.[1] The main problem is distinguishing between the response and noise in the recording.

Figure 4–2 shows examples of ABRs recorded at the same stimulation level. In each panel the recording has been repeated (hence, there are two lines). Repetitions are commonly done in clinical

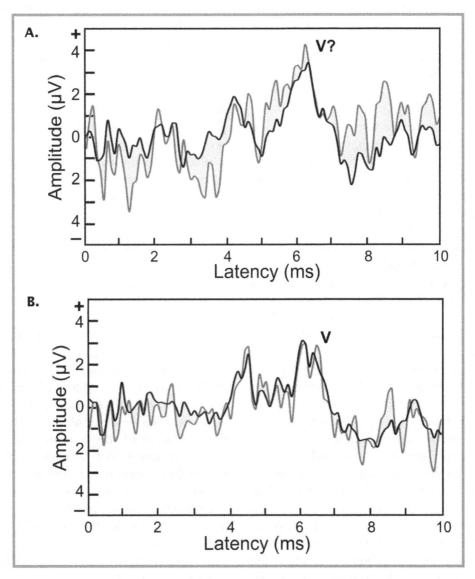

Figure 4–2. Two examples of an ABR being recorded at the same stimulation level—above the subject's hearing threshold. Test (*black*) and retest tracings (gray) are shown, with light gray fill between them to emphasize differences by both amount and direction (+/–). **A.** Example wherein there is a lot of noise in the recorded background, so wave V (which occurs at around 6 ms) is hard to identify confidently. **B.** Much less measurement noise and the repeatability of the recording of wave-V is much clearer. The two test–retest tracings are more interleafed/symmetrical overall and areas of difference are much tighter.

testing to check repeatability of the response. In panel A, as shown by the substantial variation in and/or between the two lines, repeatability is seen to be very poor. In panel B, the noise is much less; it now is easier to see that the two waveforms are quite similar. For instance, the prominent peak just after 6 ms is repeatable and not an artifact of the noise in the recording. In this application, for a given sound level, the key question is: Is there really a response from the brain to the sound presented or just *random background activity* (whether physiological or nonphysiological). Only by reducing background interference as much as possible can the examiner be confident of obtaining a reliable evoked response.

Two main methods are used to reduce noise in electrophysiological recordings: (1) reduce the noise at the source and (2) use technical approaches to reduce noise. If the noise is nonphysiological— such as a piece of equipment in the room—the simplest solution is to turn the equipment off. For example, turning off lights, computers, and mobile phones may help to reduce interference. Unfortunately, it is not always possible to do this. In many cases the equipment will be in a separate room or cannot be reached. Alternatively, such equipment may be critical for the safety of a patient, such as a ventilator or syringe pump, when beside-testing in a hospital.

If the noise originates from the muscles of the patient (physiological)—*electromyographic (EMG)* interference, getting them to relax may help to reduce interference. Strategies include having a comfortable chair or a couch that the patient can lie on, as the large muscles of the neck can produce large electrical signals. Supporting the neck/reducing neck tension may well reduce physiological interference. It simply could be a case of asking the patient if they can stop moving so much. Also asking the patient to close their eyes can help reduce interference from eyeblinks, if compatible with the test protocol for the AEP under examination (to be discussed later in this book).

Figure 4–3 shows an example of a subject who is relaxed (A) and one who clearly is not (B), along with the corresponding background activity recorded from electrodes on the head. It is also evident that if a subject is not relaxed, the noise that is measured is much higher, and it may be a real problem to record/see reliably an evoked response. Therefore, the former often yields acceptably low background interference (panel A). The nature of the ABR permits testing patients sleeping or awake, as will be a recurrent subject of interest in upcoming episodes. For now, it will suffice simply to characterize the big picture. Reliable results are possible with adequately cooperative, awake patients. However, crying/screaming patients (panel B) are impossible to test adequately, due to intolerable levels of background noise.

On most EP test equipment, it is possible to see the raw signal being picked up by electrodes attached to the patient, namely background EEG and whatever other activity is coincidentally picked up. On such displays, it may be possible to see how a particular interference changes when a piece of equipment is turned off or similarly when the subject relaxes. Indeed, inspection of the raw signal can often betray origin(s) of interference. For instance, interference from power lines will be continual and sinusoidal, with a period related to 20 ms for 50 Hz or 16.7 ms for 60 Hz, whereas muscle activity is usually more variable and nonsinusoidal.

In the following text, four technical methods to reduce effects of noise on recordings are introduced: (A) coherent averaging; (B) artifact rejection; (C) filtering; and (D) differential amplification. These four methods are generally present in EP measurement systems. Some are adjusted/set from protocols in the equipment and some, such as differential amplifiers, may be built into the hardware of the systems. The order of presentation here is not necessarily of signal "flow" (as might be shown in a flow chart), rather it covers key recording advances that made EP testing broadly clinically adaptable. Their consideration is a friendly reminder that "recording" starts in the analog world and that fundamental signals-and-systems principles (as presented in Chapter 2) must be observed.

Noise reduction method A: *coherent averaging* is based on the principle that the brain response to each sound played to the ear is fundamentally identical/invariant. This is certainly an oversimplification, but it is the assumption for averaging. Another assumption is that the background noise is random. Consider, for example, presentation of

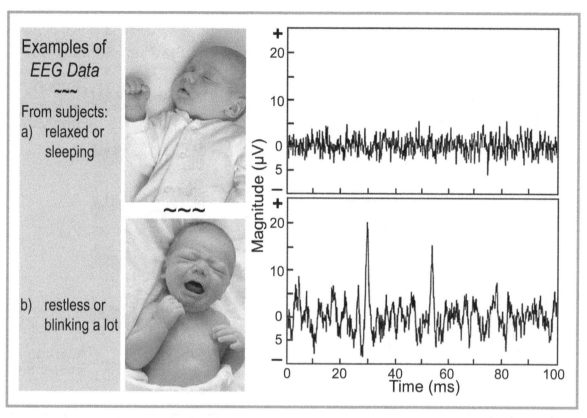

Figure 4–3. Examples of the effect of subject state on raw EEG data, which in turn is always lurking in the background of the response of interest.

3,000 stimuli (such as acoustic clicks; recall Episode 2.3) at a rate of 45.1 stimuli per second (for demonstration purposes), which takes around 90 s to record. Were only ideal (noise-free) responses averaged together, the averaged responses would faithfully represent the original response of the brain. With noise in the background, averaging can improve greatly signal quality for the examiner.

Figure 4–4 shows the steps in averaging. Panel A shows data analogous to that recordable from the brain to sound stimulation, as in this scenario. The train of ongoing stimuli (top) connotes a series of clicks in this case. The middle graph shows an idealistic response that the brain might produce (one component of the overall short-latency AEP from this level of the auditory pathway); thus, identical responses to each click (assuming indeed invariant responses). The bottom trace shows what might be recorded more realistically from the brain, now with random background noise overwhelming the response. In this demonstration, some hint of presence of the response is evident, but not discernment of its actual waveform. Panel B shows how the responses to each stimulus are aligned in time—*synchronized* or *triggered* effectively by each click. All are digital "snapshots"—brief epochs of time—of the recorded activity, with each started when the individual click stimulus is presented. Consequently, their analyses are coherent with the start of the stimulus. As digital samples of each time epoch per stimulus, a matrix of data points is stored in the computer's memory to permit high-speed computation of an average of the samples (point by point) over all repetitions. The average of the noisy individual responses per click is shown in the bottom trace of panel B. The averaging process has reduced the noise greatly (relative to that on the individual responses), revealing the evoked response more clearly in the coherent average. That is the good news. A bit of bad news is that the averaged response—though looking pretty good in this demonstration—still has some

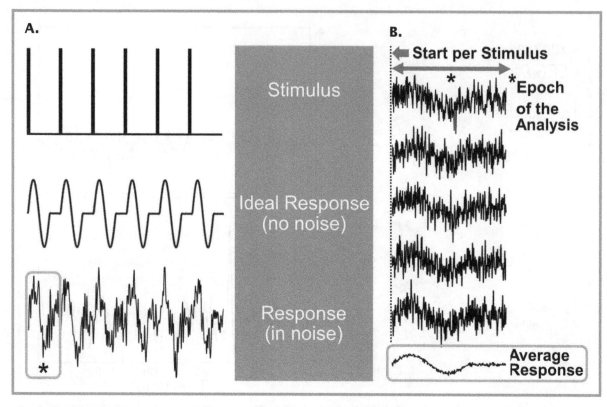

Figure 4–4. A. The top graph shows input signals that are presented through headphones when making a recoding (a series of acoustic clicks). *Although overall a steady-state presentation, the analysis is "single-event" oriented, with analysis thus being stimulus by stimulus within the pulse train. The middle function models the auditory brainstem response (for demonstration purposes), as both a simplistic and idealistic signal—identical to every click and measured in a noise-free background. The bottom graph represents more realistic data that might be recorded from the scalp, wherein the responses are buried in interference/noise from the brain, body, and/or extraneous sources. **B.** The epochs recorded are aligned in an array in computer memory, time based and synchronized to when each stimulus was initiated. The average of the samples is taken—the coherent average of the signals is computed point by point, coincidentally reducing the background noise on the final average.

residual noise. Nevertheless, the improvement is quite impressive and such results in practice could be more than adequate (see again Figure 4–1, bottom panel and inset display).

For stationary and completely random noise (more to this point momentarily), the average level of the noise reduces with the square root of the number of epochs or **sweeps** taken. Figure 4–5 illustrates the nature of this type of reduction in noise/noncoherent random signals. For example, with responses of 1 µV and presumably random EEG noise of 10 µV, the signal is only one-tenth of the noise and impossible to see. If averaged over 10,000 sweeps (taking averaging to the extreme of common practice), the noise will be reduced by 100 times (square root of 10,000). The same signal of 1 µV now has a residual noise level of only 0.1 µV. The signal is much larger than the noise—a substantially more favorable **signal-to-noise ratio (SNR)**—in this example 10. This should give the examiner a high degree of confidence that a response is genuinely present.

The inset of Figure 4–5 illustrates the "rule" in more detail—amount of noise reduction that may be counted upon (ideally) with increasing N of stimulus repetitions (thus, numbers of epochs averaged). Based upon the square root of N, the underlying function is important to bear in mind in practice. The range of N represented in the main figure is typical of processing for the featured AEP of this episode, often using averages of 1,000, 1,500, or more in multiples. A N = 4,000 epochs is generally the upper limit that is practical for clinical measurements due to diminishing gains in noise reduction and/or test efficiency. Even at the fastest stimulus rates appropriate for a given AEP, this is quite time consuming. Use of such a high N is dedicated to situations like stimulating near the limits of response detection (in general, at low hearing levels for the given stimulus in the given subject). Some points of interest are highlighted on the inset graph, as follows. Simply doubling N (2^1) is expected to yield a reduction of only ~30%, which is also the result obtained using the "trick" of averaging test–retest trials. Increasing N to 2^2 = 4 could lead to a 50% reduction. Jumping to 2^4 = 16 portends a reduction of 75%; 2^8 = 256 for nearly 94% reduction. An exponent of 12 is required to just surpass N = 4,000. However, the "payoff" in proportion is becoming diminishingly small. The good news is that tests of the SLRs often can be made at relatively high stimulation rates. Even better, the longer latency potentials can be measured handily with much lower Ns. Using 256 and test–retest trials per stimulus condition can serve well the measurement of some cortical AEPs. Such nuances will be considered along the time-space coordinates of AEPdom, as the book progresses.

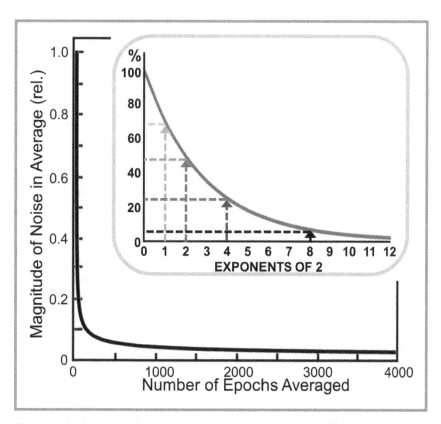

Figure 4–5. The effect of averaging on white stationary noise. The relative (rel.) noise level is plotted against the number of averages taken. The actual noise would depend on the individual test subject, filter settings, and any extraneous interference, and the predicted reduction is idealistic (see text). Inset: A closer look at the "rule"—percent reduction predicted as a function of the powers of two in the number of epochs averaged, 2^0 = 1 being the unaveraged signal (see text).

At this juncture, it is sufficient to reassure that N is still the examiner's friend but to note also that it is not the only ally/option by which to improve the SNR of the recorded response, starting with several matters to be scrutinized in the rest of this episode.

The *stationarity* of the response and/or background noise is an important factor at play in real-world AEP testing. A stationary signal is one that does not change properties over time; the amplitude remains roughly the same throughout its measurement. When a subject is in a fairly constant state such as being asleep or very relaxed, the data from the subject should be fairly stationary. However, when their state changes, such as if the subject starts blinking their eyes or crying, then the noise becomes nonstationary and the averaging process may not work so effectively. Thus for the previous example, a 100-fold reduction in the noise cannot be expected and/or is not readily predictable. This is one reason why it helps if subjects are as relaxed as possible during recording.

Rather than simply averaging all the data together with the same weight, some systems use **weighted averaging**. This is a procedure wherein blocks of data that have a higher noise level are weighted less in the final average, compared to those blocks with low noise levels. This procedure is called Bayesian weighting[2] and can reduce effects of nonstationary, as when a subject is noisier for one part of a recording than the rest. However, this technique brings no benefit if the noise is consistent in time.

Noise reduction method B: **artifact rejection.** As noted previously, averaging many repeated stimulus-response epochs/sweeps (potentially thousands) can reduce the noise/interference in evoked response recordings. However, where some of the epochs recorded are particularly noisy, it is not helpful to include them in the final average, as they are unlikely to "average out" and may only decrease the SNR of the response. This is the rationale for selectively removing unusually noisy epochs from computation of the final average (rejecting them)—hence artifact rejection.

The classical method of artifact rejection in EP measurement is shown in Figure 4–6, a replot of the "unhappy" baby's data in Figure 4–3b. This is a sample of EEG data for 0.1 s of recording (for illustration only, showing partial coverage of the total sweeps from the continuous recording). The signal of the ABR, if present, is buried within the noise and can only be seen by averaging. A couple of peaks in the data demarked by arrows are likely from eyeblinks. The noise level on the final average will only increase by allowing in sweeps bearing such artifacts. The vertical dotted lines show the length of an individual recording epoch. It may add or subtract from the final average, but there is a good chance that some such noise bursts ultimately will remain in the final averaged response, unless some countermeasure is applied. The horizontal dashed lines show an example of setting an artifact rejection level by which to exclude such epochs, in this case between −8 and +8 μV. Sweeps that are accepted in the final recording will not have peaks or troughs that exceed the artifact rejection level. Epochs that contain such peaks thus would be rejected by the evoked response system and not included in the final average. However, should a patient become increasingly noisier and/or remain longer in an agitated state, the longer it will take to complete the test. In addition, most modern test systems also reject any sweeps where the peak-to-peak voltages of the input signal exceed the limit of the A-D converter that receives the analog recording (output of the recording amplifier, discussed later in this chapter).

In the previous scenario, the exclusion of artifacts is accomplished without likely excluding sweeps bearing the targeted AEP, in this case the ABR, which is not expected to exceed +/−1 μV. It usually is possible to adjust the artifact rejection parameters based on reasonable limits for the particular AEP targeted and other considerations (for instance, the subject's own overall noise level). Most test systems show the "raw" brain data being recorded from the subject (virtually in real time) along with the artifact rejection levels so the examiner can get a rough idea of how the data amplitudes compare to the artifact rejection thresholds. A restless subject will tend to have more artifacts than a relaxed subject (as seen in Figure 4–3). During averaging, most systems will show the number of epochs that are being accepted versus rejected from the average. If rejecting high numbers of epochs—particularly more than 50%—the examination is becoming quite inefficient. The rejection rate for relaxed subjects is often ≤10%. Thus high

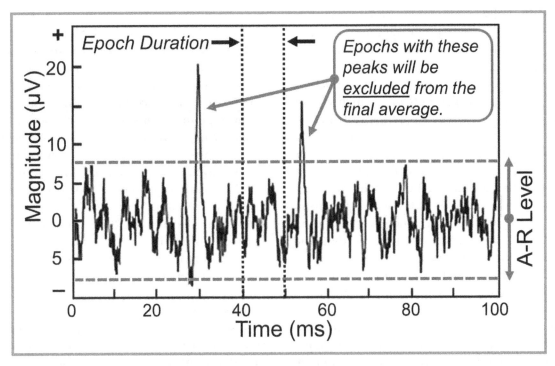

Figure 4–6. The principle of artifact rejection (AR); replot and further scrutiny of the example of EEG data for 0.1 s of a recording from Figure 4–3B. The EEG data might have an evoked response signal buried within it, yet can only be seen by averaging many repeats of the stimulus response. The vertical dashed lines show the length of an individual recording epoch. The horizontal lines depict examples of artifact rejection levels as might be chosen—in this case between −8 and +8 μV. Epochs that would be accepted in calculating the coherent average thus would have to fall before/after either of the overshooting artifacts indicated (in this case, those typical of eye blinks). Test systems typically indicate the number of epochs accepted versus rejected; the sum being the total number of stimuli actually presented.

rejection rates demand steps to try to get the subject to relax, after first determining no technical issues are the cause, like a recording electrode having a too-high impedance. Alternatively, the artifact rejection limits could be relaxed. However, many noisy epochs are then let into the final average and the final quality of the recording may be unacceptable. Inevitably, this tactic will reach a point of diminishing returns. When rejecting high numbers of epochs—particularly more than 50%—the examination becomes inefficient, literally to a fault. It is a good idea to start with low artifact rejection levels to ensure only recording good quality epochs and to only increase them if there are excessive artifacts. For example, the recent guideline[3] of the British Society of Audiology on ABR testing in babies recommends artifact rejection levels for ABR recording in infants with an initial value no more than +/− 5 μV. They also suggest not exceeding +/− 10 μV for testing babies, so if the subject is too noisy to proceed, the baby may need to return for follow-up testing.

Simply setting a threshold to exclude artifacts exceeding plus/minus certain voltages is, nevertheless, the simplest and probably the most common method of artifact rejection. More advanced methods include trying to identify artifacts with a known shape and to cancel them from the recording, rather than excluding the whole epoch. This procedure might include having a template of the shape of a known artifact (eyeblink, heartbeat, etc.), finding where part of the data matches a scaled or filtered version of the template, and then subtracting it from the data.[4] (The nature of such artifacts and their treatment will be taken up again in the next episode.)

A type of electrical artifact, as mentioned in Episode 2.3, is **stimulus artifact,** which occurs when the earphones transduce the signal. Stimulus artifacts can occur in the course of generating high-level sound stimuli—for example estimating the hearing level of profoundly deaf patients. As the driving voltage is turned up, the voltage can induce currents in the electrode leads. Hence pickup of the interference can occur where the stimulus' waveform (in effect) is added to the recording and may obscure the true waveform of the targeted AEP. The interference will likely worsen when the electrode leads are placed near the headphones/transducers or wires leading to them.

Stimulus artifacts tend to be initiated at the start of the evoked response recording for most (but not all) test paradigms; for example, using a click might produce a big voltage spike in the first millisecond or so of the recording; stimulus artifacts from tone bursts or speech stimuli will typically be longer. Recognition of the artifact and its origin (the earphones) may be sufficient to avoid confusing it with a true response such as a prominent ABR wave component (for example, as seen at 6 ms in Figure 4–2). One phenomenon that can help to separate a stimulus artifact from the true neural response is the natural delay of sound propagation down the ear canal, which is augmented by tubal-insert type earphones. Artifacts will often start in the averaged response at or near time zero, whereas neural responses should have some delay. Use of alternating polarity clicks (to be discussed in more detail momentarily) can largely cancel the stimulus artifact, although the cancellation may affect the true waveform or cancel some wave component(s), as discussed in subsequent episodes. However, in some cases, an unsuppressed stimulus artifact can be a substantial distraction in determining the true response. Most test systems permit blocking out some milliseconds of the display/printout, but it must be borne in mind that the artifact did not disappear, rather simply it is ignored for practical purposes.

Stimulus artifacts can be more problematic when using longer stimuli, including tone bursts, speech, or steady-state stimulation—depending on the particular stimulus paradigm (as discussed in later episodes). For any such "long" stimulus, the artifact may overlap the part of the response of interest. Ruling out significant interference of long duration stimuli may not always be straightforward when just looking at the raw EEG and/or coherent average in the time domain. Sometimes, it can be easier in the frequency domain (especially for steady-state stimulus-response methods). Nonetheless, additional precautions may be needed to avoid confusion between artifact(s) and the true response. Stimulus artifacts incidentally can be a problem also for machine/statistical detection methods (to be discussed later).

One way to test for stimulus artifact, particularly with insert phones, is to keep the earphone leads and transducers in the same place but clamp the tubes and remove the eartips from the subject's ears, so as to block the sound, then run a retest. As the artifact generators are in the same place, any significant stimulus artifact should remain the same, but the true AEP should disappear.

The **alternating polarity or phase** of clicks, tone bursts, and others is a stimulus-based approach to help minimize its electromagnetic stimulus artifact. However, many systems today offer **alternate averaging**—also known as **split-buffer averaging**—as a way to reduce stimulus artifact and spare the examiner of running separate trials using the rarefaction (R) and condensation (C) stimuli (recall Figure 2–19). As with the alternating click, the polarity of the stimulus going to the transducers is still alternated by the computer, but the responses of each (C and R) are averaged separately. This procedure should cancel almost all of the stimulus artifact upon averaging the acquisition "buffers" (memories) of the C and R responses. Some AEPs are more or less sensitive to change in stimulus polarity—for instance, cochlear microphonic responses that largely follow the stimulus's time history (a topic of the next chapter). They invert with stimulus polarity and are abolished by alternate averaging. However, many neural responses do not change polarity with the stimulus polarity and are not affected that much with alternate averaging. Often the default setting for clinical protocols is to use alternate averaging for this reason (the average response to all C and all R stimuli combined together). Nevertheless, there

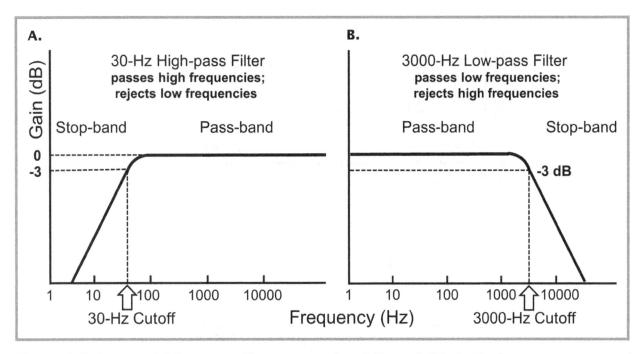

Figure 4–7. Recap and follow-up on filter concepts (recall Figure 2–6B). **A.** The frequency response of a high-pass filter. Over the stop band, the signal's gain (ratio of output to input signal amplitude) drops below 0 dB; the frequency at which the gain is −3 dB is considered often as the practical cutoff frequency of the filter. **B.** The frequency response of a low-pass filter. Overall, the illustration is representative of a basic, "classical" filter function with parameters frequently used for measurement of the ABR. As such and given a roll-off rate of −6 dB/oct, the negative gain (attenuation) by the bottom of graph would represent a reduction of the output of more than 20 dB (100-fold) in the stop-band.

can be small effects of alternating polarity. It thus can be useful to be able to view the subaverages to C and R stimuli independently; the individual polarity-based responses are protected in the digital record and are accessible independently. Indeed, using alternating polarity stimuli sometimes may obscure the details of the response and lead to misinterpretation of findings, particularly for the shorter-latency AEPs (stay tuned).

Noise reduction method C: *filtering* can remove unwanted frequencies from a signal (see Episode 2.1), which is sometimes called *signal conditioning*. Specifically (technically), filters can be used for selectively attenuating frequencies of signals whether above, below, or in some band of frequencies, relative to the filter's cutoff frequencies (recall Figure 2–6B). To recap and elaborate interests in filters for clinical electrophysiology, the idea generally is to keep the range of frequencies that are believed to contain an evoked response but remove those likely not to contain a response, yet can contain noise. Figure 4–7 shows further examples and relevant terms for frequency responses of *high-pass* (a) and *low-pass* (b) filters, as commonly are incorporated (for instance) in the design of the differential/recording amplifier.

In the case of evoked responses, the filter that typically has the most effect is the high-pass filter. This filter rejects much of the resting EEG activity of the brain, which is dominated by very low frequency components—especially below 20 Hz. Generally EEG noise power increases as the frequency decreases (sometimes called a 1/f distribution), so it helps to remove the lowest frequencies from the EEG. The high-pass filter also may reject some portion of artifacts/other noise discussed previously, including myogenic activity, which is also encountered substantially below 100 Hz. These considerations underlie common choices; for example, for the ABR of 30 Hz or even 100 Hz

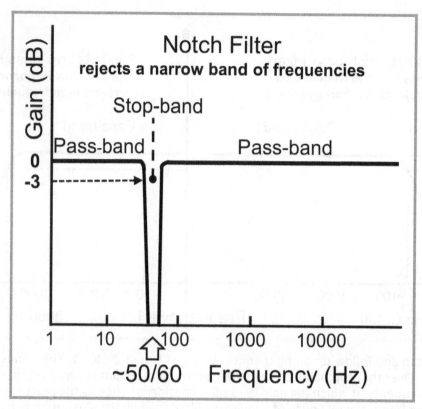

Figure 4–8. The frequency response of a notch (or band-reject) filter. The center of the stop-band is aimed sharply at 50 Hz or 60 Hz, pending the line frequency of the AC power of the test facility.

for the high-pass cutoff frequency. Historically, much research has been devoted to finding the best filter settings for different AEPs.[5] The detailed examples in this episode are especially effective for the ABR, yet are not optimal for all AEPs. Appropriate parameters applicable to others will be discussed in subsequent episodes, especially with respect to their clinical application.

AEPs with few exceptions tend to have little energy at frequencies above 2 kHz. The low-pass filter setting is mainly intended to prevent higher frequencies from causing *aliasing*, which can arise in the digital sampling of signals. Recall the rule (Episode 2.1): signals that are more than half the sampling rate of the analog-to-digital converter can be distorted by the sampling process and appear incorrectly as low frequencies in the data (recall Figure 2–9). The low-pass filter cutoff frequency should therefore be set well below half the sampling rate used in the system to avoid this.

The high- and low-pass filters combined (as commonly employed) in tandem make a **band-pass filter** (again, recall Figure 2–6B). In the example of Figure 4–7, this means sampling primarily a band of frequency of only about 30 Hz/100 Hz to 3000 Hz. As a distortion of the input signal (by definition, although not being nonlinear distortion), the critical issue in choice of the filter parameters is whether a significant portion of the targeted AEP may be substantially attenuated by band-pass filtering. This is a matter of the risk of throwing out (effectively) some of the "good" of the response's signal, as pursued further in the upcoming episode.

One other type of filter of interest for AEP measurements is a **notch filter**. This filter can attenuate a very small region of frequencies from a signal, thus leaving a notch in the frequency response. Figure 4–8 shows an example of the frequency response of a notch filter. Most commonly, this is used to "get rid of" frequencies where the most prominent electrical interference occurs: 50 Hz throughout much of the United Kingdom, Europe, Africa, and Asia; 60 Hz in North American and roughly half of South America. Under some conditions it can be difficult to get rid of all of such interference on recordings without using a notch filter. However, the use of notch filtering should be weighed carefully against its inherently negative attributes—the possible consequences of having introduced a hole into the spectrum of the recorded AEP and possible phase distortion of frequencies in the signal near the notch frequency.

Filters can be and, to some extent, often are implemented in the hardware of the EP test system. These are *analog filters*, typically built into the recording amplifier via electronic components to directly condition the recorded signal in real time, such as integrated-circuit amplifiers and discrete-circuit components (capacitors, resistors and inductors). Therefore, analog filtering can be applied before the recorded signal of the response is converted from analog to digital form. However, this does not permit an "undo" of the effects of the filter. Filters also can be implemented via computer software—digital filters comprising computational algorithms and subroutines—and applied to the digitally converted recording of the response. Once converted to digital form, a variety of digital filters can be applied to the AEP to see their effects on the data. As long as the original digital recording is protected (as is commonly automatically done), digital filters can be applied and undone. Also especially important in clinical testing, digital filtering can be applied offline.

In practice, some analog filtering is usually applied before the signal gets to the computer of the recording system. This initial filtering can prevent the amplifier from being overloaded with large signals. The filter settings today (as in the previous ABR-filtering example) are typically set in the recording system via the test software (thanks to digitally controlled analog circuits). It is prudent to keep the analog passband fairly wide. Digital filtering can be applied by the examiner for additional narrowing of the passband when the signal is analyzed further (as when preparing the report of the findings). Again, filters distort signals by definition, yet a balance of distortion versus quality of signal extraction often can be struck favorably.

Digital filters often provide choices not only of cutoff frequencies but also different roll-offs of filter attenuation and other details that affect both the shape of the frequency response and the transient response of the filter function, for instance, causing more or less ringing (recall Figure 2–18). This can apply to responses too, not just stimuli. The risk of applying a given filter to an AEP is the potential for selectively attenuating some peaks in the AEP waveform and/or delaying them. Analog filters are particularly prone to introduce delay due to phase distortion, whereas in digital filters it is possible to use filters with no phase distortion. This issue is pursued further in the upcoming episode.

Noise reduction method D: ***differential amplification.*** As noted earlier, when electrodes are applied to the subject and leads connected to the electrodes, the leads can act as an aerial and pick up nonphysiological electromagnetic signals, such as the fields given off by equipment. The interference occurs through electromagnetic induction. This is the phenomenon that when a changing electromagnetic field passes through a loop of wire, it will induce an electric current in the wire (this is how radio/television aerials work). The current will be converted to a voltage at the evoked response amplifier. Even voltages associated with minute, induced currents will be amplified many times by the recording system and thus potentially compete with the AEP voltages that are to be measured. The recording amplifier of the system is a special type, called a ***differential amplifier***, and can greatly improve AEP quality.

The differential amplifier is similar in intention to a hi-fi or a hearing aid amplifier but is designed particularly to cancel out interference, as illustrated in Figure 4–9. Given two electrodes attached to a subject, a conductive loop is formed—in effect, a loop of wire—since the electrodes on the skin will conduct some current (recall Episode 3.1). If a changing electromagnetic field passes through a loop of wire, it too will induce an electrical current in the wire, namely alternating current. The magnitude of the interference relates to the area of the loop, proximity to the source of interference, and other factors. Whatever the specifics, such an induced signal will be amplified in the evoked response recording system and appear as noise

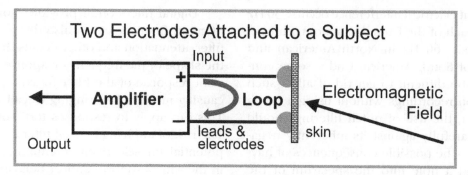

Figure 4–9. A loop is formed when two electrodes are attached to a subject. This can pick up interference through electromagnetic induction.

in the recording. Because the AEPs are very small and will be amplified tens to hundreds of thousand times in testing AEPs, even minute interference signals indeed will be amplified enough to substantially degrade quality of the recording.

The solution to reducing such interference is the introduction of a second recording loop into the system to cancel out any interference that is introduced in the first loop. This principle describes the function of the differential amplifier. The top part of Figure 4–10 shows two loops of wire with the same area. The signals A and B that are caused by induction are thus similar in the two loops. If one is subtracted from the other, they will mostly cancel out. The diagram below shows how this is implemented in a differential amplifier. A third electrode, called a *ground electrode*, is attached to the patient. In the old days, the ground electrode was sometimes attached to the ground of the electrical supply, but now there is complete *electrical isolation* between the electrodes and the power lines to avoid any possible cause of electric *shock* to the subject. This safety function is essential for any system that is used with patients.

Given the two loops of wire, one goes from positive to ground (+ve, voltage from an electrode connected to the *plus or noninverting amplifier input*) and the other goes from ground to negative (–ve at the *negative or inverting amplifier input*). Again, the electromagnetic induction will produce similar currents in both loops. The differential amplifier subtracts the noninverting signal from the inverting signal. This subtraction should substantially diminish any common signal in the two loops, such as 50 Hz/60 Hz interference from electrical wires. This will leave just the difference signal from +ve to –ve to be amplified, ideally the signal of interest. For example, the +ve might be from an electrode on the high forehead of the patient, the ground somewhere else on the forehead or on the nontest ear, and the –ve from the mastoid of the test ear (one of several montages commonly used for testing the ABR). The signal recorded is the voltage difference between the +ve and –ve electrodes. Depending on the relation of the electrode montage and the underlying position of the generator(s) of the AEP, this method generally works well and excludes nonphysiological noise generated by induction.

The **common mode rejection (CMR)** of a differential amplifier indicates how well it is able to remove the signals that are the same in the two loops and generally are unwanted. CMR is often expressed in decibels; for example, a differential amplifier with 100 dB common mode rejection will reduce common signals by a factor of 100,000. It should be noted that differential amplifiers work most efficiently when the impedances of electrodes are similar. Hence it is important to obtain low impedances when making evoked-response recordings (recall Episode 3.1). For example, obtaining impedances of 2 to 5 kOhms generally makes a differential amplifier work efficiently for most AEP tests/applications. Substantially higher impedances caused by poor electrode preparation or electrodes losing contact during testing are

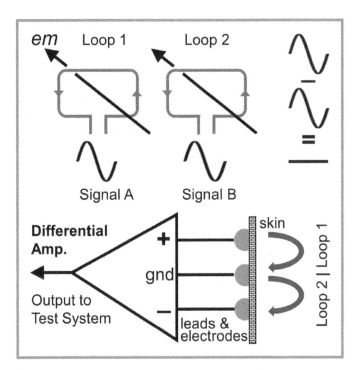

Figure 4–10. Having two similar loops of wire (top left), as typical in clinical electrophysiology (single-channel recording), is a significant game changer. Similar signals will be induced in the two loops, yet they require only one more connection to the differential amplifier (*bottom*) to form two loops. (Amp.—amplifier; gnd—ground; em—electromagnetic interference, such as 50/60 Hz.)

likely to cause imbalance(s) of impedance, resulting in noisier recordings.

Not all interference is caused by induction; an alternative mechanism is capacitive coupling between the patient and (for example) wires carrying electricity in the walls of the building or lighting (especially fluorescent) overhead. Some EEG amplifiers use a "driven right leg" circuit to reduce interference that occurs from such capacitive coupling.[6] There are also potential sources of *electrostatic interference*; for example, a DC charge can build up on a subject when they walk across a carpet. Sometimes this or similar effects can be enough to saturate the amplifier connected to the subject.

Most common evoked-response test systems have differential amplifiers built in to reduce interference from induction. It is also possible to design rooms with a metal mesh embedded in the walls, windows, and doors, called a *faraday cage*, in order to exclude electromagnetic/electrostatic energy from the room, but this is quite an expensive modification to make. Alternatively, shielding can be applied to the recording leads and stimulus transducer to help augment control of electrical interference.

Assume all has been done to improve the quality of the AEP signal using methods A to D, to the extent possible. To recap, subject relaxed, potential sources of interference turned off, good preparation to obtain good electrode impedances, use of differential amplifiers, use of appropriate artifact rejection and filters in the recording equipment, and averaged lots of responses to improve signal quality. The question then that always must be addressed is, how certain is it that there is a response present in the data? This is the key question in trying to estimate hearing thresholds. For diagnostic testing, the interest is in the waveform, although even then it is imperative to be sure that the response is of good quality before making a decision on its shape. The following approaches can be used to determine if there is really a response in the data.

1. Establishing good test–retest repeatability. Recall that for visual inspection of the repeatability of recordings, as practiced extensively in clinical and research applications, the response is replicated at a given stimulation level. Figure 4–2 gave examples of ABR recordings that had high versus low levels of noise. In panel A, the difference between the two "repeats" is relatively high (and in practice could be even worse). Consequently, it is difficult to know if a real response is represented or if it is simply random noise. In panel B, the waves in the recorded signal are similar/repeatable, and the size of the peak around 6 ms is characteristic of the particular response here. If the test–retest recordings are visually similar and the difference between the recordings is small, then the recording is generally considered to be of good quality. Nevertheless, this is a "judgment call," but the judgment could be made more rigorously, at least for some applications, by a "rule-based" decision. For example, the British Society of Audiology has endeavored to develop some useful guidelines for testing AEPs and especially the evaluation of ABRs in babies. Their guideline[3] prescribes using a 3:1 rule to indicate when a response is likely present in the data: The peak-to-trough amplitude in a recording (by this rule) should be at least 3 times larger than the average difference between two recordings. There also can be more than one rule for a stricter requirement. In this same guideline, the BSA recommends finding the lowest stimulation level with a clear response meeting the 3:1 rule and where the noise floor on the recording is less than 40 nV.

   Visual inspection of waveforms is only practical for recordings assessed in the time domain; for example, transient-evoked AEPs like the ABR where the emphasis is on waveforms. Steady-state responses generally are not viewed for measurement purposes in the time domain, but rather via spectral analysis and results presented primarily in the frequency domain. Both approaches to AEP measurement, nevertheless, can make use of statistically based detection methods.

2. Use a statistical method to detect that a response is present. Various methods have been proposed to try to detect evoked responses in recordings; some of the more prominent ones in the literature are summarized in Table 4–1. A few are highlighted in principle here. Additional details on some will be given in later episodes for particular AEP tests. For all applications, ultimately, the question asked is, is the evoked response signal statistically different from random noise? An early approach to answer this was the F_{sp} method,[7] which has been used fairly widely. Various other methods have been proposed with names such as the Hotelling T^2 and the Q-samples tests,[8,9] and there are still others more recently reviewed.[10] Generally, such methods give a number that increases as the response amplitude and/or quality improves. Ultimately, it helps to be able to produce statistical ***p-values*** based on the resultant measure of the test that can be considered indicative of a response being present. In early methods, a *p*-value was not always given, but more recent methods tend to yield a *p*-value directly. The examiner then can choose a cutoff such as $p < 0.05$ or <0.01 in order to score the response as "present." The choice is not arbitrary, but instead is made with consideration of the ***false positive*** rate. For example, there is only a 1 in 20 or 1 in 100 chance, respectively (given *p*-values of 0.05 and 0.01), that the signal recorded is merely random noise. On the one hand, choosing a lower *p*-value as the

Table 4–1. Some Statistical Detection Methods Used in Evoked Response Recording

METHOD NAME	COMPUTATION	APPLICATION EXAMPLE(S)
F_{SP} (F-value at single point)[7]	Signal strength (variance) of AEP vs. background noise	Potentially any AEP: first developed for ABR (time domain)
F_{MP} (F-value at multiple points)[16]	Similar to F_{SP} but noise variance estimated over multiple poststimulus samples	Potentially any AEPs (time domain)
HT^2 (Hotellings T-squared)[17]	Multivariate t-test comparing average time-voltage values across multiple epochs	Initially auditory LLR; broadly applicable to AEPs: transients or steady-state (time or frequency domain)
F test[18]	Analysis of variance of power in signal frequency bands vs. noise frequency bands	Steady-state responses (frequency domain)
Phase coherence[19]	Analysis of variance of phase (or could be phase and amplitude) across epochs	Steady-state responses (frequency domain)
Q samples test[20]	Nonparametric test of consistency of phase or both phase and amplitude	Steady-state responses (frequency domain)
Template cross-correlation[21]	Cross-correlation of a known-response template with a possible evoked response	Potentially any AEPs (time domain)

cutoff point can make the examiner more confident that a signal is really present in the data, but at the risk of having to average over more epochs to reach that value. On the other hand, using a higher *p*-value for detection is at increasing risk of a ***false negative*** outcome (a detection made when no response is present in the data). This topic will be discussed further and in still other contexts in subsequent episodes.

A combination of statistical detection and visual inspection may be the most robust approach for "time domain" assessment of responses: visual inspection to see that the waveform looks as expected and statistical detection to be confident of the response. For responses evaluated in the frequency domain—although relying on statistical detection—it still is advisable to keep an eye on the time history of the background EEG.

It also is important to bear in mind that a statistical method does not "know" if it is detecting a real response, a stimulus artifact, or other interference, but rather evaluates the odds of a response like the signal being present in the data. The examiner still bears the responsibility for the results. The advantage of including statistical detection methods is that, at least, the scoring of the signal recorded as a response is no longer just based on subjective judgement by visual inspection.

It can also be helpful to measure the residual noise level of the recording, akin to that from the BSA guideline discussed previously. Therefore, if the data is too noisy in reference to a specified number of nano- or microvolts, the examiner can decide whether or not to trust the data or (for instance) to bring the subject back for more testing at a later date. The question then is how to estimate the noise level?

3. Estimation of measurement noise. The average difference between **test–retest** recordings (again, see Figure 4–2) is potentially a useful indicator of the background noise. A numerical metric also could be computed, for example, the RMS of the difference between the data in the stored records of epochs collected and averaged during test and retest trials. Estimates of residual recording noise are available on some AEP test equipment. As touched upon earlier, some systems use alternate averaging and record separate responses/averages to interleave R and C stimuli. The difference between these "subaverages" (the root mean square value of the difference between them) can be used to indicate the residual noise level. Alternatively, detection methods such as the F_{sp} or F_{mp} can be used to estimate how much a point, or points, in an epoch vary across multiple repeats (for example a point 5 ms after the stimulus). If there was no noise on a recording, then all points in an epoch would be identical across multiple repeats. As the recording noise increases, there will be more variability across the repeated epochs. This variability can give a noise estimate for the recording. There is a question as to what constitutes an acceptable noise level on a recording. This will depend on the response being recorded and the application. For example, when recording the ABR for "threshold" estimates, a residual noise below 40 nV might be an indication of good data quality.

Running a "control" trial is an alternative way to test the residual noise. The classical approach was to turn the sound level down to 0 dB nHL or perhaps turn it off while still running the trial. An alternative method is to unplug the headphones/transducers and run a test recording, although this still fails to deliver the same stimulus-driving voltage to the transducer (specifically that characteristic of the highest test level and maximum radiation). The most rigorous approach requires the use of tubal-insert earphones: present the highest level used after removing only the earplug and clamping the tubing, then compare recordings at various levels to see if the peaks and/or their amplitudes look like the real stimulus-related responses (with headphones in place). For no-sound trials, the hope is not to see anything in the response time frame of interest that is substantially different from the noise floor. If peaks still appear in the data that look like a response, then there is a problem! Sometimes running control trials may be viewed as wasting time compared to testing with stimuli of interest. However, including control trials, even the most rudimentary, can be a useful tool for troubleshooting equipment and/or checking noise levels. This can be particularly useful in more "demanding" test environments, such as newborn nurseries or operating rooms.

This episode has discussed different sources of interference/noise that may be seen when making an evoked-response recording and has introduced the key challenge of the response targeted to be measured being many times smaller than the noise obtained overall in the recordings. Noise can be physiological or nonphysiological. If possible, then it is best to reduce such noise at the source by turning off interfering equipment (reduce nonphysiological noise) or asking a subject to relax (reduce physiological noise). Even then there typically still will be a lot of noise present on a recording. There are a variety of technical methods that can help to improve response quality, such as averaging, artifact rejection, filtering, and noise reduction. Finally, once everything that has been done technically to reduce the level of noise in the recording, there remains the critical decision: Is there really an auditory evoked response in the data and/or an acceptably low amount of noise on the recording? Ultimately, if it is concluded that the recordings are of good quality, then subsequent clinical decisions can be made with confidence. The principles described in this episode underpin a number of clinical AEP tests. However, considerations of some additional tools and features of AEP recording is worthwhile before fully jumping into specific clinical applications, as follows in the upcoming episode.

Episode 2: The Good, Bad, and Ugly—Optimizing Response Extraction From Background Noise and How Signal Processing May Become Too Much

The last episode emphasized more basic, yet powerful, tried and proven "tools" to ensure extraction of a response in the face of considerable background noise. One of the AEPs was favored for demonstration purposes for its particular nuances and "signature waveform"—the ABR—which had a cameo appearance in Episode 3.1 as well. The same methods are applicable broadly in AEPdom, whenever/wherever in time or space, as also was demonstrated in Episode 3.1. A much longer latency response that is a cortical potential was seen to have its own signature waveform—the *P_1-N_1-P_2 complex*. Such breadth of utility of the method of analysis in extracting the given potential from background noise—coherent (or time-ensemble) averaging—follows from its basic definition and broad applicability in statistics. It serves to find the central tendency by reducing sample variance, in this case due primarily to background noise.

The average does not know the signal from the noise; by extrapolation, it also does not know shorter from longer latency responses. That responsibility is on the shoulders of the examiner. The examiner sets the parameters for the analysis as well as for those of still other processing and/or statistics applied. It now will be useful to further test basic approaches already discussed and/or their consequences in still other aspects, as can be anticipated looking forward to more applications in practice or of promising clinical utility. This starts with a broader understanding of the need for "more tools" and, at the same time, a greater understanding of both the power and limitations of signal-processing methods that have come to be applied to evoked-response measurement.[5,11–13] A demonstration then is in order, and that starts again (in effect) from the "noise floor" up. This is another look at what happens with progressively averaging the recorded signal in noise.

The approach here will be a bit in contrast to the method primarily considered in the last episode—simply digitally "grabbing" epochs per stimulus presented and averaging all for the (final) coherent average. Even though it took a long train of stimuli (like clicks) to extract the signal of the response, the stimulus was treated and the response was analyzed as if a single event. As shown in Figure 4–11A, the acquisition now is extended over recurring blocks of *N* stimulus repetitions—trains of eight stimuli in this demonstration and in the response as analyzed initially. Also, for this demonstration for the sake of simplicity, the number of blocks (B) is limited to only five. It thus is possible to see all the data and to watch the response arise from the noise background in a stepwise manner.

So here it goes. The time history of the recording at this stage (Figure 4–11A) reveals nothing repeatable in the background. An initial coherent average (panel B) is taken to keep an eye on the stability of the apparent background. The diagrams at the bottom of panel A and top of panel B map out how many and when all of the stimuli will have been presented, 8 × 5 = 40. However, the first "processing" step will be to have the blocks repeated and the data averaged, in this case twice—call this M = 2. Not much of an average and just looking across trains. In practice, M could be increased; but also in practice, this step might only be intended for quick peeks simply for some idea of the apparent stability of the recording or even on-the-fly noise floor estimate. This then is the beginning of the display in panel B, block 1. The average shown with the black line is presented in the light gray "shadow" of the unprocessed "EEG" from panel A. Little improvement is realized, as expected. More extensive averaging thus will be needed to reveal reliably the targeted AEP and to further demonstrate the power of signal averaging. The remainder of the sequence of processing is also summarized in panel B, where the overall train average has been updated with completion of acquisition and initial averaging block-by-block, as follows: 1/1; (1+2)/2; (1+2+3)/3; and so on. The interim averages are shown as the acquisition and process progresses and are projected again on the backdrop of the raw EEG from panel A. At the very least, by "all 5" there has been impressive noise reduction. However, due to the compression of the time axis (to show the whole sequence of blocks acquired), a

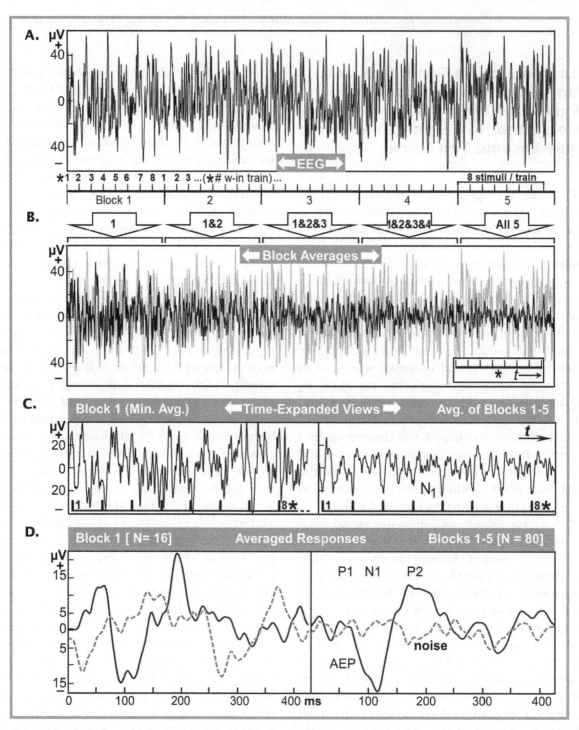

Figure 4–11. Computer-model-based demonstration: "Seeing Is Believing." Please see text for detailed description of manipulations of the signal in panel A through iterations in B–D. Test response: A simulated long-latency (cortical) response approximating that observed with moderately loud sounds like clicks and tone bursts. It is "buried" in background noise synthesized using low-pass filtered, quasirandom noise with the 1/f spectrum typical of the EEG—thus strongly low-frequency emphasized. Analog filtering was applied in analysis, 0.1 Hz to 100 Hz half-power bandwidth with –6 dB/oct roll-offs. Note: Unless qualified otherwise, "EEG" hereafter means raw EEG, namely recorded/portrayed as seen through whatever filter is used in the analog recording of the targeted AEP but not computer processed and including any incidental physical or physiological interference.

considerable amount of squinting at panel B likely is still needed to fully appreciate what has been gained in SNR, specifically with regard to "S"—the signal/response of interest. As this perhaps is at risk of not seeing, so not believing, expanded time histories are provided in panel C and by simply focusing on the cumulative results of the fifth block's versus the first block's results (minimal averaging). In panel C, the five-block average is seen to have extracted the response nicely. The distinctive N_1 component of this particular AEP now is evident for all eight stimuli and seen to be in sync with each stimulus presented. The time marks of the stimulus train have been shifted a tad in time (thus in latency) for ease of scrutiny of the coherence of this event-related potential to the events of the stimuli presented per train. Within the first block, in contrast, "bumps" may be seen that look more or less alike, yet they are not necessarily tightly synchronous with the stimuli. The filtering applied to the recording is for a "better look" at the real response (even when using signal averaging), but it also inevitably biases some of the noise to look a bit like a response. Consequently, there is a good chance of a falsely judged presence of the response (at least), likely providing a less than critical assessment of response waveform.

At this stage of processing, the overall/final train average could be used for analyses, for instance, as a quasi-steady-state signal for spectral analysis. By block five, that stimulus train clearly has evoked responses with the same rhythm. In other words, the repetition rate is providing a "signature" readily testable in the response's signal by some of the statistical methods summarized earlier in Table 4–1. For a given repetition rate (0.78/s used in this demonstration), spectral components are expected at this modulation frequency (in effect), precisely at that frequency and its integer multiples (recall Figure 2–15). This can be an excellent basis by which to test for the "good" (the signal) versus the "ugly" (the noise). However, the classical methods of clinical electrophysiology in audiology have favored more of a transient-response view of AEPs and the use of applicable methods of analyses and representation that are generally in the time domain, again treating the stimulus response as a single event. From this perspective, the measurement is akin to testing the impulse response of a system. This too is readily accomplished by further computer processing in this demonstration, that of overlapping all the individual responses. This is no problem as they are inherently synchronous within the trains and with each other by synchronizing the blocks. Results of such are illustrated in panel D of Figure 4–11. Considering the right-side panel first, the overall coherent average faithfully represents not only the robust N_1 component of the targeted AEP but also the prominent positive components of this response complex (P_1 and P_2).

In the first episode of this chapter, 1,000 or so stimulus repetitions were needed to demonstrate an AEP of adequately high/clinical quality. Here, an impressive extraction of the response was realized from what at first appeared simply to be nothing but noise—a mere $N_{Total} = M \times B \times N = 2 \times 5 \times 8 = 80$ stimulus repetitions collectively. The five-block average compared to the one-block provided a substantial increase in the number of repetitions (as single events), $80/16 = 5$ times, so a more than twofold expected enhancement of the SNR. Comparing the results in the left and right parts of panel D shows the remarkable difference in overall quality of both signal waveform and noise reduction. The response is manifest on the left, but not the sort of results that would be adequately reliable in practice.

Incidentally, it mattered not that between demonstrations of the two episodes that two different modes of acquisition were employed, as the averaging demonstrated in both is a linear process, although there are others that are not so (such as weighted averaging, mentioned in the first episode). Consequently, the same average would be obtained from applying the simpler approach. Still, **block-mode averaging** has additional benefits and not only for purposes of demonstration. For now, back to the demonstration and what seemed (by comparison) a rather little amount of averaging. This simply reflects the remarkable difference in the responses targeted. There are two ways to a better SNR—reduction of the noise and also a bigger signal. Recalling Figure 1–1 and moving up the auditory pathway in space and time, the AEPs "grow," even if "slowing down" (longer latencies). The growth side of the story is all good news, as the simpler way to beat the noise, in principle, is with a bigger signal. Simple in concept, yet not necessarily easy in practice. The slow part (noting time bases of the LLRs to be in the hundreds of milliseconds versus tens of milliseconds and less for the middle and short latency responses) is about waves building up with coverage of more generators along the expanding pathways. This is no problem for analysis, except that these slower waves are like lower frequency signals (recalling that frequency is the reciprocal of period). As hinted earlier, these potentials cannot be filtered using the same settings of the differential-amplifier (preamplifier) stage of the test system that is applied (for instance) to the ABR. The bad news is that the EEG and other interference often grow with decreasing frequency in their spectra. Nevertheless, back to good news, N_1 and such components of the LLRs still have a relatively better SNR than components of the shorter latency potentials, thus requiring far less numbers of stimulus repetition from reliable results. This indeed is good news in that a much slower stimulus rate was needed. Consequently, the total time to acquire comparably reliable short- versus long-latency responses is roughly the same.

Now it is time for a more practical demonstration using a real-subject recording: Ladies and gentlemen, readers everywhere, time to play, "The Game of Waves!" Please play honestly (namely, no peeking further into the text) as follows: The same paradigm has been used to acquire and analyze the data to be scrutinized, but simply focusing on two stages of processing. The first is the final average of the response train (as in Figure 4–11C, right), thus permitting a view of background noise overall with partial averaging. The other is an extraction of the fully averaged, single-event response (panel D, right). Now, please cover the left panel of Figure 4–12 to allow viewing of only the right panel. A fairly substantial amount of noise is evident at a glance from very low frequencies and beyond. Based on these data alone (for the moment), formulate an opinion, #1: For how many of the test levels can a decision be made with confidence that there is a repeatable, event-related response present—something looking like it is going "bump, bump, bump..." rhythmically in the otherwise random and fluctuating background? Now uncover the left-side panel, providing the overall coherent averages of the individual responses and form another opinion, #2: At how many stimulus levels would a *judgment* of clear and repeatable responses be rendered with confidence based on these results?

It would not be unreasonable—and entirely likely to be true—to render opinion #1 as "none." Although some of the stimulus levels, by a probability substantially greater than zero in the entire population, would evoked a response that should be detectable. However, there is simply too much noise competing with the AEP of interest to permit "seeing" coherent signals. For opinion #2, it would not be unreasonable to say all levels. Yet, is this entirely true? To make the game more interesting, suppose in reality the "patient" by conventional audiometry demonstrated (behaviorally) consistent responses at 40 dB HL? Yet, are the results at 40 adequate to predict this level precisely as the subject's true hearing threshold?

The lessons are several from this exercise. Again, simply looking (in effect) for responses in the ongoing EEG, even with some signal averaging, often is quite difficult. This was largely the fate of most early efforts to see auditory-/other sensory-evoked responses in raw EEG tracings (not digitally processed). EEG technology was developed over nearly a half century before compelling demonstrations of AEPs. In this case under examination, even 10 blocks averaged failed to reveal an evident recurrent response (per the stimulus train) at even the highest stimulus level. In contrast, averaging over all the stimuli presented yielded signals that can be interpreted at nearly all test levels with confidence. Returning to the right panel's view, though at the highest test level there arguably are some "response-ish" looking signals, it is important to bear in mind that this also is possibly purely by chance!

Knowing what to look for certainly helps but does not change the "odds" of a real (versus false) response in the "roll of the dice" of random noise. Only if the observed signal that is presumed response-like is truly repeatable can it be interpreted as a true response! Test–retest—provided by the lower overlaid tracings per stimulus level in Figure 4–12 (left panel)—is a very useful strategy to help the examiner judge repeatability, is broadly applicable, and is used extensively. This need not necessarily add substantially to test time and/or lead the patient to think that there are twice the trials per

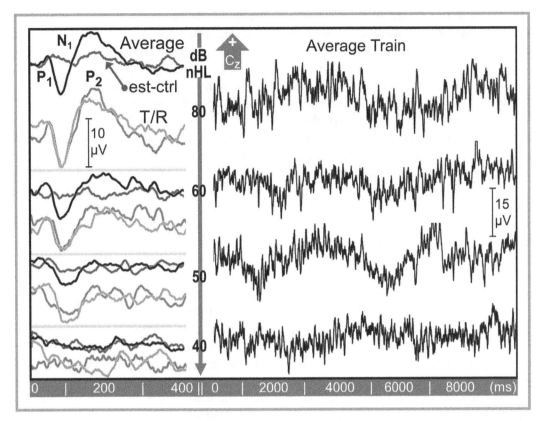

Figure 4–12. Playing the "Game of Waves" to evaluate results from a real subject (see text). Note: If seeing this figure and not having first read the text, please stop reading this and start from the text—play fair. Right panel: Similar paradigm as the demonstration in Figure 4–11, but this time simply plotting overall averages of the evoked responses to an 11-stimulus response train (N) in natural noise for B (blocks) = 10, averaging M = 2 repetitions per block. Left panel: From averaging over both numbers of blocks and repetitions, $N_{Total} = M*B*N = 220$. Stimulus repetition rate of 1.1/s, popular for testing the AEP evaluated. The subject was a male of advanced age with bilateral sensory neural hearing loss. In addition to extraction of these equivalent single-event responses, overlays of test and retest estimates (T/R, by way of split-buffer averaging) are shown. The average is also overlaid on an estimated nonstimulus/control recording (est-ctrl, computed as the split-buffer difference), effectively estimating the residual noise floor of the response epoch.

test level (that is, taking more of their time). One of the oldest "tricks of the trade" is again the use of **split-buffering** (a rudimentary form of block-mode averaging) during response acquisition, generally built into the measurement software of modern AEP test systems. As sweeps of the recording are being taken into computer memory, half are directed to one "buffer" (block of memory) and every other into a second buffer. They then can be compared or averaged together for the best overall estimate of the patient's response. The difference is also useful as a noise-floor estimate, an approximation of a nonstimulus or "control" trial, as previously proposed to help judge response presence/absence (see left panel, "est-ctrl" tracings).

The use of a nonstimulus "control" trial is molded in the foundation of knowledge in this field and still well valued. However, this use of control trials literally suffers from being time consuming—especially in the clinical real world—but time is even a luxury in research. It is an "expense" of time spent to use a test condition that (by design) clearly cannot contain a true response. The alert subject also can become less relaxed in the time gap(s) of not hearing the stimulus. As classically developed, test and retest trials were separate. Still, this is not a rigorous test of reliability, since this paradigm opens the door to differences in stationarity of the signal and/or background noise between the two trials. Split-buffering of interlaced samples is generally expected to avert this problem and, again, is not perceived by the subject to be another test condition. It also is more efficient for the examiner and/or avoids possible errors of setting the R versus C parameter of the stimulus as intended for a given trial.

Also a well-established nuance of noise during signal averaging is the expectation statistically that it should decrease systematically with increased number of sweeps over which the average is computed, namely by the square root of the N of stimulus repetitions (recall Figure 4–5). The SNR of the response similarly should increase systematically. This is demonstrated in Figure 4–13 using again a mathematically modeled real-world potential in a background noise characteristic of EEG–the major and most consistent contributor of interference on AEP recordings/measurement. Again, the spectral power of the resting EEG is inversely proportional to frequency—1/f noise. These data also were acquired via block-mode averaging, so each "block" averaged over just one-tenth of the overall N permits tracking the noise level for each and (hopefully) the ensuing reduction of the noise as averaging progresses across blocks. Panel A, left provides corresponding snapshots of the background noise (essentially as in Figure 4–11A) and the initial block average (as in panel B, block 1). On the right are the actual signal (model) and resulting average (calibrated in effect to a real response).

The residual noise is estimated and tracked over all blocks (again updated toward the final/overall average after 10 blocks in the current demonstration), using the RMS magnitude of the split-buffer's difference over the epoch analyzed. In this demonstration, it is also desirable to have an estimate of actual signal-to-noise enhancement. On the one hand, a "pure" noise estimate (strictly sampled where no stimulus-related signal is likely) is reasonably taken using the preceding one-third epoch—thus a prestimulus interval—and computing its RMS magnitude. On the other hand, the presumptive response is expected to dominate the first one-third epoch. Conversely, if the RMS value is not different for the comparable poststimulus interval, the response's presence—or more precisely, detectability—is less likely. (Note: there are more sophisticated and rigorous approaches, but the "tricks" here are confined to more basic concepts for purposes of the demonstration.) Both sets of results are provided in Figure 4–13B. In this idealistic modeling, the "laws" are expected to be observed and why such modeling is useful for both didactic purposes (to get the principles across first and then deal with reality later) and "test driving" any AEP system. Here, it is expected and indeed does demonstrate both noise reduction and SNR enhancement that abides by the square root of N rule of thumb. As more and more blocks are averaged (thus N_{Total} increased substantially), noise systematically decreases and SNR correspondingly increases. In the real world, such "performance" can be observed, yet not necessarily always by the "rule" and/or even observed throughout a given test. Such results necessarily are sensitive to state of the subject (remaining completely relaxed and quiet versus otherwise). This again is an issue of violation of stationarity. There also is no guarantee that the response/signal is itself stationary (although broadly assumed to be far more so than background EEG/noise). Also, and as a general truism, intersubject differences can be substantial. Humans simply are neither perfectly stable signal nor perfectly stable noise generators.

At the same time, the practical reality for the evoked response examiner is that interference is potentially everywhere, some more worrisome than others. Hence, the justification in the last episode to apply an artifact-rejection algorithm to the signal processing (recall Figure 4–6). The question is, Are such events all that bad and/or that ugly so as to worry that much about them? If the question is worthy of consideration, it then begs having more of an idea of the noisy "culprits" lurking about the recording.

How, for example, might the *electrocardiogram (ECG*; a.k.a., EKG*)*, originating so far away from the scalp, possibly interfere with testing AEPs? Answer (in one word): magnitude. Even well away from its origin, the ECG can be several or more orders of magnitude of the recorded AEP. Whether

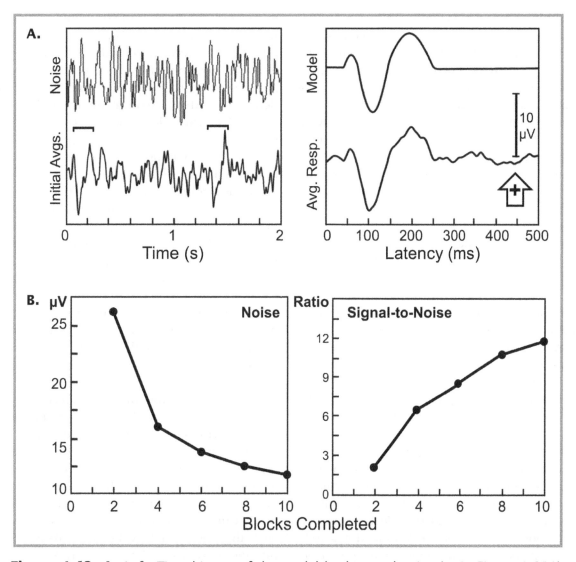

Figure 4–13. A. Left: Time history of the model background noise (as in Figure 4–11A). *Right*: Model response and overall average of model in noise. **B.** *Left*: Tracking residual noise via block-mode acquisition (split buffers' difference) over blocks acquired. This begins from block 2 (a system limitation to manage initial analyses effectively "on the fly"). *Right*: Tracking of an estimated SNR (see text).

it will interfere significantly depends on such factors of the recording as electrode montage and filtering applied. The potential ally against significant interference is coherent averaging itself. The heartbeat generally should not be synchronous with the stimulus presentation, even by chance. If fairly prominent in the recording, nevertheless, it still will be perturbing stationarity of both the target signal and/or background noise, compromising reduction in variance realizable per N sweeps averaged. Although long known as a potential culprit, a recent investigation of ABRs recorded in newborns demonstrated nuances of such interference.[14] At a period of the ECG (1/pulse rate), the fundamental frequency is well below the stimulus repetition typical of tests of transient ABRs (for example). Yet, presence of incidental occurrences were found to destabilize/slant the response's baseline. Although potentially leading to sweeps bearing the artifact via artifact rejection, asymmetry at times of the

ECG within the rejection limits was seen to be responsible. The only completely satisfactory measure of prevention was suggested to be completely removing the artifact, but is that even possible? Treatment of other artifacts from more nearby origins can shed light on that question.

The eyeblink is especially "scary" for examiners in general, but for recordings of LLRs in particular. It pretty well mimics a major component the LLR featured in this episode, as shown by demonstration in Figure 4–14A. Again, this interference is very unlikely to be literally synchronous with the AEP, as artificially overlaid in this figure. Still, it is adding to the noise background, occasionally overlapping the targeted AEP, so it is deleterious to the clearest distinction between the response's signal and the overall background noise. Fortunately, artifact rejection can be fairly effective in excluding the most "infected" sweeps from the final average. However, prevention is the "best policy" when possible. In many protocols, subjects simply can be asked to keep their eyes closed. The *electroculogram* (reflection of the corneo-retinal potential) can be similarly contributory to the background but also treated and/or controlled similarly. Other culprits include swallowing, chewing, frowning, and general bodily movements. If not excessive, any related artifactual signals likely can be controlled via the artifact-rejection algorithm. However, excessive occurrences of such artifacts greatly extend the collection time per test condition. The promise of continued research and development is still better and more-systematic approaches, such as portended by results of recent work, examining further the eyeblink[15] (see Figure 4–14B). Here the computer is effectively trained to recognize this signal's signature, suppress it, and provide an essentially unperturbed background. It however would be naïve to assume that all sorts of interference simply can be cut out of the response's record. Quality of recordings are first best served by at least enough cooperation of the patient to remain relaxed and reasonably quiet. Failing that and still for other patients for a variety of reasons (such as immaturity), they may have to be tested while sleeping or otherwise sedated, as discussed later.

So what if some artifact does "gets in"? First, it is important to bear in mind that the goal of the recording in auditory clinical neurophysiology generally is to sample uniquely **neurogenic** responses. The likes of the eyeblink, again, derive from activated muscles. These too are bioelectric but their sources in recordings from the scalp derive from compound muscle potentials and thus are **myogenic**. To recap, when picked up, reliable detection and/or accurate interpretation of the targeted neurogenic response is at risk. Even if considerably reduced by averaging (since such artifacts likely will not be coherent with the auditory stimulus response), they still add to the overall noise background and/or compromise the assumption of stationarity. As with the ECG, here too is the possible effects being manifested predominantly as destabilization of the recording, even for the likes of the ABR which is typically recorded using relatively narrowband filtering. Not only might this cause adverse effects in displaying the response, it may also compromise the validity of the measurement, for example, by distorting the true baseline of the evoked potential of interest or selectively attenuating one or more component waves of the true response.

As noted in the previous episode, preamplifiers in modern AEP test systems provide the first opportunity to "condition" the signal before "going digital" so as to let through mostly only a prescribed bandwidth of signal that is believed to provide the most reliable measurement of the targeted AEP. So when artifacts are unavoidable, filtering can be helpful to reduce their effects. However, this should not be taken to justify extreme filtering, perhaps under the impression that it is a completely harmless treatment of the recorded response.

Figure 4–15 demonstrates the results of a normal ABR recording, thus returning to the stage for its signature waveform, particularly at sound levels in the middynamic range of hearing (well above limits of hearing, considered for speech to be conversational levels of sound). The effects of progressively narrowing the filter bandwidth are witnessed in this figure in both time (panel A) and frequency domains (panel B). The same response is successively filtered more aggressively. Tracing #1 presents the ABR as often witnessed in conventional audiological practice, especially for differential diagnostic purposes, wherein the waveform itself is the primary interest. The full set of peaks potentially observable are labeled I–V,

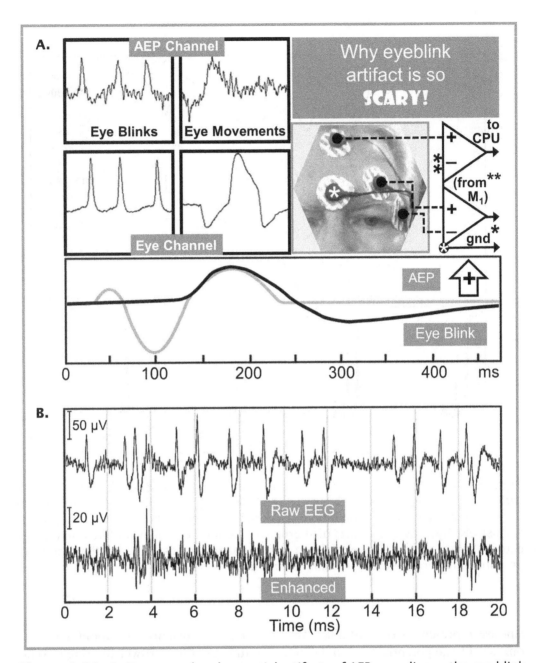

Figure 4–14. A. Two eye-related potential artifacts of AEP recordings—the eye blink (a predominantly muscle/myogenic potential) and eye movement (combination of myogenic and predominantly electro-ocular potentials, as the eyeball itself is like a movable battery). Featured in further analysis (bottom subpanel) is the eye blink for its compelling time history, not unlike one of the LLR component waves (overlaid for comparison, but not synchronized to the AEP itself and/or an acoustic-stimulus related response). Although the AEP was recorded using a $C_z - M_1$ montage and thus essentially recording such artifacts in their far field, the "AEP channel" is still readily "seeing" such artifacts, if not as reasonably faithfully as these potentials are observed in their near field (eye channel). **B.** Sample results of a recently developed algorithm to "clean up the baseline" (ostensibly background EEG, but "contaminated" by excessive eye blinks), namely by on-the-fly modeling of the eye blink artifact and re-computing the EEG via an adaptive method of signal matching and suppression. (Courtesy of Dr. J. T. Valderrama-Valenzuela.)

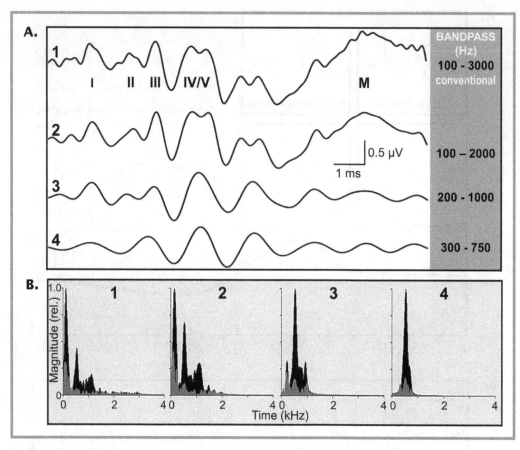

Figure 4–15. A. Tracing 1: ABR typical of those of older children and young adults with normal hearing when click-elicited in the vicinity of 70 dB nHL. Recordings are filtered with a bandwidth commonly used clinically for multiple purposes, yet not exclusively. Tracings 2–4: Effects of alternative filtering of #1 using different frequency cutoffs/bandwidths. **B.** Corresponding spectral analyses. Black areas—the brainstem potential; gray areas—the residual noise on the average.

and the response represented is "textbook." Also seen is a somewhat large potential toward the end of the recorded epoch that proves not to be neurogenic but rather myogenic, which stars in its own Heads Up (coming soon). It is sufficient here just to acknowledge its existence and simply calling it "M." Setting a narrower bandwidth (#2) nicely smooths the response of interest with still faithful representation of the primary response (#1). Still, the mysterious M remains, indeed undaunted. This signal does not interfere practically in most cases, unless it somehow were to change, particularly if getting still larger and coming to dominate the scaling of the recording (number of μV per full-screen vertical display), given that the IV–V wave complex is usually only about a microvolt in magnitude. A still narrower filtering (#3) takes care of that problem handily. However, this is not without significant distortion of the ABR waveform, having squelched the double-peak nuance of the IV–V complex. This is a very important attribute of the ABR, if considerably variable at times. Still, it is particularly important to correctly identify (at least) the wave-V peak. The resulting effective bandpass has been narrowed at the risk of inaccurate measurement of the latency of wave V—a strong benchmark indeed by which to judge normality of the response. Still more aggressive filtering (#4) goes from bad to ugly results and generally would be considered unacceptable, having fused waves II and III as well and having taken so much power out of the signal itself. Power is about the rate of energy produced or used; energy is reflected in the area under the curve (recall Episode 2.2). Also at that point, what is strongly driving the waveform is a purely nonsensory effect—that of "ringing" the filter's response (recall Figure 2–18).

The adverse effects of "over the top" filtering demonstrated in Figure 4–15 are double jeopardy in highly noisy recordings, contrary to best intentions. They potentially make noise look like a response, thus increased risk of false response detection, inaccurate waveform measures, and/or misinterpretation. The effects demonstrated in the time-domain are echoed nicely in the spectral plots (panel B) as well. While still leaving much of the lower-frequency part of this response's energy intact, the progressively aggressive filtering comes to cut both higher- and lower-frequency portions of the response, as indeed may be important for proper interpretation. This is analogous to endeavoring to judge colors of a fabric while wearing tinted sunglasses.

Filtering via the preamplifier stage is often useful to some extent, but it is an *analog*-signal treatment. A hazard of which is causing artificial *latency shifts*, again putting at risk correct interpretation of the response. In the foregoing demonstration (for sake of simplicity in generating the figure), each filter actually was configured and applied by way of *digital filtering* of otherwise matching characteristics. By way of digital processing, such delays (if inherent to the filter function) are correctable. This is evident by the lack of overall latency shifts across the tracings in Figure 4–15 (panel A), even in the face of the most aggressive filtering, rather than simply from distortion/fusing of peaks from severely limiting the frequency response of the filter's bandwidth. Furthermore, filtering at the analog stage is filtering forever—again, it cannot be undone practically. Digital filtering can be accomplished without losing the original digital record of the response. The digital filter is implemented conventionally by an algorithm computing on the digital record and storing the results as another record. Therefore, it readily can be undone by the program, akin to an "undo" command, as typically provided in spreadsheets, graphics, and other programs. Consequently, the general wisdom is to not analog filter aggressively. In some applications and/or advanced test systems, possibly not at all. In modern systems, digital filtering can be applied quite efficiently and with inherently greater flexibility than that of the analog filters.

This is particularly well demonstrated by (once more) taking advantage of a computer-simulated ABR. In this case, although simulated, it was converted to an audio "wav" file and played into the test system using a *loop-back* adaptor (intended primarily for troubleshooting the system). It actually could then be recorded by the clinical test instrument used to generate the data under scrutiny. Unlike using a human to produce the test signal, this demo benefits an invariable input signal and negligible background noise; therefore, the approach permits seeing uniquely the filter effects. Also unlike the last demo, for this virtual patient there is added to the model one of the next later waves in AEPdom, as shown in Figure 4–16. A hint of some such activity is seen in Figure 4–15A, but it is considerably obscured by both filtering and presence of the mysterious M wave. The "add-in" component is known as the SN_{10} (slow-negative wave with a latency nominally of 10 ms). In panel A, some common filter settings are represented for the high- and low-pass settings of the preamplifier's filter, in turn adjusted for different passbands. In panel B are corresponding recordings resulting from such combinations of high- and low-pass cut-off frequencies.

The bottom two tracings in Figure 4–16B present differences of effects of two band-pass settings, which are of particular interest. The clinically popular 100 Hz to 3000 Hz settings are placed under further scrutiny as well as 300 Hz to 1000 Hz, which generally would be considered as too aggressive for any clinical test of the ABR. It clearly is "unhealthy" for any waves after the IV-V complex, while also siphoning half of the energy in the I–V complex itself. Having so squelched a major complex of the overall response, great noise reduction or not, it is hard to justify. To help see (and hopefully believe) the "adverse" filter effects, areas under/over the curves relative to the actual input signal (the model response) are highlighted. In these simulated pristine recordings, the impression might be that any of these treatments would be

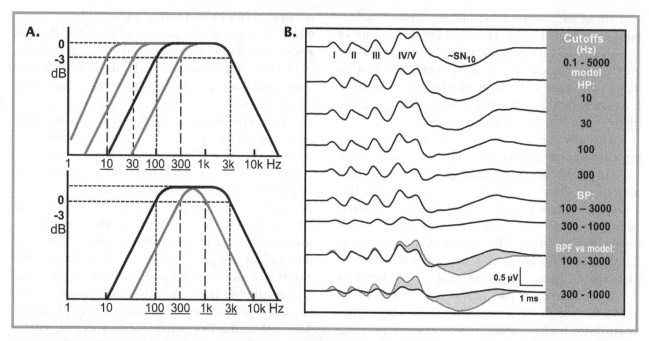

Figure 4–16. Virtual demonstration—"Seeing Is Believing—The Sequel." Model ABR with the five main positive peaks followed by a substantial SN_{10}-like component. For this demonstration, filtering was applied by actually recording the model response and applying all filtering through an AEP-test system. Examples included are effects of adjusting filter parameters of which some are in conventional use and others taken to extremes. **A.** Extending the recap of filtering principles in the last episode (recall Figure 4–7), the frequency responses intended are sketched to characterize effective bandwidths from the several sets of frequency cutoffs used. **B.** Results for actual records of the model response converted to a stimulus file that could be played to the recording amplifier at realistic voltages (microvolt range). As an aid to viewing differences from the ideal (*top* tracing; insignificant filtering for the ABR), "difference areas" are replotted at the bottom using gray fill between responses for a couple of band-pass conditions—one again that is often applied in practice versus one that is extremely narrow. Note: The narrowness of the band-pass is a bit accentuated by the scaling of the figure, attributable perhaps to artistic freedom but also an omen of the ills of excess.

acceptable as long as the examiner can see something of the response; certainly, they all are pretty. However, the important issue is not waveform "beauty," but truth in representation. The truth is that there is a present and clear SN_{10} in the actual input signal tested. This is a mere model; but it could just as well be a brain wave. Even then, this may not be an issue for numerous applications. Yet, if having been neglected by overly aggressive filtering, how will anyone ever know? Clinical applications are also dynamic, not static. A "one size fits all" mentality is barely realized in practice. The same settings that may serve well differential diagnostic applications also may serve well AEP measurement applied to the prediction of hearing thresholds—but not necessarily and generally not across maturation and/or pathologies. Furthermore, even if the SN_{10} were not the targeted AEP, what are better settings for this component could be more helpful to threshold estimation, particularly when using lower frequency stimuli (like 500 Hz). For example, dropping the high-pass cutoff down to 30 Hz or even 10 Hz. In any event, it is an incumbent responsibility of the examiner to fully understand what their conditioning of the recorded signal is capable of doing to it, as this inherently biases the actual data, if not creates misinterpretations thereof. At the very least, these issues are important bases by which to be prepared to probe further with different settings when results somehow strike the clinician as just not adding up, but not via analog filtering.

Digital filtering's strength is found particularly in offering a trail-and-error usage that is indeed nondestructive to the original-recording data file. An additional advantage is the possibility of trials of a variety of filter functions, as they are not created equally in their effects—good, bad, or ugly. Like gating functions applied to signals in the time domain, there indeed will be trade-offs among filter functions with consequences in both time and frequency domains as well as needs to consider both frequency and phase response of the filter. As in all conditioning of the recorded signal, such approaches must be well justified, as all have the potential to be overdone and/or encouraging "cherry picking" responses, rather than applied by a problem-solving approach and assurance that the chosen approach has broad validity for the given AEP in the given application. At the same time, judicious use of filtering can lead to substantially greater test efficiency. If a good "fit" to the true response and the application, the filtered version may be equal to or better than what would be realized by considerable increases in the number of sweeps averaged. Recall that while SNR is improved by increasing the N of sweeps averaged, this is a square root relationship, not merely a linear proportionality (again, see Figure 4–13).

It now would be useful, as a case in point, to play another round of the "Game of Waves." Please return first to the presentation of this exercise earlier in the episode to review issues pondered before and that are now to be applied to an alternative presentation of the recordings in Figure 4–17. The recordings have been submitted posttest to digital filtering. This is not to say that different analog filtering might not be as advantageous. However, conditioning the signal at that level on the recording side of the system also could be

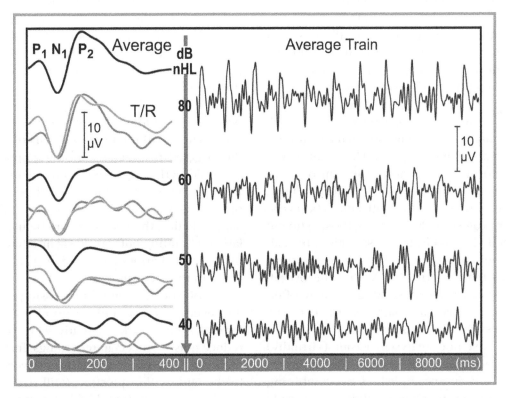

Figure 4–17. The "Game of Waves" revisited after a digital "facelift" (see text). Same paradigm and parameters as before. Postrecording signal conditioning via filtering in the frequency domain was applied to suppress all but a few hertz of bandwidth centered at harmonic frequencies of the stimulus repetition rate. It then could be inverse transformed to yield a much "cleaner" time-domain response. (Courtesy of Dr. R. E. Delgado.)

worse, and "worser" if irreparable and at the cost of additional testing. Looking at the digitally filtered results, even in the extended time domain (low-N averages in a train of responses, right panel), there is increased confidence right away of the presence of a recurrent responses at a couple of the higher levels tested. In the left panel, the N_{Total}-averages are of improved quality of waveform, as well, and test–retest overlays are improved. But what about the bottom line—is there a response or not at 40 dB? It now seems more possible to judge confidently in the "average," yet the test–retest overlay still is not entirely gratifying for making the call. The examiner might choose to repeat the condition, but it later will be learned that there is another detail of responses' behavior over decreasing stimulus levels that could be helpful. This point and the further information and illustration needed thereto is better left to subsequent episodes, including those devoted primarily to principles of **evoked response audiometry (ERA)**. What the additional filtering does help to do is give more confidence in the overall reliability of the test—all by way of a nondestructive cross-check at minimal additional time and effort on the part of the examiner and zero additional time at the patient's expense.

There are still other types of manipulations possible in post hoc processing of the recordings, especially for providing summary examples of responses for clinical reports. This again is not about waveform beauty, rather the aim of characterizing what the clinician, in good judgment, believes to best represent the truth and to best convey to other professionals, including those who are not seasoned clinical electrophysiologists. In real-time frontline work, there will be inevitable trials that are less than informative. Within the overall record of responses in real-world cases, there often can be the good, bad, and ugly records over the numerous test conditions administered during an evaluation. Post hoc analyses permit (virtually) further averaging and not just digital filtering. Commonly, this is accomplished by combining responses between two like conditions or simply overlying on the screen tracings from test–retest trials and from one side per test ear to the other. The latter can be particularly useful given the scenario of the patient becoming more or less restless for some time in their within ear and/or between ears segments of their examination. Again, adding estimated control conditions (as in Figure 4–12) to help further judge quality of the recording is useful and does not cost more test time. Lastly, comparing/overlaying ipsilateral and contralateral recordings per ear is useful, for example, to help resolve or provide greater confidence in wave identification.

Moving on, it by now should be no surprise that there are always two domains available to support decisions for signal conditioning and/or analysis—time and frequency. Spectral analysis, though not exclusively about frequency "makeup" (there is phase too!), is often available in modern test systems. Though not necessarily of routine interest for some evoked response evaluations, frequency/spectral analyses are essential to other stimulus-response approaches, such as steady state (more to this point coming soon!). It also is readily applicable and potentially useful for the sort of transient stimulus-response paradigm, as emphasized in the demonstration portrayed in Figure 4–11. There also can be neglect of use of such tools from lack of knowledge and experience or perhaps because it was not in the original or last update of the software—or worse, apropos the old adage, "old habits die hard." For instance, if observing a suddenly more noisy response (especially while working near the limits of detection of the targeted response), running a spectral analysis could perhaps provide additional insight as to any unexpected problem of interference. Because of the signature of interference from the electric supply/mains, the spectrum can be useful particularly for "sniffing out" 50/60 Hz interference, which includes any harmonics somehow generated spuriously in the recording.

Sophisticated signal-processing methods, in any event, do not replace good work up-front. Several useful "tricks" already were presented to reduce noise/artifacts in recordings; further considerations/issues are still useful/noteworthy, respectively. One is the question (still debated) of the need (or no need) for "shielded" test environments and electrical (as well as acoustical) isolation of the test subject. Shielding of the stimulus transducer and/or electrode wiring is another. The former is about controlling/reducing risks of stimulus artifact potentially arising from electrical radiation of the transducer while stimulating the ear. The latter is the issue of the extent to which the electrode leads and subjects are antennas for extraneous physical signals. The audiology clinic often provides useful electrical isolation at the same time as acoustical isolation, given test rooms constructed of metal. Still, not all and/or other contingencies are at hand, such as the need to test bedside in hospitals and in newborn nurseries. There thus are no pat answers if serving patient populations broadly or serving individual patient's personal needs comprehensively. The AEP examiner needs to bear in mind the potential issues, evaluate the test environment, and be knowledgeable and/or seek competent assistance to address issues raised.

As hinted earlier, the recording-electrode montage itself needs to be optimal for both best sampling of the targeted response while minimizing interference—to the extent possible or at least practical. Recordings are to some extent results of a compromise of goals to ensure best SNR, not necessarily the biggest response. Recording from the vertex often (yet not unequivocally) serves the former but may be noisier from greater difficulty to get best electrode impedances (for example, on hairy and/or oily skin). Fortunately, SNR is what generally is most critical for "best" recordings, as modern test systems have very low noise floors (internally). A lower signal at another electrode site thus may be preferred for patient comfort, examiner expediency, lesser noise at another site, or other considerations in a given application.

A proverbial adage that applies well to evoked response testing is, "haste makes waste" and brings the discussion here full circle to the fundamental importance of due diligence in preparation of the patient for the test. This is not only about electrode preparation. It is also about the patient's knowledge of what is to be done, why, and to whom and when results will be conveyed. Clinical electrophysiological tests can be scary to patients or their guardians. Then there are instructions/explanations essential to conveying understanding of the state of the patient appropriate to the test of the particular AEP of interest, like whether the patient needs to be awake and alert or can relax and even doze off. Circumstances will vary over patient maturity and other considerations that will be discussed in forthcoming episodes. Most are devoted in one way or the other to help limit background noise—the "poor computer" of the test system cannot do everything! Meticulous preparation may consume a bit more time, but rarely exceeds that of troubleshooting and other consequences adverse to quality results, including risk of having to disturb the patient midtest or even reschedule the examination.

HEADS UP

Interlude—And You Don't Even Have To Raise Your Hand When You Hear the Beep

Through the initial chapters, the reader perhaps has found a goodly amount of interest and understanding from the numerous lessons given by the writers thus far. There is a common expression when the intent of someone in a conversation is to impress others with a bit of knowledge: Speaker 1: "So, while working around a group of nuclear physicists, you must have learned a thing or two about the distinction between fission and fusion." Speaker 2: "I learned enough to be dangerous."

Speaker 2's reply could be alarming in more ways than one. With the chapters already in hand, enough information was presented to avoid danger, for instance, observing the caveat to use a properly grounded test system, namely with the proper configuration and hookup of the electrodes and use of instrumentation certified to be electrically safe. With Episodes 3.1, 4.1, and Figure 2–16 (recall Heads Up of Episode 2.2), the reader might manage to hook up someone to an AEP test system and obtain reasonable results. Then, with several hints about use of clinical electrophysiology to record signals from the brain, the examiner can deduce that the subject of the test likely can hear, or not. Meanwhile, the subject had nothing to do except relax and voila! The brain provided the response. The subject did not even have to raise a hand to the beep

But wait, it gets better. Do that well enough and still more deductions can be made! Nothing complicated; the examiner just carefully repeats some conditions in sequence, like turning down the stimulus level in steps until the waveform (the presumptive "response") seemingly disappears. Bingo! Now the examiner knows how good the hearing is for the given stimulus. After the protocol is repeated with sounds of different frequencies, a pretty good estimate of the audiogram is now in hand. Again, the subject did nothing while the examiner was tapping into processes of the brain. In the AEP business, this type of evaluation is called an objective test; actually, that is the whole idea. Results do not rely on conditioning/instructing the subject how to play the game; all the subject has to do is sit/lie there and be quiet. They should stay awake for cortical testing but can sleep for measurement of a brainstem response, but, regardless, relaxing to reduce myogenic noise is the key. Simple.

But wait, there is still more. The examiner can turn up the level of the stimulus and get a waveform with multiple bumps, generated from different places along the auditory pathway—what Figure 1–1 said (and skipping the gory details of Episode 3.2). Then, any recorded AEP missing a "bump" in the waveform must mean that there is a lesion somewhere. Just look at the map of the pathways; not nuclear physics or rocket science.

Conclusion: anybody can do this kind of test; what more needs to be learned? Should these scenarios fit what the reader has taken home as messages thus far and agrees with the conclusion, would likely mean having learned only enough to be dangerous!

There are several conceptions and misconceptions that will not be drawn out here exhaustively at the moment. The rest of the book is dedicated to such issues and then some. However, some points are of sufficiently great importance to emphasize with repetitious reminders. Many issues are "built" in stages—an excellent teaching tool. The risk for the reader—who is dabbling and not fully committed to the complete stories of all the episodes herein—is that of missing an important stage. This can have trickle-up consequences of a less-than-full comprehension of the foundational information being presented. This textbook then is much like a novel and needs to be read like one—from beginning to end. To be clear, the scope here is not an exhaustive AEP-neurophysiology how-to manual, but it is a substantially comprehensive coverage of the many basic principles upon which to build over time, followed up with further study and with well-mentored experiences in the respective areas covered.

Here are a few pointers to take to heart and mind and build upon. **Hearing** is a **perception**—that is, a psychological concept, most appropriately evaluated with **psychophysical methods** of testing. Audiometric evaluation is one of them. A test of word recognition ability is another. Such **subjective** tests (requiring behavioral participation of the subject) and their results are not brushed aside by clinical electrophysiology. It also is true that the inherently objective methods of AEP tests (no hand waving, etc. by the subject) may permit a reasonable **estimation** of something like hearing sensitivity. Still, only the data collection can be rendered as truly objective. Choosing the parameters of recording and stimulation, identifying the part of the epoch likely to contain the desired response, marking/measuring the peaks, and interpreting the findings overall are all subjective—"calls" by the examiner. Although intensively technological, humans still have the upper hand and responsibility here, and humans can make mistakes. Furthermore, even with great "objective tools" administered competently, the results may fail under certain circumstances to yield the best insights of the subject's functional status. Figure 1–1 is again instructive, in the opposite sense (effectively) from before. It teaches that if perception is processed in the cortex (indeed it is), then evoked response-based estimate(s) of performance of a given auditory function will be only as good as how far up the pathway the examiner tested, which depends on the type of AEP/AEP-measurement that was used. There is much emphasis in health-care on a given profession to have solid evidence bases for the tests used, namely to show good reason behind them and demonstrations of their clinical efficacy. The metrics applied similarly must be well reasoned, hence the importance of a good rationale for their use of a given test, in the given case.

Moving forward, objective tests may be seen to have some validity and reliability to sample auditory function, much the same as conventional psychophysical/behavioral tests. Equivalency, however, is another thing. There certainly are neurophysiological events along the auditory pathway that can provide measures with reasonable correlation to perceptual measurements. Yet, even simply pushing a button upon hearing a beep draws upon far more neuroanatomical resources than recording apparent excitement of the brainstem (for example). To think otherwise violates the wisdom of science 101: correlation does not establish cause and effect. Still, with informed use of AEP tests, skillful deductions and decisions can be made to move forward in the clinical management of a patient, for instance, who might be incapable of participating in conventional audiometry or heading them toward appropriate follow-up evaluations.

The presentation of the various AEPs whose measures can be useful tools is not merely about how to do the tests but to provide the bases that empower their use in various applications and to support logic in the interpretation of the results. The tests surveyed in this book are incredible tools, providing the means to peer right into activity of the brain. It is not that long ago that such an idea would have been science fiction, or perhaps, in some sectors, heresy! The reality of clinical electrophysiology today, side by side with methods of imaging, is truly a marvel. However, prudence always must temper overconfidence. The electrophysiological methods presented are functional tests of sensory or motor systems. These tests do not determine etiology and thus are not of the same nature and purpose in medical diagnosis, as generally are blood tests, biopsies, and so forth, which involve biochemical assays and/or histopathology. Nevertheless, the electrophysiological test results can help to promote better decision making in clinical management. At the same time, the use of electrophysiological tests in diagnostics is not the full picture of the utility of clinical electrophysiology. There are also important applications of monitoring treatment and rehabilitation outcome measures as well as assessments of effects of early-life maturation and late-life decline. Then, in the course of gathering information and considerations for the various AEP tests are the spin-offs of exposure to knowledge about a variety of intriguing disorders and a better understanding of brain function. Such a deal!

Bottom line: There is a choice to be made henceforth, dear reader. Learn and use the minimum base of knowledge to do the work of clinical electrophysiology in audiology, or engage in making the more challenging and intriguing decisions before and after running the machine and at times regardless of what test appeared to be in order or was requested (that is, "ordered" in common, but potentially regrettable, clinical parlance). In other words, this is a choice of whether to be simply an appliance operator or a full member of the health-care team. If the latter is the choice, please move on to the next chapter, and the next, to keep building a foundation of knowledge with a sense of fascination for the ultimate depth, breadth, and intrigue of what clinical electrophysiology in audiology can offer. Find satisfaction ultimately for having mastered a scholarly volume on the topic, not to the end but to a beginning of learning more in one of the most gratifying areas of the field in which to work. Embrace the goal of achieving ultimate clinical competency in this area. The objective is to not just "do" an electrophysiological test. It is to serve the patient's needs in resolving a potential communicative disorder and in their best interest by confidently being an actively contributing member of the team of professionals that likely will be required to fully resolve the basis for and treatment of the patient's difficulty(ies).

Parting words: There is the inevitability of change in a given field. Change can cut both ways, the most obvious being due to new methods. It is safe to say that clinical audiology has been more changed by the science and technology of electrophysiology than vice versa. Within this subarea of clinical practice adopted by professional audiologists, the "what's new is old again" effect also has occurred in the instruments and methods used and the underlying evidence bases for them. New innovations of methods under-understood and/or under-appreciated at some time earlier also have been brought again to the fore with further research and development. How to cope with such dynamics? By gaining a solid foundation in the first place and continuing education thereafter—as mandated by professional organizations in the field, per their statement of ethics and requirements to retain clinical competency. If committed ultimately to full citizenship in the community of audiologists practicing clinical electrophysiology, then onward! Up next, some really interesting stuff that the hearing organ can do to "kick-start" the ensemble of AEPs in time and space and that the clinician can put to the test!

■ Take Home Messages

Episode 1

1. A big challenge in evoked response measurement is having adequate data quality.
2. In practice, recording of the desired signal (small) requires dealing with noise (large) from a variety of possible sources, both physiological and nonphysiological.
3. Best recordings of the desired signal derive from relatively stationary signal and noise, so vulnerable to the influence of subject's state and/or noise (as in testing a crying infant).
4. Diagnosing noise sources can be helpful at the outset, like turning a nearby lamp on/off (nonphysiological) or getting the test subject more relaxed (physiological).
5. The technical approach that yields the AEP is computer processing of the recorded signal by coherent averaging (a.k.a., time-ensemble averaging) synchronized to stimulus presentation.
6. Signal averaging is robust for noise reduction, but there are "rules," such as noise ideally being random and number of epochs averaged.
7. An approach broadly applied by the AEP test system (digital stage) is artifact rejection by way of a computer algorithm to limit the magnitude of signal "let into" the computation.
8. Artifact rejection is not a "cure-all" and a special type of electrical interference is that generated by the transducer used; one fix, if appropriate, is to alternate stimulus polarity.
9. A classical and broadly used approach to condition the recording is band-pass filtering, applied at the (pre)amplifier/analog stage.
10. In AEP test systems today, the user can apply both analog and digital filtering; as the former is undoable postrecording, less "aggressive" analog filtering is advisable.
11. The particular type of amplifier used—a differential amplifier—is actually the first treatment of the signal that is aimed at

the reduction of noise on the recording, according to its CMR.
12. The amplifier and use of three electrodes (per channel) is also a part of electrical isolation of the patient.
13. Determining the reliability of the recording requires some "judgment call" by someone and/or some algorithm applied by the test system, but someone's responsibility in any event.
14. Classically and still broadly used—at least—is visual observation of test–retest repeatability.
15. The response "extraction" is a statistical estimate from an array of numbers, so the same data lends itself to further statistical testing for assurance of detection level, SNR estimation, and so forth.

Episode 2

1. Again, background noise can be reduced greatly using a combination of analog signal conditioning and digital processing, but the challenge must be understood fully.
2. In addition to recording clearly given AEP (per a nominal latency group), processing of the signal in noise must support reliably detecting it at sound levels near hearing threshold.
3. Reliable recordings require, indeed, robust reduction of background noise toward an adequate SNR, with both parameters "improving" systematically given more stimulus repetitions.
4. Interference is potentially everywhere, some more worrisome than others (like the eyeblink); again, artifact rejection is not a cure-all.
5. As in cooking, filtering/other signal conditioning can be overdone!
6. Overdone at the front end of the recording (analog stage) can be regrettable and certainly undoable, hence the prudence of adding more filtering later (digitally) than sooner.
7. Sophisticated signal processing methods do not replace good work up front, bearing in mind that, indeed, haste makes waste.

Heads-Up Special

1. The episodes to this juncture have presented the bases by which to conduct electrophysiological measurements to probe the auditory pathways—end of story?
2. There indeed are numerously more stories to be told toward a comprehensive understanding of specific methods per space and time in AEPdom, their applications, and more.
3. Of well-documented applicability to testing hearing sensitivity, the dichotomies of subjective versus objective tests and hearing versus estimations of thresholds must be understood.
4. Like conventional audiometry, ERA is also only the beginning of possible applications of AEP tests, starting with differential diagnostics requiring keen knowledge and deduction.
5. The challenge issued by the writers is that of a commitment to pursue the rest of the stories for comprehensive evidence bases by which to do the job, whatever it takes.
6. A knowledge base naturally is for the now, tomorrow will likely come to be a game changer, so solid foundational knowledge is the prerequisite for building/maintaining competence.

References

1. Vidler, M., & Parkert, D. (2004). Auditory brainstem response threshold estimation: Subjective threshold estimation by experienced clinicians in a computer simulation of the clinical test. *International Journal of Audiology, 43*(7), 417–429.
2. Elberling, C., & Wahlgreen, O. (1985). Estimation of auditory brainstem response, ABR, by means of Bayesian inference. *Scandinavian Audiology, 14*(2), 89–96.
3. British Society of Audiology. (2019). Recommended procedure: Auditory brainstem response (ABR). Testing in babies. https://www.thebsa.org.uk/wp-content/uploads/2019/04/Recommended-Procedure-for-ABR-Testing-in-Babies-FINAL-Feb-2019.pdf

4. Li, Y., Ma, Z., Lu, W., & Li, Y. (2006). Automatic removal of the eye blink artifact from EEG using an ICA-based template matching approach. *Physiological Measurement, 27*(4), 425–436.
5. Hall, J. W. (2007). *New handbook of auditory evoked responses.* Pearson Education Inc.
6. Metting van Rijn, A. C., Peper, A., & Grimbergen, C. A. (1990). High-quality recording of bioelectric events. Part 1. Interference reduction, theory and practice. *Medical & Biological Engineering & Computing 28*(5), 389–397.
7. Elberling, C., & Don, M. (1984). Quality estimation of averaged auditory brainstem responses. *Scandinavian Audiology, 13*(3), 187–197.
8. Hotelling, H. (1931). The generalization of student's ratio. *The Annals of Mathematical Statistics, 2*(3), 360–378.
9. Cebulla, M., Sturzebecher, E., & Elberling, C. (2006). Objective detection of auditory steady-state responses: Comparison of one-sample and q-sample tests. *Journal of the American Academy of Audiology, 17*(2), 93–103.
10. Chesnaye, M. A., Bell, S. L., Harte, J. M., & Simpson, D. M. (2018). Objective measures for detecting the auditory brainstem response: Comparisons of specificity, sensitivity and detection time. *International Journal of Audiology, 57*(6), 468–478.
11. Burkard, R. F., Don, M., & Eggermont, J. J. (Eds.). (2006). *Auditory evoked potentials: Basic principles and clinical application.* Lippincott Williams & Wilkins.
12. Katz, J., Medvetsky, L., Burkard, R., & Hood, L. (Eds.). (2009). *Handbook of clinical audiology* (6th ed., Chapters 11–18). Lippincott Williams & Wilkins.
13. Picton, T. (2011). *Human auditory evoked potentials.* Plural Publishing.
14. Lightfoot, G. (2017). Sloping ABR baselines and the ECG myogenic artefact. *International Journal of Audiology, 56*(8), 612–616.
15. Valderrama, J. T., de la Torre, A., & Van Dun, B. (2018). An automatic algorithm for blink-artifact suppression based on iterative template matching: Application to single channel recording of cortical auditory evoked potentials. *Journal of Neural Engineering, 15*(1), 016008.
16. Martin, W. H., Schwegler, J. W., Gleeson, A. L., & Shi, Y. B. (1994). New techniques of hearing assessment. *Otolaryngologic Clinics of North America, 27*(3), 487–510.
17. Golding, M., Dillon, H., Seymour, J., & Carter, L. (2009). The detection of adult cortical auditory evoked potentials (CAEPs) using an automated statistic and visual detection. *International Journal of Audiology, 48*(12), 833–842. https://doi.org/10.3109/14992020903140928
18. Wilding, T. S., McKay, C. M., Baker, R. J., & Kluk, K. (2012). Auditory steady state responses in normal-hearing and hearing-impaired adults: An analysis of between-session amplitude and latency repeatability, test time, and F ratio detection paradigms. *Ear and Hearing, 33*(2), 267–278. https://doi.org/10.1097/AUD.0b013e318230bba0
19. Picton, T. W., Dimitrijevic, A., John, M. S., & Van Roon, P. (2001). The use of phase in the detection of auditory steady-state responses. *Clinical Neurophysiology: Official Journal of the International Federation of Clinical Neurophysiology, 112*(9), 1698–1711. https://doi.org/10.1016/s1388-2457(01)00608-3
20. Stürzebecher, E., Cebulla, M., & Wernecke, K. (1999). Objective response detection in the frequency domain: Comparison of several q-sample tests. *Audiology & Neuro-otology, 4*(1), 2–11. https://doi.org/10.1159/000013815
21. Valderrama, J. T., de la Torre, A., Alvarez, I., Segura, J. C., Thornton, A. R., Sainz, M., & Vargas, J. L. (2014). Automatic quality assessment and peak identification of auditory brainstem responses with fitted parametric peaks. *Computer Methods and Programs in Biomedicine, 114*(3), 262–275. https://doi.org/10.1016/j.cmpb.2014.02.015

Evoking Responses of the Peripheral Auditory System

The Writers

Episode 1:	Jacek Smurzynski
Heads Up:	Wieslaw W. Jedrzejczak
Episode 2:	John D. Durrant and John A. Ferraro
Episode 3:	John A. Ferraro and John D. Durrant
Heads Up:	John D. Durrant, John A. Ferraro, and José Juan Barajas de Prat
Episode 4:	Martin Walger

■ Episode 1: First Sign Something's Going On in There: An Acoustic Response of the Inner Ear

The history of research on hearing over the last 90 years is a fascinating example that going against the established ideas might be gratifying, but sometimes seem at risk of forcing a brilliant scientist out of the field. A dramatically new era started with innovative experiments conducted in the 1920s and continued over the next several decades by Georg von Bekesy, who received the Nobel Prize in 1961 for his decades of brilliant research on the auditory system. His studies, including those demonstrating the existence of the (forward) *traveling wave (TW)*, were remarkably thorough and reflected extraordinary foresight and singularly innovative methods of investigation. However, they were mostly confined to experiments using unnaturally high-level stimuli, namely in postmortem preparations. His results proved ultimately to reflect only ***passive, linear properties*** of the cochlea. Decades later, progressively more research was conducted on the peripheral auditory system as well as in general areas of cellular and micromolecular biology, and more technological advances began to generate a new story of how this system functions. This episode focuses on measurements of what had been a seemingly improbable phenomenon, even in the face of decades of "hints" of nonlinear effects in auditory sound processing, starting likely in the periphery but awaiting vindication of a "crier" in the wilderness of unconventional thinking. What works would subsequently emerge literally can fill a book,[1] but is overviewed here as having brought forth both important scientific insights and useful tools. Discussion herein is thus both important foundational knowledge and an introduction to tools for objective assessment of the auditory system that can supplement clinical electrophysiology, in fact, considerably sharing technologies and analytical approaches to sound-evoked responses.

Shortly after World War II, Thomas Gold, a physicist best known for his work in cosmology and astronomy, started working in a biology lab at Cambridge. He applied his expertise in building radar systems, signal processing methods, and electronics to explore the inner ear, which he considered to be a superb scientific apparatus. He was puzzled by the broad peak in the TW, implying a lack of the sharpness of frequency discrimination, contrary to expectations from psychoacoustic/behavioral measures in living human subjects. Gold conducted several experiments leading to his theory of hearing incorporating an ***active transducer*** (a receiver from his perspective), namely one with its own amplifier.[2] In 1989, Gold was invited to speak at a scientific meeting on cochlear mechanics[3] and candidly described his thoughts from the late 1940s pondering that nature would not be dumb enough to put (in effect) a free nerve ending at the front end of such a sensitive system as a detector (tantamount to what is the most primitive of sensory systems.) Apparently, his discussion with Bekesy in 1948 did not convince the future Nobel laureate that the recordings made on the dead cochlea were unrepresentative. The less than enthusiastic response to several papers published by Gold in the late 1940s contributed to his decision to switch to other fascinating topics, far away from the physiology of the inner ear!

Another paper[4] had gone unnoticed for a couple of decades, presenting pure-tone threshold data that the researcher had obtained at 10-Hz intervals over a wide frequency range, showing periodic fluctuations with local minima and maxima extending over 10 dB. This "ripple effect" in the audiogram, has come to be known as the ***auditory microstructure***. The results thus were confirmed in several later studies with its frequency periodicity shown to be ≈100 Hz in the vicinity of 1 kHz. In the mid-1970s, puzzled by this periodic microstructure and reports of monaural diplacusis—perception of two tones when just one pure tone was applied at a frequency close to a local threshold minimum—David Kemp developed a standing-wave model leading to a revolutionary discovery—that of ***otoacoustic emissions (OAEs)*** from the ear. The hypothesis was based on the idea that the threshold microstructure results from multiple reflections inside the cochlea, thus giving rise to interactions between ***forward TWs***—their propagation from the base toward the apex as reported by Bekesy 40 years earlier—and ***backward TWs***. The existence of the latter was initially rejected by many researchers. More than 10 years later, having been drawn back into the hearing-research limelight, Thomas Gold charged the medical profession with (still) not having a clue as to why 15 kHz should be emitted by the ear.[5] Moreover, Kemp's standing-wave hypothesis required a ***negative damping*** of the TW or, in other words, the presence indeed of an amplifier within the cochlea, hence an ***active cochlea***. The data depicted the diminishing magnitude of the loudness microstructure (local peaks and valleys of loudness perception of pure tones measured at small frequency intervals) with an increase of the stimulation intensity. They thus supported the idea of a ***cochlear nonlinearity***, again a new concept contradicting Bekesy's theory of a linear cochlea.

To test the validity of his standing-wave model of the auditory microstructure, Kemp made a brilliant assumption that some energy of the reverse TWs reaching the base of the cochlea (1) should escape from the inner ear, (2) create motion within the middle ear (ME) including that of the eardrum, and (3) result in sounds that should be detectable by a sensitive microphone (sealed in the ear canal). Results of a series of his experiments conducted in the summer of 1977 started a brand-new area of auditory research and clinical applications of OAEs. His famous 1978 paper[6]—according to Google Scholar—has been cited in more than 3,000 publications, wherein he reported analyses of signals measured in the ear canal in response to low-level acoustic impulses. The response, observed after about 5 ms poststimulus time, included a small sound wave "echo," a ***transient-evoked response*** typically termed the ***click-evoked otoacoustic emission (CEOAE)***. The magnitude of the response in the 5 ms to 15 ms poststimulus time interval decreased with a decrease of the stimulus magnitude, yet not proportionally. Therefore, the ***input-output (I-O) function*** of the CEOAE was reported to be nonlinear. This property was later applied in commercial OAE test systems in which the linear component is subtracted and the remaining nonlinear component is treated as the true cochlear response. Kemp's first paper included preliminary data in patients with sensorineural hearing loss, indicating that their absent CEOAEs were linked to abnormal cochlear function. Already then, possible clinical applications of OAEs had been postulated.

Kemp's report was greeted with a mixture of approval and rejection. Fortunately, within the next three years, several researchers published their own data confirming the "cochlear echo" phenomenon to be real. Moreover, it had been shown that OAEs could be recorded without stimulation (spontaneous OAEs—coming soon) as well as evoked by a single continuous tone or by two-tone stimulation. When it thusly became clear that the cochlea both may create oscillations in the absence of acoustic stimulation and that the evoked oscillations last longer than a transient stimulus, the idea that the cochlea is able to produce mechanical energy was proven to be genuine.

In a now-classical paper published in 1983, Hallowell Davis described a model of active cochlear mechanics with the **cochlear amplifier (CA)** providing additional energy to enhance the TW.[7] He recognized that the OHCs might be essential elements of the active and highly nonlinear cochlea, but he admitted a lack of knowledge of how CA might work given the presumption of molecular-dimensioned motion of the basilar membrane near hearing thresholds. Then, a new discovery of a unique property of OHCs came to the rescue,[8] demonstrating that isolated OHCs are able to change length as a function of membrane depolarization causing OHC contraction, whereas hyperpolarization causes OHC elongation (Figure 5–1). The effect of the OHC **electro-motility** demonstrated in animal experiments was shown to be very fast, up to at least 80 kHz! Truly amazing, but bats are mammals too and process even higher-frequency sounds than dogs and cats. The next task in completing the puzzle of the active cochlea's micromechanics was to explain details of the biophysics of OHC motility, including a local "battery" creating changes in the OHC membrane charge and sensors that may change their conformation while exposed to a change in membrane potential. This effect was attributed to a newly discovered protein called **prestin**, which is expressed in the OHC membrane and indeed undergoes a conformational change in response to transmembrane voltage.[9] The in-vivo "battery" needed to drive the "electro" part of motility is a consequence of basilar-membrane (BM) motion. Resulting deflection of OHC stereocilia (again Figure 5–1, inset) opens mechanoelectrical transduction channels due to the difference between the endocochlear potential and the OHC's resting potential, resulting in the receptor current depolarizing the cell. Depolarization of OHCs then causes their contraction due to conformational changes in prestin molecules, in turn amplifying BM motion when all mechanisms involved are in the correct phase relationship. Simple? In fact, maybe too!

Even though the progress of explaining cochlear macro- and micromechanics has been remarkable over last 90 years, there remain several unanswered questions.[10] However, it is generally accepted that for low- to midlevel stimuli (like conversational speech), the CA represents a cycle-by-cycle injection of energy into the TW over a short distance just basal to BM peak displacements and that the TW is amplified by prestin-mediated motility of OHCs.

Since there are still several unresolved issues of the cochlear mechanics, such as the contribution of OHC stereocilia motility (the hairs moving on their own accord) and/or other details beyond the scope here, a comprehensive theory of the OAE phenomenon is still debated. Nevertheless, OAEs are only byproducts of cochlear function and mainly of the interaction between OHCs and the BM motion. While recognizing the shortcomings of OAE theories, it is clear that OAEs can provide important and clinically useful information about the cochlea of research subjects or patients. Therefore, it is essential to provide a qualitative description of OAE generation mechanisms, starting with a simple pure-tone stimulus with a frequency f delivered by a miniature speaker sealed in the ear canal. Based on Bekesy's experiments and theory of tonotopical organization of the cochlea, it is assumed that a TW would be created with its peak corresponding to the "characteristic" place for a given frequency of stimulation (recalling the cochlear/tonotopical map, Episode 3.2). A critically important modification needed for this approach is recognizing active mechanisms operating for a low-level stimulus resulting in the TW envelope with a precisely defined peak (Figure 5–2A). The forward flow of energy from the base along the cochlea will encounter irregularities in anatomic structures and in physiologic activities within the organ of Corti.[11] For example, arrangements of the OHCs, their stereocilia, and structures involved in the function of the CA are not expected to be perfectly uniform from cell to cell. The spatial variation within the cochlea, labeled arbitrarily as "cochlear mechanical properties," includes local perturbations, as shown conceptually in panel B. While the overall shape of the function is quite hypothetical and only partially linked to the gradient change of stiffness and mass from the base

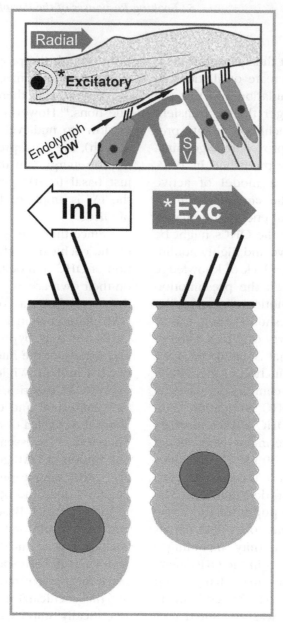

Figure 5-1. The motile response of outer hair cells. Inset: Partial redrawing of Figure 3–9B to recap the concept of excitation of hair cells of the organ of Corti (in the mammalian ear). During the excitatory (Exc) phase of vibration, the basilar membrane—not shown in the vignette of the inset figure, yet a reminder of its direction of motion toward scala vestibuli (SV)—effectively causes a rotation of the hearing organ about a pivot point situated on the modiolar side of scala media. However, that of the tectorial membrane is displaced significantly from the effective pivot of the basilar membrane (and thus the body of the hearing organ, see Figure 3–9), thereby effecting a shearing displacement of the stereocilia radially ("outwardly," toward the stria vascularis) between the tectorial membrane and hair-bearing surface of the organ. Two forces (vectors) are produced. For excitation of the inner hair cells, this is from velocity of fluid movement "pumped" past the hairs, but for OHCs—there is also the force of direct displacement by the overlying tectorial membrane, as the tallest hairs insert a bit into the underbelly of that membrane. The receptor potential subsequently generated excites a contraction of the OHCs to amplify the BM motion locally. Opposite displacement of the organ thus results in opposite directions of displacement and velocity, in turn causing an inhibitorylike effect (Inh.). That is, the alternating vibration of the organ depolarizes and then hyperpolarizes the resting membrane potential. Note: The schematic portrayals of such micromechanical events are characteristically melodramatic, with large movements of body parts involved; in reality they are miniscule, bespeaking the exquisite design and sensitivity of the hearing organ.

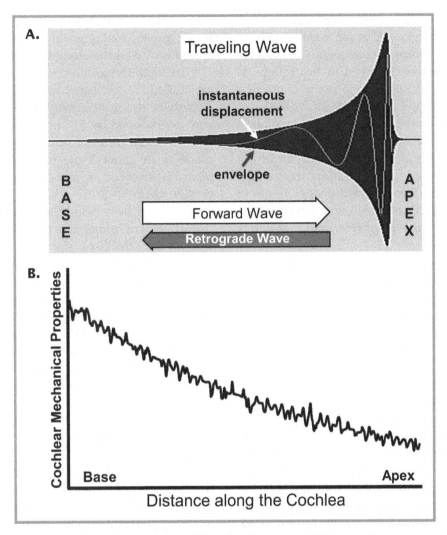

Figure 5–2. (**A**) Illustration of the development of the traveling wave—magnitude of instantaneous displacement over time and along the basilar membrane, as the TW takes time—and its temporal envelope—overall peak displacements over time, extended over subsequent cycles of vibration. The "active" properties of the cochlea enhance—in particular—the peak of the excitation at the characteristic place corresponding to the stimulus frequency. (**B**) Concept of the spatial variations of cochlear mechanical properties, based on data of Shera and Abdala (2012).[11] Intrinsic place-to-place irregularities act to scatter the forward wave's energy upon propagation along the BM, resulting in retrograde waves (not illustrated in panel **A**, but direction as indicated), again particularly around the place corresponding to the peak of the forward TW's envelope.

to the apex, a more important feature of the curve is its lack of smoothness. When a TW propagates along the cochlea, micromechanical irregularities partially reflect the forward energy, particularly around the place corresponding to the peak of the TW, resulting in the creation of a reverse wave traveling basally. A ***retrograde TW*** thus transmits vibrations to the stapes footplate, causing a tympanic-membrane motion and thus sound—an OAE—measured by a probe microphone sealed in the ear canal. Additionally, some energy of the retrograde wave is reflected at the stapes and back into the cochlear fluids. Consequently, a forward TW newly formed is expected to be "reflected" and propagated apically. This process continues, resulting in multiple intracochlear "to-and-fro" reflections between the base and apex, leading to possible cochlear resonance effects. This perhaps seems bizarre, it certainly is intriguing, but it well explains the existence of the auditory microstructure. Yet, this is not the end of the story. Some of this energy "escapes" to the ME and is transmitted to the ear canal, representing **stimulus frequency OAE (SFOAE)**.

Two fairly similar models of OAE generation mechanisms related to local perturbations act to scatter the energy back toward the stapes; they have been called **place-fixed** or **linear coherent reflection** OAEs.[12] Discussion of assumptions and details of these two models is beyond the scope of this episode. Suffice it to say simply, evoked OAEs are attributed to some combination of linear coherent reflections and distortion emissions (see the following text). At low stimulus levels, however, SFOAEs arise predominantly from a region of coherent reflection near the peak of the TW envelope. Kemp's historic paper also described the first data in patients with sensorineural hearing loss, supporting the notion that OAEs can only be generated if the CA functions properly.[6] Paradoxically, the imperfections of the cochlea are needed to generate OAEs. The first aspect of biologically inevitable irregularities already has been described. The second is related to the cochlear nonlinearity, which may sound like less than satisfactory for a very fine scientific instrument (from Gold's perspective). The OHCs are involved in the active mechanism to overcome energy dissipation (again) by injecting energy back into the TW. I-O functions of OHCs receptor potentials as a function of sound pressure, as can be measured in vivo in animals, are strongly nonlinear. Moreover, since the gain of the CA is level-dependent (like compressive, automatic gain control often used in hearing aids to limit excessive loudness), the growth of the BM motion is rendered nonlinear by their influence. Therefore, the TW can induce local nonuniformity in the cochlear mechanics, also resulting in the generation of reverse TWs. This mechanism has been called **wave-fixed** because when the stimulus frequency changes, the envelope of the corresponding TW shifts along the cochlea.

To summarize, the "reflection-source OAEs" are linked to cochlear irregularities but not necessarily to the nonlinearity. Those that arise from sources induced by TW propagation, "distortion-source OAEs," require nonlinearity but not irregularities. In general, the mixture of both mechanisms is involved in the generation of stimulus-evoked OAEs.

In an earlier episode, asymmetrical nonlinear distortion was illustrated (see Figure 2–6A), and one of the effects of any source of such distortion would be to generate difference tones—two sinusoids input to the system but more than two out, formally known as **intermodulation distortion (IM)**. From the foregoing, the hair cell system does this. One of the OAE recording methods used routinely clinically measures **distortion product OAEs (DPOAEs)**. An insert probe mounted in an earplug includes two transducers generating two "primary" tones with frequencies f_1 and f_2 and with $f_1 < f_2$. Nonlinearities within the cochlea produce numerous IM products but most prominently at a frequency in the spectrum of the response at $2f_1-f_2$. For example, in a test of DPOAE and stimulating near 2000 Hz, f_1 would be set to 2000 Hz and f_2 typically 1.2 × 2000 = 2400 Hz. The DPOAE would appear at 2 × 2000 – 2400 = 1600 Hz. A computer program, naturally, is used to run such tests, stepping the evoked response test system through desired sets of primaries and searching for targeted DPs in the spectrum, all predicted where possible to be, if measureable above the background noise, in this case acoustic noise from both the outside and the test subject.

Therefore, some energy of the retrograde waves propagates to the ear canal via multiple pathways. Because distortions occur at frequencies different than those of the primaries, DPOAEs can be easily extracted from the acoustic signal using spectral analysis, such as by the **fast Fourier transform (FFT)**. In the nonlinear cochlea, IM is expected to be the strongest when the two interacting signals (the primaries) have similar levels at the site of the nonlinearity. The TWs created by two primary/pure tones propagate to their characteristic places on the BM where they reach peaks of their activity patterns. Figure 5–3 depicts schematically half of the envelopes of these TWs (that is, the absolute values of the maxima of displacements of the basilar membrane along its length over time). Due to nonlinearity in processing stimuli by OHCs, the TWs induce local distortions in the region of overlap, mostly near the f_2 place. A fraction of the distortion energy generated in this overlap region, sometimes called the primary DPOAE source, travels basally toward the ME, representing a wave-fixed OAE; another fraction travels apically toward its characteristic place on the BM corresponding to the $2f_1-f_2$ frequency. Some of the latter wave is reflected basally, particularly around the place corresponding to the peak of the $2f_1-f_2$ TW due to local nonhomogeneities of the cochlear structure. This place-fixed OAE is known as the **secondary DPOAE source**. Therefore, there are two main and separate retrograde waves generated by the primary and the secondary source.

Noteworthy again is that DPOAEs measured in the ear canal reflect contributions from multiple sources. First, distortions created by the interaction of the primaries is not limited to the vicinity of the f_2-place, where the magnitude of the overlap is the highest. Rather, there is a region of nonlinear interaction of two TWs created by the primaries (gray-shaded area in Figure 5–3) extending from the base up to the point where the f_2-excitation dies out. Therefore, each point within that region can be viewed as a local wave-fixed source with its individual contributions to the global DPOAE signal. Second, every retrograde TW—including but not limited to wave-fixed OAEs generated at cochlear locations corresponding to the f_1-, f_2-, and $2f_1-f_2$-places—is subject to reflections. This is due to an

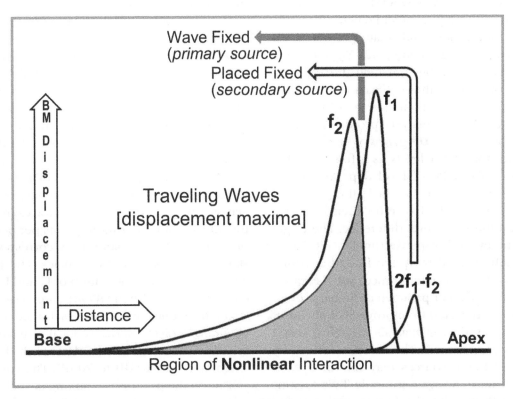

Figure 5–3. Schematic representation of the BM displacement created by primary tones with frequencies f_1 and f_2 and the resulting generation of primary and secondary sources of DPOAEs. The two forward traveling waves induce local distortions in the region of overlap (*gray-shaded area*) of their respective envelopes. A fraction of the distortion energy generated travels basally—the wave-fixed OAE—while another fraction travels apically toward the $2f_1-f_2$ frequency's place—the place-fixed OAE.

inevitable impedance mismatch at the stapes (akin to that between air and water), namely that of the ME transformer. Impedance naturally is a frequency-dependent quantity. Third, each of these newly-formed forward TWs is partially reflected while propagating apically, due to local perturbations spreading somewhat randomly along the cochlea.

In summary, the DPOAE signal measured in the ear canal is the combination of contributions provided by the primary and the secondary source as well as by multiple "elementary" sources spread over a wide distance along the BM. Waveforms generated by each of those major and minor sources can be described by their amplitudes and phases. Thus, the final DPOAE is a mixture of waveforms reflecting a distribution of both multiple self-enhancing and self-canceling signals. Any notion of destructive interference perhaps seems foreboding to have a stable signal to measure; however, these nuances prove to lead simply to ripples and dips in the net spectrum of DPOAES as the test systems scan across f_2s typical of audiometric interests, reminiscent of the side-band splatter of sinusoidal pulses (recall Figures 2–11 and 2–12). Yet, the ripple "parts" are similarly robust, making this effect of nonlinear distortion of the cochlea a reliably measureable signal of a functioning organ of Corti.

A typical DPOAE-analysis protocol used in the audiology is the **DP-gram** which depicts DPOAE and noise-floor levels as a function of f_2 (Figure 5–4). The DPOAE level depends on the parameters of the primaries, including their frequencies (f_1 and f_2), the f_2/f_1 ratio, their levels (L_1 and L_2), and the L_1–L_2 level difference. The target signal of the evoked response (unlike CEOAE) is thus precisely defined by f_1 and f_2, and anything else defined as noise/interference, yet thereafter influenced by the other parameters. Signal averaging is also incorporated to improve SNR ahead of spectral analysis, thus an analysis strongly focused on the frequency domain. The extent to which the elementary DPOAE sources may reinforce each other to produce strong retrograde TWs (again) depends on the spatial distribution of the excitation patterns created by the primaries. For a small value of the f_2/f_1 ratio (<1.05), a wave generated in the vicinity of the f_2-place is expected to be "traveling" mostly apically. The result is a low-magnitude retrograde TW, thus creating low-level DPOAEs.

For a large f_2/f_1 (like 1.5), the distribution of phases of local sources will result in largely self-cancelling waveforms and low-magnitude DPOAEs. Typically, the optimum value of the f_2/f_1 ratio is around 1.2. Making L_1 more intense than L_2 shifts the place of the greatest intermodulation, namely toward the f_2 peak of the TW and thereby enhances the output of the primary DPOAE source. A so-called "scissors paradigm" has been developed to specify levels of the primaries for optimum L_1–L_2 level differences expected to elicit maximal DPOAEs.[13] Typically, DPOAE level is calculated based on the magnitude of a $2f_1$–f_2. The background noise is estimated by averaging the magnitude of the signal over a specified band of adjacent frequencies—considered (residual) variance, thus noise—on either side of the predetermined frequency of interest. A common criterion for considering DPOAE to be "significant" is when its SNR is >6 dB. A criterion of a minimum DPOAE level is applied to ensure that the signal measured in the ear canal originates from the cochlea, rather than being generated by nonlinearity of the test system itself—***system distortion***. As with even the finest audio amplifiers, there is some level (even if inaudible) of distortion. Therefore, a criterion for acceptable system distortion may be expressed as an absolute value (DPOAE level > –10 dB SPL) or referenced to the level of the primaries (such as, DPOAE level > L_1–70 dB SPL).

A DP-gram represents a set of DPOAE data collected at several values of the primary frequencies across a wide frequency range, for example, with the interval of two or more points per octave and/or with the f_2 or a subset f_2s corresponding to standard audiometric frequencies. The f_2/f_1 ratio and the selected combination of L_1 and L_2 are kept constant over f_2. When DPOAEs are measured with small frequency intervals (as hinted earlier), a DP-gram depicts a series of local peaks (relatively broad) and valleys (sharp dips) with their levels extending over 10 dB to 20 dB. The current consensus on the processes resulting in such DP-gram microstructure is that it arises through the interference of the primary and the secondary DPOAE generation sources. Short of this type of DP-gram, the more common variety clinically will reflect the microstructure nuances haphazardly, with the sharp dip having the more emphatic and potential

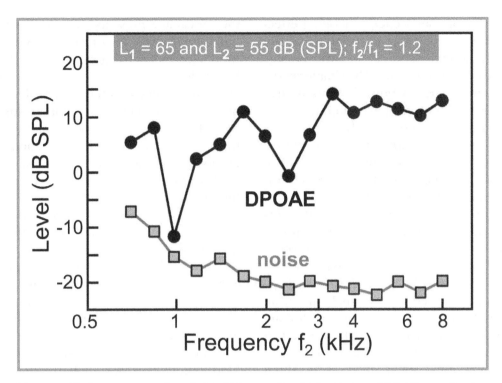

Figure 5-4. An example of the "DP-gram" which depicts DPOAE amplitudes (*circles*) and noise-floor levels (*squares*) as a function of frequency. Common practice/parameters are measuring and plotting values as a function of f_2 at multiple points/octaves (4 here), for the test parameters indicated. For example, to test at $f_2 = 1000$ Hz, f_1 must be $1/1.2 = 833$ Hz. The DPOAE then is measured by spectral analysis. In this example, the measurement would be taken at $2f_1-f_2 = 2*833 - 1000 = 1666 - 1000 = 666$ Hz. By this example, the frequency of the DPOAE itself is seen to fall below the nominal test frequency along the abscissa of the DP-gram, but to relate it to the pure-tone audiogram, comparisons are according to f_2 (rather than either f_1 or $2f_1-f_2$).

adverse effect for interpretation. An example of this effect is shown in Figure 5-4 (again, typical of a "clinical" DP-gram), wherein the DPOAE level dips dramatically at $f_2 = 1$ kHz, indeed close to the noise floor and lower than those at adjacent frequencies by more than 7 dB SPL. It is anticipated that contributions of the two major DPOAE generation sources were of similar magnitudes but almost opposite phases, thus nearly canceling each other. The upshot is that local dips visible in DP-grams measured in normal-hearing subjects are not very likely related to OHC lesions.

There is another notch around 2.4 kHz in the DP-gram of Figure 5-4. It is a typical finding of DPOAEs measured in normal-hearing subjects related to the ME transfer function. Recall that (as so hinted previously) the ME ear system is a part of acoustic impedance matching between air outside and fluid inside the cochlea. Its frequency-dependence (highlighted in an earlier Heads Up, Episode 2.3) is neither flat over frequency nor (in turn) substantially responsible for minimal auditory sensitivity/thresholds. OAEs, of whatever type, are naturally acutely sensitive to ME disorders due to effectively a "round-trip" transmission loss of sound energy. In the forward transfer, the acoustic stimulus travels from the ear canal through the ME to the cochlea. Then, energy produced by the cochlea needs to be propagated backward via the same path before reaching the ear canal and being detected there as an OAE. The tympanogram is not a very sensitive measure of the forward transfer of sound energy (looking effectively from the outside in, not at the end of the conductive apparatus). The reverse ME transfer function is heavily overshadowed by simple reflection of the eardrum. Estimation of the round-trip transfer function in humans is based on measurements in cadavers and more recently by analyzing DPOAEs and wideband absorbance/immittance data (again recall Heads Up, Episode 2.3). Those results support the hypothesis that the round-trip transfer function might have a notch around 2 kHz, consistent with a notch often reported in DP-grams in the same frequency region.[14] A strong influence of the ME status on OAEs is one of the factors contributing to a substantial intersubject variability reported for both CEOAEs and DPOAEs. The rationale is that a patient with perfectly normal pure-tone thresholds may have a subclinical ME pathology which decreases the effectiveness of the round-trip transfer function, resulting in low-level OAEs. It is obvious that obtaining ME measures is essential for the interpretation of OAE data. Clinically confirmed ME pathologies may reduce OAE magnitude in some frequency regions or more globally, or they may eliminate the ability to detect OAEs entirely, depending on the type and severity of the ME disorder.

The vast majority of the early clinical studies of CEOAEs were completed using equipment produced by a company founded by Kemp himself in 1988. Thirty years later, details of the CEOAE generation mechanisms and frequency-specific information of CEOAE data are still debated. The spectrum of the stimulus is expected to determine to a considerable extent the frequency makeup of the CEOAE. This follows from the mathematical fact that clicks are broadband signals that can be decomposed into (in effect) a sum of pure tones via the inverse FFT.

As described previously, SFOAEs evoked by low-level pure tones are assumed to arise by place-fixed or linear coherent reflections involving intrinsic irregularities. Since a click stimulus can be represented as a mixture of pure tones and under a real-life assumption that irregularities are distributed randomly across the entire cochlea partition, the reflection model portends that each component of a wide spectrum scatters rather independently. Therefore, the CEOAE signal recorded in the ear canal represents an overall contribution of multiple SFOAEs. This mechanism is presumably the major factor for generating CEOAEs evoked by low-level clicks.[12] The second model takes into account nonlinear interactions of different frequency components of a complex stimulus, such as a click. Many pure-tone components, through the TWs they create, can interact along the cochlear partition resulting in the generation of wave-fixed or distortion-source OAEs. The conclusion from this model is that CEOAEs are similar to a combination of DPOAEs evoked by wideband primaries. In light of several studies, it seems possible to assume that CEOAEs are mainly composed of reflection OAEs with some contribution from distortion OAEs, hence related and with similar vulnerabilities clinically, yet not identical.

As hinted earlier, a probe containing a miniature loudspeaker and a sensitive microphone sealed into the ear canal, akin to that of tympanometry (and simpler than that needed for DPOAE testing), can be used for CEOAE measurement. The speaker generates a series of clicks. Sinusoidal pulses may also be used but have been primarily employed for research, rather than clinical interests. Analysis of the microphone output involves stimulus-locked averaging of hundreds of samples of the acoustic signal to improve its SNR. The response waveform, representing averaged acoustic pressure in the ear canal in the time domain, is analyzed (again) using FFT, characterizing indeed the signal in the frequency domain but not at the cost of analysis in the time domain. However, windowing must be applied to reject data over the first 2 ms to 3 ms poststimulus to reduce the artifact of the stimulus itself. Typically, clicks are presented in blocks of four and the response to each block is compared against a rejection threshold criterion before adding the results to averaging buffers.

In a nominally *linear protocol*, the CEOAEs are measured with identical clicks in each block. This method preserves linear components of the CEOAEs but is substantially susceptible to the contamination of the waveform by stimulus artifacts, including reflections from the tympanic membrane and the ME. Lowering the presentation level, typically to around 60 dB peak SPL, decreases the contamination effect. However, some ears may not generate robust CEOAEs for such low-level stimuli.

Via a **nonlinear protocol**, the CEOAEs are measured with three identical clicks of the same polarity and the magnitude followed by one click with the opposite polarity, but of a magnitude three times larger than that of the first three clicks. This protocol is generally set as the default, particularly in clinical applications. The nonlinear method reduces stimulus artifacts but also removes linear portions of the cochlear response to the clicks.

An example of CEOAEs is depicted in Figure 5–5 (top panel). The "echo" response returns from the cochlea with some delay introduced by the cochlea's hydromechanical processing of the acoustic input from the ME. Nevertheless, the latency is very short for high-frequency components of the CEOAE (first signals returning to the ear canal), as they are generated mainly in the basal part of the cochlea. At the same time and as a substantial technical problem, the stimulus itself makes for the stimulus artifact of transient-elicited-OAE measurement. Even for the click and as highlighted in the encircled inset of the figure, the stimulus indeed dominates the display for a few milliseconds, in this case by about a 60 dB advantage! Hence, the general practice simply is to blank the tracing (zeroing the initial data in response's display buffer/memory) for a few milliseconds. Meanwhile, the lower-frequency CEOAEs naturally are generated more apically and thus have longer latencies. This is a reflection of the growing TW-propagation delay, plus that of the retrograde TW and other subsequent events. This panel of the figure also shows (when scrutinized closely) two traces of the waveform, created by storing the averaged signals alternatively in two buffers (split-buffer averaging technique; recall Episodes 4.1 and 4.2). Consequently, the difference between the two traces can be used to assess the residual noise in the averaged recorded signal. Again, the spectrum is routinely analyzed, as well, and the results are presented in the bottom panel of Figure 5–5 for this subject's CEOAE. Both additional time- and frequency-domain-based measures provide a rich supply of information by which to assess the given transient-OAE, a few indicted as well in this figure. These and others are worthy of mention and brief discussion. As with AEPs, there are inevitably questions of both reliability and interpretation of the results of a given test.

In the time domain, the cross-correlation between two waveforms (like testing the covariance between two sets of scores on a written exam) is a useful quality indicator and typically expressed in percent, called **reproducibility**. Its value was 96% in the example of Figure 5–5. The FFT of the correlated portions of the two waveforms (frequency domain analysis, light-gray area of the chart) reflects the frequency response of the CEOAE. Due to the complex generation mechanisms of CEOAEs, it is not surprising that waveforms and spectra recorded differ substantially among individuals with healthy ears, including between ears of the same subject. The CEOAE characteristics have been idiomatically compared to the uniqueness of fingerprints. This aspect, together with the previously described influence of the ME transfer function, contributes significantly to the intersubject variances of CEOAE data and are evident (not smoothed over) by the typical resolution of the spectral analyses, ≈50 Hz. Therefore, for clinical purposes, a typical report of a CEOAE test lists levels of the CEOAE, noise, and SNR, analyzed and reported in half-octave bands yielding histogram displays.

The actual frequency-specificity of OAE test results is highly debated, especially regarding CEOAEs, returning to the issue of wideband characteristics of clicks. The CEOAEs depicted in Figure 5–5 actually were recorded in a patient with normal pure-tone thresholds up to 2 kHz but then sloping to mild and moderate hearing loss in the high-frequency region. The customary blanking of the initial time window aside, the amplitude of this CEOAE waveform immediately afterward is still minimal for nearly a millisecond around 4 ms. This indicates absence of measureable CEOAE responses of short-latency emissions, corresponding to the basal region of the cochlea. At the same time, the initial blanking (a necessity or not) is "blinding" the examiner to possible activity much above 4 kHz. Still, the CEOAE spectrum in this case is compelling as it shows, in fact, no detectable response above 2.5 kHz. This illustrates that at least some frequency-specific information can be obtained from transient response recordings. Several studies have provided data regarding the relationships between audiometric thresholds and the magnitude of CEOAEs in half-octave bands

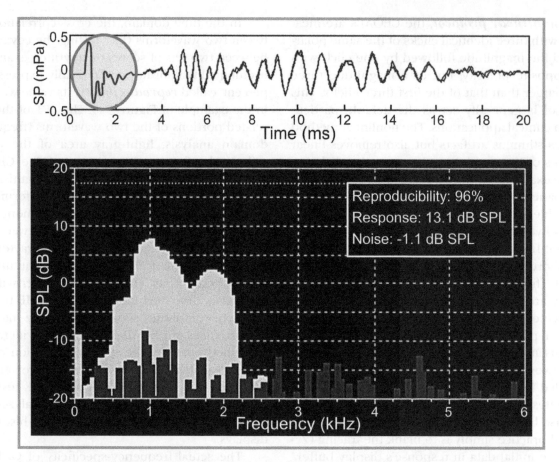

Figure 5–5. An example of an actual CEOAE. The overall appearance recalls elements familiar to many users of Kemp's systems by which OAE testing became broadly adopted in clinical practice. The upper panel displays two time-averaged waveforms overlaid in this patient with essentially perfect stimulus reliability. The encircled epoch in gray tone at the onset is routinely just a flat line (see text), but here overlaid to show the input sound. Whereas the amplitude of the CEOAE display is millipascals, namely about 0.3-mPA peak amplitudes in this case, that of the input/click is pascals—about 0.3 Pa, a 60 dB difference. Conventional test instruments thus use separate displays, yet the actual temporal relationship is important to bear in mind, as illustrated. Still, the emitted sound would be audible if played at its SPL to normally hearing listeners (given a stimulus, as here, of 85 dB pSPL). In the lower panel, the light gray is the spectrum of the response; the cityscapelike plot in dark gray is the noise estimate.

measured (regarding spectral data). Only weak correlations are manifested when univariate analyses were performed—the threshold at a particular frequency being compared to the CEOAE level in the same frequency range. Lastly, on the technical side, OAE researchers and innovators have led the way by not only paying attention to both T and F domains but also real-ear calibration. Their example has been followed only modestly in other evoked response areas. This is essential to having accurate results given the exquisite sensitivity of the test modality. Thanks to such due diligence, OAE testing can be performed being able to specify the input signal subject-by-subject—again, for both time history and spectrum—against which to compare the output measures. For example, direct comparison of the respective spectra can help to refine interpretation of nuances of the real response versus some quirk of the actual sound at the ear's input "port." The split buffering of the recorded incidental sound (windowed for the first 3 ms, the part blanked for the response display but not deleted from memory) is also tested for cross-correlation and is called **reliability** (also in percent, like reproducibility). Naturally, reproducibility can only be as good as reliability, so these numbers and the comparison between them gives the examiner objective indices to help judge quality of the recording.

Clinical applications of any objective measure, whether AEPs or OAEs, must be assessed according to a reasonable and well-supported pass/fail criteria. Some of those criteria for CEOAEs are as follows: (1) overall measure of CEOAE, for example a level greater than 0 dB SPL or 5 dB SPL; (2) global SNR greater than 3, or even 6 dB; and (3) reproducibility, greater than 50%, or even 75%. Figure 5–6 depicts normative data for a group of 100 ears of young normal-hearing adults collected using Kemp's original commercially available system, yet still illustrative of both the "challenges" of norms and overall view of (ultimately) relevant clinical limits, although no standard currently exists. The median value observed was around 12 dB SPL, and there was a substantial intersubject variability. A comparison of the data from that of the individual patient's data in Figure 5–5 to the chart in Figure 5–6 would suggest a clear "pass." The overall CEOAE level of the patient was 13.1 dB SPL, thus falling above the 60th percentile of the presumptive normal rage. Furthermore, the reproducibility was 96%. Nevertheless, there is another issue in this case; the absence of CEOAE components above 2.5 kHz. Therefore, in practice, pass/fail criteria for CEOAEs must include evaluation of spectral composition of the response. The general findings of many studies in patients with hearing levels poorer than 40 dB HL in the frequency range from 250 Hz to 6 kHz was that CEOAEs were judged as absent in almost all cases.[15] Consequently, the more comprehensive view of the results from the sample case would be "fail," and this case would be referred for further evaluation as being at risk for a clinically significant hearing loss.

The frequency specificity of DPOAEs may be viewed as potentially greater than that of CEOAEs because the stimuli are virtually pure tones (several-hundred-millisecond sinusoidal pulses), as used to elicit and measure DPOAEs. However,

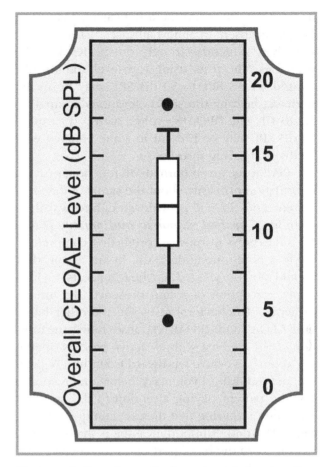

Figure 5–6. A box-whisker plot of the distribution of overall CEOAE levels (in dB SPL) measured in 100 ears of otologically normal young subjects. The horizontal line through the box—median value; the box itself—quartile range; the "whiskers"—10th and the 90th percentiles; the dots—5th and 95th percentiles. Evidence bases for clinical tests and practices, if not standards, are of great importance; these results are presented here on a virtual plaque, hopefully to vividly underscore this point.

the complex nonlinear mechanisms generating DPOAEs also should be considered when analyzing them. Even though the most important site of the generation corresponds (again) to the f_2-place, activities across a wide range of the cochlear partition (BM and all "innards" of scala media) contribute to the overall signal reaching the ear canal and measured there as a DPOAE. Results of several studies indicate that, in patients with hearing levels poorer than 50 dB HL, DPOAEs tested with the primaries corresponding to the audiometric frequencies of sensorineural hearing loss were judged as absent in almost all cases.[15] The DPOAE sensitivity depends strongly on the level of the primaries. The tests using low-level stimuli, like around 40 dB SPL to 50 dB SPL, may be useful to detect hearing-threshold elevations as small as 30 dB HL. The DPOAEs evoked with L_1/L_2 around 65 dB SPL may be present in some patients with 50 dB HL hearing thresholds.

OAE tests, given normal ME function, provide information primarily about the status of the OHC system and do not provide straightforwardly a method of *evoked response audiometry (ERA)* for the express purpose of predicting comprehensively a pure-tone audiogram. In any event, they should not be viewed as "hearing tests," which imply perception of sound presence, the unique province of behavioral tests. On the other hand, both CEOAE and DPOAE responses reflect the function of the cochlea with its active process operating about 1/3 octave basalward from the TW peak and not requiring a voluntary/behavioral response nor the patient paying attention to the stimulus (although requiring that they remain quiet during the test). Another important issue is that the OHC pathology in the basal portion of the cochlea may obscure OAEs generated more apically. Therefore, elevated hearing thresholds in the high-frequency region, for example, above 4 kHz, still may result in reduced or absent CEOAE components at lower frequencies, for example in the 1-kHz to 2-kHz region. DPOAEs provide a great high-frequency range of response. Here too, abnormal hearing thresholds in the extended high-frequency region of nominal utility (above ~8 kHz) may result in lower DPOAEs evoked at lower frequencies, for example for primaries placed below 3Hz to 4 kHz. Even though the OAE tests have their limitations, their clinical applications are important, including the following: (1) "hearing screening" (more accurately, screening for OHC dysfunction that might portend presence of a hearing loss); (2) monitoring of the cochlea function for patients exposed to ototoxic drugs or at risk for noise-induced hearing loss; (3) confirming normal cochlear function in the absence of neural activity (for instance, suggested by a "failed" test of brainstem AEPs); (4) differential diagnosis of patients known to have hearing loss, thus requiring further testing to differentiate cochlear/cochlear portion responsible for the hearing loss versus retrocochlear levels at or beyond the 8th nerve; and (5) helping to rule out malingering. Some of these scenarios will be explored along the way of presenting the electric responses and consequently along the auditory pathway (coming up!).

HEADS UP

Otoacoustic Emission Without Turning On Sound? Who Knew?

As overviewed in the current episode, the types of OAEs and their measurement are several, all have proven to be of keen research interest, and a couple have enjoyed broad clinical interests and adoption for clinical purposes. These will be explored along the way in concert with other evoked response modalities in subsequent episodes. None has been as intriguing, difficult to explain, and seemingly ripe for clinical use as *spontaneous otoacoustic emissions (SOAEs)*. Yet SOAE evaluation has not "found a home" in routine audiological assessments. Nevertheless, what can be said about the SOAE is that it is an important auditory phenomenon that has commanded a substantial volume of literature and that continues to warrant research interests (whether motivated as pure or applied research).[16] The SOAE easily provides the most dramatic testimonial to the exquisite sensitivity of the normally functioning peripheral auditory system with its unique sensory cells that almost seem to be able to dance![8]

SOAEs, like the other OAEs, are measurable directly in the ear canal.[16] They can occur however without an external sound stimulus! Initially thought to explain such effects as *ringing in the ears (tinnitus)*, they only are observed in about 4% of tinnitus cases. In other words, the vast majority of individuals with chronic tinnitus do not have SOAEs at all, although the "ringing" that characterizes SOAEs is for real, even though not perceived. Consequently, the frequencies of such ringing (oscillations) manifested in SOAEs usually are "located" at different frequencies (usually lower) than frequencies of the tinnitus (as measured by subjective pitch matching of tones presented "externally"). Finally, attempts of masking or suppression of SOAEs usually does not influence tinnitus perception. The SOAE generation mechanism is still not understood completely. Nevertheless, after years of research, it is certain that their presence generally is indicative of a healthy rather than pathologically functioning cochlea. Although not audible to the individual demonstrating SOAEs, there is evidence of some positive effect from their presence.[17] Results of a combined psychoacoustic and SOAE study demonstrated frequency discrimination (measured by difference limen) improves near SOAE frequencies, regardless of which ear demonstrates a given SOAE, thus implying a central effect and neural plasticity—the presumed upshot of its persistence.

SOAEs usually take the form of one or several tones, with some minor fluctuation in frequencies. As they approximate continuous sinusoids (effectively indefinitely!), they then are virtually "pure tones." Again, SOAEs are measured in the ear canal. However, they are much more reliably detected with the aid of signal averaging, in this case in the frequency domain by averaging the spectra of the signal recorded. They then show up as narrowband peaks that exceed the background noise. In practice, the SOAEs are more easily measured after sound stimulation (for instance, upon recording CEOAEs), as illustrated in Figure 5–7A. The idea is to use the click stimulus and measure the CEOAE with a time window extended beyond the typical 20 ms, wherein stimulus-elicited OAEs normally fade out. When analyzing the spectrum of the signal after 20 ms (thus discarding the nominally stimulus-evoked emissions for this purpose), what is expected to be left is background noise. However, SOAEs can show up, synchronized by the repetitive click stimulus of signal averaging. In other words, this technique helps to bring SOAEs above the residual noise level. This may seem like a scenario (in time) of putting the "cart before the horse." It is more like a truck pulling along a horse. The horse still can get there on its own but gets a steady tug on the reins to help keep it moving. In searching for SOAEs, spectral analysis is particularly important (see panel B). The SOAE is manifested variably, even among normally hearing subjects, seen in the results from the three cases in panel A, as follows: B(1)—none evident and B(2 and 3)—1 or more present. Furthermore, SOAEs are not always found to be synchronous, like the "sterling example" of case 2 (see insets of panel A, 1 versus 2).

That SOAE testing may not have found a place in the toolbox of clinical audiology does not imply that knowledge of the phenomenon is not important to clinical applications of OAEs overall. SOAEs may influence the evoked OAEs (that is, have consequences within those first 20 ms of the recording). CEOAEs have usually higher amplitude in ears with than without SOAEs. The spectral peaks of the SOAEs might be distinguished readily in the spectra of the CEOAEs, as shown in Figure 5–7C. Another intriguing effect of potential clinical utility (though not yet a part of routine tests of SOAEs), stimulus-elicited OAEs are subject to effects of both ipsilateral and contralateral suppression by acoustic noise by way of reflex arcs via the olivo-cochlear bundle (OCB). These are efferent nerve fibers that course between the caudal pons and the organ of Corti.

One of the challenges with possibly using SOAE testing clinically is that the incidence of detection of SOAEs in both the normal-hearing and clinical populations is variable. In adults, SOAEs usually occur in the range of 1 kHz to 2 kHz, and in newborns and children, in the 2.5-kHz to 5-kHz range. They (again) are

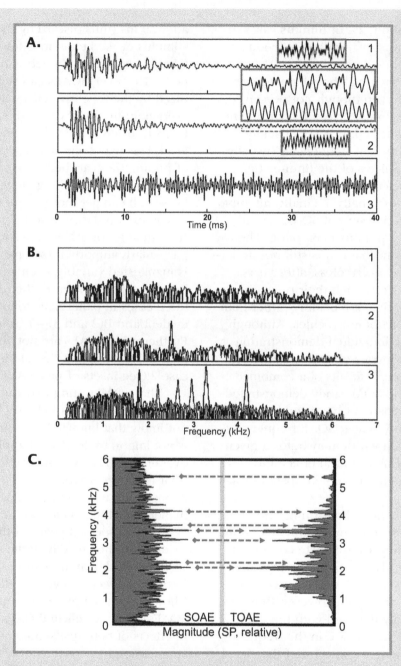

Figure 5–7. A. Forty-ms recordings of a transient-evoked otoacoustic emission (TOAE) elicited by a click (CEOAE), in cases as follows: (1) undetectable spontaneous emissions (SOAEs)—the CEOAE fades before 20 ms; (2) small amplitude SOAE—apparent oscillations seen after 20 ms; (3) multiple, high amplitude SOAEs, even after 20 ms. To better visualize the difference between case 1 and 2, a section of the overall epoch was initially amplified by 4×, and seemed highly suggestive of sustained, spontaneous oscillatory activity. To further demonstrate this, the extracted portion was amplified further (now 8×) and its time base expanded by 3×, then retraced via a quasipolynomial fit. **B.** Spectra of the 20 ms to 40 ms parts of the signals from panel A, confirming presence of SOAEs in cases 2 and 3. Magnitudes are relative, but scaled the same among the three plots. **C.** Spectra of synchronized SOAE and TOAE from the same ear. To more easily visualize here their concurrence of numerous spectral peaks, plots are presented a bit usually to provide a virtual face-off of the two data sets. (SP—sound pressure.)

narrowband (down to 1 Hz) making detection a challenge. However, over months or years, they at least are stable, within ~10 Hz. The amplitude usually is stable as well—fluctuations of less than 3 dB—yet sometimes they can disappear and reappear. SOAEs also tend to coincide with frequencies of most sensitive hearing.

The other challenge to clinical utility, ironically, is that SOAEs are highly sensitive to peripheral hearing loss—too sensitive, practically. The conventional audiogram is not only about whether the patient hears or not, but rather a metric that scales sensitivity along the dB-HL axis. Hearing screening admittedly applies a rule to effect a dichotomous classification of an individual's hearing status via audiometry (at-risk or not for clinically significant hearing loss). Still, it would not be practical to apply a screening hearing level just at the edge of the normal-hearing range in some populations, like the elderly—the failure rate would be unacceptable (as discussed in a later episode, regarding cost-benefits of screening tests). SOAEs typically are absent with hearing thresholds >30 dB, also often undetectable in cases even with hearing well within normal limits! Yet again, SOAEs are at least a "testimonial" to great hearing and are more common in children and particularly newborns than in adults. As with other properties, there is no proven explanation for this. Different researchers hypothesize that possible mechanisms behind that effect could be related to maturation of the cochlea or middle ear or even the ear canal (given that change of volume can result in change of sound pressure of the emission measured). Maturational change in middle-ear transmission currently is considered the most logical explanation, as only a slight change can result in substantial change in SOAE amplitude, if not preventing detection.

Other "fun facts" include that SOAEs are more common in women than in men and are more common in right than left ears. The higher prevalence in females is hypothesized to be related to greater release of hormones to some advantage for better hearing sensitivity, as this difference also is coincidental to females generally having better hearing than males. However, the latter is also multifactorial, given prevalence of males having other issues, starting with more significant histories of industrial noise exposure. The higher prevalence of SOAEs in right ears could be related to different specialization of cerebral hemispheres in sound analysis. The path within the CNS (implied by this theory) is that of the descending, rather than ascending, auditory pathway, "realized" as well thanks to the OCB (medially). Presumably the effect represents some sort of difference in OAE *suppression* between ears. The OAEs again are well-known to be susceptible when the listener (in effect) is placed in a noisy environment.

As indicated at the outset of this Heads Up, SOAEs are of keen research interest and theoretically of great importance, including exotic putative bases of their generation. While clinical applications have been limited—again, many clinical subjects will not have measureable SOAEs—there are interestingly cases who demonstrate large amplitude SOAEs—40 dB SPL to 50 dB SPL! Yet, SOAE frequency(ies) falls within the range of a hearing loss. The mechanism of generating these high amplitude SOAEs in such cases is postulated to be different from that of typical generation of SOAEs and only confound further any notion of value of routine tests of SOAEs.

Such unexpected revelations and the phenomenon itself still warrants continued attention by researchers and clinicians alike. Pending further discoveries, the "clinical eye" at least needs to be vigilant for possible aberrant effects of SOAEs, as potential confounds of interpretation of tests of the stimulus-elicited OAEs.

Episode 2: CM, SP, and AP: Not Alphabet Soup and First Signs AEPs Are Afoot!

This episode gives the first "blush" of an electrically generated response readily measureable using modern technology and, like OAEs, meeting both the spirit and intent of **objective auditory tests** to enhance the audiologist's toolbox. As overviewed in Episode 3.2 and explored further here, there is quite a bit of **electrophysiology** going on in the cochlea,[18,19] which is filled with ionic solutions partitioned by living cellular structures (recall Episode 3.2). It then is reasonable to assume the possibility of recording sound-elicited electric responses within or from those fluid-filled spaces. Such suspicions have been borne out over decades of hearing research, so the "buck" for testing auditory evoked electric responses starts here!

The last episode kicked off further exploration of auditory anatomy and physiology that takes Episode 3.2 both more seriously and as a literal roadmap for the natural order of issues now and henceforth to be presented. The story of the AEPdom "suburbs" in the outlying peripheral auditory system is far from over. The partial copy and adaptation of Figure 1–1 in Figure 5–8 provides, as before, a view looking into AEPdom's turf from the bottom up but explored over an even more constrained epoch involved in initiating signals destined for the central system. The time zone thus is expanded a bit more, by which to tease apart the bioelectric signals featured. The electrical signals to be explored are not only the inevitably all-important compound action potential of the 8th nerve, but also a couple of other intriguing signals that arise even earlier, sharing mechanisms and latencies of the "fastest" otoacoustic emissions. They thus originate still more distally than the first-order (primary) auditory neurons and, like the OAEs, are generated by the hair cells. These are the **receptor potentials** of the sensory cells of the organ of Corti.

As responses of the peripheral system, their origins are the only ones known in detail and unequivocally. Confirmation via research and clinical methods is inherently challenging, given that the generators (hair cells and first-order neurons)

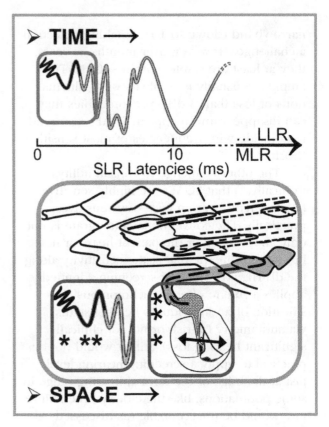

Figure 5–8. Revisiting Figure 1–1 to focus on more details of initial components of bioelectrically generated signals of the auditory system in both time and space, part of the "turf" of the short latency responses (SLRs). Associated key events and places of origin to which they are attributable are highlighted.

are buried deep within the otic capsule of the temporal bone—the hardest bone of the body. The cochlea of the primate is extremely well conceived to protect the minute and highly sensitive structures therein and in an overall system engineered by nature to survive the lifetime of the organism. Great insights—initially the only insights—evolved from decades of research in other mammals, such as feline and rodent, which have hearing ranges overlapping that of the human but are in less well "protected" cochleae. These animals have a softer bony enclosure of the overall middle-inner ear complex, permitting access with minimally traumatic surgery for recording from the round window or within the cochlea, itself a largely free-standing shell in rodents and often with more coils than that of a human.

Such anatomy is nearly ideal for pickup of receptor and/or neural potentials that are conducted through the cochlear fluids to electrodes placed in close proximity to the hearing organ. In fact, the extensive research of the mid-last century supported exploration that led to realistic estimations of electrical properties of the organ of Corti. These properties include the resistive pathways by which current flows from the generators throughout the organ and into the surrounds (Figure 5–9A). The necessary measures to fully characterize the cochlear electroanatomy could not have been accomplished by minimally invasive methods; of particular note was the discovery of the all-important resting direct-current (DC), resting potentials inside each hair cell and within the fluid space of scala media, known as the endocochlear potential (EP). Yet, "aggressive" invasion of the cochlea itself is required for their measurement and is efficacious only in animals. Fortunately, the inherently "conservative" natural engineering of evolution—thus not totally reinventing mechanisms across species (rather adapting/refining)—allows reasonable assumptions of similar electrophysiology in humans.

Resting DC potentials are the batteries powering the system. As the interior of the hair cells are negative and the EP positive, the two together impose a potential difference upward of 150 mV across the hair-bearing surface of the hair cells (Figure 5–9B, inset). The EP, rare as an extracellular polarization, thus effectively doubles the driving "force" of any change of current flow across apices of the hair cells (relative to the hair cell's resting membrane potential), resulting from deflections of the *stereocilia*. Upon acoustic stimulation to elicit vibration of the hearing organ, the resulting modulated potential difference forms the hair cell's *receptor potentials* that subsequently lead to excitation of *first-order neurons* along the peripheral portion of the auditory pathway. Collectively, these electric responses were initially coined *cochlear potentials* by Glen Wever, one of the great pioneers in hearing science.[20]

Looking at more details of Figure 5–9A, recording electrical signals of the cochlea is somewhat like recording bioelectrical signals from the skin's surface, given an underlying generator. The effective physical-electric-equivalent circuit is that of connections among batteries, resistances, and capacitances (recall Figure 3–1C). For purposes here, capacitive elements are not considered, but alternating currents (AC) sources are included. AC signals are extensively what are generated/recorded practically, starting with the hair cells. The modulation of the resting hair-cell membrane potentials produces their receptor potentials. They, in turn, drive up and down the release of transmitter substance at the synapses with the neurons at the base of the hair cells, also expressed extracellularly (dendritic and axonal potentials), which coincidentally "leak" into the perilymph from the modiolus. Therefore, the cross-sectional circuit schematic includes both DC (batterylike) and AC sources (symbolized by an encircled sinewave). Also indicated are effective test points (TPs), as common/useful in electronic circuits, for example for troubleshooting a device. "Intersections" of connections among electrical components often provide (or are even demarked on circuit boards as) test points. For minimally invasive testing of cochlear function, these are effected by physical interface to the cochlea's electrical circuit—its electroanatomy—using microelectrodes or micropipettes inserted into the perilymph or endolymph. In clinical electrophysiology, the least invasive yet most directly accessible semblance of a TP is the round window membrane. The point of the illustration is that whatever is seen of the hair-cells' receptor potentials effectively will be conducted, distributed, and influenced indeed in the measurement/recording by this elaborate combination of resistors. As illustrated, this starts with a substantial division of the generator voltages from the hair cells themselves, as the resulting current flow (like water running down hill) "seeks" a path to the system's ground. Furthermore, the cochlear circuit is actually three-dimensional (Figure 5–9B, main panel), so the electro-anatomical cross section (again, panel A) is just that, merely a slice of the cochlea's whole circuit. The "slices," in turn, are connected sequentially (in effect). Current spreads longitudinally, as well, in the salty-fluid-filled scalae. From the outside looking in, such as at the round window, the net resistive pathway will attenuate potentials more the farther away (apically) that they are generated.

Consequently, recordings need not be made in scala media or otherwise in close proximity to the

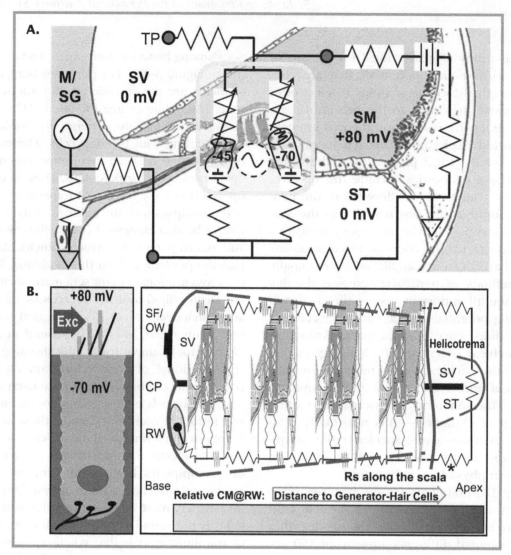

Figure 5–9. A. Simplified schematic of effective cross section of the electroanatomy of the cochlea. Nominal resting potentials of hair cells are indicated (in millivolts). For both types of hair cells, the effective wiring of these voltage sources are in series with the endocochlear potential (thus additive, as typical of the circuit of the classical multibattery flashlight), providing more driving force of ionic current flow modulated by motion of the basilar membrane. In addition to the functional importance of this electrical circuit (namely, the outer hair cells' motile responses), it is the generator of the hair cells' bioelectrical signals that drive their motility but also are key to clinical electrophysiology of the auditory system, thanks to their extracellular manifestations. They are "leaked," conducted, and distributed to/by the fluids in all three scalae and are the first AEPs. **B.** Inset, bottom left: Another hair-cell function reminder but finessed more to this context. Only an outer hair cell is shown, but points are largely applicable to the inner HCs as well. Main panel: Repetition and interconnection of cross-sectional cochlear circuit, namely along the length of the cochlea (portrayed here as if uncoiled). The views of the cross sections are oriented as if eyed slightly obliquely, having installed numerous, narrow observation windows from the basal coil up. Cross sections are seen also to be connected by resistive pathways, thanks to the cochlear fluids and thus longitudinally all along the scalae. Jumping to the apex, the helicotrema—the hole at the top—provides a final/shunt resistance between the two perilymphatic canals. The graded gray-tone bar at the bottom expresses the relative strength of the same magnitude of CM at a given distance from the base when recorded at the round window (RW) with darker shading connoting lower magnitudes. TP—test point (see text); M/SG—modiolus, with the spiral ganglia therein; SV, SM, ST—scala vestibuli, media, and tympani, respectively; Exc—excitatory; SF/OW—stapes footplate at the oval window; CP—cochlear partition (collapsing SM for simplicity); Rs—resistors (with arrow—variable); upside-down triangle—common/ground.

hearing organ (in scala vestibuli or tympani) to be useful, even for many research purposes. Rather good registration of the cochlear potentials with very low noise floors is readily accessible from the lateral (middle-ear) surface of the round window or even the medial wall the middle ear. This is also the lateral cochlear wall of the first turn—the ***promontory***. All such recordings reveal the three ***stimulus-related potentials*** that ultimately have led to clinically applicable tests. However, these (as hinted previously) do not include membrane resting potentials of the hair cells, the EP, or direct single-unit sampling of hair-cell receptors or neural ***action potentials***. The stimulus-related potentials are distributed broadly along the scalae within the cochlea, reflecting the place-frequency relation. They are most reliably sampled in relation to frequency place of strongest generation (according to the traveling wave envelope) within the cochlea. Some approaches by way of certain stimulus paradigms will be described later that permit useful approximations using noninvasive recording methods. The present focus is on what electrophysiological exploration of the cochlea and vicinity can—or cannot—reveal directly by the signals recorded. Again, the view from recordings at the cochlear base of more apically generated activity is that of a "jaundiced eye"—limited access (in effect) of the singular TP of this otherwise, on the inside, magnificent 3D-circuit of the whole cochlea.

However, the ***round-window recording*** is still quite sensitive. Unfortunately, this site is not readily available for clinical studies without at least a myringotomy or coincidentally involving a patient with a perforated eardrum. Still, although perhaps contrary to impressions from basic anatomy of the ear, a membranous lining mutually covers the lateral surface of the round window membrane and the rest of the middle ear's interior. This is like wallpapering a room with a very thin, living paper. This is because it is made up of viable cells and capillaries. These are also substantially filled with ionic fluids, so there is a good chance that the cochlear potentials will be conducted to the promontory.

Other good news is that the round window and promontory fall well within the near field of the cochlear potentials. As mentioned earlier, the near field is the electrical field within which the voltage output of the generator at the site of recording is proportional to the distance from the generator site. Recording from the promontory naturally will reflect some added resistance relative to that directly on the round window, but differences prove to be inconsequential in practice.[21] Bottom line: the promontory is easier to get to clinically, less invasive than recording from the round window, and still provides good recordings of the stimulus-related cochlear potentials. Still other methods that permit recording more laterally will be shown shortly to be efficacious as well. This too is fully predictable with the same advantages of the round window/promontory—similar sampling of the cochlear potentials versus recordings strictly from the scalp (largely far field). Nevertheless, the more lateral recording sites, further out in the near field, have the risk of ending up in the far field and suffering the worst losses of signal strength. An additional risk is that of the noise floor, which can be more or less the same. If coincidentally higher (for example, due to greater proximity to muscles), this will be double jeopardy for reduction of SNR. As demonstrated in Episodes 4.1 and 4.2, given modern technology (very sensitive and with very low internal noise), successful recording of AEPs is more a matter of acceptable SNR than any limit of the actual voltage of the evoked response of interest, however small.

At this juncture, a goodly amount of additional information about the cochlear potentials must be considered before worrying about practical recording issues and applications. Hopefully from the foregoing, there is already confidence that the means to record such potentials clinically are out there. Furthermore, regardless of the specifics of such recordings, they can provide much the same information as the more invasive procedures.

Classical experiments in testing the electrical "output" of the cochlea have favored extensive use of one of two signals for test stimuli. Certainly in the backdrop of classical/pure-tone audiometry there has been a pervasive use of at least quasitonal stimuli for their relatively strong frequency specificity. As demonstrated in Episode 2.2, a variety of underlying functions exist for the generation and utility of ***tone bursts***. Via intracochlear and round-window recordings, and especially in the "old days" predating digital signal processing, these sinusoidal pulses tended to be relatively long (≥10's of milliseconds), as exemplified in Figure 5–10A. This figure shows the electrical output of the microphone used to calibrate and monitor the sound stimulus. As pointed out earlier (recall Figure 2–18), some transducer-based and/or other distortion (relative to a pristine version of the input signal) is evident. Yet, this is minor compared to that of the recorded cochlear potentials, shown in panel B.

As to the point of departure of this exploration of AEPs from the periphery, only one of three of the stimulus-related potentials actually looks like the stimulus, namely in terms of overall (time-domain) envelope and the underlying sinusoid windowed (gated) to form the "burst" of tone—the *cochlear microphonic (CM)* (Figure 5–10B). This is also what Wever labeled as "cochlear potentials." From another school of thought, effectively led by Hallowell Davis, the originator of the model of hair-cell transduction represented in Figure 5–9, this potential was coined, "cochlear microphonic."[19] However, there is not necessarily a clear winner here. Both prove to be somewhat of misnomers. On the one hand, Wever had hoped to have identified the neural response of the cochlea but was (overall) seeing more receptor than neural potentials in his experiments. On the other hand, "microphonic" was adapted/adopted from an electronic effect of vacuum tubes, wherein amplifier circuits would sometimes demonstrate sensitivity to mechanical vibrations of the tubes. Just like "echo" being an oversimplification mechanistically for OAEs, so this is an oversimplification of the generation of hair-cells' receptor potentials. IN THIS BOOK henceforth, dear reader, please take "cochlear potentials" to imply the more general meaning of any stimulus-related potentials recorded effectively from the cochlea and CM to designate specifically the hair-cells' AC receptor potential. Avoid heated arguments thereto; just blame the authors and walk away.

Discovery of the CM created high hopes for a truly objective audiometric method. Yet, even in animal research, the utter simplicity of the pure-tone audiogram was never realized for multiple technical reasons. This fate has been the same for the "DP-gram" of OAEs. Again, in the case of the CM, the electrode placement fails to allow the examiner to realize an "unbiased view" of the response along the full length of the organ of Corti. Rather, the electrode placement provides a heavily biased view favoring the basalward end of the cochlea. Any sensitivity curve recorded is as much, if not more, about the middle-ear transfer function as about a place-frequency-specific test of the CM.[22] Although some effect of (for instance) more apical-ward lesions is possible to see, a precise representation of the effect in the audiometric sense is not possible from the round window and beyond.[23]

A particularly remarkable feature of the "electric" response (again, Figure 5–10B) is, in fact (somewhat vindicating Wever), a robust response of the 8th nerve (marked *AP*), yet it is not sustained throughout the tone burst. This response is firstly a *compound action potential* (recall Figure 3–11A). The AP thus is not an individual/single-unit spike-action potential, rather more or less of a *whole-nerve response*. Nor do action potentials just stop in a few milliseconds! Recall the primary and primarylike patterns of the poststimulus time histograms of single-unit recordings (see Figure 3–13). The underlying barrage of action potentials thus shows a form of *adaptation* during the stimulus. What then is witnessed in the "gross" recording of activity of the whole nerve is the inherently strong on-effect responses of primary auditory neurons in general and, in turn, those of the central auditory nervous system. The whole-nerve AP demonstrates a salient negative component (see left inset of panel B) known as the N_1 *component*.

In Figure 5–10B, a remaining "distortion" is observed that is not at all due to the transducer and dominated largely by the hair cells' nonlinearity of transduction, producing in effect, another (compound) receptor potential. This may beg the question, so why treat it as a separate potential? The simplest retort would be, "Because we can." That is true, yet dismissive of the possibility to see something different functionally that does not readily correlate simply from one component to the other—the CM. This component classically was demonstrated in the sort of recording shown in panel B. The CM, as an AC signal, is expected to be symmetrical between the positive and negative peaks of the response, that is, according to the

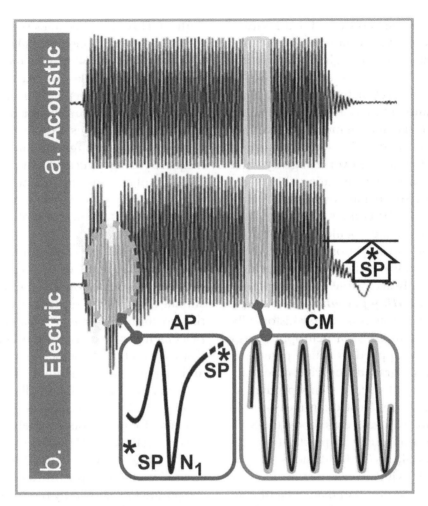

Figure 5–10. Signals typical of intracochlear recordings from scala tympani in the basal cochlear turn or on the round window membrane (middle-ear side) at moderate and higher levels of stimulation. **A.** Acoustic/input signal, tone-burst stimulus (here, signal from a monitoring/probe microphone near the eardrum; recording from a guinea pig). As was demonstrated in Figure 2–18, some ringing (temporal distortion) is seen in the acoustic input to the ear (in reference to the rectilinear sinusoidal pulse driving the transducer). **B.** More substantial effects are seen in the stimulus-related electrical response, attributable to hair cells—cochlear microphonic (CM) and summating potential (SP)—and first-order auditory neurons—whole-nerve action potential (AP, here primarily the N_1 component). Insets: Time-expanded views of the AP and CM, whereas the overall direct-current offset of the temporal envelope of the response reflects the component called "summating potential." *Left*: After N_1, other positive and/or negative peaks may be seen (suggested by undulations just outside the elliptical highlight, but otherwise the SP prevails. *Right*: The CM-electric tracing (*black line*) is overlaid on that of the acoustic (*light-gray line*) for several cycles of the expanded view, demonstrating its mimicry of the input signal; meanwhile, the CM (per its peak amplitude) and SP both follow the envelope overall. The AP lastly is only evident at the stimulus onset, essentially following the poststimulus time histograms of individual neurons, presented earlier in Figure 3–13 and often referred to as the "on-effect."

input signal. However, a notable shift is seen here—implying an underlying DC potential. Today, this DC shift is well understood as one aspect, indeed, of an ***essential nonlinearity*** of the cochlear system—an intrinsic characteristic of how the hearing organ, particularly the hair cell, works. As noted in the first episode of this chapter, this nuance of hair-cell transduction is what makes for a particularly robust DPOAE at frequencies equal to $2f_1-f_2$ for the test-frequency pairs employed in measuring the

DP-gram. It long has been observed that a saturation of the CM output will occur when the hearing organ is driven at relatively high SPLs—typically ≥90 dB SPL. This effect itself is a nonlinearity but arguably not at the level of the hair cells. However, harmonic and intermodulation distortions products are produced at even much lower SPLs.[19] Yet, the CM still "looks good" (strongly sinusoidal given a tone-burst stimulus) over a huge dynamic range. In other words, the saturating side of the nonlinearity is not so obvious by observation of the grossly recorded CM (versus single-unit hair-cell recording within the cochlea, as ultimately became possible in the laboratory). The DC offset can be observed readily, even from extracochlear sites that are clinically accessible. This component is termed the **summating potential (SP)**.

This name also has its controversy historically, indeed a misnomer in classical neurophysiology wherein it would be applied to neural potentials, such as summing of graded/dendritic potentials. After a half century of use, it seems prudent to just use it and move on. Most often measured in humans via minimally invasive methods, the SP is predominantly (if not totally in practical recordings) receptor in origin, as readily demonstrated by a simple test. Briefly, with increasing **stimulus rate** of presentation it persists, rather than "adapting" as expected of a neural response. The recorded CM also does not adapt. The same peak-to-peak amplitude continues, changing only with "interference" of the AP's component waves at stimulus onset. Therefore, the SP as well as the CM elicited by tone bursts follow the stimulus envelope. Only "fatiguing" of the ear by excessively prolonged stimulation at high SPLs tends to cause reductions in the CM and SP.[24]

While the tone burst is an attractive basic "tool" for testing cochlear potentials, it is not opportune for all applications, as soon will be elaborated. Chapter 2 presented other transient signals of interest, and in Episode 2.3, substantial interest was given to challenges of calibrating the stimulus called the **broadband acoustic click** (or "click" for short). Still, it remains a highly popular test stimulus for clinical neurophysiology in audiology. An inherent problem in electrophysiology is the possibility that transducer radiation may add to or even obscure the real AEP (also mentioned earlier). This "fear" becomes sensitized for the CM, given that the response strongly mimics the stimulus waveform. The SP may be more difficult to sort out for still other reasons, starting with teasing it out from the AP. In general, testing in a frequency-specific manner is useful for some applications, but other applications require a stimulus that generates energy throughout much of the audible frequency range (recall Figure 2–19). The click's stark simplicity and the prospect of taking a "best shot" to get a response amounts to the considerable appeal of the click to probe cochlear, as well, as neural potentials.

The approach[25] is illustrated in Figure 5–11A and takes advantage of the slight time difference between condensation and rarefaction phases of stimuli, given that the excitatory phase of stimulation in the cochlea is a scala-vestibuli-ward displacement or velocity,[26] as occurs with outward displacement of the stapes footplate. For the click and high-frequency stimuli, the time difference between the polarities is small enough not to have a substantial effect in normal ears for the AP, and not at all for the SP (as uniquely an "envelope" follower). Again, the CM mimics the microstructure of the stimulus, cycle by cycle. Combining responses elicited by the two polarities of the click tends to cancel the CM, shown by the "wave-math" cartoon inset to panel A, R+C condition, while leaving the SP and AP. Although bad for the CM, the good news is that combining the R and C responses also helps to reduce stimulus artifact (if present). In the computer of the AEP test system (recall Episode 4.1, split buffering), it is possible to store separately the R and C responses automatically, permitting computation of the R+C response and the opposite, R–C. As illustrated and for the same reasoning (it is simply a matter of phase), R–C largely cancels the SP and AP while enhancing the CM. The math here is as follows: given R and C are nominally equal but opposites, then C = –R; hence R – C = R – (–R) = 2 R. The computation performed in the computer (by default settings) likely will be the average, just as in combining separate test and retest trials to effect an average based on 2× the number responses averaged over each trial, toward a greater noise reduction. Thus, (R+/–C)/2 does the same because the noise presumably is random. Still, the first priority and justification of the

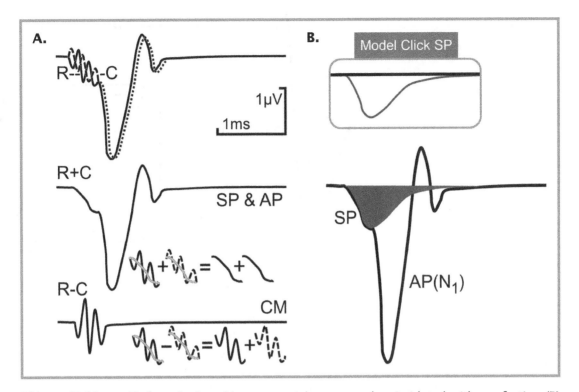

Figure 5–11. A. Click-evoked cochlear potentials: separately stimulated with rarefaction (R) and condensation (C) clicks together with computations on the responses as indicated to extract the three potentials. (Inspired by Coats [1981][25] and simplified/idealistic [noise-free] representations of the respective potentials). **B.** Computer model of a transient SP (see text), overlaid on model response (R+C) from panel A (based on data of results of Durrant and Ferraro [1991][28]). Collectively, these nuances of responses are typical of responses observed at high levels of stimulation (upward of 90 dB nHL) in otologically normal ears.

approach is that of the differentiation of CM from SP and AP. However, the risk of stimulus artifact remains a shadow over the R–C condition. If present, it is not random and (as an inherently coherent signal) will be enhanced too. Good insurance to minimize risk of stimulus artifact, in general, is that of imposing an acoustic delay to the eardrum, as does the tubal-insert earphone. The tube between the transducer and foam earplug is worth nearly a millisecond of lag time, with a few more tenths added by the ear canal's length, with respect to the excitation of the transducer versus arrival of sound waves at the eardrum. For longer-duration stimuli than the click (generally all tone bursts of practical durations), additional step(s) will be needed, such as using appropriately shielded transducers.

To its advantage nevertheless, what is expected of the tone-burst-elicited SP is more predictable than that of the click. Depending on the frequency of stimulation, the SP is either plus or minus with respect to baseline across test frequencies.[27] What the click-SP might truly be like is not so straightforward, although, a simple approximation can be made. Starting with a middle-ear-like transfer function applied to a click (recall Episode 2.3), then feeding its output to a model of the nonlinearity of the hair-cell transducers provides insight.[28] The nature of this nonlinearity can be appreciated from revisiting Figure 2–6A, demonstrating the overall nuance of being both that of a saturating input–output function of the signal and asymmetrical. Figure 5–11B illustrates such a result, a transient SP model. Surprising? Well, not really. As was seen with the click itself in Figure 2–19, while its acoustic signature is substantially different from the brief DC pulse exciting the earphone, it still did not last

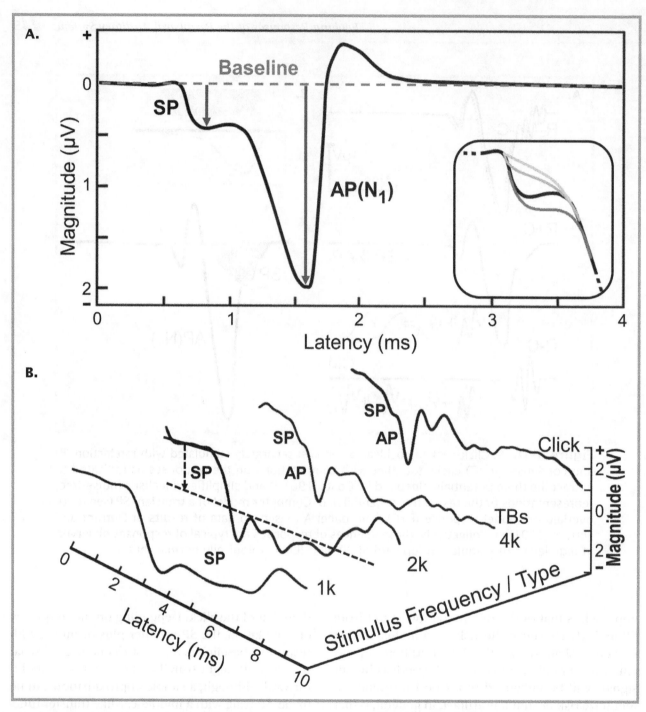

Figure 5–12. A. Model extratympanic recording, still simplified/idealistic but based directly on an actual recording characteristic of waveform that can be seen in otologically normal ears—a prominent bump/"shoulder" leads to the emergence of the AP(N_1) but in contrast to still other cases with only a slight-to-no inflection observed (pending stimulus and/or background noise levels); see inset. Additionally illustrated is the most fundamental method of magnitude measurement of SP versus AP. Under the far-less ideal conditions of clinical tests, the baseline as well as the response render both as matters of interpretation. (Courtesy of Dr. R. E. Delgado.) **B**. Comparison of click-evoked versus tone-burst-evoked SP and AP at several frequencies. These responses are characteristic of results in normal or some clinical subjects (to be discussed) using stimuli at or above 90 dB nHL and a stimulus rate of 11.1/s. The tone bursts were rectilinear without rise-fall times in gating (6-ms overall duration). However, with decreasing carrier frequency, there is an effective rise-time in the actual input signal. Hence, at this and lower frequencies (given their longer periods), there tends to be less clear definitions of the AP, but the objective is further qualifying interpretation of test findings, particularly with respect to definition of the SP. Analog filtering applied was 10 Hz to 3000 Hz.

very long. Playing the same "game" with the R and C polarities through the model effectively strips off the CM-like part, leaving a brief quasi-DC component—the transient offset of the output signal in response to a transient input signal. Lastly, while there is only the traveling wave delay in generation of CM and SP, the hair-cell transduction acts otherwise essentially instantaneously. The neurons, thanks to the *synapses* with the hair cells, inevitably cause a brief but significant delay relative to both CM and SP generation, as was demonstrated in Figure 5–10. Therefore, the SP indeed can be counted upon to present a sort of "shoulder" on the AP-N_1 waveform's leading edge. At the same time, it also is predicted to have a natural decay, normally.

This episode thus has served as a preview to practical methods of testing and measures of cochlear potentials. The SP and AP were some of the first of all electric responses in AEPdom to be employed clinically and the latter to vie for the lead in routine ERA. Figure 5–12 provides a summary (in effect) of several of the issues covered in this debut. Panel A shows again the click-evoked SP-AP complex, along with a common and most basic way to measure the magnitude of the component potentials. In the absence of stimulation, the baseline is the average through the quasirandom noise in the background, thus expected largely to average out (per the principle of coherent signal averaging, Episode 4.1). In practice, definition of the baseline can be challenging, as some residual noise is unavoidable. The baseline is thus estimated as the central tendency through the overall response and residual noise. The SP is expected to precede the AP; in effect, the AP "rides" on the SP. The SP shows substantial variability in waveform even within clinical limits of normality, in terms of size and/or form (see inset to panel A) and in proportion to the AP (it varies too, naturally). The N_1 of the AP is measured to the baseline as well, although the measure (from the foregoing) is arguably SP+AP for some portion of its time history. In Figure 5–12B are several more examples of the SP and AP, for both clicks and tone bursts. In clinical science, there is always a strong motivation to settle on a particular protocol, especially with hope that one is very efficient. Yet, it is always important to have a backup plan(s) and knowledge of various manipulations of the test parameters and their effects toward the best insurance of a successful examination. Now, it is time to take cochlear electrophysiology 101 to the next level, into the clinical arena, and see what actually works in practice.

■ Episode 3: Electrocochleography: How Do Electrical Signals Get From Hearing Organs to the "Outside" and What Good Are They?

Electrocochleography (ECochG) is a minimally invasive, clinical electrophysiological method—a technique for recording the voltage changes that occur in the cochlea and auditory nerve following acoustic stimulation. As introduced in the last episode, these potentials include both receptor potentials (CM and SP) and the whole-nerve (compound) action potential (AP) of the 8th nerve. Still more detailed information on these components is readily available in the literature, including several reports/book chapters.[29,30]

The history of discovery and research of the targeted signals of ECochG was lightly touched upon before but is worth noting in more depth, namely as essentially the history of ECochG too, given early interest/desires to be able to record these potentials in humans. That history dates back nearly a century to the 1930s when Wever and Bray[20] claimed to have recorded what they described as action currents of the acoustic nerve. As noted in the last episode, the presumptive neural potential turned out to arise largely from the hair cells—the CM. Their work was in cats, but human recordings of this "effect" were first reported in 1935.[31] Still, a practical method would not emerge for nearly four decades. ECochG for studying the cochlea and auditory nerve under both normal and abnormal conditions has now been available to scientists and clinicians alike for more than a half-century. Though several clinical applications have been reported for ECochG (described later in this chapter), the use of this technique to help in the assessment, diagnosis, and/or treatment management of *Meniere's disease (MD)/endolymphatic hydrops (ELH)* emerged as its primary application[29] and is the focus of this episode.

The technical capability to perform ECochG in humans relies on the placement of a recording electrode in close proximity to the generators of the components of interest (again, the CM, SP, and AP). There are two general approaches for achieving this goal, involving near-field electrode sites accessible via the middle ear (cochlear promontory or round window) or placements external to the tympanic cavity (ear canal, lateral surface of the tympanic membrane, TM). *Transtympanic (TT)* recordings from middle ear sites naturally involve invasive procedures that include penetrating the TM with a **needle electrode** or gaining access to the round window or promontory during surgeries that expose the middle ear cavity. TT-ECochG remains popular in some European and Asian countries, as well as Australia, but has not been well accepted in the Untied States in routine practice, where *extratympanic (ET)* ECochG is deemed preferable. Figure 5–13 illustrates both approaches.

The TT electrode is commonly a modified **needle electrode** for stimulation (for instance, as used in electromyography) or for subdermal recordings of EMG, EEG, or evoked potentials (often employed in intraoperative neurophysiological monitoring, presented later in this book).[32,33] The needle is

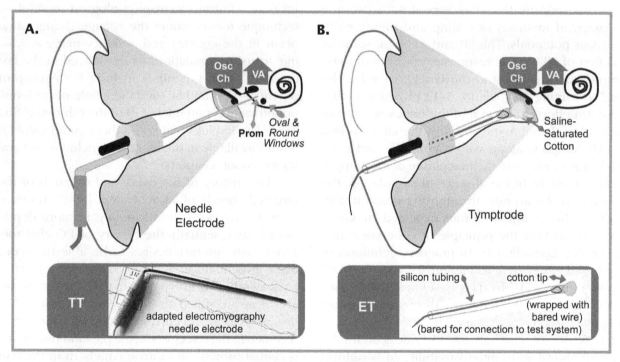

Figure 5–13. Schematic representation of the outer ear, not only the all-important "funneler" of sound energy to the middle and inner parts but also providing access to the cochlea's internally generated bioelectrical signals. Here, examples of approaches to clinical electrocochleography (ECochG) are overviewed for scenarios of using tubal-insert earphones for stimulation; only the foam tip is shown (for simplicity) but is of added significance operationally for stabilizing the electrode mechanically: **(A)** transtympanic (TT), using a needle electrode through the eardrum to the promontory (Prom), versus **(B)** extratympanic (ET), using a tymptrode—a soft-tipped wet electrode on the eardrum. Osc Ch—ossicular chain; VA—vestibular apparatus (the vestibule, into which the oval window opens, and the semicircular canals, superiorly). Insets provide close-ups of examples of the respective electrodes used, as indicated. The needle of the TT electrode is stainless steel, whereas the wire of the ET electrode is an insulated silver wire (stripped at each end), preferably salt-platted medially to form an Ag-AgCl electrode for better low-frequency pickup (recall Episode 3.1). (Photograph, inset left, courtesy of Dr. M. Walger.)

inserted through the TM with the tip resting on the promontory, by design. Akin to a hypodermic needle and as simple as a bare-metal electrode, the connection is by metal directly in contact with tissue, the membranous lining of the middle ear. Still, the contact is stabilized well mechanically by the overall approach (Figure 5–13A). In contrast, "TM" electrodes or *tymptrodes* are flexible and blunted and/or soft-tipped, designed to rest comfortably on the outer surface of the TM with minimal force holding it place. It also is well stabilized by the overall approach. The design of the tip of this electrode generally is that of a salt-bridge electrode, as effectively employed in common surface recording approaches (recall Figure 3–1) with contact through a salty solution (in effect) to avoid direct metal contact (by current methods). The soft tip is saturated with a saline-diluted electrode gel that barely leaves a residue on the TM, if any. The TM itself is not "prepared" (as described for surface electrodes, refer to Episode 3.1), unless there is excessive ear wax/other conditions. The latter scenario requires medical assistance, such as flushing the canal and/or providing whatever treatment is indicated. By the same token and as hinted earlier, electrode impedances are relatively higher in electrocochleography, although not a problem technically if not excessively high or essentially infinite—indicating poor or no contact, respectively. The only study of which the authors are aware of that employed and thus permitted a direct comparison between TM- and TT-ECochG recordings from the same subject was conducted by the first author and coworkers.[34] Figure 5–14 illustrates trends of results

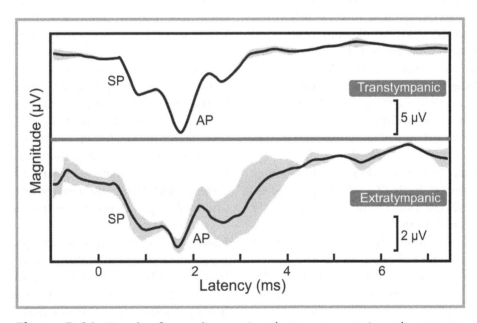

Figure 5–14. Trends of recordings using the transtympanic and extratympanic methods, as indicated (the latter using a tymptrode). Graphs based on results of simultaneous recordings by both methods in a patient demonstrating a significant enhancement of the SP while having a relatively normal AP (given the relatively high stimulus level often used in this test, 90 dB nHL). The tracings derive from computer approximations of the data to estimate the mean of test–retest trials and further reduce noise, in turn reflected in the areal differences between the original test and retest tracings (*gray-tone fill*). Note: Stimulus onset is at 0 ms. Although not always done and/or shown, in practice, some number of milliseconds (1 or more) may be added to the recording epoch to permit scrutiny of a portion of the prestimulus interval as well as to the poststimulus/response portion. This is to help better estimate the baseline. (Based on data of Ferraro and coworkers [1994].[34])

Table 5–1. Transtympanic (TT) Versus Extratympanic (ET) ECochG

	Advantages	Disadvantages
TT	**Large Signal-to-Noise Ratio** Larger component amplitudes Fewer signal averages Stable/repeatable responses	**Invasive** Medical supervision Anesthetic Subject discomfort
ET	**Noninvasive** No need for medical supervision/anesthetic Less/no subject discomfort	**Small Signal-to-Noise Ratio** Smaller component amplitudes More signal averages Responses more variable

from this study, showing that the TT recordings naturally provide a larger amplitude response and often a more stable baseline (discussed in terms of theory regarding near-field recordings, previous episode), thus providing potentially less "noisy" recordings than when using the ET approach. Nevertheless, the subject upon whose data the illustration is based was a patient with a confirmed diagnosis of MD. The critical diagnostic feature of the *electrocochleogram (ECochGm)* thus was preserved well in the ET recording—an enlarged *SP/AP amplitude ratio*. However, before jumping fully into diagnostic testing, detailing some additional technical matters will be useful.

As shown in Table 5–1,[30] there are advantages and disadvantages to both TT and ET approaches. That ET recordings can be performed strictly noninvasively and painlessly without sedation by nonphysicians doubtlessly contributes to their popularity in the United States and in a growing number of other countries throughout the world. The decision to perform TT or ET ECochG may depend on a variety of factors related to the advantages and disadvantages of both approaches. Interestingly, neither the attitude/preference of the patient nor the cost of the exam is typically taken into consideration in this decision. The TT-ECochG approach is generally more expensive to perform.

The photographs and illustrations in Figure 5–15 highlight how a tymptrode actually is placed, which involves gently inserting it along the ear canal wall inferiorly and posteriorly until the tip just contacts the TM. The electrode is then secured in place by the foam ear tip of the sound delivery tube. Placement on the eardrum can be confirmed via otoscopy or via operating microscope, acknowledged by the patient, and by monitoring the electrophysiological noise floor. With one of the two differential amplifier inputs left "floating" (the electrode tip being in air or barely touching skin), the output is quite noisy; the noise sharply decreases and becomes more stable when the tymptrode tip makes proper contact with the TM. Physically, there is negligible pressure needed for good contact. If otherwise and/or if there is excessive pressure or discomfort reported by the patient, the tymptrode is slightly backed out. If too much, loss of contact is signaled by return of high noise floor. This emphasizes the importance of scrutiny of the running/oscillographic display of the recording (sometimes referred to as the "EEG" display/mode) from the start and not counting solely upon subsequent averaged responses.

As indicated earlier, ECochG overall has a long history. Unfortunately, the parameters for recording, measuring, and interpreting the ECochGm have yet to be standardized and may vary widely among clinicians who use this test. The lack of uniformity for these features makes it difficult to compare/share results across clinics/clinicians and certainly has affected the outcomes of several studies related to the effectiveness of ECochG as a clinical tool. Table 5–2 lists the recording parameters the authors recommend when ECochG is used to study, diagnose, or assess MD/ELH. As SLRs, these settings are somewhat common to those employed for recording the *auditory brainstem responses (ABRs)*. Those details and other overlapping nuances will be taken up later.

For the moment, the focus will remain on maters specific to ECochG. First is the electrode

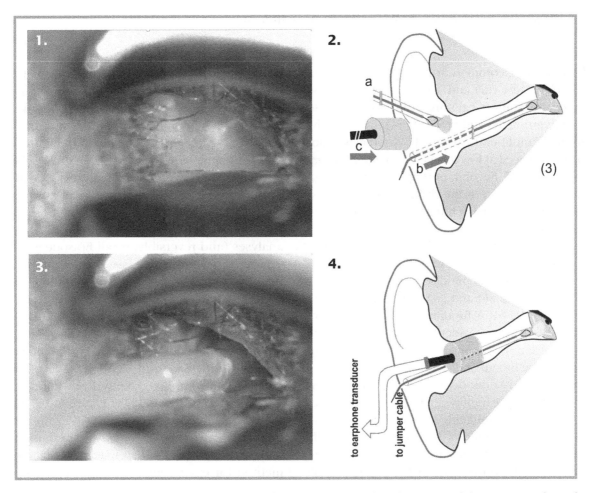

Figure 5–15. A virtual demonstration of placing a tymptrode. The point of departure is that of otoscopy (**1**). The flexible tube and lead of the electrode assembly is slowly advanced (**2a** and **2b**) to have the electrode's soft tip just contact the eardrum (**3**). While keeping the tymptrode securely in position, the foam tip of the sound delivery tube is advanced to plug the ear canal laterally (**2c** and **4**) to hold the tymptrode in place (**4**). Note: The connection of the foam tip to the tubing, in turn connected to the earphone transducer, will have been done beforehand as well as having the electrode wire clipped to a lead plugged into the recording electrode interface. (Photographs, steps 1 and 3, courtesy of Dr. P. Kileny.)

Table 5-2. TM Recording Parameters

Electrode Configuration
TM (+ input) – to – Contralateral Earlobe/Mastoid (– input); nasion (ground)
Signal Averaging
Analysis Time: 5–10 msec (click); 20 msec (tone burst)   Analog Filter Bandpass: 3 Hz–3000 Hz
Stimuli
Type: Broadband click (100 μsec electrical pulse);   Tone burst (2 cycle rise/fall; 10 cycle plateau)   Frequency: 1000 Hz, 2000 Hz   Rate: 11.1/s   Beginning Level: 90 dB nHL

configuration. A common approach is the use of a tymptrode (test ear) and a surface electrode on the opposite/nontest ear's mastoid, connected to the noninverting (+) and inverting (–) inputs of the differential amplifier, respectively. Another surface electrode is placed at low forehead/nasion and connected to ground. Second, perhaps seeming counterintuitive at a glance, is the choice of the high-pass (HP) setting of the analog filter (recording amplifier stage), optimally requiring a lower frequency cutoff than common to that of the ABR. In fact, this is more characteristic (on that side of the bandwidth) of recordings of middle or even long latency responses. To explain and as demonstrated in the last episode, the SP is fundamentally a DC potential. It still must be considered as "quasi-DC" even when recorded in response to very brief, transient stimuli like the broadband click.[28] On the one hand, it can withstand some degree of high-pass filtering through the preamplifier, namely toward better baseline stability. Simulating a click-elicited SP and submitting it to a range of high-pass-filter cutoffs demonstrates indeed that settings up to 100 Hz are workable. On the other hand, 3 Hz to 5 Hz is still preferred. This is because the pathological SP not only is enlarged in amplitude but also often broadened. The response can look like a substantially lower-frequency transient than the "normal" click-elicited SP-AP complex, as shown in Figure 5–16A. Consequently, more conservative (analog) filtering is preferred to avoid risk of untoward distortion of the true SP, especially in cases of suspected or confirmed MD/ELH and given that more aggressive filtering can be applied digitally in subsequent analyses (and reversibly; recall Episode 4.2).

So important is this issue and an understanding of what might have happened to the ECochGm recorded with a 150-Hz cutoff of the HP, more scrutiny and information will be useful to consider before moving on to clinical interests. This will be another virtual demonstration, a sort of mini-sequel to the "Good, Bad, and Ugly" episode of the last chapter and jumping directly from good to ugly. The first step (see panel B of Figure 5–16) wherein the two tracings, for a more critical examination of their respective time histories, are overlaid in reference to their respective baselines. This time-honored method for examining similarities/differences be-

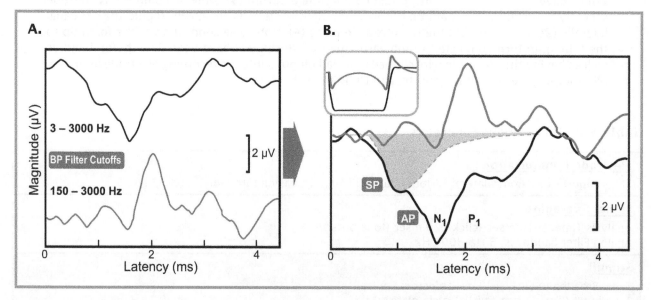

Figure 5–16. A. Examples of ECochG tracings using two different filter bandwidths, particularly with regard to the high-pass (low-frequency) cutoff: top—appropriate settings; bottom—excessive filtering, leading to unacceptable distortion of the SP-AP complex and results not permitting valid interpretation of the recorded response. **B.** In-depth analysis (see text).

tween tracings of responses takes a radical, yet enlightening, twist. "Overlay" is perhaps an overstatement, more like back to back. Nonetheless, it cannot hurt to check it out; it certainly suggests that there is more going on than readily meets the eye, yet not necessarily mysteriously. Reminder: the acoustic click is the result of a kind of band-pass filter, having been elicited by a DC pulse, even a very brief one at that. Remarkable changes are seen in the time domain for the frequency-domain "shaping" of this input signal (recall Figure 2–19). Recall also Figure 4–15; the brainstem response was substantially "deflated" with the use of a similar and still more extreme HP cutoff frequencies.

The model-transient SP from Figure 5–11B suggested a clear trend if that component presents in its "native," nonpathological form. That model has been fitted here (back to Figure 5–16B) to what looks otherwise like a typical onset ("shoulder") of the SP. At the same time, there is a lot of something more going on and looking also like a quasi-DC component or extension, which the 150-Hz cutoff has deflated markedly. However, this is where meeting the eye is a tough call, because the AP has been distorted profoundly too and is adding to the complexity in still other ways. An idea of the nature of an underlying distortion of such filtering that is predictable from the math of the underlying transfer function is given by the inset figure of panel B. Suppose, indeed, something like a more persistent DC component is involved, perhaps nearly 3 ms of duration. The black line is a test signal of this sort, filtered minimally, as in the 3-Hz- to 3000-Hz condition. The gray-line function is the result of imposing the filtering like that involving the 150-Hz HP cutoff. Such heavy-handed filtering can be expected to bias remarkably the representation of such a real response, namely on both ends and the middle! These results nicely demonstrate just how bizarre the effects can be in actual practice, as follows: The initial SP and largely AP N_1 have both been nearly flip-flopped from negative (N)-like to positive (P)-like components at the outset. Again, the middle of the waveform is clearly at risk for severe distortion (the deflationlike effect); meanwhile, the AP N_1, by this same bias, has been dragged up nearly to baseline. In contrast, on the far side, the actual slight P_1 of the more conventionally recorded response is now a behemoth, and a secondary positive peak thrown in at the end.

Bottom line: most of what the ECochG examiner is seeking to measure, for practical purposes, is gone—according to conventional interpretation. However, a supposition was hinted previously, made here, and must be and shortly will be pursued. For the moment, the point of argument is still at the more fundamental level of signals and systems. A signal is a signal, regardless of origin (electrical, bioelectrical, electromagnetic, etc.). Relative to its true time history and given a signal with both DC and AC components in the complex's makeup, heavy-handedly filtering can make it very difficult to disentangle effects of multiple influences expressed in a given recorded response, whether stimulus, recording, normal phenomena, and/or pathological factors are involved. For example, simply stimulating a normally functioning ear with a 3-ms tone burst could produce much the same ECochGm; however, the stimulus in this case was a click presented to a pathological ear. Now off to the clinical realm of ECochG that has been its iconic place in medical audiology, namely in differential diagnosis of MD/ELH.

Idiopathic ELH has indeed a long history of interest in relation to clinical neurophysiology, dating back to the mid 1970s.[35-37] Although the literature is rife with manuscripts dealing with the nature, causes, diagnoses, and treatment of MD, the true pathophysiology of this disease remains elusive. The drawing in Figure 5–17 illustrates the classical viewpoint—the distention of Reissner's membrane in the face of endolymphatic hydrops that is postulated to lead to the symptoms associated with MD. Unfortunately, there is neither a cure nor an effective treatment for MD that works for all patients. Classically, MD presents with symptoms that include recurrent spontaneous vertigo, hearing loss (often beginning in the lower frequencies), aural fullness/pressure, and tinnitus (American Academy of Otolaryngology-Head and Neck Foundation, Inc. Committee on Hearing and Equilibrium[38]). However, the presence, severity, and prevalence of these symptoms tend to vary among and within patients, making the diagnosis of MD with a high degree of certainty challenging at best.

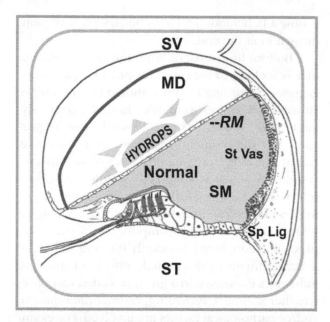

Figure 5–17. Concept of distention of Reissner's membrane, gray line in this quasischematic illustration, as has been documented by results of temporal-bone histological study (postmortem). Normal—normal position of the RM—Reissner's membrane; SV, SM, and ST—scala vestibuli, media, and tympani respectively; MD—Meniere's disease; St Vas—stria vascularis; Sp Lig—spiral ligament. (Adaptation of Figure 3–8B.)

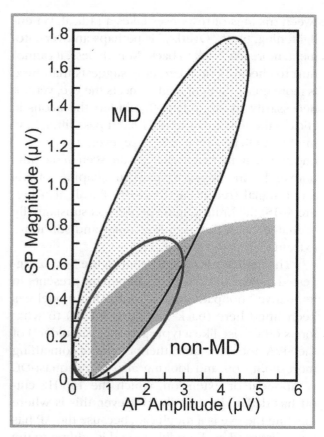

Figure 5–18. Given populations of patients, bivariate normal distributions might be assumed (as a common statistical model upon which to base establishment of diagnostic criteria). Normal variability of the SP and AP includes ranges of values, but not varying necessarily together, defining elliptical areas of confidence (statistically) of presumably clinically nonsignificant findings. Results outside this area are then suspect as pathological findings, as modeled in this figure (estimated based on samples from a clinical study). Elliptical areas drawn fit the vast majority of the values reported for cochlear/non-hydropic cases (*open, gray outline*) versus patients diagnosed as having Meniere's disease (*stippled area outlined in black*). While substantial overlap (given low values of both parameters in both subgroups), the considerably larger dispersion of SP-per-AP amplitudes of the MD patients sampled is evident. Light gray area: reference confidence limits (the "clinic's norms") for presumptive nonpathologic subjects for the particular extratympanic method used. Based on data of Coats [1981].[25]

A valid and reliable test that is both sensitive and specific to MD/ELH thus has been sought for decades, namely as a component of research and development in audiological/otological applications of clinical electrophysiology. A truly valid and reliable test has not been easy to come by, no thanks to a disease that is characteristically dynamic throughout its course. A given effect of ELH is thus, at times, a "moving target." Research in the senior author's and others' laboratories and clinics has come to refine ECochG to the level of high sensitivity and specificity—proficiently and correctly detecting ELH. In particular, as shown in Figures 5–18 and 5–19, it is well documented that the ECochGms of patients with MD/ELH often show an enlarged SP, especially when compared to the AP.[10,12,36–45]

Although never proven, the conventional rationale for this finding is that excessive endolymph production creates abnormal pressure on the organ of Corti—theoretically biasing the vibration of the basilar membrane, in turn offsetting the hair cell's transfer function. Recalling Figure 5–10, presence of the SP was seen as a temporal distortion—an AC signal was input to the transducer, but the response appeared as a "lopsided" CM (nominally an AC signal), so it is a change in such distortion that is manifest in the altered form of the measured SP (a gross/multicellular recording of hair-cell receptor potentials). This begs the question of whether an

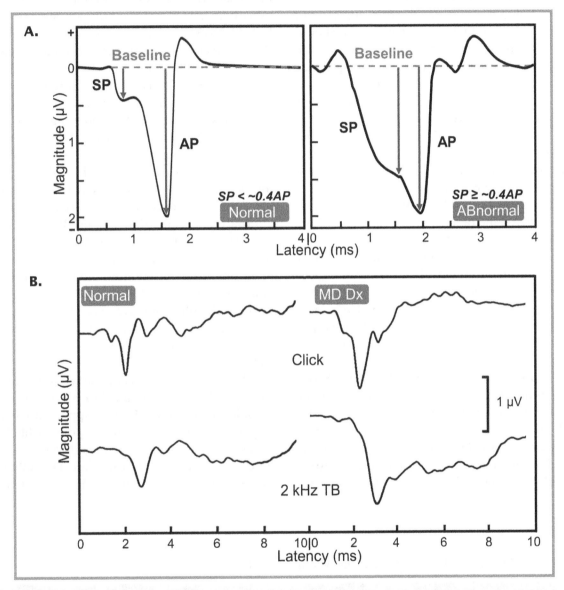

Figure 5–19. A. SP and AP measures in cases without (replot from Figure 5–12A) and with MD/hydrops, and the determination of the SP/AP ratio. Based on actual recordings (courtesy of Dr. R. E. Delgado). **B.** Follow-up to results in Figure 5–12B, comparisons between click and tone-burst responses, here focusing on the contrast of recordings in cases with and without otological diagnoses of Meniere's disease. In the latter, as the click-elicited response is only marginally abnormal, although suspicious by the apparent widening of the SP-AP complex (as hinted earlier and to be discussed further), adding the tone-burst trial provided another level of confidence to interpretation, confirming the working diagnosis of hydrops.

enlarged SP is due to mechanical bias.[36] This is a matter of whether hydrops literally lead to a biased motion of the basilar membrane, as presumed the effect of a distended Reissner's membrane (a hydromechanical effect). If the outer hair cells remain viable at some level, then at least any such bias must be considered electromechanical;[46,47] this opens the door wider to possible underlying mechanism(s), including vascular and/or biochemical. The details have yet to be resolved.[35,42] Still, the mechanical-biasing theory remains a popular perspective. As true in some other areas of hearing science, it at least is a useful heuristic model that has served research well. It is parsimonious (as science "loves") and is didactic, facilitating some level of learning and comprehension that is generally consistent with effects of idiopathic hydrops, whether or not the right mechanism.

Enlargement of the SP/AP amplitude ratio has been considered the benchmark of an ELH-positive ECochGm for decades. As revealed in Table 5–3, patients with a positive ECochGm are almost always diagnosed with ELH. However, nearly 50% of suspected ELH patients from whom ECochGms were negative for this disorder also received a positive diagnosis.[41,48] Thus, while the SP/AP amplitude ratio alone enjoys excellent specificity, its sensitivity to ELH is relatively low.

Several studies in the first author's laboratory have been devoted to improving the sensitivity of ECochG while maintaining high specificity. The first of these were focused on the association of test outcome of ECochG exams and the symptoms reported by patients at the time of testing.[41] Results indicated that suspected Meniere's patients who reported hearing loss and aural fullness at the time of testing were the ones most likely to have an enlarged SP/AP amplitude ratio. However, testing patients only when they were symptomatic proved to be challenging, at best. These challenges led to examining the utility of measuring the *duration of the SP/AP complex* in addition to the amplitude ratio between these two components. The bases for this investigation were reports of "widening" of the SP-AP complex in suspected Meniere's patients when evoked by click stimuli presented in alternating polarity.[39,49] This effect, hinted earlier, is illustrated further in Figure 5–20A (upper panels). The likely reason for this widening is an abnormally large latency difference between N_1 components evoked by rarefaction- versus condensation-polarity clicks that manifested itself as a widening of the SP/AP complex when alternating polarity clicks were used as the evoking stimuli.[49] An alternative computation to the SP/AP ratio thus was proposed, based on estimations of the *area of the SP-AP complex*. Areas under the curve of functions are more complicated to measure mathematically, requiring the help of a computer algorithm and, still, some judgment by the examiner. In-depth discussion is beyond the scope here but the main principles are illustrated by Figure 5–20A, as follows.

The first step, indeed, starts with estimating the overall area (specifically) of the SP-AP(N_1) complex (see Figure 5–20A, upper panels). This requires a judgment of the response's likely true baseline, as residual noise "plays" equally with the baseline and potential of interest. This initial step in the algorithm is as if testing a null hypothe-

Table 5–3. Chi-Squared Results for ECochG Versus Diagnosis for EH/MD

	Positive Diagnosis of EH/MS	Negative Diagnosis of EH/MD	Total
Positive ECochG	51	2	53
Negative ECochG	24	26	50
Total	75	28	103

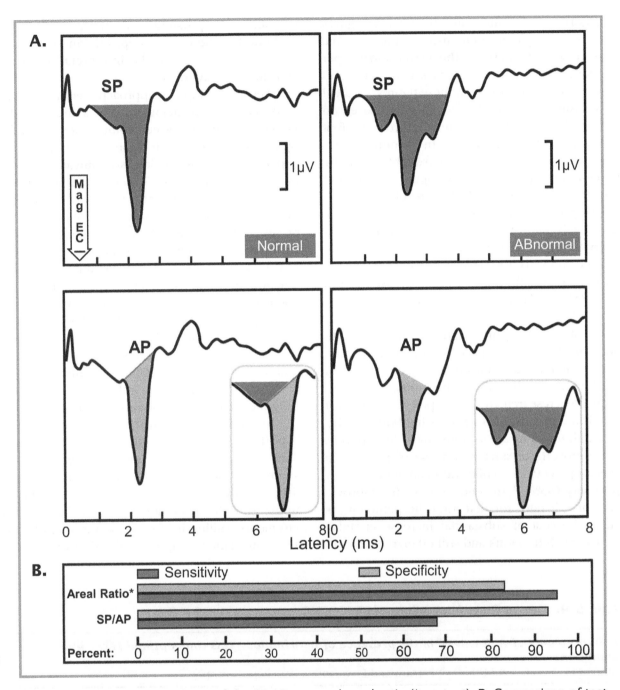

Figure 5–20. **A.** Measurement of the SP-AP area and areal ratio (*see text). **B.** Comparison of test performance (per sensitivity and specificity measures) between the two measures. The numbers used from the conventional SP/AP ratio were computed from Table 5–3.

sis, in this case, that the complex might be all SP! The next step is then to estimate that of the AP alone, as shown in the bottom panels. Why? This is because the AP(N_1) proves—both in concept and practice—to be the more consistent component in terms of waveform. Even in the face pathology, its morphology is fairly consistent, and it is that of the SP that is "suspect" here—the victim of significant morphological changes resulting from hydrops. Overlaying top to bottom graphs as virtually what the algorithm does, illustrated by the inset figures of the bottom panels, demonstrates the outcome measure sought. These are the areal estimates per component—SP and AP, demarked by dark and light gray fill, respectively, in these figures. An areal ratio is then computed by the algorithm based on the (nominally) "SP" area estimated from the first step and "AP" from the second. In the normal case, this estimate approximates reasonably well the model-transient SP (compare Figure 5–20A, bottom left, to Figure 5–11B). The resultant ratio is naturally a number ≥ 1.0; the larger the ratio, the more likely indicative it is of a significant abnormality (panel A, bottom right). This measure demonstrates improved performance as a clinical test, but most recent findings support the use of both the SP/AP and areal ratios in making the diagnostic "call."

As shown in Figure 5–20B, combining amplitude and durational features in the interpretation further enhances test sensitivity,[50] again the side of past findings of clinical-ECochG studies left wanting, despite research and development toward best technical methods. Measuring/using both the SP/AP amplitude and areal ratios, most importantly, has improved the sensitivity value of ECochG in detecting MD (95%) while still maintaining a high specificity (83%).[51] In other words, the improvement of "hit rate" for detecting the pathology is not at the cost of substantial increase in "false alarms." Such tradeoffs and still other/related considerations are pursued in a subsequent chapters. As hinted in the previous episode and evidenced herein, they pertain to the interpretation of any clinical test (stay tuned).

The extratympanic approach has been shown to be entirely efficacious; at the same time, ET-ECochG can be performed competently and safely by nonphysicians—with appropriate training and experience—using a painless/noninvasive recording approach. TT-ECochG indeed can help assess, diagnose, and/or monitor the treatment of MD/ELH. Correct detection of EHL with low false positives can be realized. Unfortunately, and as indicated earlier, the various protocols used to perform and measure ECochG continue to vary considerably among both practitioners, who use this tool in their clinics, and scientists, who study it in their laboratories. Efforts are ongoing in attempts to address this concern via some more recent studies with the aspiration to standardize ECochG recording and measurement protocols.[52,53] This goal remains an important one for future clinical research, indeed essential to realizing the most robust evidence-based practice.

In summary, ECochG has proven to be an important clinical test of inner ear/8th nerve function especially in the diagnosis, assessment, and treatment monitoring of MD/ELH. It is most sensitive to these disorders when both the SP/AP amplitude AND area ratios are included in the measurements. Failing to do so is at the risk of missing confirmation of upward of half of the patients

Table 5–4. Current Other Applications of ET-ECOCHG

Enhancements of ABR wave I in the presence of hearing loss/less-than-optimal recording conditions   Ruth et al.[44]; Yanz and Dodds[54]; Ferraro and Ferguson[55]; Bauch and Olsen[56]
Intraoperative monitoring of inner ear/auditory nerve function   Ferraro and Durrant[29]; Ruben and Sekula[57]; Koka et al.[58]; Kileny[59]
Diagnosis of auditory neuropathy/auditory neuropathy spectrum disorder   Rance et al.[60]; Starr et al.[61]; Riazi and Ferraro[62]
Diagnosis of "hidden hearing loss"   Bramhall et al.[52]; Stamper and Johnson[63]; Liberman et al.[64]
Diagnosis of superior semicircular canal dehiscence (SSCD) and monitoring the surgical repair of this condition   Ferraro et al.[53]

who are indeed likely to have MD/ELH. Although this clinical application continues to be its best-established conventional application, several other uses for this test have been reported over the years and continue to emerge and/or be refined. Current applications are summarized in Table 5–4 with relevant citations per evidence bases. Some of the applications listed will be discussed subsequently, starting with the feature up next and the episode to follow.

HEADS UP

Intriguing ECochG App: Sensing Weakened Wall of Semicircular Canal

The panlike bottom of the cranium naturally supports the brain. The skull bone is pretty tough, but how tough is it? Apparently, not always quite tough enough to fully isolate the intracranial volume of matter and fluid from the cochlea's close relative and neighbor, the *peripheral vestibular system* or *vestibular apparatus*. What has this to do with the continuing saga of ECochG? A clue is the effect of hydrops, but not hydrops. The moral to the story is that indeed, electrophysiological tools, like ECochG, are functional tests (rather than etiological tests); press certain "buttons" physiologically, related results can occur. This is such a story, but also a retrospective, looking back a half-decade ago at research findings that potentially support/validate the use ECochG in yet another application.

A portion of the cranium separates the brain from other nearby neurophysiological and cranial vascular systems in the head, including the vestibular system's *superior semicircular canal (SSC)*. Any adverse effects to this important part of the balance system can lead to debilitating dizziness. The SCCs and other parts of both the vestibular and cochlear parts of the inner ear generally are protected well by the tough petrous bone (pyramid). Although fortunately rare, SSC *dehiscence (SSCD)*—a thinning of the overlying bone—occurs in some patients.[59,65,66] Hard to think of bone becoming so thin that it is flexible, but that apparently is what happens. This allows the bone to give enough to act as a sort of third window into the inner ear, in reference to the normal two—the oval and round windows.

There is considerable discussion in the literature about both the variety of functional effects possible on both vestibular and auditory sides and the possible detailed underlying mechanisms.[66] The vestibular and auditory sides of the inner ear naturally share common fluid systems. Although much goes on differently between them functionally, they certainly cannot be viewed as isolated systems. The possibility that the SP would be sensitive to hydromechanical effects, as postulated to be the basis of the effect of cochlear hydrops, suggests that it might have something to say about introducing ad hoc another pressure valve to the system. In fact, the SP has been shown to be affected acutely by SSCD and dramatically can demonstrate changes during surgical repair of a SSCD.[67] As mentioned earlier and to be overviewed later, ECochG (whether ET or TT) is a tool readily applicable to *intraoperative neurophysiological monitoring (IONM)*. Illustrated in Figure 5–21 (see overlaid models of recordings) are the sort of changes that can be tracked in the course of such surgery, in this case, a remarkably abnormal SP/AP ratio that equally remarkably returned to within normal limits upon completion of the surgical repair.

The anatomy involved and comparable effects of SSCD to those of cochlear hydrops on the SP/AP certainly offer strong validity to the theory attributing the enlargement of this ratio to a hydromechanical bias, yet this is not exactly how this may be happening.

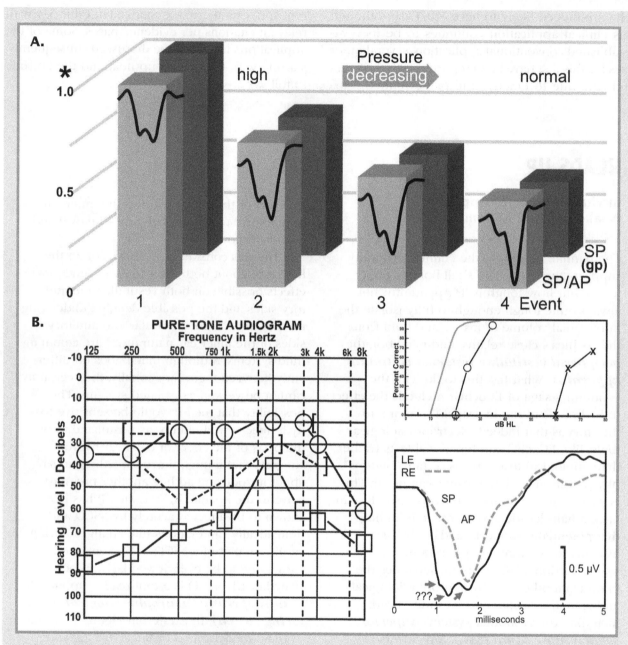

Figure 5–21. A. Events compared in the course of putative changes in perilymphatic pressure mechanically biasing hair-cell transduction of sound eliciting summating potentials. Foreground: Characteristic, human surgical case: sequential tests of SP/AP in the course of repair of a semicircular canal dehiscence (taken here to effectively decrease the source of bias—pressure.[68]) Background: Animal surgical case, guinea pig (gp): intracochlear-recording of the SP in the basal turn of the cochlea; measurements at different phases of a very low-frequency bias to which a high-frequency sinusoidal pulse was superimposed to elicit SPs at from 90° down to 0° hence at different times within the cycle of the bias signal, effecting relatively high-to-low bias pressure, respectively.[69] Modeled from data from reports cited. **B.** Clinical workup of a related case. Question marks: the challenge of wave form interpretation, yet not necessarily always a question of response abnormality (see text).

Where is the empirical evidence of cause and effect, literally? The tricky aspect is that of where this secondary pressure valve is inserted into the combined hydraulic systems. It is not immediately obvious that the third window is positioned well to bias the vibration pattern of the cochlear partition (scale media contents and both the Reissner's and the basilar membranes). It is not necessarily enough to just apply pressure to perilymph to affect the SP, in the case demonstrating an apparent enhancement of the potential. The cochlea generally is expected to balance static and even very low-frequency pressure difference between the two perilymphatic scalae—vestibuli and tympani—by way of the movable stapes footplate in the oval window and the round window membrane, respectively, via the helicotrema at the apex (permitting fluid flow between them). In any event, effective biasing of basilar membrane motion must favorably move the nominal operating point ("resting position") of the hair cells' input-output functions in the vicinity of the traveling waves actually eliciting the recorded SP. Results of IONM have been useful at times to test/confirm notions of the generation of AEPs, but are not conducive (ethically or practically) for undertaking the sorts of studies needed to fully test theories in humans.

Research in species like the guinea pig have permitted important experiments on the likely functioning of the human peripheral auditory system. Both species are mammalian with inner ears that share the mechanisms of a coiled cochlea, but that of the guinea pig is relatively freestanding, rather than buried deeply in one of the toughest bones of the body. As noted earlier, more of the cochlea is readily accessible in this animal and other rodents versus primates, even cats or dogs. In the pioneering days of cochlear electrophysiology, this animal model proved to be a great ally to hearing scientists. Excellent electronic and computational technology progressed to enable highly sensitive and reliable recordings of potentials from within the cochlea (such as in Figure 5–10). Taking their lead from an earlier research group—literally drilling a hole in the cochlear wall to infuse fluid to manipulate static pressure applied to scala tympani[68]—an approach was developed in Peter Dallos's lab to confirm those findings. Furthermore, the interest was to increase the scope of study comprehensively to the SP, which at that time was under intense scrutiny in his lab. However, this renewed interest was not that replication; rather it was the idea to test effects of mechanical bias on hair-cell transduction under strictly normal physiological conditions, namely by biasing basilar displacement dynamically and specifically without the surgical risk of perfusion.[69] This was accomplished by superimposing a relatively high-frequency stimulus for the SP on the basalward skirts of traveling waves headed to the apex, namely elicited by a much lower frequency carrier. A subset of the results are represented in Figure 5–21A. Therein, the SP/AP values taken from the surgical case are represented in parallel to data from the experimental case, simply as two sets of sequential events theoretically attributable to the same effects—both manifestations of changing perilymphatic pressure biasing of hair-cell transduction.

Another case in point and a prequel to differential diagnosis (coming soon) is that of a middle-aged male patient who presented recently at coauthor Barajas' clinic complaining of vertigo with a spinning sensation, particularly upon getting up from lying down in bed and/or with head movement, mainly to the right. The episodes of dizziness could last several hours, but without loss of consciousness at any time. He also reported tinnitus in the left ear. Audiological evaluation (Figure 5–21B) demonstrated hearing loss bilaterally, but substantially worse on the left. The loss on the right presented as purely sensorineural and of mild degree except above 4000 Hz. The audiogram for the left ear was more complicated, including a largely rising configuration up to 2000 Hz, so overall worse hearing sensitivity at lower frequencies. The configuration also included an unusual/inverted notch. Last but not trivial, there was an apparent conductive component.

At first impression, it might be supposed that the patient had already a bilateral SN loss much like that of the right ear. If so, another pathology or two—as a mixed loss affecting the left ear must be afoot. Results of speech audiometry (speech recognition tested in this case at several levels above the detection limit in each ear) also potentially support the impression of a mixed loss, as conventionally defined. The patient seemingly did not demonstrate benefit of recruitment as expected in purely SN pathologies of cochlear origin, rather indeed behaving potentially more like a conductive loss. Still, there was the symptom that most compelled the patient to come to the clinic. He was dizzy. What gives!

Further differential diagnostic testing certainly was in order, and the next step taken was ET-ECochG with a sample recording shown in Figure 5–21B (black-lined function). It is shown overlapping (for reference, gray-lined function) the grand-average TT-ECochGm from a series of patients' recordings from this clinic and typical of normal click-ECochGm morphology. So which little bump in the patient's waveform is what? The first impression is the slight shoulderlike inflection near the overall waveform maximum (most-negative value) together with the next peak defining the AP(N_1) onset and it maximum. However, this begs the question, what is the second bump—an N_2 (secondary neural-firing component)? This impression is wrong, as it defies realistic timing of the AP(N_1) relative to what it is—a compound action potential. Per the reference signal, the first nuances are just that, noise or whatever in the SP signal's detailed temporal characteristics in this case. Rather, the second bump (which proved to be repeatable) is the most likely candidate for the AP(N_1). This perspective is supported on the grounds of both the agreement with timing issues just summarized as well as the "experimental"

human subject's sequence of recovery of the normal response complex (again, panel A). That sequence starts from a nearly identically "bloated" waveform before surgical intervention began to take effect, having started with an overall envelope containing hair-cell and neural activity—broadened waveform but with two slight bumps. In time and progressive improvement in the response, they then "roll out" to be SP and AP components in their natural waveforms and respectively normal proportions.

As an aside, yet important reminder, are issues of interpretation. The last episode established the limitations of the more basic convention of ECochG and thereby clinical decisions—that of reliance soley upon the SP/AP ratio. Still useful, but to improve sensitivity of the test in cases of MD, required another analysis, based on presumptive areas of the waveform attributable to SP versus AP. Interpretation remains the judgment and responsibility of the examiner; no computer algorithm will likely fix this. On the one hand (here) and taken in isolation, the observed response is more challenging to assign peaks and/or areas with confidence. On the other, the point is moot for a precise decision that (a) it is abnormal and (b) the abnormality is attributable of an "enlarged" SP. The reference tracing makes it evident why this must be so. Much of the "corpus" of the recorded response initially must be SP by latency considerations alone (as a presynaptic potential) as well as magnitude! So large is the SP in this case as to obscure what area is truly AP(N_1). As these two components are adding in both magnitude and time, voila—the broader overall appearance of the complex. This is not the only example of arriving at a moot point by less-than-perfect (in effect) peak picking. In lectures over the years, the authors have often been approached by disgruntled clinicians complaining of not always being able to clearly identify the SP, even in known normal cases. Click-ECochG may not readily demonstrate the SP, especially if optimal electrode placement and a fully acceptable, residual noise floor are not realized. Nevertheless, if the subject of the test is a patient being evaluated to help rule out MD/hydrops and the clinician at least has observed a normal AP (or acceptable for degree of cochlear-SN hearing loss), a minimal/undetectable SP means an SP/AP ratio approaching zero. Conclusion: a negative finding. Now back to the story.

A massively abnormal SP was observed in the case at hand, wherein the SP dominated the ECochGm. Meniere's disease? Not compellingly from the overall picture, including (on the audiometric side) that mysterious conductive component and especially since the rest of the patient's history and findings by otoscopy were negative. Even the issues of balance system involvement (as seems likely from reported symptoms) are not characteristic of attacks that bring those MD patients to the clinic (often days later because they were so sick from vertigo, per the last episode). The primary suspicion soon gravitated to SSCD; indeed, this patient's ECochGm resembles well that appearing on the #1 bar in Figure 5–21A (essentially the "prepressure relief" condition of this virtual experiment). The patient thus was referred for an imaging study which confirmed the tentative diagnosis—presence of an SSCD—and was followed up by further medical management.

So, what about that conductive component—for real? Yes, in its way but just not literally (as commonly assumed) to reflect a site of lesion in the outer or middle ear. Following up the earlier background, it must be borne in mind that the oval window is in the vestibule, a "chamber" common to both the auditory and vestibular parts of the inner ear also with "plumbing" substantially in common. Messing with this elaborate fluid-filled system mechanically—whether on the hearing or balance side—potentially can change the effective mechanical load on the stapes footplate's vibration.[70]

In a historical meeting in the 1970s, key basic and clinical researchers from around the globe working in cochlear electrophysiology congregated to share their insights from both the laboratory and (then just emerging) clinical findings of ECochG.[71] The question, in effect, was as follows: Was ECochG in humans truly ready for "primetime" in the clinic? Battles ensued about what role ECochG would play. Inevitably, this remains debatable, but overall the rest indeed was history. ECochG is a method that has kept on giving, both didactically and practically, and the saga continues.

Episode 4: What More Can Electrocochleography Teach, Including About What to Expect Later?

Electrocochleography has had varied interest clinically, yet a recent resurgence overall, including TT-ECochG and in any event remains of fundamental interest. The development and "classical" application of ECochG in the differential diagnosis of Meniere's disease (as discussed extensively in the previous episode) played a substantial role in the development of ERA and such applications in the early years wherein it was performed via the transtympanic approach under local anesthesia.[72-74] Historically, ECochG was demonstrated to provide a sensitive method of ERA, which provides some of the best estimations of thresholds, excellent evaluations of ABR wave I magnitude and latency, and an objective basis of assessing a recruitmentlike effect at the level of the cochlear amplifier and the auditory nerve of the auditory periphery (see Figure 5–22, comparing results between cases—normal hearing on the left and sensory hearing loss on the right). TT-lessons learned until the 1960s together with fundamental work in animals have continued to give ECochG the foundational importance in the clinical knowledge base. Newer applications have breathed new life into both extratympanic and transtympanic approaches to the very early AEPs, the evoked responses of cochlear origin.

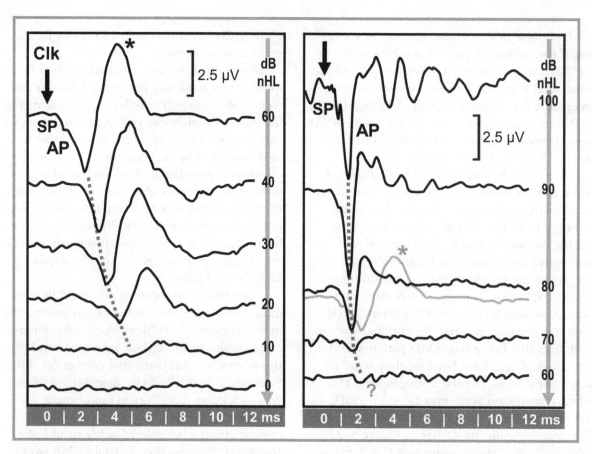

Figure 5–22. *Left*: Transtympanic ECochG results in a normal hearing subject, demonstrating click-evoked APs down to a limit of visual detection of 10 dB nHL. The dotted gray curve is fitted to the trend of N_1 peak latencies (to be revisited later in this episode). Right: Results in a subject with sensory hearing loss wherein the response is evident only down to 70 dB (that is, proving in the full analysis to be reproducible at this level, versus questionable/absent in fact at 60 dB). Yet, full-blown responses are observed within +20 dB of this detection limit, thus demonstrating the recruitment behavior of the N_1 component. The sharp growth toward a nearly normal response at high stimulus levels is further underlined by the different/minimal curvature of the dotted line. The "normal" response at 60 dB on the left is overlaid (*gray-line tracing*) on the right at 80 dB, which best matches between cases. This again underscores the dramatic growth in response in the face of such an elevation of sensitivity in this case, typical of the loudness recruitment effect often observed in patients with sensory hearing losses.

The interest and indication criteria for ECochG have increased in the last decade, and in addition to testing patients for possible endolymphatic hydrops in MD, the application has expanded to very young and older children, as well as adults, who are cochlear-implant (CI) candidates. These are patients lacking any other evidence of residual hearing, patients with inner ear malformations, temporal bone fractures, aplasia or hypoplasia of the 8th nerve, or cases of auditory synaptopathy or neuropathy. TT-ECochG is the most sensitive instrument for the clinical evaluation of the peripheral auditory system, which provides the best understanding of pathologic changes of the cochlea, including the auditory nerve, and delivers the most accurate indication for cochlear implantation in a given ear. TT-ECochG provides similar but more sensitive information compared to ET-ECochG, thus offering access to cochlear pre- and postsynaptic near-field potentials of the outer and inner hair cells and afferent fibers of the 8th nerve. Amplitudes of potentials recorded via TT-ECochG are 4 to 5 times higher compared to those from more distal near-field or upward of 10-fold toward far-field recording sites (lateral ear canal, ipsilateral earlobe, or mastoid). Excellent SNRs are often realized without disturbance of responses from the contralateral ear. It always has to be qualified, however, that TT-ECochG can only be performed under local (adults) or general anesthesia (children), as the needle electrode has to be placed through the tympanic membrane precisely onto the promontory.

As revealed in the last Heads Up feature, there are also important applications of the TT approach in intraoperative monitoring, where the 8th nerve may be affected (again, a topic of a later episode). Suffice it to say here that, due to the excellent SNR, it takes just a few seconds of averaging to evaluate the functional status of the 8th nerve during surgery (likely under general anesthesia, so in a patient who is quite sedate). In some surgical procedures, for example, acoustic (nerve) tumor surgery, recording also can be made with another type of electrode (e.g., a cotton wick or ball electrode) placed in the round window niche, but again requires a myringotomy or a posterior tympanotomy.

The placement of an electrode on the promontory or the round window offers another interesting clinical application: the combination of ECochG and preoperative testing electrically elicited ABRs, where the needle electrode can be used for electrical stimulation of the auditory nerve prior to cochlear or brainstem implantation. This area of interest too will be discussed in a later episode (dedicated to testing AEPs overall in CI patients). Issues noted here are simply to demonstrate the increasingly broad applications of ECochG.

The recording of AEPs is essential for many preoperative assessments, and TT-ECochG should be considered when other tests, like ABR and/or ET-ECochG, provide inadequate information. Results from earlier works at the very least have provided important foundational information toward research and development of purely noninvasive approaches, like threshold estimation using chirps for ABR or ASSR tests (coming soon). This includes subsequent results across tests that concur or reveal still better threshold estimates than expected, which is important (for example) in outcomes anticipated from such treatments as cochlear implantation. Such results may be indicative of remaining viable fibers of a likely damaged/malformed 8th nerve in the CI candidate. Figure 5–23 shows the conventional audiogram (panel A) in a patient and results (panel B) of both click- and frequency-specific threshold estimation using narrow band chirps in an 8-month-old child via ABR and TT-ECochG testing. The patient was considered a CI candidate. The threshold estimates from these tests have been plotted as well on the audiogram (panel A), confirming the treatment to be justified—a viable population of neurons with which to work. The results at the same time provide evidence of a potentially better prognosis to offer the parents, as the estimated hearing thresholds via ERA are significantly better than the behavioral audiogram would suggest. This portends indeed a better functional status of the 8th nerve than expected and even though the 8th nerve is still likely to be severely underdeveloped.

Though not up to expectations historically, the CM has enjoyed a considerable level of renewed interest as well, thus not just the SP. Together with OAE testing, this potential can provide a useful presynaptic test of hair-cell function. To recap, the origin of the CM is the activity of hair cells mainly (as commonly recorded via noninvasive methods) from the basal turn of the cochlea.[75] At audiometric frequencies, the CM inherently reflects the time history of the stimulus. The CM amplitudes reflect partially some active mechanisms of the cochlear amplifier, as noted in Episode 5.1. Recordings of the CM in a child with a history of profound hearing loss are shown in Figure 5–24. They thus can show, seemingly illogically, higher amplitudes in some hearing-loss cases, commonly in cases suspected of an auditory neuropathy spectrum disorder (ANSD). Such results potentially implicate an involvement of the olivo-cochlear bundle (OCB). The response is often so robust in such cases as to give it some special attention and discussion of a now-common way to look at the CM.

To explain, first a recap regarding rarefaction and condensation clicks/stimuli, with the aid of the inset in the top panel of Figure 5–24 (adapted from Figure 2–19, panel A). The predominant initial

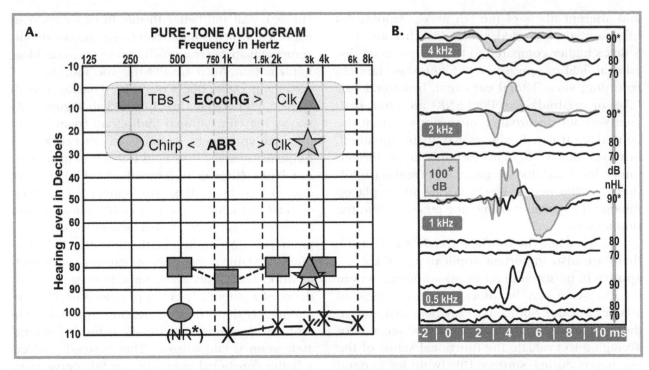

Figure 5–23. Hearing threshold estimates in an 8-month-old child with a profound loss of hearing. **A.** Plots of several measures as indicated, in addition to those based on tests of auditory brainstem responses and electrocochleography. TBs (tone bursts)—estimations using frequency-specific stimuli; Clk—click stimuli; NR—no response. X—X: left-ear, pure-tone audiometric findings; at 500 Hz, NR at 110, although a response was observed at 115 dB. **B.** TT-ECochG measurements using tone bursts at different frequencies (as indicated). For 1 kHz to 4 kHz, 90 dB trace in black (as will be all others) is shown overlaying the gray-line tracing and fill for the response also tested at 100 dB nHL (to increase confidence in the data). A relatively high stimulus rate was used (37.3/s) to enhance test efficiency. Magnitude of responses relative with the same scale factor across all conditions.

"polarity" (phasing) of the resultant response of the transducer to the brief DC pulse is nominally rarefaction (R) versus condensation (C). Yet, there still is some oscillation, thus in reality some amount of R and C regardless of polarity of the pulsatile input signal. The CM follows accordingly, so it is interesting to overlay the respective responses as shown, highlighted here correspondingly with gray shading for R- and C-dependent phases (top tracings per panel). This approach makes the waveform observed even more compelling to be attributable to a receptor, rather than neural, potential. Nevertheless, there also is increased risk of contamination by stimulus artifact. A check when using the tubal insert earphones is to clamp the sound delivery tube to see that (at least in good part) the recorded signal greatly diminishes, if not totally disappears. In this figure, a more direct assurance of a largely, if not totally, real response is the substantially prolonged activity, not expected from the relative brevity of the click. Results in the bottom panel are compelling as well. Here the CM was tested at the relatively low-frequency of 500 Hz, reflecting an increased latency of onset attributable in part to additional traveling wave delay of the lower-frequency stimulus. In both examples there is negligible latency-intensity shift but, again, faithful phase following. Consequently, use of overlaying recordings from two or more test conditions (starting with simply a test–retest comparison) provides an excellent cross-check, in this case in endeavoring to distinguish between the CM and AP, as the AP does not follow the stimulus phase in this manner (recall Figure 5–11).

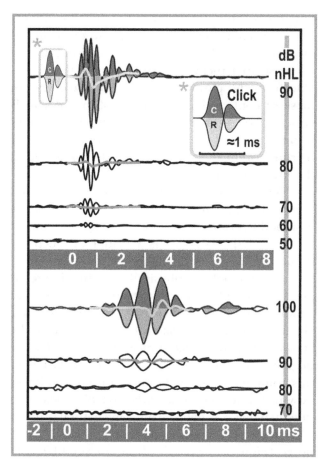

Figure 5–24. Cochlear microphonic recording in a child with profound hearing loss proving to be due to neural dysfunction. *Top*: CM to clicks are robust; nevertheless, (*see light-gray overlaid segments*) they demonstrate some level of neural synchrony, sufficient for a detectable AP, although minimal with a highly elevated sound level for detection. Rarefaction and condensation responses are overlaid for a sort of back-to-back plot of the two phases to enhance identification of the CM (see text). *Bottom*: Tone burst elicited responses at 500 Hz. Magnitude of responses relative, with the scale factor for the tracings in the top panel being about 5× that of the bottom tracings.

The SP should enlighten clinicians further apropos underlying pathological mechanisms of cochlear damage, as again a largely presynaptic response of hair cells. It is generally relatively straightforward to identify and quantify, as discussed and presented thus far. To recap: the SP is mostly seen in clinical recordings as a negative deflection, initiated prior to the AP and thus appearing first as a sort of shoulder of the AP(N_1). Nevertheless, there are some notable variants worth mentioning. First, the SP at relatively higher frequencies than involved in the conditions of recording presented/discussed to this juncture can have a positive peak at times. Thus caution must be taken not to misinterpret the apparent reversal polarity.[43] The SP's polarity is only fully represented and understood from recording inside the cochlea—not by any clinical method—as this requires measurement of the potential difference between the two perilymphatic scalae or from within scala media, to better sample local hair-cell receptor potentials. Their magnitudes and polarity are seen to reflect the underlying hydromechanical events—effects of traveling waves as their peaks move past the recording site with changing frequency.[27] This effect is only somewhat evident in the scala tympani or its effective extension laterally to the round window and beyond. In practice, using the popular tubal-insert earphones makes seeing a polarity reversal less likely, especially with testing only using a click. This is due to its substantial roll-off of frequency response (recall Figure 2–19B). Sound-field stimulation with a loudspeaker may permit adequate high-frequency stimulation to see the effect in subjects with normal hair cell function, an approach which has been practiced more (and initially always, historically) in TT-ECochG. However, whatever the method used, this effect has been reported more commonly in MD cases.[43]

Second, the SP's time history—that is, its wave morphology—can be more complicated too in some cases and/or under some test conditions. In-depth discussion is beyond the scope here, but the "bottom-line" nuance is characterized readily. It may not always be monophasic—unidirectional in its deflection—rather, possibly showing both initial positive and subsequently negative maxima.[76,77]

Third, as described before, the whole-nerve AP with a strong negative deflection (N_1) is the summed postsynaptic response among the cochlear potentials, arising indeed from the primary auditory nerve fibers themselves. Synapses take time to operate, hence the natural delay by which the AP is seen after the initiation of SP. It too has some added nuances, also/especially at relatively high stimulation levels; a second negative deflection (N_2) often is observed. This is typically attributed to a second rarefaction phase of the stimulus. The overall take-home message is that it is sometimes difficult to distinguish between the SP and AP or easy to somehow be misled by the variants just summarized.

Fortunately, at least in many cases and working with tubal insert earphones, testing progressively at lower frequencies generally does not present the polarity reversal dilemma (recall Figure 5–12B). Also, in any case, the most important characteristic of the SP for its identification is the constant latency (0.8–0.9 ms for click stimulation), in other words independent of stimulus level, unlike the AP. This is also true of the effect of stimulus rate, and this is the basis of a good added test condition (if time permits)—a retest at upward of 90 clicks/s. The AP will be adapted heavily while the SP is pretty much invulnerable. In contrast, the latency of the AP increases generally, while the amplitude decreases, with either decreasing stimulus level and/or increased repetition rate. These nuances prove to be good bases to not only resolve the two responses but also serve as a test for validity of interpretation of one or the other, particularly in the cases like ANSD.

The (conventional) SP-to-AP ratio was shown earlier to be a powerful tool toward diagnosis of MD. A further improvement of the assessment has been realized with the advent of SP/AP areal ratio.[50,51,78] Although research and development of the method was carried out using ET-ECochG, it is equally applicable to recordings via TT-ECochG, as this is a matter of the computation applied in the measurements, rather than how the potentials involved are recorded. It also shows promise to be informative in patients suspected of ANSD.[76,77]

It is important to remind here that the early AEPs recorded via TT-ECochG (see Figure 5–25, inset vignette) are sampled in the nearer near-field that extends essentially from the ipsilateral cochlea out to the earlobe or mastoid—but not without a "cost" (Figure 5–25, panel A versus B, respectively). The cost, as learned in the last episode, is the substantial reduction of signal strength toward the surface of the skull. Although the AP(N_1) is still clearly evident at the mastoid, this approach is not sufficient for differential diagnostic purposes of ECochG (as in the diagnosis of MD) because the cost is too severe to trust having an adequate SNR for reliable definition of the SP-AP complex. If also wishing to use tone bursts to elicit the SP, even with ET-ECochG (panel C), caution must be taken so that pickup of other potentials recordable from the particular scalp's surface does not mask or confound the definition of the SP. This is typical of recordings between the eardrum (tymptrode connected to noninverting input) and CZ or hairline forehead (surface electrode connected to the inverting input).

The apparent polarity of what is measured versus actual polarity (+/– μV) and the convention assumed—positive up or down in the tracing of the recorded response—is a matter of electrode hookup to the recording amplifier and preference. The absolute polarity physically is defined in reference to "ground." Practically, it suffices to reference simply to a point of contact at which the electrical signal of interest can reasonably be assumed to be zero (such as the nasion; recall Episode 3.1). The negativity of the AP recorded via ECochG has to this point in the chapter followed the convention of downward deflections as indicative of a measured potential that is negative. This is the natural primary wave of the compound potential generated by the nerve (Figure 5–25A–D). The most popular convention today in audiology, however, is not "tied" to the AP, rather to waves from beyond. These are peaks in the response complex generated in the brainstem. As seen in panel E, popular "demand" has the electrode on the mastoid connected to the inverting (–) input of the amplifier; consequently, two negatives make a plus! Nevertheless, this is not always the case in the literature, and the reader must be cautious to confirm the montage to verify that the lead of the electrode placed at C_Z or a similar site was connected to the positive input of the differential amplifier. In any event, in conventional ABR nomenclature, wave I = N_1 of the AP.[79]

There are no untoward effects of this flip-flopping "trick," indeed an advantage ultimately for some important measurements—to be discussed in the upcoming episode. Nevertheless, the examiner needs always to be mindful of the trick. Meanwhile, also mindful of the last episode: ET-ECochG, again, can be combined with recording of brainstem responses (see Figure 5–25, panel C and what the conventional ABR recording amounts to, with sim-

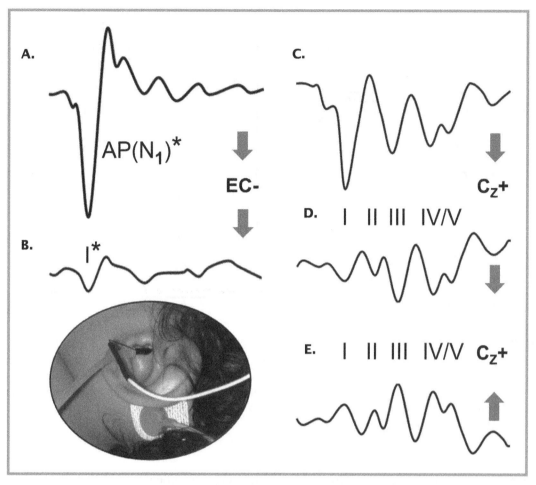

Figure 5–25. The "ups and downs" of the AP(N_1)/ABR(wave I) among recording sites and convention of polarity reference and preference (see text). Inset photograph: Simultaneous recording from the promontory and a surface electrode on the mastoid.

ply a less sensitive pickup of the first wave). Consequently, the "flip-flop" of the hookup either way does not change the waveform otherwise (see panels D and E). Conversely (in a manner of thinking), combining ET-ECochG with ABR testing (whether plotted "up" or "down") is a good way to improve the measurability of wave I (in "brainstemese"), as may be needed in the face of an impaired hearing organ and/or 8th nerve that has caused a substantial loss of hearing sensitivity.

There are still other aspects of what happens in the cochlea but do not "stay" in the cochlea, in effect. In Figure 5–26 panel A, the schematically represented cochlea, with respect to the prevalent concept of how the sound stimulus is conditioned for a primary frequency code, provides an appropriate input signal to the ***central auditory nervous system (CANS)***. The basilar membrane "looks" like a delay line. In addition, timing information—from neural synchronization to the sound, particularly for lower frequencies and lower-frequency modulation of higher-frequency sounds—is also well encoded. By the place of origin of the ascending nerve fibers, time of place-frequency information across the nerve is represented by the single-unit spike-rate plots in panel B; high-frequency information literally arrives at the brainstem earlier than low-frequency-evoked activity.[80] As discussed in a subsequent episode, this effect can be revealed as well by testing the click-elicited AP in a manner that permits producing frequency-specific responses (Figure 5–26, panel C).[81] Following the negative

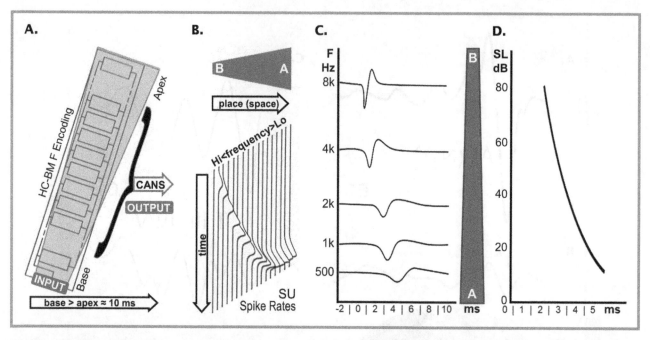

Figure 5–26. Origin of latency-intensity shifts of the AP. **A.** Schematic illustration recalling the cochlear receptor wiring of the 8th nerve along the basilar membrane (Episode 3.2). **B.** Consequences expressed in spike rates (for a transient stimulus) across time and cochlear space. **C.** Computer models of responses of the AP approximately for octave-audiometric intervals. **D.** Function of stimulus level-dependent shifts (a.k.a., latency-intensity function) plotted on its side to illustrate relation to frequency-dependent (thus place-dependent) behavior of responses in panel **C**.

tip of the AP in time or *latency* per frequency clearly reflects a curvilinear trend, as confirmed by a function fitted to actual ECochG results. However, in this analysis, AP-peak latencies are tracked for different stimulus levels in panel D. The upshot is as follows: stimuli concentrating sound energy at different frequencies will produce responses of different latencies—yet another "time–space thing"—up front! The *latency-intensity (L-I) function* (as the more conventional presentation of such data) expresses a shift toward longer latencies at lower sound levels. These shifts are attributed to a spread of excitation effectively toward the cochlear base with increasing sound levels, another nuance of the traveling wave envelop (recall Figure 5–2A).

The parting words of this episode and chapter are dedicated to a peek further into time and space of AEPdom. The latency-shifts of both stimulus level and frequency—although all natural!—beg several questions if indeed effectively carried forward to the CANS. As a preview to what comes next, time to play, "Guess that L-I Function." The reader is asked not to look beyond this paragraph and only at the next figure—Figure 5–27. The modeled L-I functions in this figure now are presented conventionally with latency as a function of sound level. These functions can be supposed to be overall realistic and lend themselves to consideration of several possible issues of clinical interest. The overall theme of questioning is that of what might happen in reference to the AP's L-I function, A1. Incidentally, A1 is essentially the same function as that presented by the dashed line in Figure 5–22 at the beginning of this episode, but having been transformed a bit further (rotated and rescaled for purposes here), yet still deriving from results of an actual clinical recording. Questions: Will at the next level of the auditory system (second-order neurons arising from the DVCN) the next AEP-wave's peak latency follow simply in parallel (function B1), if not, how will it follow? What will be the overall time delay involved (recalling Episode 1.1), like version B1 versus B2? What about functions for subsequent waves like C1? Simply another shift

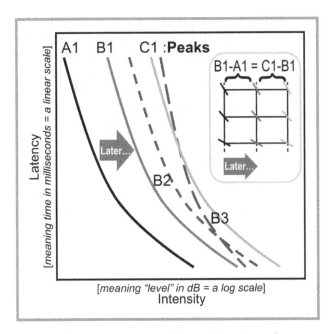

Figure 5-27. Hypothetical L-I functions of potentials, upon pondering possible subsequent effects "looking ahead" centrally (see text). Inset: Grid for considering parallel shifts of such functions upon testing at several stimulus levels.

of latency of the same or a "quantum leap"? Same curve? Or might it have a different tilt or even a different configuration? For reference, what all three being essentially parallel functions mean is illustrated by the inset figure—equal jumps in time when tested at different levels. The results of such measurement would yield an array of numerical interpeak differences. New subset of questions: Now suppose that for whatever AEP peak, B1 represents the norm for a test. What might function B2 (compared to B1) imply, if observed? What about B3? Indeed, supposing both to be beyond the statistical confidence limits of this norm, would B2 and B3 (intuitively) seem likely to be about the same or different etiologies of these abnormalities?

Possible answers can be seen best by example, but for now, only to the point of whether any of the scenarios queried are realistic clinically. So this is just a preview for the upcoming chapter but not to be a spoiler, of course. This is also a matter of closure of affairs between ECochG and ABR forthcoming, which enjoys far broader clinical interests and use. At the same time, it serves to underscore

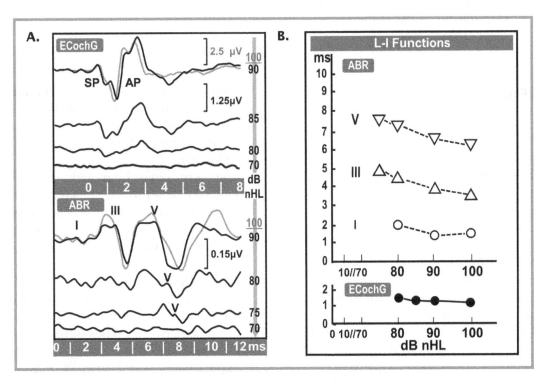

Figure 5-28. **A**. ECochG (transtympanic) and ABR testing with same stimuli (clicks) in an 8-month-old child presenting with a severe sensorineural hearing loss. **B**. More comprehensive analysis yielded the results for plotting L-I functions for the major wave components.

the importance of not leaving ECochG behind. It is always there; simply a matter of how far to go with it for a given clinical purpose. The results summarized in Figure 5–28 derive from both ECochG and ABR testing using the same acoustic stimulation in an actual clinical case. An 8-month-old child was seen, presenting (as turns out) a severe sensorineural hearing loss. This is reflected in both series of recordings, TT-ECochG and conventional ABR testing (panel A, top and bottom, respectively). Latency measurements are summarized in panel B accordingly. Essentially the same "absolute" latencies of N_1 (panel B, bottom) and ABR wave I (panel B, top) were observed, as expected, but ECochG provided the clearer definition of the AP overall, plus the SP. All waves are seen to have prolonged latencies that never converge substantially toward the normative ranges—except wave I. The L-I functions for waves III and V overall resemble more B2 of Figure 5–27. In reference to the inset of that figure, the latency interval of wave III – I (unlike B1 – A1) is not equal to that of V – III (like C1 – B1, per the scenario for the initial subset of questions). The latter is actually a bit longer, although overall parallel between III and V. All are significant findings clinically. So what does it all mean? Well, this was only a preview; please tune in to the next chapter! Happy peak picking.

■ Take Home Messages

Episode 1

1. The "season premiere" spotlighted again the remarkable microanatomy of the hearing organ and the miraculous outer hair cell that is not just along for passively riding the waves.
2. Before electrophysiological signs of activation of the auditory periphery are acoustico-mechanical signals radiated back to the ear canal from the cochlea.
3. OAEs are created by linear reflections from passive hydromechanics (traveling waves in the cochlea)—also known as "place-fixed" OAEs—but that is not the only source!
4. DPOAEs are generated by two sources: place-fixed and wave-fixed—nonlinear distortion arising from active micromechanics added to traveling waves (thank you OHCs!).
5. DPOAE tests readily offer audiometriclike results; sharp valleys in DP-grams are not necessarily pathological, rather reflecting multiple sources (in normal/near-normal ears).
6. CEOAEs provide some frequency-specific information about the cochlea, more limited in frequency range and resolution, yet clinically useful.
7. Clinical use of OAEs begins with normative data from young adults and evaluations of SPLs of both the presumptive otoacoustic emission and the noise floor.

Heads Up

8. Spontaneously occurring OAEs are a dramatic "testimonial" to the exquisite sensitivity of the auditory system.
9. Incidence of detection of SOAEs in the normal and clinical populations is variable, rare though with less than clinically normal hearing and/or rarely observed in cases with tinnitus.

Episode 2

1. "Blowing up" the overall AEP (in time) reveals the first electrophysiological signs of activation of the hair-cell transducers and neurons of the 8th nerve (that is, in space in AEPdom).
2. The cochlea must be thought of as an elaborate 3D circuit through which currents flow associated with receptor and action potentials and with some/limited access from outside.
3. AEP measurement begins in the near field of two types of signals observed, again the receptor potentials reflecting hair-cell transduction and action potentials of the distal 8th nerve.
4. There are also two types of hair-cell potentials—CM and SP—the latter being another expression of nonlinearity of transduction but still of diagnostic importance.
5. In sum, both sensory and neural potentials readily can be recorded using minimally or

noninvasive methods and elicited by clicks or tone bursts.

Episode 3

1. ECochG takes advantage of the spread of cochlear electric potentials away from the round window, although at the cost of decreased response per distance in the near field.
2. For extratympanic recordings, with skill, an extratympanic electrode like the tymptrode can be placed comfortably deep in the patient's ear canal or (preferably) on the tympanic membrane.
3. As with any test, ECochG must be used purposefully and with due consideration of need to know, what to measure, and appropriate methods—case by case.
4. AEP tests are largely functional indicators, not like some imaging tests and biopsy, but the SP does show a keen sensitivity to cochlear hydrops.
5. The strength of ECochG is that it adds to symptom-based diagnosis (subjective) an objective test result, frequently an elevated SP in patients with Meniere's disease.
6. The SP/AP ratio is a broadly used metric but one-dimensional (magnitudes); incorporating measurement of widths of components (areas) enhances sensitivity of the test.

Heads Up

7. The SP has long been known from research in animals to be sensitive to fluid pressures effectively applied to the cochlea and consequently offsetting basilar membrane motion.
8. The case of semicircular canal dehiscence is both intriguing clinically and confirmative through surgical treatment (namely via intraoperative monitoring).

Episode 4

1. ECochG has had varied interest clinically—yet recent resurgence overall, including TT-ECochG—and is always of fundamental interest.
2. In ECochG-ERA, TT-ECochG is the most sensitive electrophysiological test for directly evaluating the peripheral auditory system.
3. ECochG and/or other AEP testing is essential to preoperative assessments, and TT should be considered when other tests (ET/SLR-brainstem) provide inadequate information.
4. CM and/or SP can enlighten clinicians about specific underlying mechanisms, for instance in cases suspected of auditory neuropathy (one of the "revival" areas for ECochG).
5. Moving the recording electrode to the "surface" (again) reflects much the same ECochG "picture" but—reminder—with some important consequences.
6. Equally important to ECochG's value is what results thereof teach beyond the periphery, starting with latency shifts in component potentials.
7. Cochlear mechanics and wiring sets the stage for latency effects that well can be expected to be more or less passed along to higher-order neuronal responses.

References

1. Robinette, M. S., & Glattke, T. J. (Eds.). (2007). *Otoacoustic emissions: Clinical applications* (3rd ed.). Thieme.
2. Gold, T. (1948). Hearing II. The physical basis of the action of the cochlea. *Proceedings of the Royal Society of London. Series B-Biological Sciences, 135*(881), 492–498.
3. Gold, T. (1989a). Historical background to the proposal, 40 years ago, of an active model for cochlear frequency analysis. In J. P. Wilson & D. T. Kemp (Eds.), *Cochlear mechanisms: Structure, function, and models* (pp. 299–305). Springer.
4. Elliott, E. (1958). A ripple effect in the audiogram. *Nature, 181*(4615), 1076.
5. Gold, T. (1989b). New ideas in science. *Journal of Scientific Exploration, 3*(2), 103–112.
6. Kemp, D. T. (1978). Stimulated acoustic emissions from within the human auditory system. *Journal of the Acoustical Society of America, 64*(5), 1386–1391.

7. Davis, H. (1983). An active process in cochlear mechanics. *Hearing Research, 9*(1), 79–90.
8. Brownell, W. E., Bader, C. R., Bertrand, D., & de Ribaupierre, Y. (1985). Evoked mechanical responses of isolated cochlear outer hair cells. *Science, 277*(4683), 194–196.
9. Zheng, J., Shen, W., He, D. Z. Z., Long, K. B., Madison, L. D., & Dallos, P. (2000). Prestin is the motor protein of cochlear outer hair cells. *Nature, 405*(6783), 149–155.
10. Guinan, J. J., Salt, A., & Cheatham, M. A. (2012). Progress in cochlear physiology after Békésy. *Hearing Research, 293*(1–2), 12–20.
11. Shera, C. A., & Abdala, C. (2012). Otoacoustic emissions: Mechanisms and applications. In K. Tremblay & R. Burkard (Eds.), *Translational perspectives in auditory neuroscience: Hearing across the life span—Assessment and disorders* (pp. 123–159). Plural Publishing.
12. Shera, C. A., & Guinan, J. J. (1999). Evoked otoacoustic emissions arise by two fundamentally different mechanisms: A taxonomy for mammalian OAEs. *Journal of the Acoustical Society of America, 105*(2), 782–798.
13. Kummer, P., Janssen, T., Hulin, P., & Arnold, W. (2000). Optimal L1–L2 primary tone level separation remains independent of test frequency in humans. *Hearing Research, 146*(1–2), 47–56.
14. Keefe, D. H. (2007). Influence of middle-ear function and pathology on otoacoustic emissions. In M. S. Robinette & T. J. Glattke (Eds.), *Otoacoustic emissions: Clinical applications* (3rd ed., pp. 163–196). Thieme.
15. Robinette, M. S., Cevette, M. J., & Probst, R. (2007). Otoacoustic emissions and audiometric outcomes across cochlear and retrocochlear pathology. In M. S. Robinette & T. J. Glattke (Eds.), *Otoacoustic emissions: Clinical applications* (3rd ed., pp. 227–272). Thieme.
16. Bright, K. E. (2007). Spontaneous otoacoustic emissions in populations with normal hearing sensitivity. In M. S. Robinette & T. J. Glattke (Eds.), *Otoacoustic emissions: Clinical applications* (3rd ed., pp. 69–86). Thieme.
17. Norena, A., Micheyl, C., Durrant, J., Chéry-Croze, S., & Collet, L. (2002). Perceptual correlates of neural plasticity related to spontaneous otoacoustic emissions? *Hearing Research, 171*(1–2), 66–71.
18. Durrant, J. D., & Feth, L. (2013). *Hearing sciences: A foundational approach*. Pearson Publishers.
19. Dallos, P. (1973). *The auditory periphery: Biophysics and physiology*. Academic Press.
20. Wever, E. G., & Lawrence, M. (1954). *Physiological acoustics*. Princeton University Press.
21. Durrant, J. D., Burns, A., & Ronis, M. L. (1977). Electrocochleographic studies in animals. *Advances in Oto-Rhino-Laryngology, 22*, 14–23.
22. Dallos, P. (1971). Comments on "Correspondence between cochlear microphonic sensitivity and behavioral threshold in the cat." *Journal of the Acoustical Society of America, 50*(6B), 1554.
23. Durrant, J. D. (1979). Comments on the effects of overstimulation on microphonic sensitivity. *Journal of the Acoustical Society of America, 66*(2), 597–598.
24. Durrant, J. D. (1979). Changes in summating potentials and related electrophysiological manifestations of overstimulation. *Journal of Auditory Research, 19*(3), 183–200.
25. Coats, A. C. (1981). The summating potential and Meniere's disease. I. Summating potential amplitude in Meniere and non-Meniere ears. *Archives of Otolaryngology, 107*(4), 199–208.
26. Dallos, P., Billone, M. C., Durrant, J. D., Wang, C., & Raynor, S. (1972). Cochlear inner and outer hair cells: Functional differences. *Science, 177*(4046), 356–358.
27. Dallos, P. (1975). Electrical correlates of mechanical events in the cochlea. *Audiology, 14*(5–6), 408–418.
28. Durrant, J. D., & Ferraro, J. A. (1991). Analog model of human click elicited SP and effects of high pass filtering. *Ear and Hearing, 12*(2), 144–148.
29. Ferraro, J. A., & Durrant, J. D. (2002). Electrocochleography. In J. Katz (Ed.), *Handbook of clinical audiology* (pp. 249–273). Lippincott Williams & Williams.
30. Ferraro, J. A., & Durrant, J. D. (2006). Electrocochleography in the evaluation of patients with Meniere's disease/endolymphatic hydrops. *Journal of the American Academy of Audiology, 17*(1), 45–68.
31. Fromm, B., Bylen, C. O., & Zotterman, Y. (1935). Studies in the mechanisms of Wever and Bray effect. *Acta Otolaryngologica, 22*, 477–483.
32. Eggermont, J. J., Odenthal, D. W., Schmidt, P. H., & Spoor, A. (1974). Electrocochleography: Basic principles and clinical application. *Acta Otolaryngologica, 316*(Suppl.), 1–84.
33. Schwaber, M. K., & Hall, J. W. (1980). A simplified technique for transtympanic electrocochleography. *American Journal of Otology, 11*(4), 260–265.
34. Ferraro, J. A., Thedinger, B., Mediavilla, S. J., & Blackwell, W. (1994). Human summating potential to tonebursts: Observations on TM versus promontory recordings in the same patient. *Journal of the American Academy of Audiology, 5*(1), 24–29.
35. Eggermont, J. J. (1976). Summating potentials in electrocochleography: Relation to hearing disorders.

In R. J. Ruben, C. Elberling, & G. Salomon (Eds.), *Electrocochleography* (pp. 67–87). University Park Press.

36. Gibson, W. P., Moffat, D. A., & Ramsden, R. T. (1977). Clinical electrocochleography in the diagnosis and management of Ménière's disorder. *Audiology, 16*(5), 389–401.

37. Ferraro, J. A., Best, L. G., & Arenberg, I. K. (1983). The use of electrocochleography in the diagnosis, assessment, and monitoring of endolymphatic hydrops. *Otolaryngologic Clinics of North America, 16*(1), 69–82.

38. American Academy of Otolaryngology- Head and Neck Foundation, Inc. Committee on Hearing and Equilibrium. (1995). Guidelines for the diagnosis and evaluation of therapy in Ménière's disease. *Otolaryngology-Head and Neck Surgery, 113*(3), 181–185.

39. Morrison, A. W., Moffat, D. A., & O'Connor, A. F. (1980). Clinical usefulness of electrocochleography in Meniere's disease: An analysis of dehydrating agents. *Otolaryngologic Clinics of North America, 13*(4), 703–721.

40. Kitahara, M., Takeda, T., & Yazama, T. (1981). Electrocochleography in the diagnosis of Meniere's disease. In K. H. Volsteen (Ed.), *Meniere's disease, pathogenesis, diagnosis and treatment* (pp. 163–169). Thieme-Stratton.

41. Ferraro, J. A., Arenberg, I. K., & Hassanein, R. S. (1985). Electrocochleography and symptoms of inner ear dysfunction. *Archives of Otolaryngology, 111*(2), 71–74.

42. Staller, S. (1986). Electrocochleography in the diagnosis and management of Meniere's disease. *Seminars in Hearing, 7*(3), 267–277.

43. Dauman, R., Aran, J. M., de Sauvage Charlet, R., & Portmann, M. (1988). Clinical significance of the summating potential in Ménière's disease. *The American Journal of Otology, 9*(1), 31–38.

44. Ruth, R. A., Lambert, P. R., & Ferraro, J. A. (1988). Electrocochleography: Methods and clinical applications. *The American Journal of Otology, 9*, 1–11.

45. Ferraro, J. A., & Krishnan, G. (1997). Cochlear potentials in clinical audiology. *Audiology and Neurotology, 2*(5), 241–256.

46. Durrant, J. D., & Dallos, P. (1972). Influence of direct-current polarization of the cochlear partition on the summating potentials. *The Journal of the Acoustical Society of America, 52*(2B), 542–552.

47. Durrant, J. D., & Gans, D. (1975). Biasing of the summating potentials. *Acta Oto-Laryngologica, 80*(1–6), 13–18.

48. Pou, A. M., Hirsch, B. E., Durrant, J. D., Gold, S. R., & Kamerer, D. B. (1996). The efficacy of tympanic electrocochleography in the diagnosis of endolymphatic hydrops. *The American Journal of Otology, 17*(4), 607–611.

49. Margolis, R. H., Rieks, D., Fournier, E. M., & Levine, S. E. (1995). Tympanic electrocochleography for diagnosis of Ménière's disease. *Archives of Otolaryngology-Head & Neck Surgery, 121*(1), 44–55.

50. Ferraro, J. A., & Tibbils, R. P. (1999). SP/AP area ratio in the diagnosis of Ménière's disease. *American Journal of Audiology, 8*(1), 21–28.

51. Al-momani, M. O., Ferraro, J. A., Gajewski, B. J., & Ator, G. (2009). Improved sensitivity of electrocochleography in the diagnosis of Meniere's disease. *International Journal of Audiology, 48*(11), 811–819.

52. Bramhall, N. F., Konrad-Martin, D., McMillan, G. P., & Griest, S. E. (2017). Auditory brainstem response altered in humans with noise exposure despite normal outer hair cell function. *Ear and Hearing, 38*(1), e1–e12.

53. Ferraro, J. A., Kileny, P. R., & Grasel, S. S. (2019). Electrocochleography: New uses for an old test and normative values. *American Journal of Audiology, 28*(3S), 783–795.

54. Yanz, J. L., & Dodds, H. J. (1985). An ear-canal electrode for the measurement of the human auditory brain stem response. *Ear and Hearing, 6*(2), 98–104.

55. Ferraro, J. A., & Ferguson, R. (1989). Tympanic ECochG and conventional ABR: A combined approach for the identification of wave I and the IV interwave interval. *Ear and Hearing, 10*(3), 161–166.

56. Bauch, C. D., & Olsen, W. O. (1990). Comparison of ABR amplitudes with TIPtrode and mastoid electrodes. *Ear and Hearing, 11*(6), 463–467.

57. Ruben, R. J., & Sekula, J. (1960). Electrical potentials of the organ of hearing. *Laryngoscope, 15*, 401–406.

58. Koka, K., Saoji, A. A., & Litvak, L. M. (2017). Electrocochleography in cochlear implant recipients with residual hearing: Comparison with audiometric thresholds. *Ear and Hearing, 38*(3), e161–e167.

59. Kileny, P. R. (2018). *The audiologist's handbook of intraoperative neurophysiological monitoring*. Plural Publishing.

60. Rance, G., Beer, D. E., Cone-Wesson, B., Shepherd, R. K., Dowell, R. C., King, A. M., . . . Clark, G. M. (1999). Clinical findings for a group of infants and young children with auditory neuropathy. *Ear and Hearing, 20*(3), 238–252.

61. Starr, A., Sininger, Y., Nguyen, T., Michalewski, H. J., Oba, S., & Abdala, C. (2001). Cochlear receptor (microphonic and summating potentials, otoacoustic emissions) and auditory pathway (auditory brain stem potentials) activity in auditory neuropathy. *Ear and Hearing, 22*(2), 91–99.

62. Riazi, M., & Ferraro, J. (2008). Observations on mastoid versus ear canal recorded cochlear microphonic in newborns and adults. *Journal of the American Academy of Audiology, 19*(1), 46–55.
63. Stamper, G. C., & Johnson, T. A. (2015). Auditory function in normal-hearing, noise-exposed human ears. *Ear and Hearing, 36*(2), 738–740.
64. Liberman, M. C., Epstein, M. J., Cleveland, S. S., Wang, H., & Maison, S. F. (2016). Toward a differential diagnosis of hidden hearing loss in humans. *PLoS One, 11*(9), e0162726.
65. Minor, L. B., Solomon, D., Zinreich, J. S, & Zee, D. S. (1998). Sound- and/or pressure-induced vertigo due to bone dehiscence of the superior semicircular canal. *Archives of Otolaryngology–Head and Neck Surgery, 124*(3), 249–258.
66. Ward, B. K., Carey, J. P., & Minor, L. B. (2017). Superior canal dehiscence syndrome: Lessons from the first 20 Years. *Frontiers in Neurology, 8*, 177.
67. Adams, M. E., Kileny, P. R., Telian, S. A., El-Kashlan, H. K., Heidenreich, K. D., Mannarelli, G. R., & Arts, H. A. (2011). Electrocochleography as a diagnostic and intraoperative adjunct in superior semicircular canal dehiscence syndrome. *Otology and Neurotology, 32*(9), 1506–1512.
68. Butler, R. A., & Honrubia, V. (1963). Responses of cochlear potentials to changes in hydrostatic pressure. *Journal of the Acoustical Society of America, 35*(8), 1188–1192.
69. Durrant, J. D., & Dallos, P. (1974). Modification of DIF summating potential components by stimulus biasing. *Journal of the Acoustical Society of America, 56*(2), 562–570.
70. Rosowski, J. J., Songer, J. E., Nakajima, H. H., Brinsko, K. M., & Merchant, S. N. (2004). Clinical, experimental, and theoretical investigations of the effect of superior semicircular canal dehiscence on hearing mechanisms. *Otology and Neurotology, 25*(3), 323–332.
71. Ruben, R. J., Elberling, C., & Salomon, G. (Eds.). (1976). *Electrocochleography*. University Park Press.
72. Gibson, W. P. R. (1978). *Essentials of clinical electric response audiometry* (pp. 59–106). Churchill Livingstone.
73. Picton, T. W. (2011). *Human auditory evoked potentials* (pp. 189–212). Plural Publishing.
74. Schoonhoven, R. (2007). *Responses from the cochlea*. In B. F. Burkard, J. J. Eggermont, & M. Don (Eds.), *Auditory evoked potentials. Basic principles and clinical application* (pp. 180–198). Lippincott Williams & Wilkins.
75. Durrant, J. D., Wang, J., Ding, D. L., & Salvi, R. J. (1998). Are inner or outer hair cells the source of summating potentials recorded from the round window? *Journal of the Acoustical Society of America, 104*(1), 370–377.
76. Stuermer, K. J., Beutner, D., Foerst, A., Hahn, M., Lang-Roth, R., & Walger, M. (2015). Electrocochleography in children with auditory synaptopathy/neuropathy: Diagnostic findings and characteristic parameters. *International Journal of Pediatric Otorhinolaryngology, 79*(2), 139–145.
77. Stuermer, K. J., Beutner, D., Streicher, B., Foerst, A., Felsch, M., Lang-Roth, R., & Walger, M. (2016). The correlation between ECochG parameters and early auditory behavior after cochlear implantation in children. *International Journal of Audiology, 55*(7), 412–418.
78. Grasel, S. S., Beck, R., Loureiro, R., Rossi, A. C., de Almeida, E. R., & Ferraro, J. (2017). Normative data for TM electrocochleography measures. *Journal of Otology, 12*(2), 68–73.
79. Jewett, D. L., & Williston, J. S. (1971). Auditory-evoked far fields averaged from the scalp of humans. *Brain, 94*(4), 681–696.
80. Kiang, N. Y. S. (1975). Stimulus representation in the discharge patterns of auditory neurons. In E. L. Eagles (Ed.), *The nervous system: Human communication and its disorders* (Vol. 3, pp. 81–96). Raven Press.
81. Eggermont, J. J. (1976). Analysis of compound action potential responses to tone bursts in the human and guinea pig cochlea. *Journal of the Acoustical Society of America, 60*(5), 1132–1139.

Evoking Responses of the Central Auditory System: Testing the Brainstem

> **The Writers**
>
> Episode 1:   George A. Tavartkiladze
> Heads Up: Cynthia G. Fowler
> Episode 2:   David Purcell and
>   Viji Easwar
> Heads Up: Ananthanarayan Krishnan
> Episode 3:   Maria C. Perez-Abalo
> Episode 4:   Susan A. Small
> Episode 5:   Cynthia G. Fowler and
>   Jun Ho Lee
> Heads Up: Jun Ho Lee and José Juan
>   Barajas de Prat
> Heads Up: Suzanne C. Purdy

■ Episode 1: Brainstem Auditory Evoked Potential: General Interpretation—Its Nature and Peripheral Versus Central System Aspects

This episode is a debut dedicated uniquely to the various aspects of eliciting, recording, and clinically applying the most extensively studied and widely "used" AEP in clinical audiology, from the early days of research and development in the early 1970s to date. This AEP already has been featured in various ways and was presented substantially in Chapter 4 for its combined nuances of a nearly iconic waveform, broad clinical appeal, and size—diminutive in a background of not so diminutive noise. Still, highly efficacious and practical methods rapidly emerged to reliably record this potential, the basics of which were presented. This of course is the **short latency response (SLR)** that is called the "brainstem response." It has been labeled by various names by users among and within disciplines. Most popularly, it is known in audiology as the **auditory brainstem response (ABR)**. The advent of broad clinical acceptance and coincidentally continued research and development of AEP-related technology overall have both ensured continued roles for "ABR apps" and benefits also applicable to other AEPs. This episode focuses on tests of the transient-elicited ABR that remain a mainstay of clinical electrophysiology in audiology and allied areas of health. The focus then is to provide a more substantial foundation of understanding of the ABR and upon which to build throughout this chapter.

Since Jewett and Williston first described the brainstem response as such,[1] it has become a valuable tool for investigating the development and function of the auditory system. Sohmer and Feinmesser[2] also described SLRs earlier, potentials recorded with surface electrodes in humans but which subsequently proved to be the same wave components. However, they were recorded with the opposite-polarity hookup of the electrode montage to the recording (differential) amplifier (recall Figure 5–25). Sohmer and Feinmesser sought to maintain the negative downward plotting of the first wave as recorded with their electrode montage which proved to be N_1 of the ***whole-nerve or compound action potential (AP)***. It soon became clear that both laboratories had made the remarkable observation of the same potentials, despite the minute electrical signals that barely reach a microvolt in magnitude.

The pointing up or down of the waves is simply a convention (again, Figure 5–25), as noted earlier. The vertex-positive peaks of the ABR, soon to be shown the most resilient of them, are what Jewett and Williston decided should dictate the convention of their plotting, namely graphed in reference to their natural polarity as positive at/near the vertex (C_Z), hence positive up. Following Sohmer and Feinmesser's logic, given the principle of differential amplification (Episode 4.1), this meant connecting the vertex to the inverting amplifier input. Their practice also happened to be consistent with the prevailing convention observed for the EEG (positive down), still the convention preferred by some workers to this day—but that's another story. The "majority rule" in audiology is that of Jewett and Williston. In any event, it is always good form to specify the electrode montage and which way (up or down) is C_Z+, as failure to do so may lead to erroneous interpretation with serious consequences.

Measurement of ABRs is a useful and reliable means of examining the lower-central auditory pathway but with the understanding that wave I indeed is generated by the 8th nerve distally. As illustrated in Figure 6–1A, it often is seen to be followed by a smaller component, wave II, generated before the proximal portion of the 8th nerve enters the brainstem at the ***pons-medulla junction***. The term "ABR" thus is a bit of a misnomer; only waves III–V are generated from the pons-medulla junction and up to the inferior colliculi at the upper border of the pons (recall Figures 5–8 and 5–25). The ABR thus reflects firstly activity/function of the peripheral auditory system, being in effect a form of ECochG! As will be seen, it is quite useful to have both nerve and brainstem potentials conveniently in one "package." The typical/basic test system was presented earlier (see Figure 2–16).

Interpretation of ABRs requires first defining what constitutes "normal" responses. This often commences with endeavoring to observe at least some of the characteristic waves of the ABR, but for reliable identification this requires an adequate stimulus level, typically in the middynamic range of hearing for the full-blown iconic waveform (see Figure 6–1A). As learned in Episode 4.1, adequate signal averaging (as the critical digital signal conditioning/processing) is essential, as demonstrated further by Figure 6–1B. Following the Jewett wave nomenclature, the peaks of these waves are commonly labeled by Roman numerals from I–V (sometimes VI and VII thereafter). In practice, ABRs of adequate/repeatable quality require 1,000 or more stimulus repetitions and more when stimulating at low stimulus/sensation levels. Generally, test–retest trials are completed to help judge reliability of the recorded response (panels A and B). Therefore, with the ever-popular click stimulus presented at 60 dB nHL to 70 dB nHL, the major waves (I, III, and V) are expected to be demonstrated reliably in the normal ABR and with reasonably good test–retest overlay of tracings. Nearly perfect overlay though is rare and/or can require upward of 4,000 sweeps for each trial, especially in "nosier" patients. (Note: often the numbers of repetitions, as in examples in panel A, will appear such as 1,024 rather than 1,000; the former is a binary-based number, like 2, $4 = 2^2$, $8 = 2^3$, . . . $64 = 2^5$, . . . $4096 = 2^{12}$, thus related to how computers count naturally, rather than the 10-based system favored by most humans.)

In clinical practice (even often in research), test–retest with a high number of trials (two trials × 4,000 = 8,000 sweeps) is quite time consuming—about 2 × 8 minutes for test–retest trials together. As discussed in Episodes 3.1, 4.1, and 4.2, additional improvement of SNR of the response may be realized by means other than more averaging and with considerably more efficiency. To recap, attention always must be given to good patient preparation and an appropriate electrode montage, appropriate filtering/other signal conditioning, effective artifact rejection, and ensuring that the patient is comfortable and quiet/cooperative, all devoted to optimizing SNR of the recording. Still, if more averaging seems the only way to tease out a responselike signal, the square root of N rule for chances of significant improvement must be borne in mind. For example, if the starting number of sweeps is 2,000, then 3,000 sweeps is predicted to provide only a marginal improvement: 3000/2000 ~ 1.2×. An increase in the number of sweeps to 4,000 allows

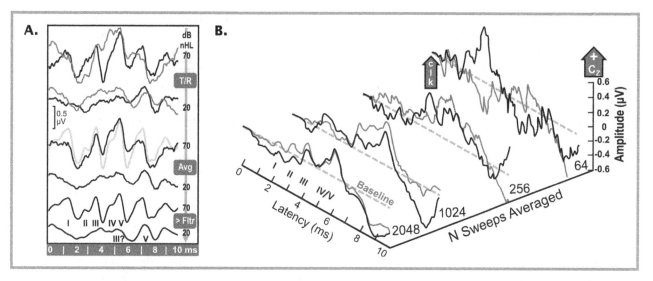

Figure 6–1. A. Normal auditory brainstem response at a moderately intense level versus one approaching the limit of normal hearing sensitivity for the acoustic click (for example, as typically seen in a young adult subject). Also included is demonstration of a practical sequence of signal processing beyond the initial response acquisition: inspection of test–retest trials (T/R, *black versus gray tracing*); average of T/R trials (Avg, *black tracing*); additional/digital filtering (>Fltr) and subsequently replotted and rescaled for direct comparison with Avg at 70 dB nHL (*light gray tracing*). **B.** Dependence of test–retest overlay on number of sweeps averaged per trial for a click (clk) presented at 70 dB nHL.

a more substantial and justifiable improvement to 1.4 ×. Consequently, it takes 8,000 sweeps to double the SNR. Conventional wisdom suggests that 8,000 sweeps or more are not likely to lead to significantly improved outcomes. A valid response is thus assumed unlikely to be detectable for the given test condition and/or patient.

The effects of both recording montage and test parameters can be substantial, even though these are far-field potentials. The recording montage and hookup to the test system was illustrated earlier in Figure 3–2 and in Figure 2–16 regarding the connection of the subject to a modern AEP test instrument for a single channel of recording with differential amplification of the signal. Recall in Episode 4.1 discussion of principles/advantages of differential recording (two active inputs, nominally + and –, and isolated from ground [Figure 4–10]). In general, the ABR is measured optimally between the vicinity of the vertex (C_Z) and the ipsilateral earlobe or mastoid.[3,4] Typically in clinical practice, instead of C_Z, placement of the electrode at midline hairline is used (approximately halfway between F_Z and F_{PZ}; again, Figure 3–2). By convention, this electrode is connected to the "+" (noninverting) amplifier input to yield positive-up waves that are generated in the pontine brainstem. This configuration favors the virtual view of the response from the same side of the head as the ear of stimulation. This location (recall Figure 5–25) is chosen because it yields the strongest wave I (again, equivalent to the AP, N_1 component when observed in extratympanic and transtympanic electrocochleography).

As shown in Figure 6–2, a faint-to-no wave I as such (no clear initial, upward peak) is evident in the recording from the contralateral side of the head, though a negative-going peak or "trough" often is observed. This is reasoned to be an ipsilateral versus contralateral difference favoring quasi-near-field versus purely far-field recordings of the whole-nerve action potential on the surface of the scalp. Fully competent recordings of the ABR often require bilateral/two-channel recordings for differential diagnostic applications (coming soon) and can be useful for other applications as well. When used, this also minimizes test time and reduces possible errors by having the earlobe/mastoid electrodes in place for both ears/sides from the outset, namely by not having to disturb the patient midtest to reconfigure the ipsilateral-only hookup. As pondered and turned out to be possible in recording the ABR in the virtual demonstration presented in Figure 3–6, the ipsilateral and contralateral views can be expected to be different for the later ABR waves as well. This too is evident in the example in Figure 6–2. However, individual variability cannot be underestimated. For instance and as illustrated by the inset tracings, the ipsilateral recording may yield separate or more or less fused waves IV and V, potentially confounding precise measurement of latency of the all-important wave V. Using simultaneous recording of the ABR ipsilaterally and contralaterally provides the chance that the two different angles of view of the space-time distribution of its electrical fields will give the examiner greater opportunity to separate peaks IV and V or to confirm wave V.[5]

The ipsilateral recordings, nevertheless, are favored for most test purposes. However, the pathways underlying the ABR's generators must be understood to be largely crossed after the dorsal-ventral cochlear nucleus (recall Figure 3–12A). On the one hand, binaural stimulation nearly doubles the response. On the other hand, there is an interesting twist to this story that will be featured shortly and is a nuance that further characterizes the ABR (stay tuned).

In Episode 5.3, principles and considerations for reliable ECochG recordings were presented. Specific test parameters that were exemplified in Table 5–2 are largely similar for ABR recordings, as summarized in Table 6–1, specifically for evaluating the transient-elicited ABR (stimulated by a click or brief sinusoidal pulse). Yet there are some differences worth noting. For the ABR recording a higher low-frequency cutoff is typical toward greater suppression of background noise (since recording the SP is not a priority). Use of a time window/epoch for best scrutiny of the ECochGm can be too brief for ABRs/other AEPs of longer latencies. The choices thus are dictated both for optimizing the recording of the target response as well as minimizing extraneous interference/noise (for example, in using excessively broadband filtering) and test efficiency (for instance, unnecessarily low stimulus repetitions rates). They are also dictated by the particular application, as will be elaborated further in this and subsequent episodes/chapters.

The effects of the stimulus' characteristics are profound, but not necessarily intuitive, nor obvious in the testing of the ABR for a given application. Unlike the CM, though an exception (soon to be revealed), classical transient-ABR does not mimic the stimulus's waveform. It might be argued that the response is a transient and thus dictates that the optimal stimulus must be a transient as well. What is predictive or **deterministic** about a true response— especially a normal one—is that it is expected to be initiated at a certain time, +/− confidence limits (statistically) in a normative data set ("norms") derived from testing an appropriate cohort of subjects. However, that is about it, and that prediction was empirical—revealed by experimentation, not readily predicted from a known transfer function of the auditory system. It thus is based on observation and scientific research leading to statistical estimations of typical response onset latencies (in reference to that of the stimulus)—all good infor-

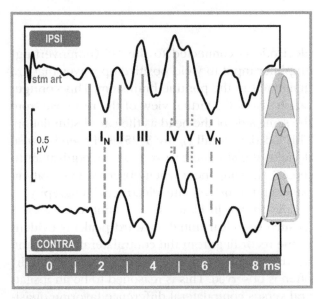

Figure 6–2. Model responses representing the sort of ipsi- versus contralateral differences that may be observed in recordings of brainstem responses, with the general trend in the contralateral view of clearer separation of waves IV and V or wherein wave V may be more apparent, even if IV and V appear "fused" into a singular peak. Some such variants are sketched in the inset panel to illustrate wave morphology of distinct peaks (line drawings) versus a fused IV–V complex (*gray fill in background*).

Table 6–1. Common Recording Parameters for Recording the ABR

Parameter	Recommendations
Transducer	Tubal insert or supraaural earphone; bone vibrator
Stimulus	Click: 100 μs (DC pulse input) Tone pip: 2-1-2, Blackman, etc.; brief tone bursts (AC/sinusoidal pulse input) Chirp
Polarity	Rarefaction/condensation/alternating
Stimulus Rate	≈17.1/s
Intensity	Variable (dB, generally referenced to a standard pending stimulus and purpose)
Electrodes	Channel **Ipsilateral (test ear side)** Noninverted input: C_z or forehead at hair line Inverted: ipsilateral mastoid or earlobe **Contralateral (opposite of test ear)** Jumper CZ or forehead lead to serve both channels of recording Inverted: contralateral mastoid or earlobe Ground: nasion; forehead if using C_z; opposite mastoid if single channel
Filters	High-pass: 30–100 Hz Low-pass: 3000 Hz
Window	10–20 ms (pending purpose)

mation—yet only one parameter of this response. In other words, there is no practical way by which to excite the auditory nerve and brainstem with an impulse and predict parameters of the characteristic ABR (if taken to be the impulse response of the underlying system to the given input signal). In particular, it is difficult to know from the stimulus' spectrum what the ABR should "look like." Considering the neuroanatomy and neurophysiology from which the ABR's component potentials are generated, its morphology is not the result of just one transfer function—a singular function (again) by which the output is readily computed from knowledge of the input/stimulus' function—if fully deterministic. The effective "buildup" of the ABR waveform over time and space is a complex sum (mathematically); consequently, this involves ***phasor summation***. Such complexity thus clouds a straightforward association of specific peaks to a singular anatomical generator site, after wave I.

Nevertheless, there are aspects of the stimuli that have well-known effects apropos spectral consequences of temporal parameters of stimuli. The two broadly useful stimuli are clicks and brief tone bursts) and for the latter, the gating (windowing) functions employed (recall Episode 2.2). The most effective temporal envelope combines brevity—which promotes good neural synchrony with very low energy spread beyond the main spectral lobe—thus energy that is well centered at the intended stimulus frequency. Both frequency (panel A) and stimulus level (panel B) are also very influential, as illustrated in Figure 6–3, based on actual recordings in normal-hearing, neurologically intact subjects.

Full understanding of the overall behavior of the ABR for a click or tone burst at various stimulus levels also is essential to competent assessment and interpretation of ABR findings. It was speculated in the last episode (recall Figure 5–26) that there should be a particular outcome of the mechanics and wiring of the peripheral auditory system; that is, there should be parallel ***latency-intensity (L-I) functions*** for subsequently elicited, compound potentials arising at the brainstem level

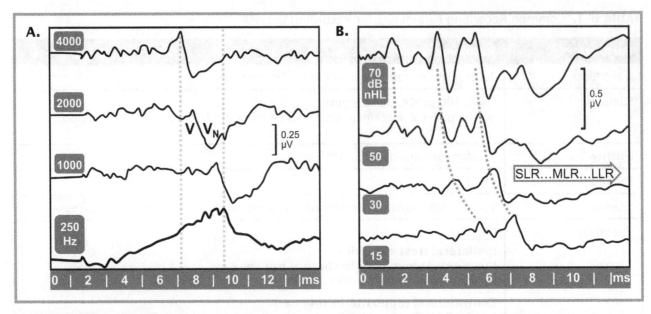

Figure 6–3. A. For demonstration purposes, ABR recordings in a normal-hearing subject at very low levels of stimulation—20 dB nHL for brief tone bursts with carrier frequencies indicated. This is to minimize possible bias of latency shift occurring with upward spread of excitement as stimulus level increases (that is, in frequency, thus basalward in place along the basilar membrane). The wave V peak is seen to shift to longer latencies according to the place dominating the response apically with decreasing frequency. Attention is also drawn here to the negative peak of wave V (V_N), which is often useful to help identify the presence of a response, even if the positive peak is uncertain. **B.** ABR latency-intensity (L-I) effects in a normal-hearing subject, highlighted for the three major ABR components (I, III, and V). Comparing results between panels A and B well supports the notion of bias of basalward spread of excitation as the primary basis of the L-I function and trends portended by way of Figure 5–26 earlier (particularly panels C and D).

(perhaps beyond). This proves to be so, as demonstrated in Figure 6–3B). In the case of ABRs in normal-hearing, neurologically intact patients, the L-I shifts tend to be nearly parallel, exponentiallike functions. Systematically, latencies of the waveform peaks demonstrate increased latency as the stimulus level is reduced toward the *visual detection limit (VDL)* of the response.[6] The detection of wave I is limited in these recordings and, in general, is more reliable with the addition of extratympanic electrocochleography (recall Episode 5.3). However, it is noteworthy that in following wave I at lower levels, it is normal behavior that wave I latency tends to shift relatively more than that of wave V.[7,8] There thus is the need to consider this nonpathological nuance in interpreting intervals among ABR peaks for purposes of differential diagnosis (the focus of a subsequent episode).

The VDL was introduced in concept in Episode 4.1, visual inspection of the recording's tracing and "scoring" it as to whether there is a reliably detectable response. The VDL of the ABR is commonly found to permit prediction of the behavioral threshold of the given stimulus, if not the pure-tone audiogram. The VDLs of ABRs recorded in a clinical case were plotted in the summary results in Figure 5–23; further examples will be presented in subsequent episodes. As the stimulus level decreases, the amplitudes of the component potentials are seen to diminish systematically. The earliest waves, I–II (also seen in Figure 6–3B) or even III and usually IV, more quickly disappear in the noise background than wave V, typically at some decibels above the ultimate VDL. Nevertheless, wave III is still usually larger (therefore easier to detect) than wave I. Still, it is wave V that is the most robust wave component overall, well persevered to nearly the behavioral limit of hearing of the stimulus. Consequently, the IV–V complex appears to fuse into a singular wave approaching the VDL.

Heading back up in stimulus level (moderate to high) and using the conventional recording montage, wave V is often seen to be about twice the size of wave I (again, Figure 6–3B), or at least demonstrating an *amplitude ratio (V/I)* ≥1. With decrease of the level of the click from higher to midlevels (≈60 dB nHL), the amplitude ratio dramatically increases, thus often doubling or more, approaching infinity toward the VDL (that is, the result when dividing by 0—no wave I response). The wave V amplitude thus changes more gradually with stimulus level and at different rates for different age groups. This is just a preview of such changes in the ABR, as will be considered in more detail shortly. Some more clues as to the potential scope of variables are still needed to fully appreciate the nature and importance of this AEP.

Even the stimulus polarity—condensation (C) versus rarefaction (R)—can have visible effects (Figure 6–4, top tracings). Wave I demonstrates the most sensitivity latency-wise to the polarity of the click stimulus with wave V latency being the least sensitive to polarity. This effect also originates from cochlear hydromechanics in reference to the phase/polarity that is excitatory (recall Figure 3–9 and further discussion in Episode 5.2). In sum, a rarefaction click initiates earlier discharges in the afferent auditory nerve fibers than condensation clicks, as the rarefaction phase of the sound at the eardrum is that which leads to movement of the hearing organ toward scala vestibuli—the excitatory phase.[5,9,10] The timing difference appears to get pretty much lost in the statistics of neural discharges that add up to the longer-latency components. Still, the majority of the research indicates a general trend for rarefaction clicks eliciting slightly earlier components for I–IV, while minimally influencing wave V.[11] Nevertheless, the use of rarefaction clicks may help to separate the IV–V peaks (again, see upper tracings). Low frequency tone bursts, on the other hand, can show some significant morphologic and latency differences between the responses to rarefaction and condensation stimuli.[12]

Clinically, it is popular to use alternating (A) polarity stimuli (Figure 6–4, lower tracings), as this helps to ensure minimal stimulus artifact by way of cancellation of the radiated electrical interference (due to destructive interference between the R and C phases). However, it is not uncommon for rar-

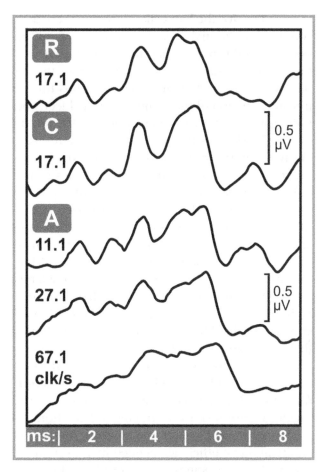

Figure 6–4. ABRs to rarefaction (R), condensation (C), and alternating polarity (A) clicks. Also shown (using alternating clicks) are effects on the ABR's waveform as a function of the rate of stimulation, as indicated (clk/s—clicks per second).

efaction click stimuli to yield a rarefaction response with a clear wave IV and less distinct wave V, and the opposite turn of events for condensation click stimuli, as also seen in Figure 6–4. Should the exact latency of wave V be needed (for example to measure the I–V latency interval), alternating click stimuli might merely confound the interpretation. Ideally, results of stimulation by both rarefaction and condensation polarity stimuli should be considered. The good news of the modern test system is that they offer the facility to view the separate R and C responses when alternating polarity stimuli are used (an application of the split buffering of acquisition; recall Episode 4.1). Furthermore, using only rarefaction clicks is also popular on the assumption of this being the polarity/phase that ultimately is excitatory for the hair cells. However, there are a couple of additional variables: accuracy of calibration of stimulus polarity and possible differences in the actual polarity/phase of the motion of the stapes in the given individual's ear, apropos the net transfer function of the combined transducer, coupling via the outer ear, and response of the middle ear (recall Heads Up of Episode 2.3). Therefore, it always is more prudent (if time permits) to examine responses to both R and C stimuli at a substantial suprathreshold level to see if stimulus polarity has a substantial effect on the ABR waveform.[13,14] After all (thanks to computing), the two records (R and C) always can be combined computationally to derive the alternating-stimulus response off-line. Not obtaining polarity-specific responses risks misinterpreting findings in differential diagnosis, possibly by having missed important observations of changes in the ABR waveform between polarities that could signal possible 8th nerve or more central pathology or merely cochlear based effects.

A more profound influence is that of *stimulus rate*, which has systematic effects on the ABR (again, Figure 6–4, lower tracings). The choice of stimulus rate is a compromise between response clarity and test efficiency needed in a given application. A slower stimulus rate produces the most clearly defined waveforms, but at the same time, it increases the time required to obtain a single-trial average. A higher stimulus rate reduces test time but it decreases the amplitude of the ABR components, particularly the earliest components, and affects other, more subtle features of the waveform.[4,5,15] In adults, rate associated changes in wave V are independent of stimulus intensity. That is, latency shifts at increased rates are essentially constant for different stimulus levels. The stimulation rate similarly affects latencies of both peripheral and central ABR wave components. With increased stimulus rate, the latencies of wave I, III, and V consistently and progressively increase and are more pronounced for wave V than waves I and III. As a result, the *interpeak (latency) intervals (IPLs)* also increase with the stimulation rate, which can be interpreted as being predominantly a central-system effect but still nonpathological.

As stimulus rate increases, the *interstimulus interval (ISI)* correspondingly decreases, and this ultimately will lead to overlapping of the ABR waves. For the conventional test of the transient ABR (the focus of this and earlier episodes), this overlap is to be avoided. The effects of rate are taken to be a form of *adaptation* of the response and thus are a neural effect. The concept of adaptation derives from the notion of stimulating neurons' responses without enough time between stimuli for their repolarization—so to speak, to "recharge their batteries"—and fundamentally reflect the refractory period of neurons after discharge (Episode 3.2). The normal resting-intracellular potential is not fully immediately recovered but may be close enough for another action potential with adequate stimulus intensity, but then still at the cost of increased latency. For the stimulus-rate effect and given compound potentials that make up AEPs, this explanation is certainly an oversimplification on three counts. First, some contributors to the components comprising the brainstem end of the ABR are potentials that do not arise uniquely from spike-action potentials generated by neural tracts (rather, also dendritic field potentials; again, Episode 3.2). Second, recurrent stimulation inherently tends to synchronize neuronal discharges, as fundamental to coherent signal averaging. Third, the auditory system is quite efficient at extracting frequency information apropos time (as well as place cues via cochlear mechanics). The more straightforward demonstration of adaptation, as classically defined, is a paired-click paradigm (for example), allowing a relatively long ISI between each pair presented per trial (for signal averaging). Then the ISI of the click pair can be varied to explore adaptation as dependent upon the time interval between the paired clicks.

Incidentally, the specification of the stimulus rate in Figure 6–4 may look strange, namely being given with decimal point numbers. Such numbers are commonly used to help discourage synchronization of the signal averaging to other than the intended responses, perhaps accidentally "locking in" on some external quasiperiodic interference. The most common such problem is that of interference from the power lines/mains, namely 60 Hz/50 Hz. A stimulus rate of 10/s literally invites trouble; a preferable rate would be 11.1/s, (see middle tracing in panel B). In general, when something seems to be interfering with the recording (perhaps ECG on the side of physiological noise), mak-

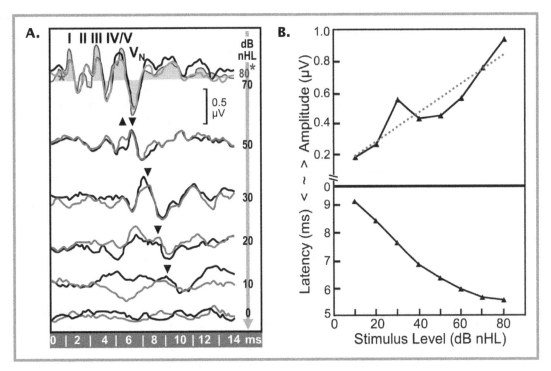

Figure 6–5. A. Latency-intensity effects, focusing primarily on wave V, observed in another normal-hearing subject. Test (*black*) and retest (*gray*) tracings are overlaid from 70 dB nHL and down, and for 70, overlaid on the average of test–retest responses at 80 dB (*lighter gray with gray fill in the areas under/over the curve*). The latter further demonstrates the good stability of this subject's recordings overall, permitting tracking responses to a visual detection limit well within normal-hearing limits. **B.** Both input-output (*top*) and latency-intensity functions of wave V derived from these recordings. Response amplitude is seen to be considerably more variable (less systematic dependence on stimulus level) than latency.

ing small fractional changes in stimulus rate are also appropriate, as they do not significantly change the overall rate, but possibly do enough to defeat untoward synchrony with the interfering signal. Some of the more sophisticated test systems provide rates with a ***jitter***—stimulus rate varied from trial to trial randomly—to discourage spurious synchronization of unwanted signals, whatever their origin.

All the effects discussed to this point are important for appreciating nonpathological variances in the ABR waveform. For completeness, the effect of stimulus level is of such importance as to deserve a bit more consideration. Another set of ABR recordings across stimulus level are shown in Figure 6–5 panel A, this time with graphs in panel B of both wave V ***input-output (I-O)***—response amplitude versus stimulus level—and L-I functions. The I-O function is more erratic than the L-I function. These are single-subject data, so the "erratic" part may be attributable to the inherently proportionally higher variability of amplitude of potentials and/or increased interference of background noise on amplitude observed among the respective trials per stimulus level (compared to means of data from groups of subjects). Consequently, amplitudes of the short-latency responses tend to be considerably more variable than latencies of the peaks of the component waves[16] and generally are considered less informative clinically. Yet, the I-O function shows overall a clear trend of increase of this component's amplitude with increasing stimulus level. Furthermore, in some cases, the V/I ratio (expected normally to be ≥1) may prove useful. In general, pending time considerations for the examinee and purpose of the exam, the ABR test is initiated at a level reasonably expected (from the patient's history and any available audiological information) to yield a repeatable response. The examiner then proceeds from there to test at other levels and with respect to other matters of protocol, as will be considered in a subsequent episode.

Although later episodes are devoted progressively to more issues/information apropos clinical testing, some overall trends of pathological findings can be contemplated in reference to this subject's data. Questions were posited in the previous episode (Episode 5.4) as to what might be expected, particularly regarding the relationship of the L-I functions among components/potentials generated more peripherally versus centrally along the auditory pathway. This is a question of behavior of relatively shorter- versus longer-latency components. Extensive research providing examples of L-I functions in patients with various types, configurations, and degrees of hearing loss from the audiometric findings as well as (ultimately) sites of lesion have taught clinicians much about the power of ABR measures as a clinical tool and how to interpret the findings.[17,18] Although wave V is generated well into the pontine level of the brainstem, this subject's L-I function clearly follows the trends suggested in Figure 5–27. The recordings in Figure 6–3B from the earlier subject also demonstrated an overall trend of parallel shifts of the subsequent components' latencies. Both sets of data were from subjects characteristic of those who commonly serve in cohorts for establishing clinical norms for ABR (and other AEP) latencies. By inference, deviations from these trends in some fashion(s) are expected to reflect a possible abnormality of function, but at what level of the system? It is also reasonable to deduce that since the L-I shifts of the ABR peaks are seeded in the peripheral system, then there should be nuances that are more indicative of a problem beyond. Conversely, might the relationships trending in the normally functioning system be benchmark(s) of a more or less likely peripheral-system-only involvement in a given diagnostic group? The answers will have to be left to upcoming episodes, as there still are more basic considerations for the near term, but with the promise of intriguing revelations by way of various demonstrations of the effects of pathology on the ABR. Nevertheless, a fair practical question at this juncture is how extensively must the L-I function be evaluated in routine practice? The answer is that, the L-I and/or I-O functions tend not to be explored routinely in such detail. Still, the data in Figures 6–3 and 6–5 form pictures that must be borne in mind, namely of what underlies the behavior of the ABR, regardless of the number and order of stimulus levels tested. The examiner certainly is exploring portions of these functions one way or the other, and the proper interpretation of the findings is dependent upon knowing and understanding them.

After the cochlear potentials, the ABR is most "vulnerable" to effects of the transducer used—another nonpathological aspect (Figure 6–6A). First, both the cochlear potentials and other SLRs are the most at-risk for interference by stimulus artifact. Second, latencies for supraaural versus tubal insert earphones are substantially different and must be taken into account. The latter yield latencies 0.8 ms to 0.9 ms longer than the former, due to the length of the standard sound tube (Figure 6–6B). Potential advantages of the latter are that they provide more flexible positioning of the transducer—including moving it further away from electrode leads as well as improved patient comfort (no pressure on the auricles), greater isolation of the ears from ambient noise, and greater interaural isolation.[19] Returning to panel A, as noted in Episode 2.3, the net spectrum of the sound stimulus reaching the inner ear reflects a combination of effects, including frequency response of the transducers. Illustrated here are frequency responses for several earphones that commonly have been used clinically and in research as well as conventional audiometry. These are results of sound analyses on a manikin called KEMAR,[20] which provides real-ear-like acoustics. Some of the effects may be subtle among transducers, although overall levels are intended by standards to yield more or less identical pure-tone audiometric results. The standard specifies calibration tables for each accordingly, yet in practice, they demonstrate somewhat different frequency responses in detail. Therefore, latency norms for ABR measurements must be established per device (and per clinic) as these nuances can bias significantly the latency results, which risks inaccurate interpretation.

Two of the three sound transducers used in general audiometry are fundamentally two versions

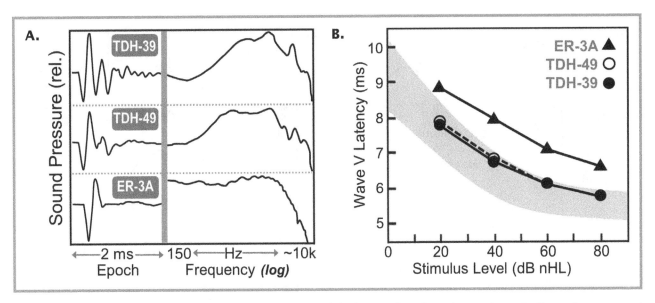

Figure 6–6. A. Time histories (*left*) and spectra (*right*) obtained with each earphone indicated, measured on KEMAR (100 μsec clicks at 75 dB nHL). **B.** Acoustic-delay-based latency shift of the tubal-insert type earphone (ER-3A) versus supraaural type earphones (TDH-39 and TDH-49).

of the same design of their electromechanical transducer elements, with only a difference of intentions; these are the earphone versus the loudspeaker. Loudspeakers also can be used in some AEP work. Both are designed to vibrate air, thus conveying sound energy by the vibration of the diaphragm/speaker cone to the eardrum via air conduction (AC). The third, while employing a similar transducer element as in earphones, is intended to couple energy generated by the transducer element to the skull of the examinee by way of vibration, hence bone conduction (BC). As in conventional audiometry, use of BC in AEP tests has the same objective, that of substantially bypassing the conductive apparatus of the outer and middle ear. However, and especially for ABR measurements, the use of BC stimulation has had a stormy past. As with earphones and loudspeakers, frequency response of the transducer must be considered (again, recall Episode 2.3). Applied to eliciting ABRs, conclusions initially fell upon impressions from data from measurement of these transducers on their respective couplers, as specified by calibration standards (Figure 6–7A). These are acoustical measurements yielding remarkable differences of apparent earphone versus bone-vibrator response characteristics, yet questionably representative of effective frequency response in practice.[21] However, the modes of calibration prove to be less than a fair comparison, starting with the remarkably different designs of the couplers specified by audiometric calibration standards. For the earphone, the coupler used merely represents a volume of air between the earphone diaphragm and the eardrum (on average). In reality, it is barely representative of real-ear acoustics; for one thing, it does not present the typical acoustic load of the real ear on the transducer. For the bone vibrator, the artificial mastoid is designed to reflect engineering considerations to substantially model the mechanical load of the head (at mastoid) on the bone vibrator, although historically with its own shortcomings.

Therefore, there was an inherent confound facing early workers seeking an understanding of outcomes of BC- versus AC-elicited ABRs. Work from another approach using psychoacoustical methods subsequently provided findings demonstrating a more favorable comparison in practice, as shown in Figure 6–7A, functions labelled psychoacoustic AC and BC.[22] These data derive from evaluation of relative effective masking of broadband noise via the acoustic versus vibratory device excited with (essentially) pure-tone probe stimuli. Two aspects of the results are compelling. First, there are not nearly the differences between AC and BC as portended by calibration results, although AC does

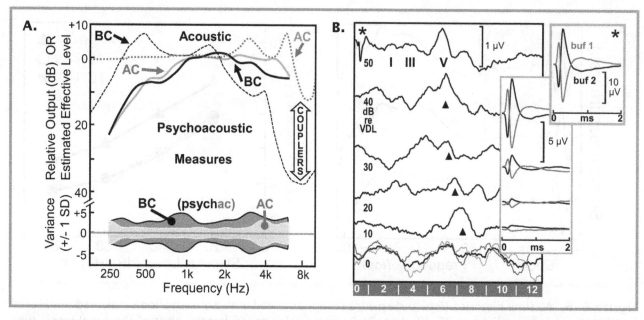

Figure 6–7. A. Overall frequency responses typical of an earphone measured in a 2 cm³ coupler versus a bone vibrator measured on an artificial mastoid, in turn compared to frequency responses when estimated from psychoacoustic (psychac) measurements using masking levels of broadband noise presented by air (AC) versus bone (BC) conduction on pure-tone (AC) thresholds. (Means [*top*] and standard deviations [*bottom*], as indicated; based on data of Durrant and Hyre [1993].[22]). **B.** Electromagnetic artifact in recordings of click-elicited ABRs. Main graph—responses for alternating clicks; insets—artifacts of single-phase clicks, thus no cancellation at the beginning of traces.

have a slight advantage of effective output over BC above 2000 Hz. Second and probably the more troublesome for precise estimations of "air-bone" gaps is the variance data at the bottom of the graph in panel A, showing BC effective levels to have twice or so the standard deviations across frequency relative to those of AC. Nevertheless (overall), these results can be taken to favor the assumption of validity of use of BC stimulation in tests of the ABR.

There is no question that the bone vibrator can be an effective stimulator for the ABR (for that matter, other AEPs), within its output limits. However, these devices require a substantially larger driving voltage from the stimulator side of the test system to achieve the same AC HL in pure-tone audiometry. This also will be the case for its use in testing ABRs/other AEPs. Toward 60 dB nHL to 70 dB nHL in the midfrequency range (even lower below), output comes to reach unacceptable distortion by saturation. The other issue is stimulus artifact from electromagnetic radiation, again as happens with earphones. Stimulus artifact is worse for BC testing from the higher driving voltage per dB nHL and, in general, closer proximity of the transducer to the skin of the subject and the mastoid/earlobe electrode. The latter reduces the benefit of differential amplification (the first stage of possible reduction of interfering signals up-front in the recording; recall Episode 4.1). The stimulus artifact is readily evident in the insets to Figure 6–7B. Therein the data from individual split buffers have been plotted and time expanded to reveal artifacts for the two stimulus polarities. This need not be intimidating, as the alternate polarity works well to minimize the artifact even at the top level tested and much of the ABR is well isolated from contamination by way of latency of most response components. Meanwhile, the results otherwise follow expected trends from earphone-stimulated responses presented earlier, including the anticipated latency-intensity shift with stimulus levels descending toward the subject's VDL.

Having returned to the latency-intensity effect, it will be useful to recall the direction in frequency that is associated with the shift. Relevant data (from Episode 5.4) were taken to bespeak—when going from lower to higher stimulus levels—a ***basalward shift*** in the spread of excitation along the basilar membrane (thus, from lower- to higher-frequency places), thus most responsible for the sum of neural activity reflected in the ABR. This is akin to the asymmetrical spread of masking demonstrated psychoacoustically. It is well known from this effect that relatively lower frequencies better mask higher frequency (probe) tones than vice-versa. As discussed and substantially illustrated in the last episode (recall Figure 5–26), cochlear hydromechanical delays are manifest in neural responses (starting with the primary auditory neurons) in good part due to the tonotopical organization of wiring of hair cells along basilar membrane, in turn "mapped" centrally. Mechanical and neural estimates of cochlear delays agree in that they are typically shorter for high frequencies compared to low frequencies.[23–25] The sensory-neural system is effectively riding the traveling waves and thereby effecting frequency selectivity via a bank of band-pass, "cochlear" filters (recall Figure 5–26A). Thus the peripheral sound encoder includes both passive (traveling waves) and active mechanisms (hair-cell amplification of vibration of the basilar membrane). Effects of the cochlear delays thus are manifested, as well, in otoacoustic emissions (recall Figure 5–5) and thereafter in the AP/wave I and subsequent ABR wave components.

The consequences of the peripheral system's encoding of the stimulus is not entirely revealed by stimulus paradigms, such as in measures of click-elicited versus tone-burst ABRs. It is particularly puzzling that the L-I shifts occur with both types of stimuli. That the click-elicited ABR should come to correspond strongly with the hearing sensitivity over the audiometric 2 kHz to 4 kHz frequency range can be attributed in part to the strong boost of the peripheral auditory system's frequency response. With earphones this is due to standing waves in the ear canal (recall Figure 2–7B; with loudspeakers, there is also such ear canal resonance plus head- and pinna-baffle effects. With either, there is the middle ear's band-pass filter effect (with greatest efficiency, midaudiometric frequencies). However, this is neither the complete story, nor the most important side of it!

The sound-level dependence of tone-burst-evoked ABR latencies include both acoustico-mechanical and neural contributions via confounds of overlapping of the traveling waves, all of which start from the cochlea's base regardless of frequency and relative timing/phase differences of these stimuli that also influence the neural synchrony. The upshot is that the neural responses forming the compound action potential will have done so, not by simple math, but with phasor summation. Consequently, both magnitude and phase count and the resulting effect is that of a ***phase dispersion*** that adversely affects the overall AP/ABR, wherein contributions from the more apically activated neurons is progressively delayed. This consequence is a sort of destructive interference, even for frequency-specific stimulation, given that stimuli for SLRs needing to be very brief and in turn still splattering of energy over a bandwidth (= place-width along the basilar membrane), rather than discretely stimulating precisely one frequency (place). Yet, certainly this effect is most dramatic for the broadband click. Without a more elaborate stimulus paradigm and increasing the sound level, the examiner literally loses sight of the relatively lower-frequency-elicited activity, and AP/ABR latencies gravitate to the 2 kHz to 4 kHz range.

Various ways have been tried to work around issues of frequency specificity of the stimulus toward more frequency-/place-specific estimates of the ABR. The most trusted way involves a clever masking technique, first employed to analyze the whole-nerve AP in animal research then adapted to ECochG/AP measurement in humans. Returning to Figure 5–26, it was the results of such measurement upon which panel C was based. The method subsequently and equally successfully was applied to the ABR. The click is used for its two strengths: temporal abruptness for excellent synchronization of neural responses and broadband stimulation to permit estimations for any frequency band of interest. The approach makes use of high-pass noises to more or less mask portions of the overall click response. The high-pass cutoff from trial to trial is moved up a frequency band with each trial. Across these trials, the difference potential is computed between the first and second, second and third, and so on to obtain each band-specific-response component of interest.[25] Although this method has been used extensively in research, it has not received adoption clinically, as it is a considerably time-intensive protocol with considerably long exposure of the subject to near-/uncomfortably loud noises, as required for the maskers.[26] Over the same history and technological advances, sinusoidal pulses have become more sophisticated, hence permitting similar specificity in many practical applications, using the likes of the Blackman window[26,27] (recall Figure 2–12). On the other hand, the derived-band paradigm remains the irrefutable approach and virtual "gold standard" for validation of any other approach to "so-called" frequency-specific stimulation, and further research and development did not stop with fancy tone bursts. Thought was given to compensate for the cochlear delay itself, wherein each response is delayed according to place frequency by time shifts in the computer to remove the relative delays (effectively to neutralizing the cochlea's natural phase dispersion). For example, aligning all according to the wave-V peak for a band centered at 4 kHz; then stack them up in memory and add them all together. Such a "stacked" ABR[28] proves to be efficacious, enhancing the response's magnitude to the maximum that it can be. This approach will be explored further, subsequently, in the context of differential diagnostic applications of the ABR.

For the moment, it will be useful to look more on the other side of the stimulus-response relationship. The subtractive masking approach, though depending on an elaborate stimulus paradigm, is thereafter more of a computational game of response-side analysis.[25,28] Results of using simply sinusoidal pulses and doing the same math on the response thereafter was found to obtain comparable results (regarding the original/pioneering work[28]).[26] There also was some modest time savings realized, and the paradigm was "voted" to be kinder to volunteer subjects and patients alike.[26] However, what if the cochlear delay could be compensated by the stimulus itself, namely by a singular stimulus (as was the original method, using the faithful click), but without the masking paradigm to tease out the frequency-/place-specific information? At the same time, no math in processing the response! This clever new idea was to start with the click, for the same good reasons as before but thereafter thinking in both time and frequency domains. Intuitively, the idea is to create a pulse whose energy across frequency is systematically delayed as a function of time (akin to phase dispersions/delays per frequency in the cochlea). In other words, an increasing lag with increasing frequencies. This is doable computationally and results in the generation of a *chirp*. The chirp is a transient variant of frequency modulation (the term connotes the birds' vocal utterances, which often are characterized by both transients and FM).

The chirp stimulus potentially compensates for the traveling wave by coordinating the arrival time spectral component by spectral component (or place by place along the hearing organ), apropos the inverse of the place-frequency map along the basilar membrane.[29,30] Consequently, great progress, yet the chirp may still not be quite ready for "prime time" in all potential areas of clinical application. Some challenges remain toward broad deployment of the technology. As will come up in another context shortly, basilar membranes vary among individuals in the lengths, which naturally makes the place-frequency mapping somewhat variable. Then there is the cochlear hair-cell system. As underscored in Episodes 5.1 and 5.2, nonlinearity of cochlear function is natural, not bad, and essential to normal function of the cochlea. However, its effects are also strongly stimulus-level dependent (by definition). These issues thwart the optimization of parameters of the chirp to make it work throughout the auditory response area. With that, further discussion is left to specific applications (coming soon).

Back to basics, one of the largest variables in ABR waveforms is simply idiosyncrasies of the individual subject's responses commonly observed. The technical discussion earlier regarding limits of coherent signal averaging (Episodes 4.1 and 4.2) focused primarily on trying to deal effectively with background noise, especially in deference to its likely nonstationarities in real-world tests. The tacit assumption is that variance of background noise and any perturbations are likely far greater than that of the ABR itself, at least within subjects. Suppose for a moment a small sample of subjects whose peripheral auditory systems and brainstem pathways are functionally identical. For a given test protocol, environmental conditions, and cooperative subjects, what would be a reasonable expecta-

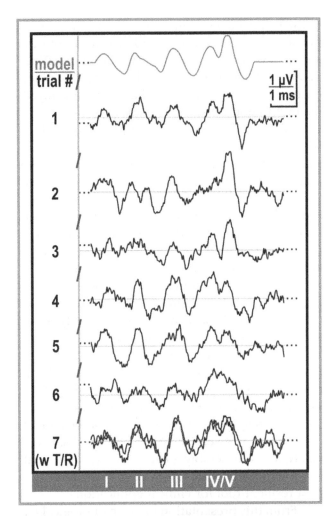

Figure 6–8. Variances of an ideal/modelled ABR in a realistic but truly stationary random noise background (trials 1–6). Plus, further demonstration of how test–retest results (trial 7) add confidence to the interpretation.

tion of their collective results? Computer simulation permits such an ideal experiment. Traces 1 to 6 in Figure 6–8 from such a hypothetical group were generated using a realistic model of the ABR in realistic background noise, but both signal and noise being stationary. All 7 subjects' results would likely be judged as clinically normal by expert examiners. Yet, these pseudoresponses emphasize the incredible differences that are observable simply at the "mercy" of the limited signal-to-noise ratio that, at best, is realized in practice. Added to this demonstration is a test–retest comparison (bottom tracings, example of split-buffer–like comparisons),

especially useful when in doubt. Here, the result is nearly optimal. In practice (real-world subject, conditions, and time available), overlays of any two of these responses might be as good as it might get within the confines of the test session. Still, it is that examiner's call. For instance, would the overlay of waveforms like #2 and #6 (if in fact the test-retest trials in question) be good enough to be judged as reliable results?

Individual-subject differences are inevitable and certainly play a role in applying any test. Indeed, the sort of variances demonstrated by Figure 6–8 is equally characteristic of data that would be observed in a sample of seven normal-hearing, young adult subjects. Indeed, intersubject variability is compelling. But wait, there is more. Results of ECochG and ABR evaluations can be influenced by a variety of specific factors. Core body temperature is quite important. Changes in core temperature affect the pre- and postsynaptic activity and possibly the receptor activity involved in the ABR. Temperature exceeding ±1°C from 37°C (normal) must be considered as a possible factor in ABR outcomes, especially for the latencies.[31] With a 1°C decrease of body temperature, the latency of wave V can increase by about 0.2 ms.[32]

Sex and/or stature have been considered possible sources of variance across subjects, initially on the notion that taller persons and the prevalence of taller males than females should be associated with longer pathways overall. If so, presumably for the ABR, head size would matter.[33] Despite largely overlapping distributions for the individual data, the mean latencies and amplitudes of ABR demonstrate significant differences between male and female, wherein females commonly show shorter latencies and larger amplitudes than males. However, the relationship between the head size and the ABR measurements is not so pronounced. An equally plausible theory is that physiologic and biochemical differences between sexes could influence neurotransmission. At the same time, a more compelling explanation is that of length of the basilar membrane. Females demonstrate smaller latency shifts between high- and low-frequency responses than male subjects, thus presumably less dispersion of phase of vibrations across place (thus frequency), that tend to affect response amplitude adversely. In other words, each frequency band

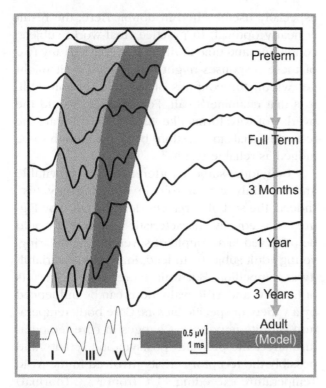

Figure 6–9. Trends of early maturation—age-related changes in the ABR (based on data of Salamy and coworkers[36]). Shaded areas behind the ABR plots approximate wave I–III and III–V intervals. These trends in particular are interpreted generally to reflect a more rapid maturation of the lower/peripheral part of the auditory pathway than that within the brainstem. Inset at bottom: model adult response from Figure 6–8 rescaled and replotted for comparison.

is distributed over a shorter length of the basilar membrane and thus has greater synchronization in the nerve fiber discharges.[34,35]

Early maturation and advanced aging also have received considerable attention as causal factors. Both can be shown to have significant effects on ABRs, but early maturation is by far the more dramatic, as reflected in Figure 6–9. Generally, only waves I, III, V are observed reliably at birth, and interwave latency values are initially prolonged.[36,37] During the first 18 months after birth, other wave components emerge and waves III and V progressively shorten in latency. Therefore, wave I–V latency interval also matures. The amplitude measures and the V/I amplitude ratio are more variable than latency measures, but certainly an evolution of wave morphology is occurring. Wave I reaches normal adult latency values by age 2 to 3 months,[38] but wave V does not attain adult values until the age of 2 years.[27] The scalp distribution of ABR in neonates differs from that of the adult. This difference could be explained by the incomplete myelination of neonatal auditory pathways.

The first 12 weeks of life present a golden window of opportunity to test infants in natural sleep and thus near-ideal test conditions for this group. Beyond that age, practically, testing younger/younger-mental-age patients may require drug-based sedation, some of which can have adverse effects on the ABR. However, the ABR is one of the most resilient AEPs for testing under sedation or even anesthesia.[39] The ABR even remains robust in comatose patients. Fortunately, in general, the timing of the ABR's dominant peaks (I, III, and V) demonstrate only small variances normally under a variety of conditions. These issues are discussed in detail in a later chapter of this book; so for the moment, it is the fundamental principle that bears reinforcement, as virtually the point of departure in Episode 4.1. Although the ABR does not require volitional responses or participation of the patient, cooperation is essential for the best results. Fortunately, the considerably greater stability of the peak and interpeak latencies allow ABR measurement to be a resilient tool for clinical applications.

From this presentation of nonpathological parameters of the ABR and further development of understanding of this intriguing SLR, clinical applications can now be pursued with greater dedication toward knowledge-based clinical competency. The focus here was the transient ABR and rightfully so, again given the great amount of research and development invested in tools of its measurement and evidence bases of their use in practice. The ABR test primarily paved the road to the routine offering of clinical electrophysiology in audiology and otorhinolaryngology clinics and ultimately private practices. The transient ABR, at the same time, represents only one perspective on the ABR. Another technological advance more recently has led to a steady-state stimulus-response approach to enhance clinical applications, particularly for estimation of hearing sensitivity. But hold that thought for another fascinating nuance of the ABR, toward the general truism that two ears are better than one and what the ABR has to say about that.

HEADS UP

Binaural Interaction in Auditory Brainstem Potentials

Binaural hearing is typically taken for granted in everyday experiences, including allowing individuals to localize sounds and converse with friends despite ubiquitous background noise. Some individuals—including those with hearing loss, advancing age, or auditory disorders—find this feat difficult. At least part of this difficulty is attributable to reduced binaural function. Although binaural function has been explored in a multitude of behavioral studies, relatively fewer studies have focused on neurophysiological changes in humans that may underlie the behaviorally manifested impairment of binaural function. This Heads Up will serve as an introduction to the electrophysiology of binaural hearing, namely starting in the pontine brainstem, recognized as the initial "hotbed" of binaural processing (recall Episode 3.2).

Several ways are available to investigate the neurophysiological bases of binaural function. The one discussed here is by way of a special protocol applied to measurement of the ABR. Several types of stimuli can/have been used, including clicks, tone bursts, and chirps.[40] The method in question requires three test conditions: monaural left ear, monaural right ear, and binaural. All are tested with replications, with the stimulus presented at a moderately intense level (like 70 dB nHL) to ensure both a reliable response of the subject and a well-defined waveform. In the computer, the left (L) and right (R) monaural responses are added. (Note: the computer must be set to simply summate the two ABRs selected, rather than average responses.) This computation is to form a theoretical response, the L+R ABR, as expected to occur were the responses for each ear (E) of stimulation to arise from completely separate neural pathways through the pontine brainstem.

It might be interesting enough then to just compare these several ABRs on the screen (L, R, and L+R). What might be reasonable expectations here (at least for subjects of no known neurological disorders and bilaterally normal hearing sensitivity)? Certainly, one expectation is that L = R. The trends of ABR norms is that given essentially equal sensitivity, the LE and RE ABR responses are pretty "symmetrical," both in terms of detectability and wave morphology. The next prediction is that L+R = 2L = 2R. Short of some unexpected ear-dominance effect, especially without using a more elaborate stimulus paradigm (like competing noise and/or more "exotic" stimuli than the click or a sinusoidal pulse), this supposition seems clear enough. Two alternating-current signals pretty much alike in magnitude and latency (in effect, in phase spectrum) should just add up to 2× the monaurally stimulated response.

What about L+R then when compared to an actually binaurally elicited ABR—call this the BIN? By way of the elaborate wiring of the CANS, there conceivably are three possibilities: (1) BIN = L+R (and if so, end of story); (2) BIN greater than L+R, if real BIN somehow adds new activity to the potentials making up the ABR; or (3) BIN smaller than L+R, if somehow the net effect is a reduction of the combined activity of the pathways on both sides. In Figure 6–10 is the answer: at a glance, it appears to be the last effect. However, just looking at these tracings does not make a uniform statement of outcome across the entire set of wave components of the ABR. Hence, the question is how best to evaluate what is actually happening and how best to measure the effect? After all, the responses are groups of potentials that can be treated like any other voltage measurement (bearing in mind that underneath will be consequences of phasor summation).

The solution: subtract the BIN ABR from the L+R ABR. Again, consider the possibilities. Were the computation simply applied to the test-retest-trial responses, the resultant would

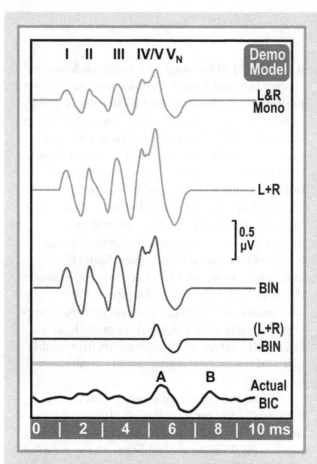

Figure 6–10. Computational basis of the binaural interaction component of the auditory brainstem response (see text). Key trends are modeled here per the computation and assumptions of negligible binaural interactions from waves I to IV, thus primarily an effect particular to V–V_N, if not beyond (to be considered in a subsequent episode). The resultant difference potential—(L+R)-BIN —obtains (*black-line trace*). *Bottom*: An actual BIC from a neurotologically normal subject. It is evident that the initial assumptions are about right (little to nothing before the BIC, yet that there is more to the difference than obtained by the most basic model of signal generation or perhaps by the most basic underlying neuroanatomical model conceivable.[41]

be expected to be no more than an estimate of the noise floor of the recording. Recall from Episode 4.1 that coherent potentials should simply cancel, as in the case of test-retest trials. However, that there is evidently some difference between the waveforms of the BIN and L+R signifies presence of a difference potential, as illustrated in Figure 6–10. That difference signal is called the ***binaural interaction component (BIC)***. The BIC quantifies, in effect, the amount of neural resources allotted specifically to binaural function and is expressed typically as a ratio: BIC/(L+R). (Note: In some studies, the investigators chose to do the subtraction in the reverse, which leaves a difference potential in the opposite polarity and affects the numerical value; the terminology for the components has not been standardized.) As the binaural response is 16% to 25% smaller than the predicted response (L+R), this outcome is taken to suggest that a subset of neurons are shared between left and right pathways.[41] This situation happens to be true, as indicated from the neuroanatomy of the pathway.[42] The ABR-BIC centers around waves IV–VI (VIs present variably in ABR recordings as another but smaller positive peak following the wave V trough). The BIC is primarily attributed to neurons in the superior olivary complex up through the lateral lemniscus, based on their latencies and the results of animal studies.

The ABR-BIC is recorded across the audiologic frequency range, but low-frequency stimuli provide a more robust ABR-BIC than high-frequency stimuli.[43] Differences in frequencies between ears produce an ABR-BIC when the perception of the signals fuses. A disparity between ears for frequencies, such as 1000 Hz versus 3000 Hz, produces only partial fusion in perception and a reduced BIC.[44] The BIC persists with both time and level differences between ears—up to 1.6 ms and 16 dB disparities between ears for the ABR.[45] These differences agree with perception of fused signals and reflect psychophysically demonstrated sound lateralization/localization abilities.

How then is measurement of the ABR BIC used? On the one hand, the BIC is demonstrable in infants as well as adults. On the other, binaural processing in infants is not fully developed at birth.[46] Consequently, the BIC can provide neurologic measures of the maturation of binaural processing through the brainstem. Various AEP measures will be considered later in the ever-intriguing cochlear implant patient. In binaurally implanted cases, the BIC can be measured to evaluate the interaction of electrode sites within the cochlea, thus augmenting information on functional status of the implantee's binaural processing.[47] More broadly, the BIC can reveal central auditory processing deficits,[48] declining binaural function in aging,[49] and sequelae of otitis media in children.[50] The BIC also has been used to detect abnormal binaural function in neurological disorders such as pontine strokes[51] and multiple sclerosis.[52]

Is the BIC ready for prime time in clinical practice? Perhaps not quite because of some pragmatic issues, mostly impacting time—a virtual commodity which tends always to be inadequate in the clinic. The BIC is a small derived potential: requires minimally six trials, involves posttest processing, may require substantially more sweeps and/or replications, and requires a very quiet/cooperative patient for results of adequate quality. Patients typically have higher physiological noise compared to research participants, and they may become uncomfortable or restless during long recording sessions. Consequently, simpler and faster methods for recording and processing responses are needed before the BIC is finally brought routinely into the clinic. Since it apparently has clinical usefulness, the hope is that continued research and development efforts will come to serve interests toward a more efficacious adaptation of ABR-BIC testing.

■ Episode 2: Brainstem Responses to Complex Stimuli—Frequency and Envelope Following Responses

The previous episode described measuring the brainstem's response to a brief transient sound and how to assess the resulting transient response using its time history, thus emphasizing what more commonly is called the "waveform," or in evoked-response measurement "wave morphology." Transient stimuli like clicks and tone bursts are only a subset of the types of sounds listeners encounter every day. The present episode describes the brainstem's response to sounds that are inherently more complex, including even naturally spoken vowels that are of longer duration and entail inherent periodicity(ies). It also often proves more convenient to assess the brain's responses to such sounds in the frequency domain.

A given sound can demonstrate repetition or periodicity at different time scales. As a first example, consider a pair of tones that are 400 Hz and 500 Hz. The upper panel of Figure 6–11 displays the sound pressure of these tones individually for 30 ms. At this time scale, many cycles of each tone are visible because their periods are $1/400 = 2.5$ ms and $1/500=2$ ms, respectively. Most real-world sounds, as emphasized earlier (Episodes 2.1 and 2.2), are more complex than these simple tones and can be synthesized by summing many tones with appropriate amplitudes and relative phases. The exact set of tones required will change with complexity, but for short periods of time, the set can be determined from spectra using *Fourier analysis*. In the bottom panel of Figure 6–11, a slightly more complex sound has been synthesized simply by summing the two tones. The "summed" waveform still contains changing sound pressure with a period between 2 ms and 2.5 ms ($1/450=2.222$ ms). Nuances of this sort are referred to as *fine structure*.

The original tones achieved the same maximum and minimum sound pressures every cycle (again, upper panel of Figure 6–11). Limits of +1 and −1 can be imagined to define a rectangular *envelope* for the tones. For these individual tones, the envelopes are constant. In the bottom panel, the individual cycles of the fine structure achieve maximum and minimum sound pressures that vary cyclically, expressing a form of amplitude modulation (AM). This envelope has a period of $1/(500 - 400) = 10$ ms. In this case, the envelope is referred to as *beating* between two tones and occurs at the rate of their difference frequency $500 - 400 = 100$ Hz. The *envelope rate* of complex tones is referred to

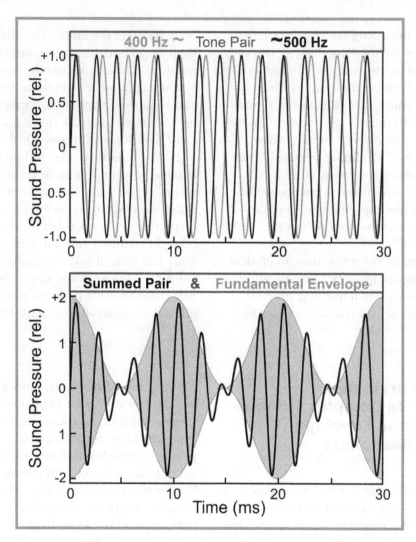

Figure 6–11. Time-domain representation of two tones (*top*) and their sum (*bottom*, with time history overlaying its temporal envelope [*gray fill*]).

as the ***fundamental*** frequency. The envelope is not quite sinusoidal, but a sinusoid of 100 Hz is gray-filled and "backlights" the two-tone complex to illustrate the slower periodicity of the envelope.

In the psychoacoustics literature, this complex tone—apropos what is heard—is an example of the ***missing fundamental***. Figure 6–12 shows the spectrum of the sum of these two tones. The lines 400 Hz and 500 Hz represent the discrete spectrum that characterizes sinusoids and other periodic functions (simple or complex), and thus the foci of energy present in these tones. Although the eye can clearly see the slower envelope rate in the time history defining the waveform, there is no acoustic energy at the difference frequency in the spectrum. Despite the lack of acoustic energy at the envelope rate, information in the stimulus is delivered by both the envelope and the fine structure, thanks to the auditory neurons' substantial ability to encode such temporal information, starting with the fundamental frequencies of individual tones. Evoked potentials thus can be elicited at the envelope rate (100 Hz) as well as the rates present in the fine structure (that is, the carrier rates or the tone frequencies).

Figure 6–13 shows a schematic of these evoked potentials as a spectrum that might be obtained from an individual with normal hearing. The spec-

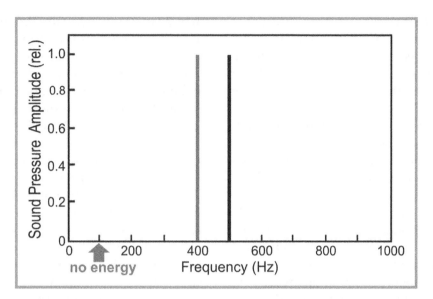

Figure 6–12. Spectrum of the tone pair in Figure 6–11.

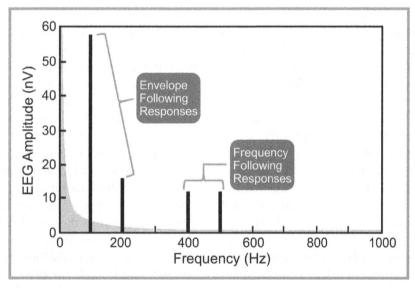

Figure 6–13. Schematic illustration of spectrum of brain responses elicited by a tone pair. (Gray fill: background EEG)

trum contains lines at both the envelope and tone frequencies that rise above the EEG noise decreasing with 1/frequency. Evoked potentials elicited by the carrier tones are labeled *frequency following responses (FFRs)*. They are generated by neurons time locked to the stimulus tones, and for practical recording durations, are detectable for stimulus tones under 1 kHz, or above but with diminishing efficacy. Evoked potentials elicited by the stimulus envelope are labeled *envelope following responses (EFRs)*. In the special but audiologically common case where the stimulus properties do not vary over time, these EFRs have been called *auditory steady-state responses (ASSRs)*. They have been used extensively for estimation of behavioral detection thresholds,[53] methodological details and clinical applications of which will be presented soon. For the purposes of discussion at the moment, the principle at hand is that such potentials are generated by neurons time locked to the envelope and its low order harmonics. In the example of Figure 6–13, a response is also shown at 200 Hz, which is the second harmonic of the envelope rate.

Many authors use the term FFR to refer to both envelope-following and fine-structure following responses. In some literature, a subscript (for example, FFR_{ENV}) or other notation is added to differentiate the two. As detection and measurement of AEPs are as much about SNR as actual magnitudes of the given response, practical/clinical interests (although not exclusively) have come to favor the EFR, which usually has a larger amplitude than the FFR.

A response spectrum in humans can be obtained that is similar to that portrayed in Figure 6–13 by presenting the stimulus at a modest level (for instance, 70 dB SPL) and recording at an adequate sampling rate (namely >2000 samples/s) with a relatively wide band-pass filter (such as 1–1000 Hz), high gain (100,000×), and for at least several minutes of signal processing. Generally, noise rejection is used to remove small segments of the recording when myogenic artifact is especially large (recall Episodes 4.1 and 4.2). The remaining data could be **synchronously (coherently) averaged** to diminish myogenic noise and background EEG unrelated to the stimulus, much like as done for the transient ABR. However, the click/tone-burst ABR is about capturing coherent activity as if it were possible to do for a single event. Practically, it is not, so multiple samples have to be averaged to extract something measureable as the presumptive response in the EEG/noise. Synchronous averaging (conceptually) means that brain activity exactly corresponding to stimulus repetitions/trains (that is, time locked) should dominate the resultant signal, and thus taken as the true response. The average recording sweep is also used for spectral analysis. For this purpose, it normally should contain an integer number of cycles of each response frequency of interest. In the example of Figure 6–13, selecting the sweep duration to include an integer number of cycles of the envelope rate (100 Hz) would also guarantee an integer number of cycles of envelope harmonics and the stimulus tones. Computing the Fourier transform of the average recording sweep then produces a spectrum like that shown in Figure 6–13. The waveform of the average recording sweep can be observed instead of the spectrum, but it is generally dominated by background EEG and myogenic noise. It can be difficult to interpret due to the low signal-to-noise ratio (SNR) of real-world recordings, unless the response is very large (more typical for responses near 40 Hz) or with additional narrowband filtering applied. This is demonstrated in principle looking back at Figure 4–12 (right panel), although having measured a different AEP elicited simply by tone bursts. Therein trains of responses were difficult to impossible to reliably identify, given minimal signal averaging. With additional filtering applied, as in Figure 4–17, the "train" was clearly revealed and consistently evident except at the lower stimulus levels.

The difference in amplitude between FFRs and EFRs could be explained in part by their initiation mechanisms. The FFRs elicited by the carrier tones are initiated from cochlear regions with corresponding characteristic frequencies plus neighboring regions due to spread of excitation at higher stimulus levels.[54] Similarly, the EFR is also initiated from cochlear regions where the carrier energy is present but the response is at the lower frequency envelope rate. Since there is no acoustic energy at the envelope rate, additional nonlinear mechanisms must be involved to introduce the envelope rate into the auditory system. Candidate nonlinearities are present within the cochlea,[55,56] and were discussed more or less in Episode 5.1 on the generation of otoacoustic emissions. At least readers who are audio-high-fidelity hobbyists may have become uncomfortable to have been told multiple times now (recalling also the summating potential story) of cochlear nonlinearities, indeed hinting of such nonlinearity to be "essential" to how the auditory system works normally. Not to worry. Nonlinearity is also about dynamic range of operation (like $\approx 10^{12}:1$ in power!) which must be compressed practically, but compression is inherently a nonlinear process.

The amplitude of EFRs is smaller for low frequency carriers, compared to high frequency carriers. The bandwidth of cochlear auditory filters increases with increasing carrier frequency.[57] Envelope rates of 80 Hz to 110 Hz are often used for eliciting EFRs that are dominated by brainstem generators (for instance, ASSR[53], up next). For carrier frequencies below 750 Hz, an envelope rate of 100 Hz may reduce cochlear interactions between stimulus tones because they mostly fall in different cochlear auditory filters. EFR amplitude is higher for carrier tones >750 Hz at response rates of about 100 Hz.[53,58]

Scalp-recorded EFRs elicited at envelope rates >80 Hz predominantly reflect phase-locked activity, indeed, in the brainstem. The term predominant is used because when recorded on the scalp, EFRs could reflect neural activity phase locked to the same envelope rate combined from more than one source.[59-62] However, since the ability of the auditory cortex to phase lock reduces as the envelope rate increases,[63] contributions from cortical sources are substantially reduced at higher envelope rates. Several lines of evidence support the predominant brainstem generation of EFRs elicited at >80 Hz. These lines include (i) source localization using multichannel EEG recordings,[64-66] (ii) response latency,[59] (iii) limited impact of sleep,[59,67] and (iv) limited impact of temporal lobe lesions.[68]

There are many other cyclical stimuli that have periodic envelopes and can elicit EFRs.[69] The top panel in Figure 6–14 shows the time waveform of a *sinusoidally amplitude modulated (SAM)* tone that has a carrier frequency of 500 Hz and an envelope modulation rate/frequency (F_M) of 100 Hz. A gray line shows the exact sinusoidal shape of the envelope. The envelope is symmetrical in positive and negative pressures. The carrier frequency and the envelope frequency can be varied independently. The middle panel shows that sinusoidal amplitude modulation requires the sum of three sinusoids that are separated by the modulation rate. This stimulus can be considered to be reasonably narrow band for modulation rates near 100 Hz and elicits place-specific responses from the cochlea.[70] The relative amplitude of the original carrier tone to the two sideband tones varies with the depth of modulation. For 100% amplitude modulation, the envelope reaches zero each envelope cycle and the sideband tones are half the amplitude of the carrier—that is, sideband tones 6 dB down from the carrier's amplitude. Increasing modulation depth generally increases EFR amplitude,[71,72] but saturation can occur above 50%.[55,73-75] Other variants of SAM include envelopes that are sine-squared and sine-cubed. They have longer-duration sections of low amplitude during each envelope cycle and steeper rise and fall slopes as the envelope increases and decreases, which may increase response amplitude.[69] The bottom panel shows example responses elicited by an amplitude-modulated tone. The largest response is usually the EFR at the envelope rate and there may be low order harmonics of that rate. Only the second harmonic is shown at 200 Hz in Figure 6–14. Smaller FFRs at the carrier and sideband rates can also be observed in reasonable measurement times if the carrier frequency is below about 1000 Hz.

Other stimulus possibilities can also elicit EFRs. As shown in Figure 6–15, SAM can be applied to complex carrier sounds, such as broadband noise and narrowband noise. In the figure, the gray line shows the sinusoidal shape of the envelope, but is plotted only on the positive side of the vertical sound pressure axis as a reminder that the envelope only exists implicitly as limits on the moment-by-moment sound pressures of the noise signal. Broadband noise more clearly illuminates those envelope limits compared to narrowband noise. The narrowband noise only irregularly approaches the larger envelope limits, but is still forced to zero in each modulation cycle. Responses occur at the envelope modulation rate and its harmonics, but there is no FFR from the noise carrier. The carrier signals discussed so far, tones and noise, are continuous and the envelope generally spends only a short proportion of each cycle with an amplitude near zero.

Following responses can also be elicited by (in effect) trains of brief/transient sounds. Figure 6–16A shows the electrical signal of a single polarity pulse train. Adapting from earlier demonstrations (in effect), here the DC pulses are 0.5 ms in duration at a repetition rate of 100 Hz. Although in the long run, this signal will be characterized by a line spectrum with lines at 100 Hz intervals; its spectral envelope (panel B) will follow the continuous spectrum's envelope for the single pulse, with nulls at every $1/0.0005 = 2000$ Hz. Only the first lobe and null are shown here in the interest of viewing spectral detail. In practice to produce acoustic clicks by transducing such a DC pulse and for a

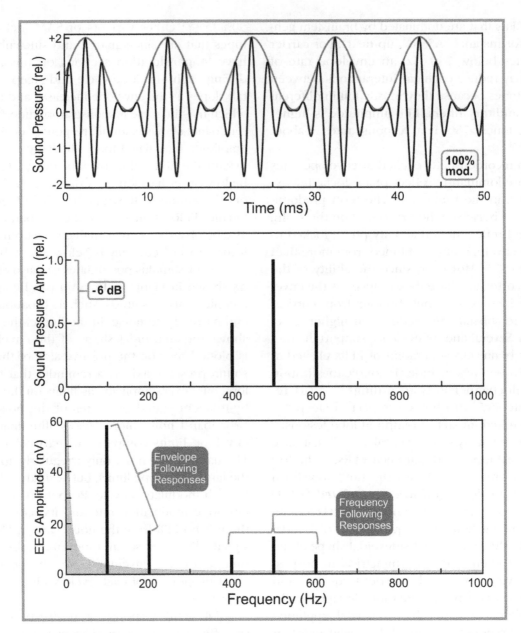

Figure 6–14. Sinusoidally amplitude modulated tone—time- and frequency-domain analyses and brainstem potentials expected from a SAM tone.

more expansive first lobe of the spectrum (recall Figure 2–17), the duration of the individual pulses used is commonly only 100 μs, illustrated in the time domain in panel C. Predicting its discrete spectrum from its continuous spectrum for the single-click response, the click train would have much the same overall nuances as in panel B, but displaying a relatively flat energy level in harmonics of the presentation rate until approaching its first spectral null at the reciprocal of the plateau duration (1/100 μs = 10 kHz [recall Figure 2–17]). While only a small set of clicks is displayed in panel C showing the time analysis of a click train, it might be played to the listener for several minutes at a modest stimulus level of sufficient data processing to generate adequate responses. The signal actually plotted in panel C is the acoustic waveform that could be recorded in an adult ear (detailed waveform and subsequent spectrum at the oval window pending actual transducer used). Unlike the electrical driv-

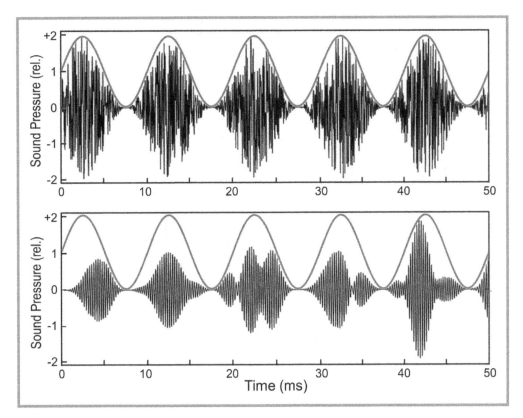

Figure 6–15. Sinusoidally amplitude modulated noises—broadband (*top*) versus narrowband (*bottom*)

ing signal, the acoustic waveform rings for a short time and the amplitude envelope reflects brief excursions to nonzero sound pressures followed by about 8 ms of silence. The silence following each click thus fills a significant proportion of the repetition period. This stimulus would elicit an "ABR" that could be partially observed as a time waveform in an analysis window of 10 ms duration that shows the average of the brain activity following more than 1,000 clicks. However, at modest stimulus levels, there could be overlapping of early and late waves (V onto I and II, etc.) and stimulus-computational-analysis techniques like ***maximum length sequences (MLS)*** would be needed to "unwrap" overlapping responses.[76] The mathematical side of the approach is to assume this overlapping is interactive, not merely something like destructive interference of otherwise unaltered ABRs, which is far from reality in fact. As discussed in the last two episodes (Episodes 5.4 and 6.1), there is some neural adaptation going on at such high stimulation rates. The result is taken to be much like what mathematically is called a convolution for which there are clever "tricks to undo"—hence, "deconvolution." Though an area aggressively pursued at one time to improve ABR test efficiency, the approach has yet to command clinical interests. More germane here and apropos current practices is the fact that the stimulus would also elicit an EFR at the repetition rate/frequency and (particularly of interest) its low order harmonics.

A train of tone bursts similarly creates a stimulus amplitude envelope with the period of the repetition rate. An example with a tone-burst repetition rate again of 100 Hz is shown Figure 6–16D. An EFR would be elicited at the tone-burst presentation rate and its low order harmonics. At moderate and low stimulus levels, the response is usually initiated near the characteristic place for the tone-burst frequency.[77,78] With enough cycles of the carrier tone in the tone burst, a smaller amplitude FFR also may be detectable at the frequency of the carrier. In addition to tone bursts, a train of chirps can also create an amplitude envelope that elicits an

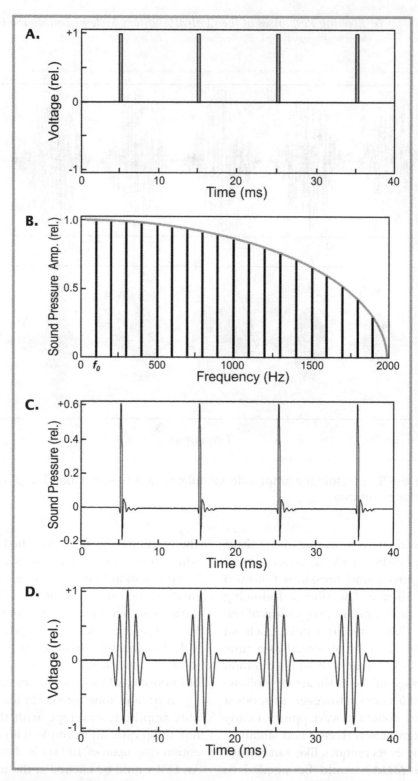

Figure 6–16. Recap illustration, recalling and adapting Figures 2–15 and 2–17: time-frequency realities by example of the DC pulses that also underlie effects of windowing sinusoidal carriers. Temporal analysis of a pulse train (**A**) and its line spectrum (**B**) with spectral envelope highlighted (*gray line*). **C** and **D**. Time histories respectively of repeated acoustic clicks and sinusoidal pulses. Still other signals, like the chirp, can be used in trains to elicit following responses.

EFR at the chirp repetition rate and its low order harmonics. Although technically challenging to extract, an FFR that follows the instantaneous frequency of the changing carrier tone may also be present. Following up on related discussion in the previous episode, the cochlear place specificity of EFRs and FFRs (that is, where in the cochlea they truly are initiated) can be verified using masking noise to desynchronize contributions to the measured following response that might be initiated from other cochlear regions, again due to spread of excitation at modest and high stimulus levels. Masking noise also can ensure place specificity in the case of a steeply sloping sensory hearing loss for the purpose of objective threshold estimation in the cochlear region of the carrier frequency.

Many systems found in nature readily vibrate at a fundamental or resonant frequency and its harmonics, such as the human's vocal tract. The relative amplitudes of the harmonics drive human perception of a complex tone during the somewhat steady-state middle part of the sound, giving it a specific timbre such as that of a trumpet versus a clarinet or versus the voice. An example was given earlier (recall Figure 2–5A). **Speech** has unmatched ecological validity for auditory assessment. Vowels are the longest duration and most energetic phonemes in speech. They exhibit spectrally prominent regions called formants wherein the harmonics associated with a formant are relatively high amplitude compared to harmonics in regions falling between formants. The first two formants contribute significantly to the perception of vowel identity.

The sample used for Figure 2–5 was that of a vowel produced by a male talker with an average f_0 of 108 Hz, calculated from the steady-state "body" of the speech token /ɛ/. It now is examined after further processing, as shown in Figure 6–17. In panel A, the signal of the vowel has been rectified to simulate the nature of the effect of processing/ encoding in the auditory periphery. In panel B is the spectrum. A robust EFR can be detected readily at the voice fundamental frequency and its low order harmonics.[79,80] The amplitude envelope being followed is the difference frequency between any adjacent pair of vowel harmonics. Each pair of vowel harmonics is akin to the tone pair shown in Figure 6–11 and Figure 6–12. The spacing between the harmonics reflects the rate of opening and closing of the vocal folds during voicing, the voice's fundamental frequency, and is ultimately perceived by listeners as ***voice pitch***.

In the cochlea, adjacent pairs of harmonics (Figure 2–5, top panel) can interact within cochlear auditory filters to introduce the ***local envelope rate*** into the auditory system. Given many pairs of equally spaced adjacent harmonics, EFRs, at the same fundamental frequency (again, envelope rate), are initiated concurrently from vowel harmonics across a broad region of the cochlea where there is adequate stimulus energy. Due to cochlear traveling wave delays, parallel responses initiated from different cochlear regions sum at the measurement electrodes either constructively or destructively (namely, unlike MLS; now back to the more basic math of phasor addition). Although EFRs from higher frequency harmonics dominate the scalp-recorded EFR,[81] low frequency vowel harmonics in the region of the first formant also contribute to the measured EFR.[81-84] In addition to within-cochlear filter nonlinearity, there may be additional nonlinear brainstem mechanisms at play that operate across auditory filter frequencies. For some vowel tokens, the net EFR at the measurement electrodes can be very small. It has been demonstrated that larger EFRs can be measured by introducing a stimulus delay to the envelopes generated in the cochlea by harmonics in the second and higher formants.[81,85] Such a stimulus manipulation can phase-align responses initiated from harmonics in different formants and produce a larger net EFR at the measurement electrodes, similar to a chirp stimulus. A second possible stimulus manipulation (to avoid EFR cancellations among components initiated by harmonics in the first and higher formants) is to slightly adjust harmonic spacing in different formants.[83,86,87] Multiple simultaneous EFRs then can be recorded at slightly different fundamental frequencies without dramatically altering the EFRs elicited by individual formants,[87] for instance, perception of the vowel or signal processing of the vowel by a hearing aid.[86]

Returning to panel A of Figure 2–5, it shows a single acoustic polarity of the time waveform for the vowel token. The detailed moment-by-moment pressure fluctuations (makeup of the fine structure) are not clearly discernable at this time scale,

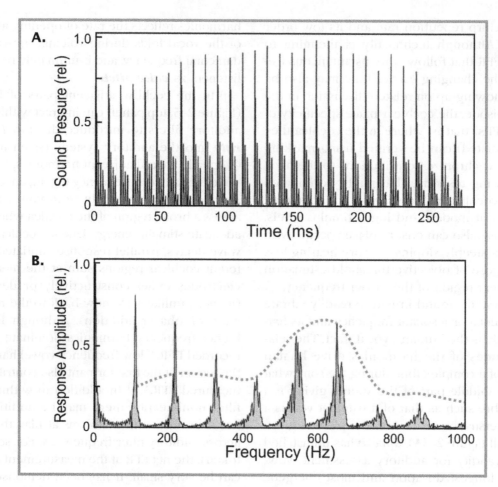

Figure 6–17. Model of overall following response for a speech stimulus presented earlier; see Figure 2–5 which presented both time and frequency analyses of the vowel /ɛ/ produced naturally by a male speaker. **A.** Time history of results from rectifying that signal, approximating effects of the nonlinearity of front-end auditory processing. **B.** Spectrum of this signal (*highlighted light-gray fill*) and approximate spectral envelope (*gray dotted line*) of the stimulus (modeled via a graphical interpolation algorithm applied to spectral peaks of the actual spectrum of the vowel). Comparable results to those of Figure 6–4 are evident, representing similar nuances overall to those of a far less complex signal (sinusoidal amplitude modulation of single carrier and modulation frequencies). Envelope following again prevails, although not to the exclusion of frequency-following response components in the vicinity of a vowel formant (midfrequency hump in analysis over the first formant near 600 Hz). Note: this spectrum is also fundamentally discrete, but "pristine" lines (used earlier to focus on principles) are not produced via this still-brief sample (relative to infinity) with varying f_0, yet also useful as more characteristic of actual response recordings.

but the repeating vocal fold cycles at the voice's fundamental frequency are visible. The overall amplitude envelope of the phoneme is also evident; the vowel begins, fluctuates a bit in overall amplitude, and then ends. To emphasize the EFR and reduce the chance of stimulus artifact, the waveforms elicited in the recorded EEG by vowel tokens of both polarities usually are synchronously averaged.[88] This approach is based on the assumption that similar EFRs are elicited by the two vowel polarities. However, the assumption deviates in the case of some vowels. The vowel envelope of /ɛ/ is asymmetrical, unlike the tone pair example in the bottom panel of Figure 6–11 and the SAM tone in the top panel of Figure 6–14. Therefore, asymmetry in the vowel envelope can have some effects on the EFR amplitude[89] and which are likely intensified or confounded by the front-end-processing nonlinearity (as portrayed by Figure 6–17A).

Smaller FFRs can also be detected in response to individual voice harmonics[88] if they are relatively low frequency and enough time has been spent averaging to reduce background noise (Figure 6–17B). Brain activity recorded in response to opposite stimulus polarities must be subtracted in an average. The FFR has been shown to follow stimulus polarity, and if ignored, the signal extracted (in reference to the true potential) will be greatly attenuated. Figure 6–13 is similar to one used[88] to demonstrate the detectability of a possible FFR at the frequency of every harmonic of the voice. Additionally, results demonstrate that a potential FFR contribution from the first harmonic of the voice can be a very small proportion of the total measured EFR.[79,88] Concurrent contributions from higher frequency harmonic pairs generate larger EFRs, thus dominating the net EFR measured on the surface of the head.[81]

The predominately brainstem-generated responses discussed in this episode have either followed the stimulus envelope (EFRs) or the fine structure of a stimulus carrier tone (FFRs). Succinctly, EFRs follow the AM of the envelope. A further look into the nuances of speech-elicited following responses and applications of their measurements is the topic of the next Head Ups, followed by an in-depth look into what is easily the most broadly clinically adapted and adopted application of EFRs to date—ASSRs.

HEADS UP

Speech-Evoked EFR and FFR

This Heads Up presents further background and potential clinical applications of FFR measurement of speech-elicited responses. For the EFR, this means **phase locking** of the evoked potential to the **envelope's periodicity**, which presumably is related to suprasegmental aspects of speech, like pitch and prosody. For the FFR, this means phase locking to the **temporal fine structure (TFS)**, which presumably is related to the representation of spectral components, like vowel formants, that play a role in speech perception. There is keen and growing interest in the clinical application of such responses in audiology. Speech is a mix of complex, quasi-steady-state/quasiperiodic and transient components.

As a stimulus, speech tokens contain a temporal structure that is characterized both by a relatively **slowly varying temporal feature** (periodicity envelope) that is superimposed on a more **rapidly varying temporal feature** (TFS). However unlike complex tones, speech is characterized by distinct time-varying spectral-temporal attributes. These are imparted by the vocal track during production, which the listener (in turn) uses as cues to identify and discriminate among speech sounds. While the use of the 80-Hz ASSR (again, an EFR to modulated sinusoidal carriers/tones) has been limited primarily to threshold estimation, highlighted here are some applications of EFR/FFR measurement wherein responses are elicited well above threshold. The results of such tests may provide insight on the nature of changes in the underlying temporal pattern of neural activity, in particular how its representation is degraded by cochlear impairment. This knowledge is paramount not only to track effective retraining strategies but also to facilitate the development of optimal signal-processing strategies that can be implemented in prosthetic devices, like hearing aids and cochlear implants. This implies that these responses potentially have a role in monitoring outcomes and in the refinement of signal processing parameters tailored to the individual patient's needs. For instance, cochlear hearing loss is known to alter/degrade the envelope and/or temporal fine-structure cues (to be scrutinized further, shortly). However, enhanced envelope representation in cochlear-impaired individuals is not particularly helpful for speech perception and even may contribute to the degradation of speech perception.

This feature story thus introduces analyses of EFRs and FFRs elicited particularly by speech stimuli and their potential application toward an understanding of the nature of degradation in the neural representation of stimulus envelope and its fine structure—namely as a potential consequence to hearing loss. Both play important roles in speech perception. The view expressed here will be that these responses do provide important fine-grained information about neural representation of certain segmental and suprasegmental acoustic features that are important for speech perception. Such information should be useful clinically, when evaluated judiciously and knowledgeably of limitations of their representation of the neural encoding of speech.

The recording methods for these responses are essentially the same as for recording an ABR or ASSR. Responses are recorded differentially between electrodes at midline-hairline (connected to the noninverting input of the amplifier) and electrodes (connected to the inverting input) as follows: electrodes placed on (1) the right and left mastoids (M_1 and M_2) and (2) the 7th cervical vertebra (C_7). The ground electrode is placed on the forehead at F_{pz}. Responses averaged from the two electrode configurations yield a response with a higher SNR than from the more conventional ABR-test montage.[90]

The paradigm of alternating stimulus onset and split-buffer averaging is used to allow the storage of responses to each polarity in a different buffer which can then be used to derive the EFR (addition of the two buffers) and the FFR (subtraction of buffers). Addition and subtraction of polarity-inverted responses have been widely used in FFR studies to obtain brainstem-level neural representations of the temporal envelope and fine structure, respectively.[91,92] It should be mentioned here that the use of magnetically shielded earphones is essential to ensure stimulus-artifact-free responses, since the stimulus largely overlaps the responses, including directly the fine structure (much like recording the cochlear microphonic to tone bursts; recall Figure 5–10).

Response analysis includes both *frequency- and time-domain-based metrics* and applying autocorrelation analysis to both responses. Spectral analysis of the EFR response shows peaks at F0 and its harmonics, which are essentially distortion products that are not phase locked with the temporal fine structure. Therefore, it is incorrect to characterize this information as a representation of TFS of speech sounds. In contrast, spectral analysis of the FFR shows robust peaks at stimulus harmonics, occurring prominently at formant-related harmonics. For time varying speech stimuli, a joint time-frequency analysis is necessary (essentially obtaining a spectrogram, as commonly used in speech science) to evaluate the response to the time-varying segments of the stimulus. This is to determine if the phase-locked activity is faithfully tracking the frequency changes. Another useful measure is the index of spectral correlation between the stimulus and the response to evaluate how well the stimulus spectrum is being represented by the phase-locked neural activity. In the time domain, autocorrelation analysis (a correlation of the signal to itself over time) is used to estimate the presence of periodicities and their strength, computed over the duration of the response. For example, a single-frequency sinusoid expressed over some cycles will have a correlation of 1.0. The reciprocal of the time lag of the response's autocorrelation peak (or the pitch period) is an estimate of the F0. The magnitude of this peak represents the *strength of neural periodicity*.

In sum, the phase-locked neural activity among neural elements in the rostral brainstem that generates the scalp recorded "FFR" has been shown to preserve information about both the envelope periodicity (EFR) and the temporal fine structure (FFR) of steady-state and time-variant speech sounds.[90,93–95] In the following, review of several studies from the author's laboratory will serve to highlight the basic science and clinical applications of the EFR and FFR to speechlike sounds and point to new areas of potential research and clinical applications.

The first report demonstrating that the spectra of scalp-recorded FFR elicited by steady-state vowels showed prominent peaks at several harmonics around the first and second formant frequencies.[94] This observation portended that the phase-locked activity preserved information about the TFS of the speech stimuli in addition to its envelope periodicity (see example in Figure 6–18A, to follow shortly). Thus, these brainstem components provide an effective physiologic window by which to examine the neural representation of these temporal cues in the human brainstem noninvasively and how they indeed may be altered consequently by sensorineural hearing loss (SNHL). Neural representation of time-varying TFS cues—represented by formant transitions in CV syllables—was explored subsequently in listeners with normal hearing (NH) and mild-moderate SNHL, using FFR measurement.[96] Results showed that the phase-locked neural activity in the SNHL group, unlike the NH group, was not indicative of the formant transition in the CV syllables presented, suggesting degraded TFS representation due to disrupted neural phase locking. Also noted was improvement in neural representation of the formant transition with increasing presentation level, potentially suggesting that the observed degradation was not attributable merely to lack of audibility.

More recently examined is the level-dependent neural representation of envelope versus TFS of steady-state speech stimuli in normal hearing and individuals with SNHL.[91] Compared were the responses at equal SPL versus equal SL to permit further scrutiny of the issue of audibility. The results showed that the neural representation of both envelope (F0) and TFS (F1) at equal SPLs was stronger in NH listeners compared to SNHL listeners and that neural representation of F0 and F1 across stimulus levels expressed in SPL versus and SL (per audibility) were different for the two groups. Their results overall showed greater degradation in the neural representation of TFS compared to periodicity envelope in the SNHL group. This suggests a disruption in the temporal pattern of phase-locked neural activity, likely arising from altered tonotopic maps and/or effectively wider filters causing poor frequency selectivity in these listeners.

In a couple of the most recent investigations, the issue of envelope and TFS encoding using vocoded speech were examined.[97,98] This is a multiband filtering channelizing of speech to simulate the effects of the speech-processing strategies of the cochlear implant (which will be taken up in more detail in a subsequent episode). The point here is that normal-hearing listeners' ability to understand such speech, inherently degraded relative to the cochlea's natural processing, permits researchers to pursue measures of interest in subjects who can also serve as their own controls. Recording and analyses of the ENV and TFS proves a useful tool for exploring such effects, indeed providing robust metrics, as demonstrated in the unprocessed speech (that is, nonvocoded control condition) in Figure 6–18A. Note in panel B the effective tracking of format transitions during the speech token /au/. Measurements are then repeated for each condition of N-channels of encoding. Overall outcomes are as expected, the fewer the channels of encoding, the more degraded is the representation of natural speech. Still, there are some "devils" in the details. In the first of these studies,[97] the focus was on the effects of systematically varying spectral and temporal cues on the brainstem's neural representation of F0 (envelope periodicity) and the formant phase-locked activity (TFS) with number of channels as the experimental parameter. The results showed that both temporal envelope and TFS cues improved when the number of channels increased from 1 to 4, followed by a plateau at 8 to 16 channels. However, a reduction in phase-locking strength occurred at 32 channels. When the temporal envelope cutoff frequency increased from 50 Hz to

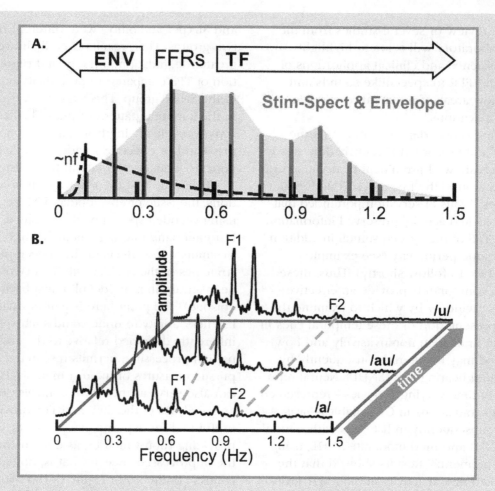

Figure 6–18. A. Line spectrum ("slice") of FFR elicited by the speech token /au/ overlaid on that of the stimulus and its approximate spectral envelope (*gray shaded area*). The approximate spectral envelope of the noise floor (nf) is traced with black dashed line. ENV/TF: nominal frequency ranges of envelope versus temporal fine structure components of the FFR. **B.** Spectra at several instances during the stimulus, thus capturing the transition from /a/ to /u/ and related shifts in respective formants, F1 and F2.

500 Hz, an improvement was observed in FFR representation, yet with no change in spectral peaks at the F1 harmonics. While the improvement in neural representation of temporal envelope and TFS cues with up to 4 vocoder channels is consistent with results reported in the behavioral literature, the reduced neural phase-locking strength noted with even more channels is less so and may occur because of the narrow bandwidth of each channel, as the number of channels increases. Meanwhile, stronger neural representation of temporal envelope cues at the higher F0 is likely due to the more prominent envelope in the 500-Hz condition compared to the 50-Hz condition.

Much about speech production and processing in the CANS in real time is naturally more about complex modulations than steady state, as such, the idea that the brainstem is refined in its design to facilitate feature detection (recall Episode 3.2). A speech token—like, a single sustained phoneme versus a diphthong, is an example (at the simplest level). Therefore, in a second study,[98] the differences in the neural representation of vocoded, time-variant speech was examined having been encoded by means of amplitude (alone) versus amplitude plus frequency modulation, namely as the spectral and temporal cues were varied. The aim was to determine if the addition of FM to AM (theoretically more cues for feature detection) improved the neural representation of envelope periodicity (FFR_{ENV}) and temporal fine structure (FFR_{TFS}). The results showed that increasing the number of channels produced a greater reduction in periodicity strength of the FFR_{ENV} for the AM stimuli than for AM+FM stimuli. FFR_{ENV} spectral peaks were consistently present at the stimulus F0 for all the AM+FM stimuli, but not for the AM stimuli. Neural representation, as revealed by the spectral correlation of FFR_{TFS}, was better for the AM+FM stimuli. Lastly, the neural representation of the time-varying, formant-related harmonics was also better for the AM+FM stimuli. These results are consistent with previously reported findings of psychoacoustic studies and suggest that the AM+FM processing strategy elicited brainstem neural activity that better preserved periodicity, temporal fine structure, and time-varying spectral information than the AM-alone processing strategy. The relatively more robust neural representation of AM+FM stimuli observed likely contributes to the superior performance on speech, speaker, and tone recognition and could potentially be a better CI processing strategy, compared to the use of AM alone.

Taken together, the studies and results overviewed suggest, indeed, that neural information preserved in the FFR may be used to evaluate signal processing strategies considered for the likes of CI treatment. In the long term, such knowledge hopefully can be built upon in further research and development of CI speech processing strategies toward better encoding and subsequent perception of specific acoustic features in the speech signal. At the same time, research and development in this area has been devoted to making the encoding of music pleasurable too, especially given that what is the best strategy for speech processing (especially for speech recognition in background noise/speaker babble) is not necessarily optimal for music enjoyment. In any event, the FFR will always be there for research and development purposes. Meanwhile in the noble cause to translate laboratory results to useful clinical tools, there certainly is the hope of increasing applications of FFR measurement in monitoring treatment and adding to outcome measures to best serve patients.

■ Episode 3: Auditory Steady-State Response—80-Hz Response

Introduced in this episode are further details of the *auditory steady-state responses*, in particular, the currently most broadly used following response. This AEP is an EFR that can be elicited by repetitive transient stimuli such as clicks, but more commonly and purposefully in audiological applications by some form of modulated tones, and all at relatively high stimulus rates. At rates of about 70 Hz and above and by virtue of typical front-end filtering of the EEG needed for excellent SNRs of ABRs, only short-latency components of the AEP are observed that result in a quasiperiodic response, largely from overlapping component potentials of ABRs. Therefore, of particular interest here is an ASSR elicited at a modulation frequency (F_M) that is nominally 80 Hz (70 Hz–110 Hz in practice)—the *80-Hz ASSR*.

Having inherent qualities of the ABR, the 80-Hz ASSR has enjoyed considerable interest for *evoked response audiometry (ERA)*. However, research and development for the application of "80 Hz" was preceded by the pioneering work of Robert Galambos and coworkers in 1981,[99] who first demonstrated a practical steady-state method based on a middle latency response (coming soon!). They used the classical transient-stimulus-response paradigm but extended the time-domain analysis to permit observation/measurement over some four stimulus cycles. The robust response observed at the relatively high rate of 40 Hz was enhanced in amplitude (relative to the transient MLR) and nearly sinusoidal in waveform. At this repetition rate, it was generated by overlapping of the MLR component waves. This all was counterintuitive at the time, yet with immediate promise of ERA applications. Vigorous research and development thereafter included production of a commercially available test system, but interest took a downturn as initial results of 40-Hz-ASSR ERA showed the response amplitude to be significantly reduced by sleep[100] and to have poor reliability in infants.[101] This was naturally a blow to one of the major sectors of clinical interest (a topic presented in-depth in subsequent episodes), having "failed" to match the ABR's resilience in deep stages of natural or drug-induced sleep and even coma.

However, this was not the case in neuroscience wherein steady-state-related research was of broader interest in sensory evoked potential work. For instance, the inherent frequency band of the EEG (like alpha rhythm) makes any oscillatory brainwaves intriguing. With steady-state stimulation using repetitive stimuli, increasing the rate effectively "pushes" the observed response caudally, descending from the cortex with their very long latencies potentials down toward the pontine brainstem.[102] In the mid-1980s and on, ASSRs to modulated tones caught the interests of other researchers who first applied spectral analysis to their measurements and performed response evaluation in the frequency domain.[103] Using rates ≈80 Hz yielded results little affected under natural sleep and drug-induced sedation[67] and research and development of steady-state AEP measurement resumed with a new vitality.

Basic and clinical research of ASSRs grew rapidly in the 1990s, producing findings particularly of the efficacy and usefulness of 80-Hz ASSR. At this time, stimuli used were **single-modulation-frequency (SAM)** carriers.[104,105] Subsequently, the use of other stimulus paradigms using multiple simultaneously presented stimuli was investigated.[106,107] By the mid-1990s, 80-Hz-ERA was validated for use in both adults and children. The overall research and development had also been impressively multinational, as the earliest test systems were developed in Australia, Cuba, and Canada and subsequently the United States and Denmark. ASSR test instruments were either stand-alone or software modules in existing general-purpose AEP test systems that became available from 1998 to 2005 with European certification (CE) and U.S.-FDA certification (Food and Drug Administration). This facilitated both broader interests and clinical use of this "new and improved" approach to **objective audiometry** via clinical electrophysiology and launched a remarkable wave of translational research.

The revelation of analyzing and interpreting ASSR results based on spectral analysis was essential to a more efficacious approach and was the step-stone to further innovations, as will be demonstrated. The fundamental concept of performing an analysis in the frequency domain was not new, even in the early 1980s, being nearly two centuries old. However, the implementation of the principle via a computer algorithm for the FFT (for spectral analysis) and computer research and development toward cost-effective systems would take nearly a decade to foster production of sufficiently economical test systems for routine clinical use. Recalling Episode 2.1, the math of spectral analysis is actually a two-way street, applying as well to signal synthesis. In practice, tools for both sides of the stimulus-response approach that is called "steady-state" are those of both generation of complex stimuli and speedy computation of high-resolution spectral analyses of the recordings. Thereafter are the sort of tools taken for granted today via the likes of electronic spreadsheets and word processing: rapid user-friendly applications at a mere "click," efficient output of results of analyses, multiwindow graphics for spectral and polar/phasor plots, audiogram-like charts, and clinical report generation.

The 80-Hz ASSR is mostly generated by the overlapping components of the transient-elicited ABR, most notably peaks V, V_N, and SN_{10}.[108] ASSR-ERA thus benefits from ABR features particularly important for ERA, including evaluation of auditory function in infants and other difficult-to-test subjects, as well as provision of some other advantages that will be described in more detail. In general, it will be revealed that the innovation of the

ASSR is not just one of putting another or even prettier face on ABR measurement, rather also providing a few remarkable capabilities/advantages.

Unlike the transient ABR, the 80-Hz ASSR is a quasisinusoidal response, virtually continuous in time and elicited virtually continuously by repeating stimuli within the acquisition epoch (again, typically at 70 Hz–110 Hz). By use of the word "epoch," there still is coherent averaging applied to capture the recorded signals (in the time domain), but the repeated epochs themselves are longer, extending over numerous repetitions of the stimulus. This is another application of block-mode averaging (recall Figure 4–11). Although a variety of stimuli can be used, much of the research and development work has favored amplitude and/or frequency modulated carriers of different frequencies (usually of relevance to the audiogram). Given their periodic nature, ASSRs indeed are best described via spectral analysis. The elicited ASSR follows the modulation frequency (F_M) of the carrier tone (recall Figure 6–14). This is energy not in the stimulus due to combined nonlinear properties of the hair cell receptor and synaptic-neural properties of underlying mechanisms of the cochlear transduction/encoding process. Some more details of such mechanisms and their effects will be (re)called upon, but consider for a bit what is evident from the last and even some earlier episodes.

Fact: The ASSR's presence is signaled around F_M in the amplitude spectrum of the recording. The full spectral representation of the response is a peak at this frequency with "sideband" components per the complex-tone stimulus (recall Figures 2–11 and 2–14). This makes for a robust package of measures that can be applied to the detection of this evoked potential in noise and which is conductive to the variety of statistical methods summarized earlier (recall Table 4–1). This facilitates objectivity of "scoring" responses (likely present versus not), and it removes the bias of examiner's subjective judgment of the VDL. Indeed, the approach has been confirmed to yield appropriate results in a range of hearing abilities, especially a frequency-specific audiogram that reasonably approximates pure-tone audiograms, with particularly good correlation in the midauditory response frequency range of 500 Hz to 4000 Hz.[109,110] Beyond this frequency range of carriers, responses are observed readily toward the conventional audiometric frequency range limits and beyond, for instance at 250 Hz and 12,000 Hz. However, correspondences with the pure-tone audiogram are not as good, and for 12 kHz were not found to be promising for ultra-high-frequency ERA.[111] ASSR-ERA also can be transacted efficiently via automated protocols. All such empowerment of the clinician by the features summarized thus far are more fundamental than simply efficiencies of computer programming, rather by virtue of a singular attribute of the approach—it is substantially ***deterministic***. Given the known spectrum of the stimulus and knowledge of the nonlinear cochlea (recall Episode 5.1), where to look in the spectrum for a response is directly predicted.

The use of 80 Hz as a nominal F_M for objective audiometry can help to resolve some problems of transient-ABR ERA. The classical transient ABR to clicks and brief tone bursts are well established in audiological practice as methods of choice for objective assessment of hearing thresholds in uncooperative subjects (to be discussed more in-depth in later episodes; the first of which will soon follow). When used appropriately and applied and interpreted competently, the VDL of ABRs often predict well hearing sensitivity with relatively small estimation errors.[112] It is timely here to have a "friendly reminder": Neither this nor any other AEP measurements are literally tests of hearing.

The behavioral and the evoked electric responses have their own neuroanatomical pathways and underlying neurophysiological mechanisms, shared to be sure, but not identical. The behavioral response adds another "layer" for the response mechanism—the higher levels of the brain/auditory system implicated in the perception of sounds and production of motor responses. Another consideration is that AEPs are extracted through averaging and this technique cannot clearly resolve/extract the smaller responses elicited at or near the behavioral hearing threshold for the stimuli—hence physiological or response thresholds are generally observed above the behavioral-hearing threshold of the eliciting stimuli. Consequently, residual differences in behavioral versus objective audiometric findings may be unavoidable. Yet if fundamentally valid and comparably reliable as well demonstrated for 80-Hz ASSR-ERA in relation to behavioral audiometry,[113] then such alternative

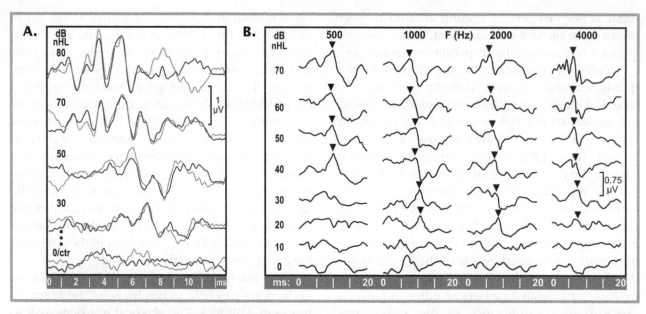

Figure 6–19. A. VDL recap: Essence of estimating the visual detection limit of the click ABR via descending stimulus levels tested. Example: Normal-hearing subject. (0/ctr: zero dB, literally or nonstimulus control trial.) **B.** Estimating the (behavioral) pure-tone audiogram using brief tone bursts in descending series for each of four audiometric frequencies. The inverted-triangle marker highlights presumptive wave V components at each level for which the examiner scored a response at or above the VDL. Example: Patient with slightly rising configuration of their pure-tone audiogram (which indicated a borderline clinically significant hearing loss).

methods are strong candidates for ERA. Overall, ABR-ERA and ASSR-ERA have been shown to be reasonably comparable, essentially equal for most clinical applications. However, in clinical practice there are other considerations that may influence choice of test in a given application. For example, what about objectivity (as hinted earlier), tester skill, and efficiency (always an issue among test methods in practice)?

To scrutinize these issues, it will be useful to elaborate further on the classical approach—a "threshold-seeking" paradigm, starting (for simplicity) with the click, recalling Figures 6–5A and 6–7B and given an example from still another subject's recording in Figure 6–19A. The responses are tested over various stimulus levels (for the virtual demonstration here, simply in descending order). The response components/peaks of the ABR are visually identified in each recording "trial" by an appropriately trained evaluator. As the stimulus level decreases, the amplitude of the elicited ABR naturally decreases, until it becomes impossible to recognize the response in the background noise. The earlier peaks being overall far less robust render ERA via click-ABR measurement primarily dependent upon detectability of the V-Vn (peak-trough) component. ABRs elicited by tone bursts of different frequencies from 0.5 kHz to 4 kHz (Figure 6–19B) can provide reasonably close estimates of audiometric thresholds, with sometimes smaller differences between VDL and BTH (behavioral thresholds) seen above 1 kHz. Data from a meta-analysis of results[78] using tone bursts in normal-hearing subjects showed the following averaged VDL-BTHs (means +/− standard deviations at 0.5 kHz–4 kHz in octaves, respectively): 20 +/−11, 17+/−12, 13+/−10, and 15+/−13 in children; and 20 +/−13, 16+/−10, 13+/−10, and 12+/−8 dB in adults. Smaller differences are typically reported for hearing-impaired subjects, likely because of a loudness-recruitmentlike effect in the input-output functions of the ABR in such cases.

Although a highly efficacious method that is still broadly embraced clinically—a "bread-and-butter" test in clinical audiology—there are inherent limitations of transient ABR-ERA beyond theoretical concepts of threshold estimation. One is an inherent problem of true "objectivity" suggested by the VDL protocol itself; it requires a judgment by the examiner. This is not all bad news though. Visual-based determination of presence versus absence of a response has been shown to provide reliable results when obtained by trained examiners. Nevertheless, the judgment being a subjective element is a **nonsensory variable**, as is the evaluator's expertise.[114,115] This places at risk the accuracy of threshold estimates, and worse conceptually, by factors having nothing to do with hearing. Routine pure-tone audiometry is performed using adaptations of methods nearly a century and a half old, but finally brought under scrutiny by more modern psychophysicists who were concerned with effects of even the subject's own bias in response to presentation of the test stimulus. The interaction of bias and estimated limits of detectability of a stimulus in behavioral tests is most critically assessed using principles of the **signal detection theory**.[116] Analyses of **receiving operator characteristics/curves (ROCs)**[117] showed similarly that accuracy of visual detection of click-ABRs for near-threshold responses (at 30 dB nHL) measuring *d'* (the **detectability index**) yielded values that varied among evaluators in relation to their relative skills and training. Highly trained and more skilled evaluators showed larger ("better") d' values than those who were lesser skilled/trained.

A variety of statistical methods (e.g., correlation between replicates, template matching, or estimating the signal-to-noise ratio) have been successfully applied for automatic "objective" detection of click-evoked ABR in both research and clinical contexts.[117,118] However, the application of automatic detection indexes/statistics for objective identification of ABR to brief tonal stimuli has not proven as effective. This in part is thanks to the changes in waveform of ABRs across sound level, frequency, and/or how the examiner filtered the recordings in the first place (Figure 6–19B and recalling Figure 4–16B, respectively). Currently, the introduction of statistical methods for objective and/or automatic detection of threshold mostly has been limited to automated screening technology (to be presented in a later chapter) and/or included in ABR test systems to provide quantitative metrics that can assist the tester in their interpretation of the waveform (again recall Table 4–1).

Another problem is the prolonged testing times required for estimating a substantial portion of the full audiogram so as to reveal reasonably well the configuration of any hearing loss, if present. Thus testing the ABR to brief tone bursts, as was illustrated in Figure 6–19B. These sample recordings illustrate VDL-seeking sequences of ABR recordings carried out at four different test frequencies (0.5 kHz–4 kHz, in octave steps), rigorously applying the same steps of stimulus level for all four test frequencies. Since each test frequency is evaluated separately, the estimation of an audiogram configuration requires a considerable number of recording trials—here, 6 stimulus-level steps × 4 test frequencies = 24 trials. Consequently, this strategy is quite time consuming, and this would be just to obtain results for one ear. In practice, a more adaptive protocol with less number of stimulus-level steps per test frequency is used, as illustrated in Figure 6–20. This would be the overall plan, but not necessarily starting with relatively high-level stimuli (like 70 dB nHL or above). Pending the clinician's knowledge of the case (history, observations of significant others, etc.), the "search" for a response might start at (for example) 40 dB and then proceed up or down in stimulus level accordingly. Still approximating something like a full clinical audiogram is quite time consuming, especially if completed for both ears, as likely required—perhaps 45 minutes to 90 minutes, given test–retest trials (if having to be done on nearly all trials per condition, for a confident decision of response/no response). The dynamics of the protocol in real time depend on the subject's state, actual hearing status, and the evaluator's expertise and efficiency. There is always the potential risk of requiring more than one test session to have complete success. Therefore, how might ASSR measurement provide an alternative approach in ways to reduce some, if not all, such variables/issues?

The answer to this question starts with the nuances of the 80-Hz-ASSR. The previous episode characterized ASSRs as fundamentally one type of "following" response—EFRs. As such, these responses are following modulations of the carrier (not the carrier's frequency), where F_M falls

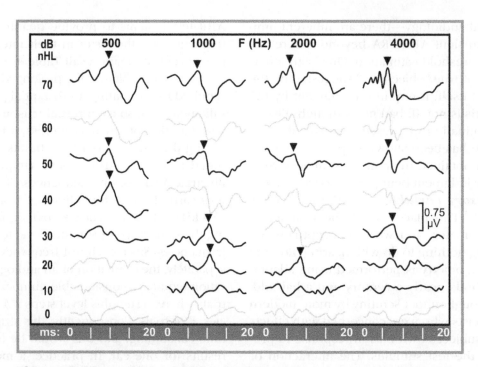

Figure 6–20. Replot of data from Figure 6–19B to portray adaptive VDL-search sequences that would be more efficient than strictly testing all frequencies at all the same levels—using fixed levels and/or continuing with steps regardless of responses observed at previous levels in a given sequence per frequency. In this case, levels per frequency that would be unlikely to be any more informative/affect overall outcomes have been "dimmed" (*light-gray tracings*).

indeed well below the carrier frequency. This does not mean necessarily that the test stimulus need be modulated exactly at 80 Hz; in fact, a variety of F_Ms are efficacious (as hinted previously). This too is an important advantage (to be considered further, shortly). At such rates of stimulation, given substantial adaptation of earlier components of the ABR and at lower levels inevitably causing their complete "loss" in background noise, the resulting response derives primarily from the wave IV–V complex (typically and simply labeled "V" in ABR-ERA).

Figure 6–21 is an illustration of the 80-Hz ASSR stimulus and response paradigm and characteristics of signals involved "coming and going" as well as underlying principles of response generation and subsequent graphical analysis. As shown in panel A, the modulated-carrier input signal to the basilar membrane (SAM at 80 Hz) is encoded at the carrier-frequency (1000 Hz) place along the basilar membrane. Panel B shows how there is a considerably lopsided transduction of the incoming acoustic signal, namely approximating *half-wave rectification*. This consequence was hinted in the initial overview previously but now warrants a more detailed summary. The stimulus encoding is initiated by the substantially nonlinear transduction of sound by the hair cells. Recall Figure 2–6A, illustrating this general type of nonlinearity—asymmetrically saturating—and Episodes 5.1 and 5.2—generation of distortion products of otoacoustic emissions and the summating potential, respectively. It is subsequently exaggerated by the synaptic-based excitation of the afferent fibers and finally the action potentials themselves—virtually monopolar "spike" potentials. Overall, excitation of the auditory neurons (largely controlled by the IHCs; recall Figure 3–10) is effectively occurring only with deflection of the stereocilia from motion of the basilar membrane toward scala vestibuli. Statis-

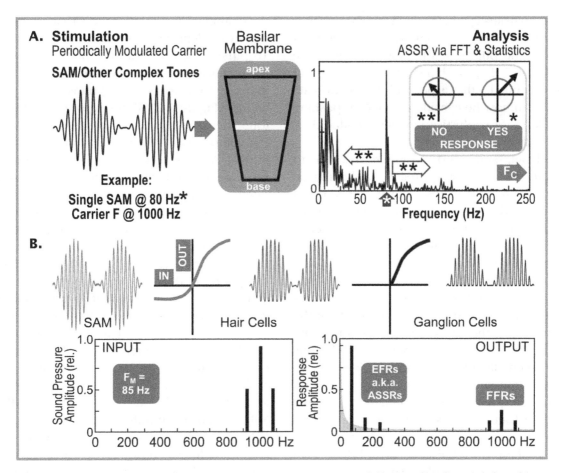

Figure 6–21. **A.** Bases of recorded response to a sinusoidally amplitude-modulated carrier (F_C) with a single modulation frequency (F_M = 80 Hz). Although from the last episode, following responses are seen at both the carrier and modulation frequencies, here the analysis is focused on the inherently more robust envelope following response. Inset to spectral analysis: Polar plots portraying both magnitude and phase of the signal at 80 Hz, significant* versus nonsignicant** responses (evaluated via a statistical detection algorithm). **B.** Concept of the hair-cell (in effect) half-wave rectification process. Note: spectral representations appear here as lines for simplicity; practical results are less than pristine (as hinted earlier); panel A provides the more practical view, namely for a substantially suprathreshold response. More important conceptually is that the results indeed approximate a line spectrum to thereby inform the examiner as to where to look for a true response (versus noise), having employed a stimulus that has a discrete spectrum.

tically, there is still a periodic pattern of stimulation of the ganglion cells and subsequently central-system neurons in step, cycle by cycle. In panel B (bottom panels) to the right is the overall spectrum of the responses, which may show some FFR from the carrier (or not, pending stimulus and noise levels), but where the "real action" of interest is found—again at F_M (in this example at 80 Hz)—the EFR robustly elicited. (Note: The bottom plots of panel B schematically show spectral analyses in the form of bar graphs for simplicity.) The illustrations in Figure 6–21 also reminds that (as before, whether or not reported) all such signals have both amplitude and phase spectra. In addition to reporting simply the essential measure of magnitude taken from the amplitude spectrum, both magnitude and phase can be represented in a ***polar plot*** (see inset to spectral plot in panel A). Additionally, statistical analyses can be applied to ensure better that the signal at 80 Hz is significantly different in magnitude and phase than the background noise in the "vicinity" of F_M. With these fundamental ASSR measures defined, other aspects of the steady-state approach can now be considered, indeed "pushing the envelope" of sophistication as engendered by this method.

The label, "single AM," in Figure 6–21A is to emphasize the simplest approach to eliciting an ASSR in a manner that best approximates, if not surpasses all others, for degree of frequency specificity. This approach thus permits response detection using ABR measurement in a manner most comparable to that of pure-tone audiometry. Recall from Figures 2–14A and 6–14 that the acoustic energy of this stimulus is concentrated in a manner to demonstrate three distinct peaks along the frequency axis—the carrier frequency and plus/minus the modulation frequency. The SAM thus has fundamentally a line spectrum. This is in contrast to the continuous spectrum or "splat" around the carrier frequency if the modulation amounts to simply a train of sinusoidal pulses, no matter how the carrier was gated to form the sinusoidal pulses (recalling from Episode 2.2 and the lesson of the uncertainty principle). This is simply the physical consequence of the functions of the various stimuli. Nevertheless, these and other variants (for instance, FM) yield close-enough approximations in frequency specificity wherein the bulk of energy is "focused" within ≃1/3 octave bandwidth. This again is approximately the width of the critical bands by which the peripheral system can effectively process and differentiate the frequency makeup of complex, multifrequency stimuli (like speech). Furthermore, any greater risk of errors of estimation of the audiogram among stimuli researched to date would likely be limited to cases of unusually sharply changing configurations of hearing loss (that is, across test/carrier frequency). The most important point is a reminder (a "spoiler alert") that no modulated sinusoid, including a SAM carrier, yields a sound that is a pure tone, as strictly defined. Nor does it have to necessarily in practice (the "good news").

There also have been further innovations of the steady-state approach realized, empowering the examiner in still other ways that are not immediately evident without a frequency-domain view. To pursue such innovations, first a recap: Due to the rectification property of the hair cells and their interface to neurons, during transduction of sound energy (Figure 6–21B), the response to the carrier tone (here 1000 Hz) will be recorded as a spectral component at the modulation frequency (here 80 Hz). After the rectification stage and given the resulting spectral components, the modulation frequency "flags" the response associated with the carrier tone, providing an "objective" index or label by which the frequency-specific response elicited by the carrier tone can be identified. Such labeling facilitates detection, including the ability—via computing FFTs and other calculations—to render an objective determination of a statistically significant signal/response (panel A). Why not, then, go ahead and label more than one carrier/test tone (as if asking the patient during behavioral audiometry to respond to two or more tones at a time and even with simultaneous presentation)? Seems a bit absurd, to be sure. No less so for ABR-ERA. Still, is it absurd if indeed the examiner would be able effectively to "tap into" the CANS (not unlike a telephone linesman or other electronics technologist in troubleshooting a multiline communications circuit)?

The labeled-line analogy was applied earlier as a classical model of sensory processing, like the skin for tactile sensation. The organ of Corti was illustrated subsequently (recall Figure 5–26A) to provide input signals to the brainstem and (in turn) with extensive preservation of the frequency-place map of the organ of Corti. Can the brainstem's responses to more than one stimulus then permit teasing apart the frequency-specific responses via AEP recordings from the scalp? The answer is a resounding "yes," using ASSR measurement with multiple (***M***) simultaneous stimuli. As illustrated in Figure 6–22A, in fact, this approach has been shown to be efficacious for ASSR-ERA.[109,119,120] Results of numerous studies have demonstrated the clinical utility of ***M-ASSR*** in both normal-hearing and hearing-impaired populations.[107,109,121] The M-ASSR is made efficacious by the ASSR being measured via a strongly deterministic method in the first place. Using distinct modulation rates (F_Ms),

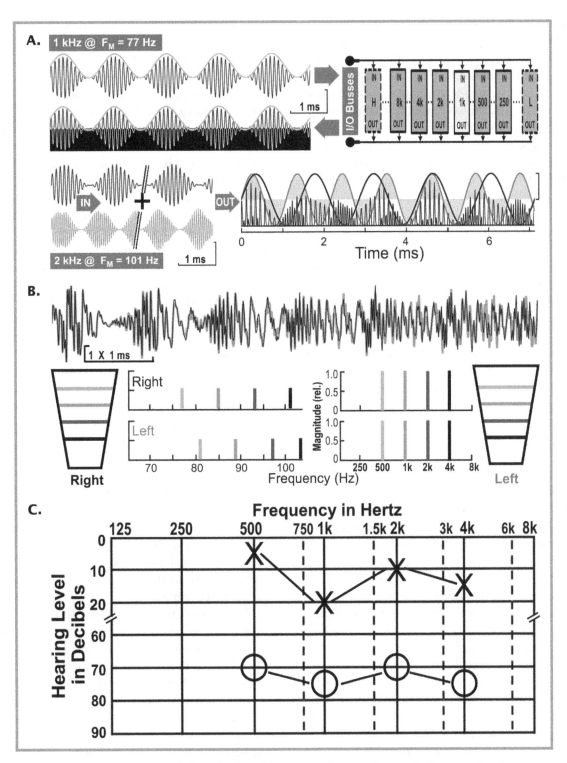

Figure 6–22. A. Principle of multiple ASSRs, tested at audiometric frequencies in octave intervals from 0.5 kHz to 4 kHz. **B.** Different modulation frequencies flag each carrier's frequency, with a different set of four per ear. **C.** Resulting data used by the computer to plot the predicted audiogram for a patient presenting with a unilateral hearing loss.

the examiner knows precisely where to look for even multiply targeted (flagged) component-responses in the spectrum. As illustrated in Figure 6–22A, the multicarrier stimulus excites motion of the basilar membrane to displace it maximally at separate places, thus optimally exciting multiple groups of neurons around their respective characteristic frequencies; in this case, for audiometric frequencies at octave intervals from 0.5 kHz to 4 kHz (panel B). Although the rectification stage is nonlinear, combined micro- and macromechanics of the hearing organ (by which individual pitches are heard and discriminated) encodes by a virtual spectral analysis the multiple frequencies with little interaction among carriers and their modulations.[122] The result is data from which to estimate a pure-tone audiogram. The results plotted (panel C) are those of an actual patient with a unilateral hearing loss.

Inherent to the method, there is the possibility to improve substantially the efficiency of estimating the audiogram by M-ASSR-based ERA. Furthermore, the same approach can be applied to testing simultaneously both ears, as also illustrated by Figure 6–22B. In this case, a spectral "code" is created for both the respective tones and ears tested. Therefore, in just one sequence of decreasing stimulus levels—about six or less trials in practice—the examiner could have a fully populated audiometric plot in the midfrequency ("speech-frequency") range of the auditory response area. Furthermore, since the responses can be detected using statistical methods, the protocol can be fully automated and the results directly plotted in the estimated audiogram, using calibration data stored in computer memory. M-ASSR-ERA has proven to be a valid and accurate means to estimate frequency-specific thresholds in normal-hearing adults, well babies, and hearing-impaired children.[106,107,109,123] The M-ASSR can be reliably recorded in newborns[124,125] and has shown prognostic value in follow-up to newborn screening, with potential advantages over ABR-ERA for identifying low-frequency hearing loss.[123,126] The extent to which such efficiency can be realized in ERA will be considered further in the upcoming episode. A possible issue, for example, is that of dealing with nonsymmetrical hearing losses between ears and/or sharply sloping losses. In such cases, time might be lost by "over-testing" responses in the better ear and/or at frequencies of better sensitivity. More adaptive testing strategies that allow switching or combined use of single and multiple stimuli would be needed. Nevertheless, the M-ASSR approach is a significant contribution of innovative research and development.

As the primary objective of this episode was to build on the foundation of the last episode, zeroing in on this broadly interesting and useful steady-state AEP tool, further considerations and/or technical specifications are left to subsequent episodes. Nevertheless, a couple of caveats and future directions for improvement are worth noting at this juncture. There is little contention that the underlying neurophysiological mechanisms are one and the same as for the transient ABR and 80-Hz ASSR. However, it is also true that given the high effective stimulus rates employed (upward of 110 Hz), the ABR sampled by this approach is not identical to that tested at rates of about 20 Hz or less. Classically, an even slower rate—down to 10 Hz—was considered ideal to optimize the transient ABR, particularly for neurodiagnostics wherein the full waveform (suprathreshold) is essential. However, near the VDL, the ABR extracted from the background has been reduced to a singular bump (nominally wave V) as adaptation will then have taken its toll; therefore, it is not surprising that the ASSR ends up being fractions of a microvolt in amplitude, often reported in picovolts (10^{-9} volts; for example, 0.1 µV = 100 pV). It follows that the classical mid-dynamic-range ABR is not recoverable from the currently conventionally recorded 80-Hz ASSR.

In practice, which response to test in a given application is one of choice. Ongoing research and development efforts are promising a future of not having to sacrifice time and/or information by having to choose one test versus the other. As well, the ASSR approach is of recent advent and its capabilities can be further enhanced through standardization of testing protocols and continued research and development to improve methods and technology that will allow more effective use and extended applications in clinics. In the meantime, many AEP test systems have come to be outfitted with ASSR-ERA software, so the clinician can move readily from one to the other test, benefiting from stored test parameters/protocols that certainly facilitate working with multiple test programs—on demand. The AEP-toolbox thus became endowed further by the quantum-leap of ASSR-ERA research and development, with great promise for further advancements.

Episode 4: Evoked Potential Audiometry Using Auditory Brainstem Response/ Auditory Steady-State Response Measurements

The main goals of *objective electrophysiological measures* of auditory function are to determine limits of detection of electric responses and to do so using essentially specific frequencies of testing to render results that are highly predictive of behavioral hearing thresholds. As for conventional audiological assessments, this information is needed to accurately establish hearing status and to set preliminary amplification-fitting targets in a timely manner. These measures are used when behavioral estimation of hearing thresholds is not efficacious or unlikely to be accurate. Candidates most commonly are young infants who cannot give reliable behavioral responses until approximately 6 months to 8 months of age[127] or older children and adults who cannot be tested behaviorally due to cognitive delays. Other clinical scenarios might be cross-checking of behavioral thresholds for medico-legal or work-related compensation cases. Both MLR and LLR measurement also are used for evoked-response audiometry; their applications are subjects of episodes in the next two chapters. This episode continues from the last to provide additional principles and considerations for the use of the *ABR* and *ASSR* in ERA, primarily for older children and adults. However, much of the work forming ERA evidence bases overall was strongly motivated by the goal of developing objective testing methods that provide for accurate assessment of auditory function in infants who may be at risk for hearing loss and wherein early identification is a mandate. Herein, their example and related research findings will be called upon freely as they inform insights and practice, in general.

As with conventional audiometry, the validity and usefulness of any tests of the auditory system starts with calibrated instrumentation (recall Episode 2.3). The use of clicks and brief sinusoidal pulses (tone bursts) requires a somewhat different method than for pure-tone audiometry. Table 6–2 gives some exemplary calibration values for brief-tone stimuli used in British Columbia by their provincial Early Hearing Detection and Intervention program.[128,129] Click stimuli will not be discussed in this episode with respect to threshold estimation using either AC or BC stimuli, as *frequency-specific stimuli* are required for the vast majority of evaluations calling for ERA. However, it should be noted that some researchers have recommended the use of clicks in combination with low-frequency stimuli. The click ABR remains of interest in differential diagnosis (coming soon!), but for patients who require objective testing to estimate their pure-tone audiogram, measurements using tone-burst stimuli are the more informative.

Typically, to save time, threshold searches are not performed for levels below the clinically significant limit for hearing loss or—in other words— the normal-limit cutoff. Some of the challenges of interpreting the presence/absence of responses are reliance on the VDL of the wave V component. As

Table 6–2. Acoustic Calibration for Air (dB peSPL)[129] and Bone Conduction (dB re: 1 µN),[78] Brief Tones at 0 dB nHL

500 Hz			1000 Hz			2000 Hz			4000 Hz		
AC TDH 49	AC ER3-A	BC B-71	AC TDH 49	AC ER3-A	BC B-71	AC TDH 49	AC ER3-A	BC B-71	AC TDH 49	AC ER3-A	BC B-71
25	22	67	23	25	54	26	20	49	29	26	46

Table 6–3. Summary of Typical Stimulus Parameters for 2-1-2 Linearly Gated Tones and 5-Cycles Blackman Tones With No Plateau for Air and Bone Conduction of ABRs Using Brief Tone Bursts (Based On Data From Small & Stapells [2017])[146]

Stimulus Parameters	AC	BC
500 Hz	4 ms rise/fall 2 ms plateau 10 ms duration	4 ms rise/fall 2 ms plateau 10 ms duration
1000 Hz	2 ms rise/fall 1 ms plateau 5 ms duration	2 ms rise/fall 1 ms plateau 5 ms duration
2000 Hz	1 ms rise/fall 0.5 ms plateau 2.5 ms duration	1 ms rise/fall 0.5 ms plateau 2.5 ms duration
4000 Hz*	1 ms rise/fall 0.25 ms plateau 1.25 ms duration	1 ms rise/fall 0.25 ms plateau 2.25 ms duration*

Note. *To reduce ringing.

noted earlier, this is the **subjective judgment** of the response's presence, its replicability, and other features, such as appropriate latency shifts with changes in presentation levels. The stimuli that are used to elicit the ABR for threshold estimation purposes are 2-1-2 cycle rectilinear (2 cycles rise/fall, one plateau—classically referred to as a "tone pip"), Blackman, or other gated sinusoids. Typical stimulus and recording parameters are shown in Tables 6–3 and 6–4. These stimuli have been shown to be reasonably frequency specific for both AC and BC stimuli and have been used for many years in the clinic to estimate hearing thresholds in infants, older children, and adults.[130,131]

More recently, **narrowband chirp stimuli** have been added to the selection of stimulus choices for this technique. Recall that there were issues for making the chirp work as desired, relative to "fixing" the inherent cochlear-mechanical issues with the classical acoustic click for an optimal response (Episode 6.1). In brief:, the purpose was/is to address the problem with the latter wherein superposition of responses from individual nerve fibers is suboptimal; this is a sort of destructive interference that reduces response amplitudes of the ABR. What perhaps is less expected from this reminder is that they pertain, as well, to the 80-Hz ASSR. This, once more, is where realities of the total time-frequency picture must be borne in mind. The addition of contributions across the population of nerve fibers innervating hair cells in the vicinity of the nominal frequency place (per the carrier frequency) is not simple arithmetic; rather, it is the net result based on phasor summations, reflecting both magnitudes and phases of contributing neural potentials. This is the neural "code" sent on to the brainstem generators of the response (recalling that a significant group of types of brainstem responses are "primary like" and others still having strong onset responses; see Figure 3–13).

Chirps thus are designed to compensate for basilar membrane traveling wave delays, wherein greater compensation occurs for low frequencies,[132–134] thus potentially improving the SNR of both the transient and steady-state brainstem responses. For example, for the broadband, "CE-chirp" delivers energy in lower frequencies preceding higher-frequencies to effectively reverse phase dispersion inherent to travel waves while still maximizing synchrony of neural firing across frequencies. For stimuli presented at levels less than 60 dB nHL, ABR amplitudes to CE-chirps versus clicks were found to be 1.5 to 2 times larger.[133–135] This is a significant advantage for screening purposes in infants.[135] However, for CE-chirps at higher intensities, there is also upward spread

Table 6–4. Summary of Typical Adult Recording Parameters to Elicit Air And Bone Conduction Brief-Tone Auditory Brainstem Responses (Based On Data From Small & Stapells [2017][146])

Typical Adult Recording Parameters	AC	BC
EEG Channels	1 channel: C_z - ipsi mastoid (most often) 2 channel: C_z - ipsi mastoid C_z - contra mastoid (only if large asymmetry between ears)	1 channel: C_z - ipsi mastoid (most often) 2 channel: C_z - ipsi mastoid C_z - contra mastoid (only if large asymmetry between ears)
EEG Filters	12 dB/oct; 30-HZ high pass; 1500–3000-HZ low pass	
Gain	50,000–100,000 X	
Artifact Rejection	Trails > = 25 µV; = 10–15 µV if low rejection rate (<10%) - Set artifact rejection starting point after the end of the stimulus to avoid stimulus artifact triggering artifact rejections	
Trails	Per replication - minimum of 1,000 - typically 2000 - can vary depending on noise levels Per conditions - 2–4 replications (may vary) - 1 replication only if very quiet and criterion for no response met (depends on ABR system)	
Recoding Time Window & Stimulus Rate	Typically 24–25 ms - allow a rate up to above ABR system - maximum rate used will depend on ABR system - as rate is increased, time windows will either shorten or stimuli will be skipped to accommodate for fast rate - this must be checked when selecting optimal rate	
Visual Display	Selection of display gain is important to avoid small-amplitude responses - peak-to-peak amplitude of largest wave should be ~1/4 of recording length - this will vary with ABR systems	

(effectively to higher frequencies) of excitation by the individual frequency components of the chirp as level increases. Again, this effect represents the inherent bias of traveling wave propagation initiated from the basal end of the basilar membrane, regardless of stimulus paradigm. Then there is again the hair cell nonlinearity up front. As a result, there may be no amplitude advantage of chirp-elicited responses over those of more conventional stimuli. However, these realities from earlier work on chirps have not stifled further research and development efforts. To remedy these problems, chirps more recently have been modeled with different delays per intensity (in principle) to optimize response amplitudes across a range of intensities needed to assess mild to profound levels of hearing loss. The most efficient design is to increase the delay for decreasing stimulus levels. Some clinical ABR-test systems now provide the option to use narrowband chirps adjusted for stimulus level. One example is the ***narrowband level-specific CE-chirp (NB CE-Chirp LS)***. These stimuli indeed elicit larger responses than traditional brief tone bursts at low, moderate, and high levels.[136,137] However, it is likely that these larger ABR amplitudes result from poorer frequency specificity, meaning that a wider region of the basilar membrane is stimulated.[138,139] Further research and development is needed to evaluate the benefits and disadvantages of these new chirp stimuli.

Effective ERA must be goal driven and systematically carried out via best practices. Clinical goals for and methods of ERA substantially differ from those of behavioral assessment. For instance, it might be assumed that because the overall ERA method is objective, by not requiring voluntary behavioral responses, that it should be more efficient than behavioral testing. That proves to be true only for certain ERA methods but, more often than not, they tend to be much more time consuming and provide less information than behavioral methods. This, in turn, leads to the need for establishment of clinical protocols with ***testing sequencing*** designed to optimize the information obtained in the first ERA assessment. In fact, it is not uncommon to need more than one test session to obtain complete audiometriclike assessments via ERA. It will be useful here to recap some basic methods (for comparison purposes) of behavioral testing. Behavioral evaluations usually begin by conducting unmasked AC-threshold searches at audiometric frequencies (minimally 500 Hz–4000 Hz, ideally 250 Hz–8000 Hz) in one ear, followed by testing the other ear. When there is more than a 40-dB difference in thresholds between ears, a ***clinical masking*** protocol is followed to obtain ear-specific AC thresholds. The need for masking depends on ***interaural attenuation (IA)*** values for the population being tested, the type of earphone used to present the stimulus, and the stimulus type. It is well established that adult IA values for pure tones vary significantly with frequency among types of insert and supraaural/circumaural earphones[140,141] and for AC versus BC stimuli. Unmasked and masked bone-conduction (BC) testing usually then follows (250 Hz–4000 Hz). Estimation of AC and BC thresholds across the audiometric frequencies in cooperative patients is easily achieved in one appointment of as little as 30 min, often including speech audiometry (testing speech reception thresholds and speech recognition scores). The rules for applying clinical masking in adults are the same whether using behavioral or ERA methods to establish hearing thresholds. However, this protocol in ERA is far more time consuming, hence the need to prioritize the sequencing of testing and reduce the number of test conditions—starting with numbers of frequencies and stimulus levels evaluated (recall Figure 6–19 versus 6–20) and focusing on the most essential information for purposes of the initial assessment.

Determination of the presence or absence of the wave V component of the ABR (as demonstrated earlier, for example, Figure 6–19) is the primary focus of the examiner when tracking responses down to the limit of detection. The wave V component occurs at approximately 6 ms to 15 ms over the range of nHL presentation levels—suprathreshold responses down to the limit of detection. As shown in Figure 6–23, the clinician needs to select where to mark the waveform to determine the amplitude and latency of wave V; typically, the latency of the response is marked at the point in the waveform just before the point at which it begins to head in the negative direction. The amplitude of wave V is calculated between this point and the largest negativity, typically within a couple of milliseconds of the peak latency marker. In this example, the clinician has marked the wave V amplitude and latency on the average waveform, initially at about 8 ms. Clinicians learn to recognize the typical features of wave V at different stimulus presentation levels and frequencies when they record responses at either "normal levels" or to threshold levels when responses are elevated. An infant case was chosen to illustrate both an example of conductive lesion (but hold that thought for the moment) and that latencies are inherently longer in such cases. The other upshot, and with hearing loss in general, is that perhaps without the examiner ever having sufficient levels of stimulation and/or the patient having an adequate range of hearing left (a greatly reduced dynamic range), it may not be possible to see a full-fledged ABR waveform. Still, an identification of the response must be made with confidence, which includes a

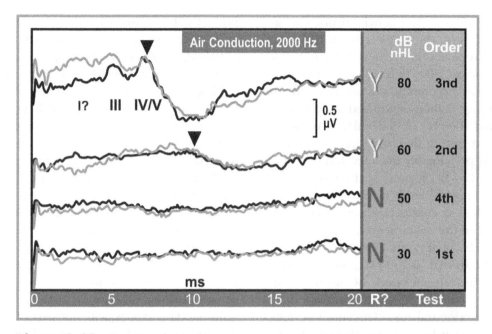

Figure 6–23. Sample of recording in a conductive hearing-loss case (infant)—search for visual detection level of the brainstem response to brief tone bursts of 2000 Hz presented by air conduction. Test order: Sequence of hearing levels tested and decisions—response (Yes/No).

measureable magnitude of the presumptive true response in reference to the noise floor (recall Episode 4.1).

As mentioned earlier, threshold estimation using the ABR represents a different approach than that of standard behavioral measures, starting with the impracticality of obtaining thresholds at all audiometric frequencies from 250 Hz to 8000 Hz and even more so with 5-dB resolution. As noted in the last episode in effect (recall Figure 6–20), an adaptive protocol is essential. There indeed are substantial time constraints involved. This is especially the case when evaluating sleeping infants but can also be the case for older children and adults, when ERA is warranted. A common clinical observation is that patients tend to have quieter baselines as the test progresses, especially if they doze off. If not, the opposite effect can occur; restlessness can increase over time (even worse, for instance in testing an adult, if the patient is looking at their watch). As luck may have, such perturbations may occur just when the sound level is low or imperceptible to the patient and (with diminishing magnitude of the ABR) just when noise levels need to be as low as possible to complete testing and to have the most reliable results. Any unnecessary movement will likely increase the background noise of the recording.

Typical protocols then are aimed at prioritizing test conditions' levels—typically steps of 10 dB nHL—and frequencies—usually 500 Hz, 1000 Hz, 2000 Hz, and 4000 Hz. Also as nHL is intended to correspond to behavioral audiometric limits, the focus initially is on testing at 25 dB nHL or greater. The choice of the 10-dB step size is commonly used in the interest of time. Occasionally, a 5-dB step may be attempted, especially when the dynamic range of hearing is more limited[142] or if a more precise estimate is desired to facilitate hearing aid fittings. However, time is usually too limited for this level of precision. Thereto, Figure 6–23 also illustrates the concept of adapting/prioritizing testing sequencing (see "test order" in inset panel) and is applicable to test frequencies as well. This all is to make the most of the testing time available. Recommended as an infant protocol[142] is to begin with 2000 Hz at 30 dB nHL in one ear; if a response is present, the test ear is switched and the process is repeated in the opposite ear. If both ears appear normal, 500 Hz is tested next at 35 dB nHL; if responses are present, one ear is tested then the other; testing is then conducted at 4000 Hz at 25 dB nHL and 1000 Hz at 35 dB nHL. If responses are not present during this first stage of testing—AC thresholds presumably are elevated at 500 Hz and/or 2000 Hz—BC testing is then conducted, beginning with normal levels to determine whether the apparent loss is conductive, sensorineural, or mixed (at least in the better hearing cochlea). If BC responses are absent at normal levels (20 dB nHL at 500 Hz and 30 dB nHL at 2000 Hz) and AC thresholds are significantly elevated, BC levels should be tested at maximum levels to confirm (now) suspected sensorineural loss. Threshold searches would then follow as time allows. Although the forgoing strategy focuses on acquisition of threshold estimates in a protocol recommended for infants, the same principles can be applied to older children and adults.

How well, then, does ABR-ERA work in practice? Correlation coefficients for comparisons of ABR and behavioral thresholds have been reported to be 0.94 to 0.97 for 500 Hz, 2000 Hz, and 4000 Hz for infants 0 months to 6 months, children 7 months to 48 months, and children older than 4 years of age.[143] Similar correlation coefficients (0.94–0.95) have been reported when comparing ABR and behavioral thresholds for 250 Hz, 500 Hz, 1000 Hz, 2000 Hz, and 4000 Hz for a sample size of 76 participants including infants, children, and six adults.[144] For AC tone bursts, mean ABR-minus-behavioral difference scores (± 1 standard deviation) for 84 to 167 adults were 13(11) dB, 10(12) dB, 8(10) dB, and 5(13) dB for 500 Hz, 1000 Hz, 2000 Hz, and 4000 Hz, respectively. In contrast, for 310 to 510 infants and children, difference scores for weighted ABR-behavioral thresholds were smaller compared to adults: 6 dB, 1 dB, 2 dB, and −2 dB at 500 Hz, 1000 Hz, 2000 Hz, and 4000 Hz, respectively.

The results in Figure 6–23 were those typical of a search for VDLs of *air conduction, frequency-specific ABRs* (subsequently followed to completion of testing at other frequencies). These results indicate the VDL at 2000 Hz to be elevated by at least 50 dB at the test frequency of 2000 Hz, in what proved to be an overall flat conductive hearing loss in this pediatric case. Sample recordings from *bone conduction, frequency-specific ABRs* testing are presented in Figure 6–24, revealing clear responses having been observed down to 20 dB nHL at 500 Hz and 30 dB nHL at 2000 Hz, indeed consistent with a conductive hearing loss. Note that these responses are from ipsilateral, one-channel recordings. For infants, two-channel recordings are made with a different imperative than in older children and adults or than in other applications, namely to help determine which cochlea actually is responding to the stimulus, as is possible in this population. This intriguing effect will be pursued in more detail in a subsequent episode. For the more mature cases, as in conventional audiometry, no assumption is made of response sidedness of unmasked responses, with one exception. That is for wave I, but wave-I measurement is not efficacious for ERA by strictly noninvasive test methods, like ABR-ERA.

Mean VDLs for bone-conduction, frequency-specific ABR in adults ($N = 14$) have been reported to be 9(8) dB nHL and 5(11) dB nHL at 500 Hz and 2000 Hz, respectively; therefore, thresholds are similar between 500 Hz and 2000 Hz.[145] More substantial data sets derived from pediatric cohorts have shown a different frequency-dependent pattern. In the same study, infants ($N = 14$) mean BC ABR thresholds were 3(10) dB nHL and 14(7) dB nHL for the same frequencies, respectively. Across six infant studies (94–140 infants at 500 Hz and 2000 Hz; 14–20 infants at 1000 Hz and 4000 Hz), weighted mean BC-ABR thresholds were 3 dB HL, 5 dB HL, 14 dB HL, and 7 dB HL for 500 Hz, 1000 Hz, 2000 Hz, and 4000 Hz, respectively.[146] Consequently, there are statistically significant adult-infant differences in BC sensitivity that have been shown consistently via ABR-ERA. Consequently, different norms are needed for infants and adults to interpret most critically how BC-ABR results relate to behavioral thresholds. Last, but certainly important, these trends hold as well for ASSR-ERA assessment of bone conduction sensitivity.

In contrast to behavioral testing, ABR testing efficiency is frequently complicated when the hearing status of the patient requires (indeed) the use of masking. This, naturally, is often the case for BC testing of ABRs due to minimal BC *interaural*

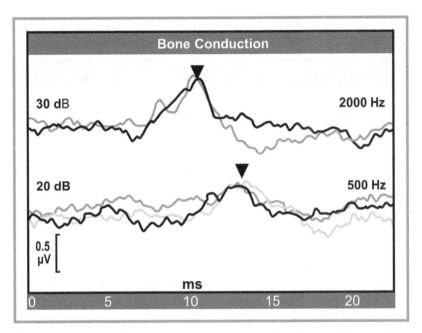

Figure 6–24. Follow-up to Figure 6–23—sample results from bone conduction testing (frequency and levels as indicated). Note here for the 500-Hz condition, use of test, retest, and (another) retest trials—at one time virtually standard practice. In any event and as time and/or patient's status permits, if any question of confidence in scoring the response, this is a good idea.

attenuation (IA), while less frequently the situation for AC testing. The latter is in good part due to much greater AC IA, particularly with the use of tubal insert earphones.[147] Masking levels needed for behavioral testing in adults for both AC and BC stimuli have been known for many years; however, it has been shown that adult masking levels suitable for behavioral testing are not the same as for physiological assessment methods. For example,[148] more masking has been found to be needed to eliminate erroneous behavioral responses than erroneous electrophysiological responses to AC-amplitude-modulated tones—7 dB to 13 dB more for the 80-Hz ASSR. Similarly, for BC-ASSR, *effective masking levels (EMLs)* were 10 dB to 17 dB greater for behavioral responses compared to ASSRs for 1000 and 4000 Hz.[149] Results of linear regression analyses also revealed that BC behavioral and ASSR EMLs were not significantly correlated for most of the stimuli presented. From these results, it can be concluded that there are significant differences between EMLs for AC and BC behavioral responses versus ASSRs, and that it is not possible to predict accurately EMLs for 80-Hz ASSRs from behavioral findings or EMLs for behavioral testing from ASSR findings.

Therefore, EMLs for BC ABR were investigated recently to determine how much binaural AC white noise was needed to mask ABRs elicited at 500 Hz and 2000 Hz in infants and adults with normal hearing.[150] Age- and frequency-dependent differences in these EMLs were found to be very similar to EMLs observed for ASSR-ERA. For adults, 10 dB less masking was needed to eliminate an ABR elicited at 500 Hz, whereas similar masking levels were observed between infants and adults tested at 2000 Hz. Based on the assumption of 0 dB IA and considering a maximum safe level for the masker to be approximately 80 dB SPL to 85 dB SPL, preliminary adult EMLs for BC-ABR-ERA were recommended, as provided in Table 6–5. It is also important to be mindful that older children and adults exhibit the occlusion effect (enhancement of BC sound level by covering/plugging the external

Table 6–5. Effective Masking Levels for Bone Conduction Auditory Brainstem Responses for Adults With Normal Hearing

Frequency	Stimulus Level dB nHL	Effective Masking Level dB SPL
500 Hz	20	72
	30	82
2000 Hz	20	62
	30	72
	40	82

ear), naturally present whether testing responses behaviorally or electrophysiologically.[151]

Several stimuli of possible use for 80-Hz ASSR measurement which were pursued extensively in research and development of this method were summarized in the last episode but deserve a recap and further considerations here, before discussing exactly how well AC and BC ASSRs predict behavioral thresholds. Figure 6–25 illustrates stimuli found commonly in the ASSR literature and in practice, such as AM, FM, AM-FM (mixed modulation), and still others. While all are basically intended to permit frequency-specific testing, they do vary in detailed spectral content and effective bandwidths (or splatter), as illustrated. Nevertheless, all also have been shown to be suitable for predicting pure-tone thresholds. Most recently, chirp stimuli have been incorporated into ASSR testing and are available in some clinical-ERA test systems. The characterization of the spectra of such stimuli has been more or less closer or equal to short-term spectral analysis even that of a single cycle of the modulator or sinusoidal pulse within the stimulus train. To this point, coverage of related issues has been toward the goals of presenting principles first and then—as time, space, and scope permit—filling in more details of practical applications along the way. The first principle was, whether on the side of analysis or synthesis, gating of the signal generated (simple tone, complex tones, speech, or noises) has consequences, namely "canning" the signal in a finite time frame; this is a transient event of sorts regardless of overall duration. Ditto for an analysis constrained to a finite duration of a train of pulses. However, in a "bigger can," (longer epoch) power builds up progressively toward the carrier frequency, yet the duration will fall considerably short of being infinitely long and the uncertainty principle will not just go away. Hence, in practice, what is termed a steady-state stimulus-analysis approach falls between the extremes of "purely" the transient's continuous spectrum and the "purity" of the indefinite complex tone's discrete spectrum. Therefore, issues of potentially limiting frequency specificity have been pursued similarly for ASSR-ERA as for conventional, transient ABR-ERA, therein seeking the same sort of balance of overall limits of spectra actually realized versus acceptable limits for practical purposes. In Figure 6–25 then, spectral envelopes simply are used to characterize the stimuli overviewed and—good news—at least should be adequately conservative for many ASSR applications. None, however, can be expected to match a pure tone. A severe-to-profound partial loss of hearing sensitivity with an extremely steep slope inevitably remains a challenge for any method; it is just a question of how much and how important the precision of measurement is. However, clinical priorities vary too, from applications in hearing screening to differential diagnosis (starting with hearing loss typing), to hearing-aid fitting. The other good news is that ASSR measurement (again) provides a straightforward approach to ERA in parallel with conventional audiometry. The carrier frequency is setting faithfully at the desired spectral "center of gravity" (per "audiometric" frequencies) with the addition of straightforward knowledge of where to look in the spectrum for the true response component(s). Furthermore, commercially available instrumentation today can provide multiple paradigms readily to support differing needs across the clinical population.

Reports of studies of BC-ASSR-ERA, as will now be considered, are based on fewer studies than

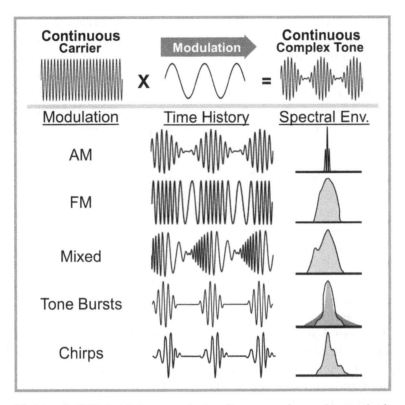

Figure 6–25. Partial recap of stimuli commonly used in evoked-response testing with time- versus frequency-domain representations, but a bit more and in the context of ASSR testing. Signal samples shown are by way of time-expanded views framed for a period of approximately three cycles of the modulation but represent ongoing signals, coming and leaving the window of view. As noted in the last episode, as commonly needed practically, signal averaging is applied to repeated trains of such stimuli for virtually a continuous complex tone for virtually a steady-state stimulus-response paradigm (even with trains of brief tone bursts or chirps). The spectra are presented essentially per spectral envelopes of the modulation function for a single cycle, burst, or chirp but can be taken as the worse-case estimate of the effective spectral splatter. Note: for tone bursts, a variety of envelopes (rectilinear, sine-squared, Blackman, etc.) are possible by choice of the gating function, and spectral differences among them will be expressed as a trade-off between a sharper central lobe versus greater spread of the sidebands/skirts of the spectral envelope (recall Episode 2.2).

those of AC-ASSR, simply by default. The use of AC stimuli have been the focus of the vast majority of published ASSR studies, as also true for ABR-ERA. In normal-hearing adults, AC- and BC-ASSR limits of detection (nominally, for purposes here to be called "thresholds") tend to be similar across frequency, as expected given that ASSR stimuli most often are calibrated effectively to the pure-tone audiometric standard, thus dB HL (recall Episode 2.3).[152] The one exception is that BC ASSR thresholds at 500 Hz tend to be greater than those at higher frequencies. Correlation coefficients for comparisons of AC-ASSR and behavioral or ABR VDLs across a range of hearing losses are 0.70 to 0.85 for 500 Hz and 0.80 to 0.95 for 1000 Hz to 4000 Hz. Across studies, average adult AC ASSR thresholds are 17(12) dB, 13(12) dB, 11(10) dB, and 15(11) dB at respective audiometric frequencies.[153] Based on data from 10 adult ASSR studies,[146] the following are recommended as normal limits for AC-ASSRs: 40 dB to 50 dB, 40 dB to 45 dB, 40 dB, and 40 dB for 500 Hz, 1000 Hz, 2000 Hz, and 4000 Hz, respectively. Preliminary correction factors to predict adult behavioral thresholds from AC ASSR thresholds have also been proposed, accordingly: 10 dB to 20 dB, 10 dB to 15 dB, 10 dB to 15 dB, and 5 dB to 15 dB at 500 Hz, 1000 Hz, 2000 Hz, and 4000 Hz, respectively.

One potential application for the use of M-ASSRs (described in the previous episode), rather than standard/behavioral audiometric testing, is found in the medico-legal sector or other compensation cases. An investigation[154] of different methods of threshold estimation for clients of a workers' compensation board revealed mean differences (ASSR minus behavioral thresholds) to be 5 dB to 17 dB for an 80-Hz-ASSR group, 1 dB to 14 dB for an 40-Hz ASSR group, and 20 dB to 22 dB for those tested measuring LLR (cortical N_1–P_2) potentials. Furthermore, of the three approaches, thresholds estimated using the 40-Hz-ASSR-ERA were significantly closer to behavioral thresholds than the other methods; both the 40-Hz-ASSR-ERA and LLR-ERA yielded threshold information more quickly than 80-Hz-ASSR-ERA. More recently,[155] from a study of adults exposed to occupational noise, analyses of ROCs for 80-Hz-ASSR-ERA versus behavioral thresholds for warble tones revealed sensitivity (proportion of true-positives) to be high (93%–98%), but the specificity (proportion of true-negatives) was frequency dependent. It improved with increasing frequency: 59%, 73%, 82%, and 99% at 500 Hz, 1000 Hz, 2000 Hz, and 4000, respectively. The investigators also found that ASSR limits more accurately predicted behavioral thresholds for greater degrees of hearing loss, compared to mild or normal-hearing thresholds, as previously reported.[105,107]

When using ASSRs to estimate audiometric thresholds, a factor to consider is the *efficiency of multiple stimuli* versus stimuli of single-frequency modulation. For normal-hearing and hearing-impaired adults (sensorineural hearing losses) and in estimating AC thresholds using monaurally-presented AM stimuli that are at least one octave apart, M-ASSR amplitudes (as hinted in the previous episode) are not reduced significantly. Frequency specificity of the response also is not affected when stimulus levels are 60 dB HL or less (compared to the single-modulation-frequency ASSRs). However, at intensities greater than 60 dB HL, amplitudes decrease due to interactions between responses to the multiple stimuli. For stimuli with broader spectra, interactions are greater for adults, even at 60 dB HL. Nevertheless, despite the reduced amplitudes at higher intensities, the multiple-ASSR technique (in adults) is still more efficient, but only by 1.5 to 3 times rather than 4 times faster to complete the evaluation than in ERA based on single-frequency ASSR measurements (over 4 frequencies).[156,157]

For infants, interactions have been reported for the M-ASSR measurements with stimuli presented at 60 dB HL. On the plus side, when efficiency is considered, the multiple-carrier approach is still more efficient than ASSR-ERA using a single-carrier frequency.[158,159] Nevertheless, as stimulus level increases and/or when stimuli with broader spectra are used to elicit the M-ASSR, whether in infants or adults, efficiency starts to decrease. Therefore, it is likely most efficient to use M-ASSRs for low-to-mid hearing levels but consider switching to the single-carrier paradigm to continue ERA at high hearing levels.

For BC ASSR-ERA, this approach (again) has yet to be studied nearly as extensively as for AC testing. Across four studies, average BC ASSR thresholds for normal-hearing adults appear to be 26(13) dB, 19(13) dB, 18(8) dB, and 13(10) dB (HL) for 500 Hz, 1000 Hz, 2000 Hz, and 4000 Hz, respectively.[146] The mean data are provided in Figure 6–26 for direct comparison to those for AC ASSR-ERA noted earlier.[146] For BC ASSR-ERA, still fewer data are available regarding threshold estimates in adults with hearing loss. Results from a study in adults comparing sensorineural hearing loss and hearing loss simulated using masking noise[160] yielded results demonstrating reasonably

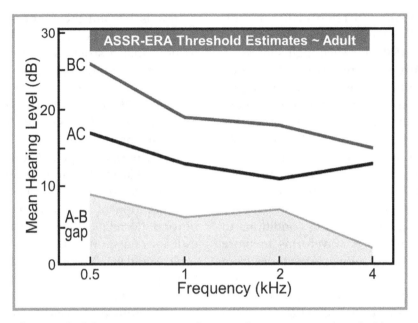

Figure 6–26. Comparison of AC and BC average thresholds in adults obtained by 80-Hz-ASSR-ERA. Overall similar trends are seen, although a bit of an "air-bone (A-B) gap" to consider in practice. (Based on data reported in Tlumak et al. [2007B] [AC][153] and Small and Stapells [2017] [BC].[146])

good correlations between ASSR-ERA estimated and behavioral thresholds for bone conduction (in adults). Correlations again were higher for 1000 Hz to 4000 Hz (0.84–0.94) than for 500 Hz (0.71–0.82). Also reported correspondingly, the investigators could accurately classify hearing losses at 2000 Hz and 4000 Hz (93%) but otherwise only 86%. The results thus are promising overall; this method would most commonly be used to assess infants.

Another technical detail to consider is the possibility of eliciting *artifactual responses* via the steady-state approach, namely to high-level AC or BC stimuli. On the one hand, the possibility of transducer-radiation artifact must always be considered, potentially more so for the steady-state stimulus-response paradigms, given virtually continuous stimulation. On the other hand, as long as the transducer behaves reasonably linearly (not pushing the respective devices to their extreme limits), the ASSR (as an EFR) is not particularly vulnerable to contamination by electromagnetic radiation; the targeted response's spectral components fall well below those of the test carrier. Still,

there is an artifact lurking for relatively high levels of stimulation (again, per the HL-range limits of AC or BC, as the case may be). This is one that is both physical—sound evoked—and physiological—from the inner ear too! This is a vestibular response. It is well established that the vestibular system does react at times to intense sound stimulation, also more so to BC stimuli (as will be taken up in a subsequent episodes, ultimately in a more positive light of clinical interest). It is common to think of the stapes pumping sound energy directly into the cochlea—not so—rather, into the vestibule, with nothing to stop it from affecting the otolithic organs as well. For instance, it is possible to elicit a negative wave in the ABR at approximately 3 ms in response to AC stimuli at 95 dB nHL or higher due to such vestibular stimulation. However, unlike the ABR that is analyzed in the time domain, the same vestibular responses can manifest in the frequency-domain ASSR analysis and cannot be distinguished from an auditory response. The proof is that such spurious responses have been recorded in adults with profound hearing loss at only 50 dB HL to

60 dB HL for BC ASSRs and 118 dB HL to 120 dB HL for AC ASSRs[161,162]; therefore, caution is needed when interpreting ASSRs for such high stimuli.

Putting the diagnostic pieces of information together can sometimes be difficult, depending on the quality of the ABRs recorded and the experience of the clinician. It is generally accepted that the most reliable interpretation of clinical threshold ABR data is done by skilled experienced clinicians (recall Episode 6.3). New clinicians and/or clinicians with low ERA caseloads (thus less time in the "school of hard knocks") often face challenges knowing which testing conditions to prioritize, how to interpret waveforms in more complicated cases, and teasing apart sensory from neural deficits. Examiners in countries or regions with fewer resources for training face still greater difficulties. ***Telehealth-enabled ABR (TEABR)*** technology is being pursued to mitigate this situation. For example, in the province of British Columbia, audiologists at the largest pediatric hospital conduct ABR-ERA assessments for infants and families who live hundreds of kilometers away from audiology facilities. This has decreased wait times as well as addressed potentially poorer quality of the services due to the issues mentioned.[163] Another solution is to offer threshold estimation methods that require less training and skill, such as ERA using ASSRs; as highlighted before, there are inherent methodological advantages to techniques that are less reliant on VDL judgments.

What are these advantages? To recap, for threshold estimation, ASSR-ERA relies on evoked potentials that are repetitive in nature and are analyzed in terms of their frequency components rather than their waveform characteristics, taking advantage of a more substantively deterministically relation between stimulus and response—thus, purely objective bases for where in the spectrum to look for and objectively detect presence of the response. Potential clinical uses of ASSR testing were thoroughly overviewed in Episode 6.3. The upshot was to suggest that for ERA using modulation rates greater than 70 Hz—often called the ***"80-Hz ASSR" or "brainstem ASSR"***—ASSR-ERA from the start passed quickly the "litmus test" of applicability in sleeping infants and subsequently to have demonstrated broad clinical utility.[67,103] The relevant literature is expansive and an in-depth review is beyond the scope here (but has been submitted to meta-analysis).[153] It will suffice here to note that a strictly empirical study was done using masking noise to induce a temporary hearing loss of a relatively challenging configuration of varying degrees.[113,164] The results confirmed a problem with 80-Hz-ASSR-ERA for utmost accuracy in estimating the pure-tone audiogram within the clinically normal range at 500 Hz. This "quirk" was confirmed in another study at 250 Hz.[111] Still, results of ASSR-ERA represented very well the degree and configuration of losses from mild-moderate and beyond. Correlations with behavioral and LLR-ERA estimates (again measuring N_1-P_2, virtually another "gold standard" historically) were excellent, confirming both validity and reliability of 80-Hz-ERA, as portrayed herein.

The numerous issues considered in this episode, both technical and practical, should not be taken to speak negatively about the methods presented, simply informatively by which to both build insight and foundational knowledge toward (ultimately) clinical competence in ERA. Research and development of the ASSR "suffered" double jeopardy on its journey to becoming broadly accepted for routine clinical use; ASSR technology experienced the usual trials of research and development but also pushback from devoted users of ABR-ERA. Historically, ABR-ERA had "earned" respect as the winner of a war between great minds with remarkably different perspectives—ABR-ERA versus TT-ECochG-ERA. ABR-ERA as a strictly noninvasive approach won out to a broader good of leading to efficacious methods suitable for routine clinical use, especially in the hands of nonmedical professionals, as is essential to having sufficient manpower to meet demands. More ASSR data (particularly BC-ASSR data in individuals with hearing loss) are still needed, even for the widely used ABR-ERA (such as EMLs for AC and BC testing). All further work needs to be done with the same attention as given to issues of behavioral pure-tone audiometry and for both adults/older children and infants.

In summary, there are a number of physiological tools that can be used to estimate hearing thresholds when behavioral measures cannot be used reliably or to verify behavioral findings. These methods are largely equally applicable among older children and adults, indeed having emerged from research and development strongly motivated by interests in objective audiometry in young children, even infants. The ABR-ERA has been used the most extensively and remains a commonly and considerably reliably used method for clinical electrophysiological assessments. A natural "offspring," the 80-Hz-ASSR-ERA came onto the clinical scene in somewhat of a troubled research and development era, but since has commanded keen clinical interests and enjoyed continued research interests and refinement. Its well-demonstrated methodological advantages are difficult to match fully on the counts of improved efficiency and objectivity for ERA; however, still more research is needed, particularly for BC testing, for utmost implementation in this ever-important clinical application.

■ Episode 5: Differential Diagnostic Applications

Differential diagnosis is the process of determining which, among a set of diseases/disorders that share similar signs and symptoms, a particular patient might have. For audiologists, that typically requires the use of ABR measurements and other audiological tools to differentiate among conductive, cochlear, and retrocochlear pathologies. The goal of the differential diagnostic workup in these cases is to tease apart respective effects of the pathologies, which includes how to deal with one to get to the other and how to determine the level(s) of the auditory pathway of the probable site(s) of lesion. Any conductive or cochlear pathology affects the information transferred to the 8th nerve. As demonstrated later, a high-frequency hearing loss effectively will reduce or remove high-frequency elicited responses while passing along the lower-frequency-elicited activity to the neural system, thus causing longer latencies and smaller amplitude ABRs compared to the normal responses. This episode is devoted to the application of ABR measures to differential diagnosis; specifically, the purpose is to demonstrate how to differentiate the characteristics of the ABRs among conductive, cochlear, and retrocochlear pathologies.

The logic behind the interpretation of the ABR is founded on the substantial knowledge base (in the literature) of the time and space coordinates of the generators and the documented effects of a variety of pathologies on the ABRs. The characteristic clinical results for peripheral, as well as neural pathologies, will now be discussed starting with a pure conductive loss at the front end of the peripheral system, together with knowledge of nonpathological factors presented in earlier episodes. The first step is to revisit the normal ABR and the reference latencies and amplitudes of the component waves of primary interest—I, III, and V—as well as the interpeak intervals and the ratio of wave V to I amplitudes. These metrics are the standard against which the clinical ABR measures will be compared.

However, ***norms*** for evaluating the response currently are not a part of a standard. Each clinic must develop a normative data set by testing at least 20 individuals, ideally young adults with normal hearing and negative histories of CNS disorders. These subjects are tested with all the stimulus and recording parameters that are expected to be used in diagnostic protocols. Some clinics obtain individual sets of norms for men and women, but most compile one set of norms for use with both sexes. The typical stimulus for the basic ABR is a 100 µs click presented at rates between 10/s to 20/s at approximately 70 dB nHL. In the absence of a standard, it is incumbent upon examiners to have reviewed their data in light of comparable results published in the literature to confirm that theirs reasonably approximate the central tendencies and confidence limits of the published data. Any departures from the routine protocol anticipated require their own norms. The values commonly used to evaluate the ABR for differential diagnostic purposes are discussed in the following text, along with their strengths and weaknesses.

The basis for interpretation for differential diagnosis depends on several specific characteristics of the ABR waveform. The most important measure is latency. Recall from earliest discussions of this measure, the practical and most reliable measure of latency is defined as the time from stimulation onset at the earphone input (compensated for added sound propagation delay for tubal-insert type earphones) to the peak of a given wave. Also of critical importance is that wave I marks the start of transmission of the neural coding of the sound stimulus via the 8th nerve to the CANS. At this time, the stimulus already has gone effectively through multiple *transfer functions* (spectral changes) via the earphone, ear canal, middle ear, and cochlea—all before activation of the 8th nerve fibers (recall Episodes 3.2, 5.1, and 5.2). The wave I component of the ABR to the sound stimulus is shaped by the filtering properties of all the peripheral transforms. Consequently, the response at the 8th nerve is likely to be different for normal and disordered peripheral auditory systems and even before the "signal" reaches the 8th nerve itself. It, therefore, is important in differential diagnosis first to consider the ways conductive and cochlear presynaptic pathologies (that is, before the hair cells synapse with the neural fibers) can affect the interpretation of neural function in the brainstem. Effects of neural pathology cannot be considered in the absence of knowledge of the peripheral effects on the ABR.

Latencies do not tell the whole story. Amplitudes of waves I, III, and V as well as their presence or absence matter, as do differences between ears. As noted earlier, wave V is the most robust wave normally; earlier waves can be reduced or absent with hearing losses and/or advancing age. Absolute amplitude of the waves is not nearly as reliable measures as are latencies.[165] The overwhelming pickup of background noise in electrophysiological recordings from the scalp (EEG, etc.) with the great amplifier gains required for measuring the ABR also can be exacerbated by physical interference and/or poor electrode placement/contact.[166] The residual noise simply never is suppressed enough by the net signal conditioning applied (differential amplification, filtering, and averaging) to yield an truly optimal SNR. Fortunately, the timing of wave peaks proves to be statistically more resilient. Nevertheless, the general trend of growth of the response normally from the 8th nerve into the CANS is that of dramatic increases in wave amplitudes along the auditory pathway (by way of neural arborization; recall Episode 3.2). Consequently, a possible red flag for a lesion beyond the peripheral system is an amplitude ratio, V/I, which falls below 1.0.

Amplitude and latency are both dependent upon effects of stimulus parameters (recall Episodes 2.2 and 2.3), recording parameters (recall Episodes 4.1 and 4.2), and not just a given pathology. The test protocol and any variances must always be considered first. Thereafter, differential diagnosis starts in the periphery and then moves step-by-step along the auditory pathway. As a framework of reasoning are considerations of several possible peripheral-system lesions, starting with involvement of the conductive part of the peripheral system. A *pure conductive lesion* often is not too problematic if the stimulus level is sufficient to overcome the air-bone gap. Such lesions thus effectively attenuate the sound, and this *effect is linear*. Hence, the loss is readily compensated by increasing the signal level in dB to match the elevation of the hearing threshold.

Cochlear hearing losses typically include loss of outer hair cells for even mild degrees of hearing loss, whereas more severe losses may include a sizable population of inner hair cells.[167] In the latter case, the associated neurons innervating the hair cells may not be entirely available, either not stimulated or lost through retrograde degeneration.[168] The result (in effect) is filtering of the input signal at the cochlea but with the added effect of *stimulus-level dependence*. Accordingly, at relatively low sound levels for a particular degree of loss, compensation is similar to that of simple conductive losses but with the configuration of the hearing loss included. Thus, the response is shaped by the frequency response of this *cochlear filter*, complicated by the *nonlinearity* of the cochlear system. The resultant signal through these initial stages of the peripheral system naturally affects the measured response from the 8th nerve and brainstem. The 8th nerve and/or subsequent retrocochlear lesions can block, partially or wholly, neural conduction to or within the brainstem, creating and/or adding to the filtering effects of any presynaptic hearing loss. These general issues dictate changes in test strategy and/or interpretation in order to determine the condition of the auditory neural system, which is the ultimate goal in the differential diagnostic application of ABR measures.

These general expectations can be summarized by manipulation of a given brainstem response by applying the foregoing concepts to a model ABR, as in Figure 6–27. The figure shows the effects of four hearing conditions: first—normal hearing, second—conductive loss, third—sensory hearing

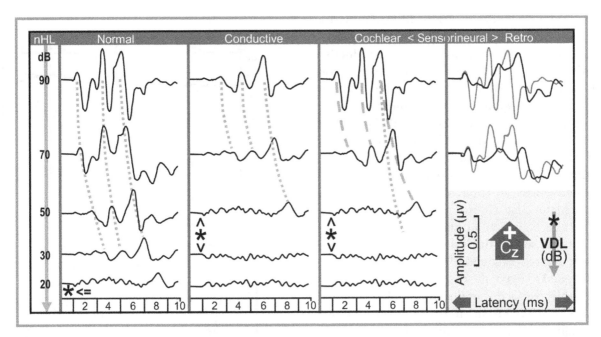

Figure 6–27. Illustration of general principles of interpretation of auditory brainstem responses in cases of classical types of hearing loss of primarily end-organ or more peripheral (nominally presynaptic) origins as well as an example of the sort of change in ABR wave morphology that raises suspicion of more central sites of lesion (Retro—retrocochlear). Shifts in latency with intensity are seen to be nearly parallel (recall Episode 6.1) for conductive or cochlear disorders, but the latter also shows a remarkable "catch-up" toward normal/more-normal latencies at upper hearing levels (*dotted line at wave V versus dashed line copied from that of the "normal" data set*). This recruitment effect is neither typical of conductive nor retrocochlear losses, but the latter typically presents additional latency issues. Variants all modeled from actual recordings (normal-hearing young adult) but are trends seen in many actual clinical cases. (Now please keep reading as one figure does not a competent diagnostician make.)

loss, and fourth—retrocochlear pathology. The nHL of clicks are represented as levels from 10 dB to 90 dB and the subsequent ABR waveforms develop to the right panels. For the first condition, the normal hearing individual shows only wave V at 10 dB nHL; waves III and V at 30 dB nHL; and waves I, III, and V at 50 dB nHL to 90 dB nHL. At 70 and 90 dB, all five waves are present and easily distinguished. The expectation for an individual with normal hearing thresholds is this pattern of responses—again, only wave V near thresholds and the full sequence of waves when stimulus levels are in the mid- to upper dynamic range of hearing, as seen with stimuli at/above 70 dB nHL. However, as discussed further shortly, such results would not fully rule out an 8th nerve/retrocochlear lesion.

The second waveform in the figure portrays the effect expected from a 45-dB conductive hearing loss. Note that only noise is present at 10 and 30 dB nHL, but at 50 dB, a small late wave V is present and looks much like the wave V seen in the normal response at 10 dB nHL. Then at 70 and 90 dB, the ABR in the conductive case appears similar to the normal waves at 30 and 50 dB nHL, respectively—a 40-dB difference for each signal level that is explained by the degree of the conductive hearing loss. Raising the signal level is enough to allow the underlying normal cochlear/neural function to be observed, appearing as normal for the sensation level (dB SL).

The third and fourth waveforms in Figure 6–27 also show effects of cochlear (sensory) versus retrocochlear (neural) pathologies. The 45-dB cochlear hearing loss also shows only noise for the 10 and 30 dB stimuli, and at 50 dB nHL, a small wave V is present. At 70 dB, waves I, III, and V are present with latencies about the same as for the waveforms of the normal response but earlier than for the response in the case of conductive loss. Also notable is the difference in the wave morphology at 70 dB nHL for the normal and cochlear responses. The response in the cochlear case only has waves I, III, and V, rather than all five waves as in the normal response. The reduced cochlear input reduces the amplitudes of the waves, until the stimulus level is increased substantially above the effective loss. In contrast, the response in the retrocochlear case (fourth tracing) shows more variable effects, which are dependent on the type, location, and size of the lesion. In the figure, note that only high-level stimuli (70 and 90 dB nHL) are used/needed to make the case, and the waves show significantly reduced amplitudes and prolonged latencies compared to the normal response, shown by the light gray waveforms. In other words, merely increasing the stimulus level does not resolve the abnormality of this pseudopatient's ABRs.

The case of purely **conductive hearing loss** was shown largely to increase latencies and decrease amplitudes commensurate with the hearing loss. More severe conductive hearing losses may reduce some ABR components to levels below the noise floor. The larger the air-bone gap is, the smaller the amplitudes and longer the latencies will be. The former is the input-output (I-O) function and the latter the latency-intensity (L-I) function at work; hence, they are normal but shifted by stimulus level. An example of an ABR in an actual clinical case of a conductive loss is shown in Figure 6–28. This case presented with an ossicular malformation in the left ear. The findings of pure-tone audiometry (panel A) were consistent with the diagnosis. An ABR test (panel B) revealed prolonged latencies and overall reduction of amplitudes of the waves in the pathological ear. The left ear wave V at 90 dB nHL was about the same as the right ear wave V at 70, although the audiogram reflected a 40-dB difference between ears. At higher stimulus levels, latency-intensity shifts are not as dramatic, and overall, the results are consistent with the model-response prediction. The interwave latency differences vary slightly with signal level but should not be significantly different, and were interpreted as normal. Had wave I been undetectable, however, the information from two

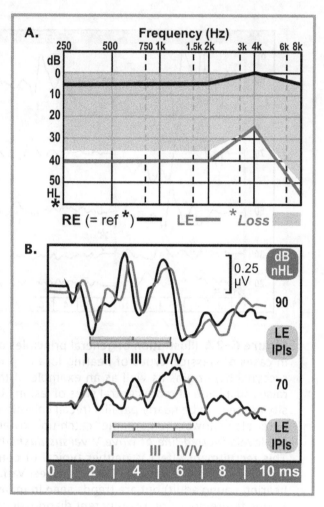

Figure 6–28. **A.** Conventional/behavioral audiometric results in a case of a unilateral conductive hearing loss, left ear (LE). If purely conductive indeed, then the defect is acting much like an earplug (simply attenuating the input sound)—a very good one in this case. The equivalent insertion loss is highlighted in light gray, estimated by the interaural difference. **B.** ABR findings in this case are typical of conductive pathology. Also demarked are the major interpeak intervals (IPIs: I–III, III–V, and I–V for the LE), seen not to be significantly different from those of responses for the right/normal ear (RE).

(of three) important interwave latency differences would be lost as well, thus rendering the interpretation of the ABR more challenging. Useful further tests may include ECochG,[169] combined ECochG and ABR, or a retest with BC stimulation[170,171] to enhance the amplitude of wave I. The tentative concern of possible retrocochlear lesions in cases such as this one will become more evident later in this episode.

All conductive losses are not that simple. For conductive losses that are not flat or are mixed, the actual level or spectrum of the stimulus reaching the cochlea may not be as expected. This situation is responsible for the fact that identification of conductive pathology using the L-I function is only correct about half the time, and in some cases, L-I functions are steeper than predicted for conductive losses. These conductive cases can look very similar to some sharply sloping, high-frequency sensorineural hearing losses. Mixed losses are more complicated and results tend to be more variable. Indeed, substantial mixed hearing losses may cause ABR results to be uninterpretable for differential diagnostic purposes.[172–174]

The best way to evaluate any patient who reports for a diagnostic ABR is to determine if there is a conductive component and, if so, whether it is transient or permanent. As always, preliminary otoscopy can identify excess cerumen, debris, or foreign objects in the ear canal or may give evidence of middle ear pathology. Acoustic immittance tests can identify middle ear pathology, and an audiogram can provide basic information about the type, configuration, and degree of loss. If the loss is transient, the best approach is to determine if the pathology causing the loss can be treated prior to testing, if delaying ABR testing is medically acceptable. Again, BC-ABR testing or ECochG may provide more insights. In general, the more knowledge about the patient the clinician has before the ABR test, the more efficient the testing and the stronger the interpretation of the results will be.

The influence of **cochlear sensorineural hearing loss** is not straightforward. The effects of cochlear pathology on the ABR depend on the degree and configuration of the hearing loss and the extent to which the hairs cells and nerve fibers are intact. Two nonlinear factors are potentially involved—that of the initial transduction of sound energy (recall Episode 5.1) and the density of subsequent neural discharges elicited per dB (recall Episode 3.2). The neurons encode sound intensity as density of discharges; central connections of these neurons are ramified along the auditory pathway until they reach the cortex and ultimately "produce" the loudness perception. It is this pathway that is responsible for the behavioral loudness recruitment commonly associated with cochlear losses. The phenomenon is one of an individual not hearing well at low sound levels, yet perceiving virtually the same loudness at high levels as that perceived by normal-hearing individuals. Cochlear/neural manifestations strongly correlated with that perception occur in the acoustic reflex, the $AP(N_1)$, and the ABR. This recruitmentlike effect is not present in purely conductive or (typically) in retrocochlear pathologies. Consequently, cochlear function must be considered along with the effective spectrum of the input sound to the inner ear (recall Episode 6.1).

The combined effects of the cochlea and the spectrum of a common stimulus, such as a click, can be appreciated by way of the contrast of outcomes of ABR tests among three configurations of cochlear hearing losses: low frequency, moderate flat or high-frequency, and sharply sloping high-frequency.[175] The hearing loss effectively filters the signal at the transduction level of the hearing organ and changes the ABR morphology in predictable ways.[176,177] Mild to moderate low-frequency cochlear hearing losses generally have no appreciable effect on the click-ABR, as shown in Figure 6–29. The high frequency bias of the cochlea,[178] derived from the strong representation of neurons excited toward the base of the cochlea and at substantial suprathreshold sound levels dominate the click-ABR in the same way as in the normal ABR. Correspondingly, the latencies and amplitudes fit the norm, and the VDL of the click ABR typically falls within normal limits. Hence, the value of the click is limited for purposes of auditory threshold measures in these cases.

A substantial range of outcomes are possible in cases of sloping/high-frequency hearing losses, as shown in Figure 6–30A. The ABR data characterizing this type of hearing loss (group P2) complicate the differential-diagnostic decision by the examiner. Yet, with adequate understanding of the interplay of stimulus, presynaptic sensory, and postsynaptic neural effects, enlightened decisions can be made. The best news is that flat or gently sloping cochlear hearing losses (group P1) have mild effects on the click ABR[177] measured at suprathreshold stimulus levels. Because the loss is relatively flat across frequencies, the stimulus spectrum

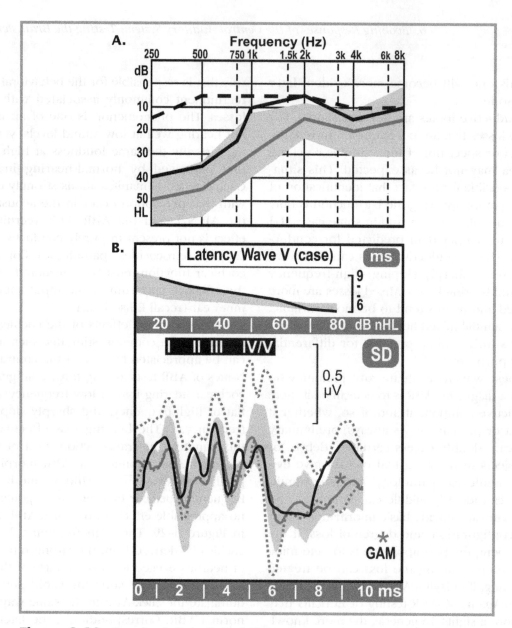

Figure 6–29. Trends of click-elicited ABRs given predominantly low-frequency sensorineural losses. **A.** Summary audiogram for a group of patients with similar unilateral sensorineural hearing losses (*mean—gray line* and *+/– standard deviation [SD] area—gray fill,*); mean thresholds for contralateral ears (*dashed black line*) fell essentially within +/–5 dB for the group (not plotted for simplicity). Thresholds of an exemplary individual patient (affected ear) from another clinic shown by the solid black line. **B.** Upper subpanel: This case's latency-intensity function for wave V (*black line*) is shown to be within that clinic's norms (*gray area*; standard deviation). Main subpanel: This case's ABR (*black line*) also plotted for comparison with several data sets from the group study, results based on grand average ABRs—pointwise mean of potentials (GAM) computed across individual ABRs within the group sampled, as follows: +/–1SD results for the normal ears (gray fill) versus the affected ear (*area between dotted lines*); GAM*/means (*solid gray line**) for affected ear (normal ear data not shown, as very similar). Note: The substantially greater variance of data for the affected ear was attributable to one outlier, but this clearly was more related to variance of amplitudes than either latencies or overall wave morphology. (Alternating polarity clicks presented at 85 dB nHL, rate of 17/s; based on data of Fowler and Durrant [1994].[175])

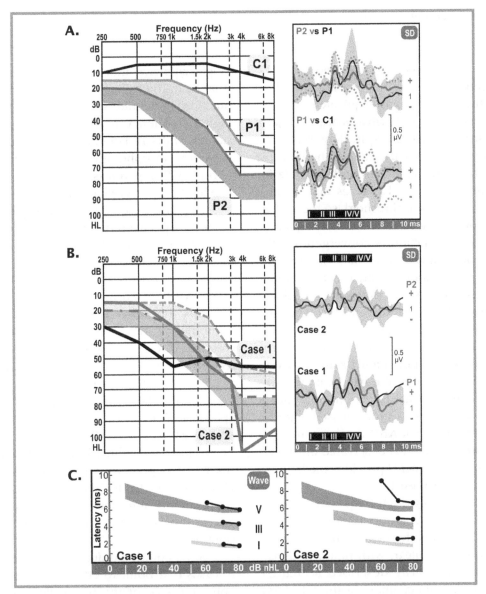

Figure 6–30. Trends analyses (as in Figure 6–29), here for sensorineural hearing losses of relatively moderate—group P1—versus moderately severe, high-frequency losses—group P2, all unilateral. **A.** Mean thresholds for the unaffected ear also are shown (*black line*), but only for the P1 group (designated C1), as results for the better ear of P2 was nearly identical (per both means and variances observed). Here, means and only +1 standard deviation areas are shown in the audiogram panel as severity of loss primarily accounts for any differences of effects on the ABR between groups. Plots in the ABR panel contrasts (again) grand averages and +/− 1SD areas of responses (as indicated). Mild-moderate, high-frequency sensorineural losses (P1), while not inconsequential, are still seen to permit ABR waveforms and latencies to fall closer to results in normal-hearing subjects and often more robust responses than in cases of more severe losses (P2). **B.** Results for two cases from another clinic are shown (as in Figure 6–29) and who presented with similar losses in the high frequencies to groups P1 (Case 1) and P2 (Case 2). Their ABR results (*black line*) are overlaid on the respective SD areas from the grouped data analyses, respectively (*gray lines/fill*). **C.** Latency-intensity functions of the two cases are overlaid on that clinic's norms. (Alternating polarity clicks presented at 75 dB for P1 and 85 dB nHL for P2, rate of 17/s; based on data of Fowler and Durrant [1994].[175])

is changed little by the cochlear filter and/or can be largely overcome by way of the recruitment effect. Latencies of the ABR waves are equivalent on average to those measured in normal hearing subjects when they are assessed at equivalent sensation levels. As a rule of thumb, the stimuli should be at least 20 dB above thresholds around 4000 Hz for adequate stimulation.[179,180] Latencies may be prolonged for responses near threshold, so the VDL of the click response may be elevated. Consequently, the underlying L-I function is convergent on the normative latencies at adequate sound levels. Typically, wave I is measurable and the I–V latency interval is normal in cases of presynaptic cochlear losses.[181] These effects are driven by the recruitmentlike growth of the amplitude of the 8th-nerve response (recall Episodes 5.3 and 5.4) and approximate or match norms at the higher stimulus levels. Furthermore, in such cases, the interpeak intervals should be normal. In panel B, data from a patient (Case 1) approximating P1-group losses where it most counts for the click-ABR demonstrates the effects just summarized, thus observable indeed on a case-by-case basis. Panel C provides the latency-intensity function for Case 1.

The sharply sloping, high-frequency cochlear loss (see Figure 6–30A, group P2 and panels B and C—Case 2) thus is the most difficult hearing loss to confirm as cochlear, with multiple departures from the previously described scenarios. Although lower-frequency fibers of the 8th nerve can be excited by the click, the effects of suprathreshold bias toward high frequencies normally make the configuration of the hearing loss more consequential as the effective filter function imparts a steep slope. Effects on the click ABR are demonstrated in Figure 6–30. Waves before V may be reduced in amplitude or lost, at least without use of ECochG or combined ECochG-ABR (recall Episode 5.4), or, inevitably, if the hearing loss is too severe. Latencies of all waves likely will be prolonged beyond norms, reflecting additional travel time on the basilar membrane to reach an adequately healthy part of the cochlea that is capable of eliciting sufficient density of neuronal firing in the pontine brainstem. Virtual elimination of the basal end of the cochlea is like deactivating fibers with the shortest response times in the normal cochlea. Consequently, the L-I function is shifted to longer latencies, much as in a conductive disorder (that is, to the right in the typical graph of the L-I function). Moderate-severe, or worse, losses in the higher frequency region do not only cause substantial shifts in latency; in many such cases, the waveform morphology is poorer than that of the normal ABR regardless of stimulus level. The VDL inevitably is elevated as well.

The more severe high-frequency cochlear losses indeed may have differential effects on wave components of the ABR. Given a truly cochlear loss of such degrees, the effect is expected to be a slight shortening of I–V interval. This effect also occurs in the ABRs of normal-hearing subjects, although perhaps the effect is more readily seen with a combined ECochG-ABR[165] or elicited with low frequency tonal stimuli.[181] Wave I may be prolonged more than wave V because wave I requires greater synchrony to stimulus onset for optimal elicitation, rather than envelope following or even "phase locking" to the fine-structure (recall Episode 6.2). In some ABRs, the I–III interval may be prolonged slightly, but I–V should be within norms.[176,181] pending an adequate stimulus level. Otherwise, if the I–V interval is also prolonged, the examiner must be suspicious of pathological effects involving nerve fibers of the 8th nerve or pontine brainstem.

Some additional details are important to note in cases that point to effects not beyond the synaptic interface of the hair cells to the 8th nerve fibers. High-frequency hearing losses may exaggerate latency differences between ABRs elicited by R- versus C-click polarities (recall Episode 6.1), and thereby could be misconstrued as a sign of a neural pathology. This situation is another consequence of steeply sloping high-frequency hearing losses that create sharp roll-offs of the cochlear-loss filter. The normal effects of polarity depend on lower frequency stimulation. In this scenario, the high-frequency response is absent and the lower-frequency contributions to the net ABR are exposed.[13,182,183] The bottom line is that the R–C latency differences emanate from presynaptic processing in the cochlea.[184] As discussed earlier, the R phase is nominally the excitatory phase in general; this polarity is relative to the stapes motion (the cochlear input signal). In general, the best practice is to test with both click polarities and to base the interpretation of the ABR on the response that is closest to normal if there is a discrepancy (recall Episode 6.1).

The typical patient referred for differential diagnostic testing of the ABR is frequently one who has unilateral or asymmetrical hearing thresholds. It follows from the foregoing considerations that different hearing losses in the two ears often yield different ABR waveforms and latencies. The dilemma regarding the origin (cochlear or retrocochlear) of the latency differences may be difficult to resolve if wave I is abnormal or absent. Several options are available to address these cases. Overall, these options are motivated by the desire to obtain at least a trend of physiological recruitment in the responses, which is a cochlear function.

Norms for ABRs (again) are based on response parameters assessed in normal-hearing individuals with clicks at about 70 to 80 dB nHL. However, if the hearing loss at 4 kHz approaches/exceeds 70 dB, the need for a 20 dB overhead puts the starting level at 90 dB or more. If the clinic has developed norms at the higher levels and the results fall within those norms, the interpretation is straightforward. In any event, given a more substantial hearing loss, the L-I effect may still help with the interpretation. If the physiological recruitmentlike effect is not complete, the convergence of the L-I functions in the two ears should still manifest trends toward the normal function. A two-point function using, for example, 70/75 and 90 dB nHL is typically adequate to demonstrate some recruitment (if present). The use of higher-level stimuli ideally would permit observing waves I, III, and V. If the interpeak intervals are reasonably symmetric and within the norms, the lesion can be identified as cochlear, regardless of the absolute latency values.[185]

To reiterate, only in the cochlear case (not conductive or retrocochlear) does such convergence toward the normal L-I function occur. Unfortunately, wave I is highly vulnerable to reduced effective stimulus levels in the cochlea. If wave I is not apparent, the best solution is a follow-up with ECochG or combined ECochG-ABR—for two reasons. First, in general principle, AEP measures concern both SNR and actual magnitudes of a targeted potential. If wave I seems to be absent despite adequate recording parameters, then seeking a better SNR is the most straightforward approach. Second, the clinician needs to avoid increasing the stimulus to a level that poses risks to the patient's test ear(s), such as discomfort, auditory fatigue (temporary threshold shifts), posttest tinnitus, or even permanent threshold shifts. Peak SPL at 90 dB nHL is over 120 dB peak SPL!

Another approach is to use a brief tone burst, such as at 1 kHz, namely where hearing thresholds may be better and more symmetrical between ears. This procedure, however, has had limited success. A full complement of waves is not typical with this stimulus and a high frequency bias is still present within the band of frequencies stimulated. Symmetry of the ABR still may not occur with steeply sloping configurations. The question of how much a given retrocochlear lesion affects high and low frequency fibers has not yet been answered. Nevertheless, this approach is useful in some cases.[186,187]

If these approaches fail, another approach is that of estimating latency corrections to compensate for the degree of hearing loss. One example[188] allows a normal interear difference of 0.2 ms plus 0.1 ms for each 10 dB increase in the hearing loss at 4 kHz above 50 dB HL. For example, should the hearing loss at 4 kHz in a given case prove to be 80 dB HL, an *interaural latency difference* of as much as 0.5 ms (= 0.2 + 0.3 ms) might still be considered to be consistent with a "cochlear" interpretation. Admittedly, this correction is rough and works better on average than with individual patients. The weakness of the approach is that it ignores the effects of hearing loss below 4 kHz and any conductive components (again, always a potential confound of the differential diagnosis). Still, if absolute latencies and interaural latency differences fall within normal limits for the degree of hearing loss, a cochlear interpretation is reasonable. However, all of these efforts fail with enough hearing loss, permitting only the conclusion that a retrocochlear pathology cannot be ruled out and the patient should be referred for medical follow-up. If the case was a medical referral, the patient would be asked to return to the referring physician.

In summary, several rules of thumb guide the interpretation of ABRs for differential diagnostic purposes. For a diagnostic ABR, the stimuli are presented at same suprathreshold levels as if the patient had normal hearing, given that the level is reasonable in reference to the audiometric data. The pattern of stimulation on the basilar membrane is important, not the sensation level of the stimulus. At suprathreshold levels, the latencies should be essentially normal if the cochlear hearing loss is low frequency or mild-moderate flat or of gently sloping configuration. At signal levels near thresholds, latencies may be slightly prolonged, but interpeak intervals should remain unremarkable. The effects of more severe, sloping high-frequency losses likely will require these considerations and more, but in many cases, the recruitmentlike growth of the ABR strongly suggests cochlear pathology. If the ABR is still difficult to interpret, hearing-loss compensation of latency measures may be invoked but must be done so judiciously and with due consideration for additional testing (like ECochG). High-level stimulation also must be respected from what it really is, not just nHL rather peak SPL, as safety first is always the best policy.

Retrocochlear pathology is an "umbrella" term for any pathology that occurs after the cochlea. Although it has long been used as such, it proves to be a bit of a misnomer on anatomical grounds. The bigger and more basic anatomical picture is that the 8th nerve courses distally from the hearing organ and for some distance until the internal auditory meatus opens into the 4th ventrical, across from the brainstem (see Figure 3–12). The proximal portion then is a retrocochlear structure, yet still very much a peripheral nerve. There are finer points distally to be recalled as well. Neural lesions can occur at the synapse, dendrites, spiral ganglia, and distal portion of the 8th nerve (within the petrous pyramid). On the one hand, "retrocochlear" (the term) has continued to work categorically in practice in deference to the huge part of the auditory pathway that literally is beyond the cochlea. On the other hand, a considerable game-changer in the differential-diagnostic applications of AEPs has been the revelation of a neural disorder/spectrum of disorders[189] that can affect the 8th nerve, mentioned earlier (ANSD; recall Episodes 5.3 and 5.4). A characteristic defect of this disorder is desynchronization of neural discharges, which in some cases may be caused as far distally (laterally) as the 8th nerve synapses with the hair cells.

For simplicity, "retrocochlear pathology" will be used here, given the qualification earlier of "cochlear" to pertain to presynaptic function. By way of the nuances just summarized, retrocochlear pathology inevitably can have variable effects on the ABR depending on the type, size/extent, and location of the lesion.[190,191] The most common effects—regardless of the specific type of pathology—are delayed latencies beyond wave I, prolonged interwave intervals, delayed latencies in the suspect ear compared to the better ear, and/or absence or reduction in size of any of the ABR components. In other words, these abnormalities are not explained readily by concomitant cochlear (end-organ) and/or more peripheral dysfunction (both sensory and/or conductive components of a given loss of hearing). Meanwhile, retrocochlear pathology as thus defined cannot be expected necessarily to be expressed in basic measures of hearing sensitivity.

The approach to identification of a retrocochlear pathology is to obtain the ABR with the same protocols that were discussed for the peripheral hearing losses. The difference broadly between cases of conductive/cochlear pathology and retrocochlear pathology is the expectation of abnormal results in the latter. The ABR measures most commonly found in 8th-nerve tumors, for instance, are prolongation of the wave I–V interpeak interval, the absolute latency of wave V, and/or the interaural wave-V-latency difference.[192] Wave amplitudes and the V/I ratio may be reduced. Absence of some or all of the component waves is possible in any retrocochlear pathology.

Comprehensive interpretation of ABR findings can rarely be made without a thorough patient history and information from other tests. Important red flags in the case history include complaints of unilateral or asymmetrical hearing loss and/or tinnitus, difficulty with speech understanding, and possible dizziness. These symptoms require further investigation because they suggest the possibility of a neural pathology, but not specifically an 8th-nerve tumor (for instance). Patients with these symptoms are typically candidates for ABR diagnostic tests. Conventional audiometry is still useful but may/should be supplemented by tests of acoustic immittance (including acoustic reflexomety), otoacoustic emissions, and/or other tests from the audiologist's toolbox.

For decades, testing the ABR was in high clinical demand as an audiological tool for possibly detecting tumors of the 8th nerve. **Acoustic (nerve) tumors** histopathologically are typically vestibular schwanommas, often seated within the internal auditory meatus (described as intracanalicular) and thus pressing on the 8th nerve. This tumor is is ostensibly an adult disorder, and it tends to be slow growing. Consequently, many patients presenting with this lesion are middle-aged or older, which means that their victims probably have suffered the hazards of a lifetime of hearing in noisy surroundings and/or "ravages" of aging—presbycusis.[193-195] The point is that rarely do such patients present with just one pathology, namely other pathology(ies) lateral to the 8th nerve. The goal of the differential diagnostic workup in these patients thus is to tease apart the respective effects of the pathologies in order to determine the level(s) of the auditory pathway of the probable site(s) of lesion that is involved. As discussed earlier, any conductive or cochlear pathology affects the information transferred to the 8th nerve. To reiterate in particular, high-frequency hearing loss effectively will reduce or prohibit high-frequency elicited responses while passing along the lower-frequency-elicited activity to the neural system, thus causing longer latencies and smaller amplitudes of the ABRs compared to the normal responses.

Basic categories of pathology that affect the 8th nerve and/or auditory brainstem include space-occupying lesions (indeed including acoustic tumors), neural degenerative disorders (such as ANSD and multiple sclerosis), viral disorders (such as HIV/AIDS and measles), and cardiovascular disorders (such as sickle cell anemia, strokes, and infarcts).[196-199] Space-occupying lesions can disturb neural impulses by compressing the nerve, which slows or blocks the neural transmission. If the nerve is not completely blocked, the remainder of the neural pathway still may support some normal interpeak intervals; for instance, an abnormally prolonged I–V interwave latency still may have a normal III–V interval. If the pathology completely blocks 8th-nerve conduction, then essentially no waves will be detectable. In other words, the peripheral system has been rendered incapable of passing information on to the CANS at that point. Neural degenerative diseases also affect efficiency of neural conduction, but by different means, such as causing demyelination of axons, thus interfering with saltatory conduction (see Figure 3–11B).

A few representative cases follow as examples of the diversity of ABR findings in etiologies that follow expectations according to the possible functional effects just overviewed. Acoustic tumors and multiple sclerosis (MS) are particularly instructive because these disorders represent two remarkably different etiologies and underlying histopathological mechanisms. Yet, their functional impact can be quite similar or different, pending other factors, such as extent and site of lesion. Historically, the most common neural pathology evaluated with the ABR was the space-occupying lesion of the acoustic tumor. Often referred to as an acoustic neuroma, again most such tumors prove to be vestibular schwannomas. They thus arise typically from the vestibular branch of the 8th nerve; this etiology explains the dizziness that sometimes is a presenting or accompanying symptom to patient's auditory complaints. All such tumors are distinguished from tumors of the CNS because they involve Schwann cells that form the myelin sheath of axons in peripheral nerves. The 8th nerve then is insulated mostly by the Schwann cells, but not exclusively. When the neural fibers enter the brainstem, astrocytes take over the job of insulating the remaining proximal portion of the 8th nerve. In contrast, MS is a progressive, neural degenerative disorder of the CNS that also can affect both the auditory and vestibular systems. Possible symptoms include dizziness and progressive or sudden-onset sensorineural hearing loss. At times, hearing sensitivity also may recover, although not necessarily to completely normal function.[200] MS plaques that form along the central auditory pathways can cause abnormalities of the ABR. The etiology is demyelination of the nerve fibers, thus interrupting rapid conduction along the nerve tracts involved. If the disorder involves multiple plaques, the neural pathway may be impaired extensively, and the subsequent ABR waves may be progressively prolonged or become undetectable. Equally important,

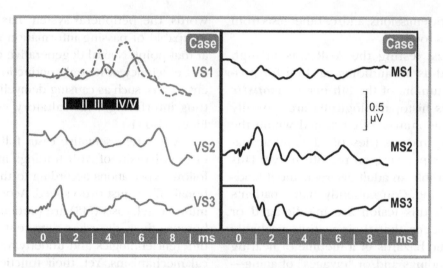

Figure 6–31. Contrasting ABR evaluation findings for cases of lesions due to vestibular schwannomas (VS 1–3) versus multiple sclerosis (MS 1–3), thus both considered to be retrocochlear lesions. The dashed line in results for VS 1 represents that patient's ABR with stimulation of the unaffected ear, essentially a "model ABR" for reference. Cases VS 3 and MS 3 show similar click ABRs that are particularly interesting. Their ABRs are suggestive of an effective "disconnect" of the 8th nerve from the brainstem, yet from two different etiologies—acoustic tumor versus a root-entry plaque, respectively.

a patient presenting with a history of MS may not demonstrate abnormal ABRs. MS plaques thus may occur anywhere in the brain or spinal cord and may or may not affect AEPs. Nevertheless, in patients with new symptoms suggestive of MS, the ABR can help in the differential diagnosis of MS. In patients with a history of MS now presenting with exacerbations of auditory and/or vestibular symptoms, the ABR can assist in the differential diagnosis of those symptoms. In both types of patients, the ABR can help define the extent of functional impact of the disease and determine if more than one pathology is present. An example is an MS patient with complaints of aural fullness and dizziness. It is possible to have the misfortune of two diseases like Meniere's disease and MS. In this particular example, combined ECochG-ABR again becomes useful to sort out the pathologies.

Some effects of these disorders are demonstrated in Figure 6–31, with the uppermost panel showing a normal ABR for reference. The left column contains three ABRs from individuals who were diagnosed as having vestibular schwannomas (VS; 1–3); the right column pertains to individuals with MS (MS; 1–3). VS 1 and VS 2 have prolonged absolute latencies of waves III and V and interwave intervals I–III and I–V. Nevertheless, III–V is within norms. The difference between the first two cases is that for VS 1, wave I also is delayed substantially, likely because of concomitant involvement of presynaptic cochlear loss, secondary to the tumor putting pressure on the cochlear artery and/or preexisting cochlear involvement. Case VS 3 has a nearly solitary wave I, suggesting the pathology affecting wave I extensively has blocked propagation or caused desynchronized neural impulses to the CANS. Incidentally, at times, an examiner may endeavor to assign wave numbers to what in the likes of VS 3's and MS 3's tracings are minimal "bumps" after wave I. Wave identification ("peak picking") is moot here given that wave I is clear and the latencies of any other bumps are ambiguous—clearly abnormal. Therefore, nothing is added to prediction of the site of lesion. The word "prediction" is used here in contrast to a definite statement of location of the lesion. What can be reported (after detailing the findings in a comprehensive report) is that these results are consistent with a retrocochlear pathology with a site of lesion at the level of the 8th nerve.

Corresponding waveforms for the MS cases in Figure 6–31 serve to demonstrate both similarities and differences in functional presentations of the two disorders represented therein and underscore another important reality of the ABR interpretation. The ABR patterns are evidence supporting the two caveats raised earlier: (1) the same pathology can result in different ABR morphologies (compare waveforms within each vertical column) and (2) different pathologies can result in similar ABR morphologies (compare waveforms in horizontal pairs). Thus, VS 1 and MS 1 both manage to have near-normal III–V interwave intervals in the face of prolonged I–V intervals and (consequently) an overall delay, yet for remarkably different etiologies. Site of lesion is more difficult to deduce precisely without a case history and other test results. Nevertheless, in the absence of cochlear and/or more peripheral pathology to explain the results, a retrocochlear decision certainly is supported. VS 2 and MS 2 both have prolonged I–V interwave intervals, yet VS 2 has a I–III prolongation, whereas MS 2 has a III–V prolongation. Both results are consistent with expected effects of the respective pathologies—compression of the proximal 8th nerve (VS 2) versus plaque before or at the level of the ipsilateral DVCN (MS 2). Why DVCN and same side as ear of stimulation, given crossover of the ascending pathways? Wave III itself is affected and, thus, must be ipsilateral to the side of stimulation. The ABR for MS 3 is quite remarkable as it suggests emphatically a very similar functional impact and level of site of lesion. How or where is this possible? Consider first a feature of the ABR not often closely considered—a clear wave II. This component is typically not as robust as I and III, but when it is clearly evidenced it should not be ignored either. Whereas wave I is understood to be generated at the distal end of the 8th nerve, this view of wave II is evidence of the proximal compound AP.[201] Wave II of VS 2 and VS 3 are only vaguely suggested, if indeed they are true responses. For MS 2 and MS 3, an excellent wave II bespeaks a functioning proximal portion before entering the brainstem but for MS 3 compared to MS 2 a more complete disconnnect of the nerve from the brain by the lesion (in effect). Again, although technically situated within the CANS, these still are lesions of peripheral nerves in both cases. So how in such cases of MS to frame the report accordingly? In deference to the neuroanatomical reality, the results may be said to suggest retrocochlear pathology at the brainstem level with a root-entry site of lesion of the 8th nerve.[200] Meanwhile, the cases illustrated in Figure 6–31 keenly remind of another reality of ABR/AEP tests—they indeed are functional tests not direct tests of etiology of the lesions manifested.

The ABR results shown in Figure 6–31 are presented in isolation. Other tests in the audiologic test battery and any previous ABR and audiometric findings need to be considered before the whole picture emerges in any patient. Another evoked-response test particularly worthy of inclusion in the audiologist's routine test battery applied in differential diagnosis is the OAE. Examples for the same diagnostic contrast featured previously are shown in Figure 6–32 for the two cases whose ABRs were shown in Figure 6–31—VS 1 and MS 1. The interpretation of site of lesion was left (purposefully for didactic purposes) a bit vague in consideration of the ABRs in isolation. Figure 6–32 now provides distortion-product results (DP-grams), respectively, for these cases that help to refine/reinforce the prediction of site of lesion. Each subject's ABR for the nonaffected ear (in these unilateral-retrocochlear cases) and the pure-tone audiograms are shown in panels A and B. Panel A also reflects the fundamental importance of potentially nonpathological variables, one of the greatest being individual variability of AEPs (recall Figure 6–8)—they are not all "textbook." Yet, the examiner still has a differential diagnostic decision to render!

The challenge, indeed, in any test is to determine what the individual's "normal" is and in diagnostic practice, what the statistically optimal criteria are appropriate for the examiner's decision. A false-negative decision is always possible for the presumptive nonpathological ear, just as is the possibility that a MRI may fail to detect plaques in a patient's brainstem pathways that might cause a documented hearing loss. At face value, the ABRs in cases VS 1 and MS 1 are substantially different for their respective better ears, although not substantially so apropos the hearing in their better ears (Figure 6–32B, upper panel). In these two

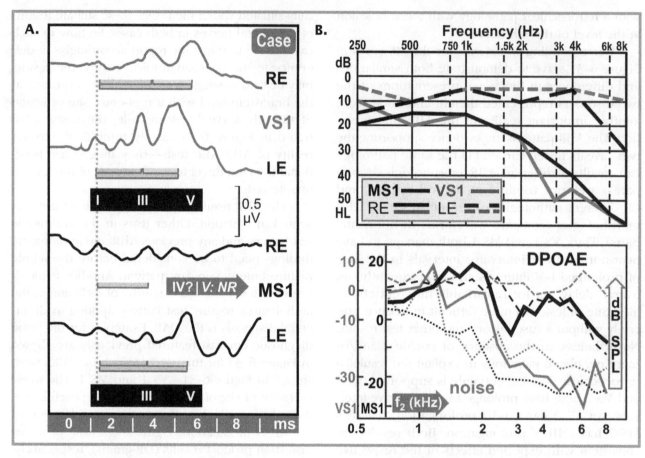

Figure 6–32. Further details of results from cases VS 1 and MS 1 presented in Figure 6–31, as cases presenting similar ABRs for the "pathological ear" and wherein distortion product otoacoustic emissions were also evaluated to further inform the interpretation. Indeed, VS 1's results bespeak combined sensory and neural dysfunction (the former presumably from compression of the cochlear artery by the tumor), whereas MS 1's DP-grams bespeak a purely neural lesion.

cases, the most comprehensive diagnostic decision comes down to the respective DP-grams for these patients (lower panel). VS 1 exhibits a variant of effects of an acoustic tumor, wherein the tumor is likely to be substantially compressing both the nerve and the cochlear artery and causing a high-frequency cochlear hearing loss, which would explain the absent DPOAEs for those higher frequencies. In contrast, MS 1 has completely normal DPOAEs, suggesting that the cochlear hair cells are functioning normally. Overall, only about 20% of acoustic neuroma patients have OAEs, with the loss either secondary to the neural lesion or from a preexisting condition.[202] Postoperative loss of outer hair cell function is worrisome with respect to growth of the tumor or as a surgical complication. Debulking or removing the tumor may inadvertently lead to interruption of the cochlear blood supply, to which the hair cells are quite sensitive. However, absence of OAEs does not preclude 8th nerve or brainstem involvement. MS 1's DP-gram supports the interpretation of brainstem site of lesion because the OAEs are reasonably normal in the face of slight (although clinically significant) high-frequency hearing loss.

Lesions beyond the DVCN are progressively more likely to impact crossed pathways, although not necessarily (recall Figure 3–12A). This possibility is the reason that a single ABR peak is neither uniquely attributable to a particular site of generation nor indicative of a singular site much beyond the DVCN. Nevertheless, relatively limited lesions have been reported to cause relatively focal functional events. Recall the Heads Up of Episode 3.2. The damage of the "nail in the head" was bilaterally focal having violated both sides of the brainstem with relatively sharply defined lesions. Although miraculously not fatal, it still was consequential functionally. One of the waveforms used to further support the interpretation of residual functional impact of these lesions was a tracing approximating findings from another clinical report. In that case, an inferior colliculus had been inadvertently necrotized unilaterally during neurosurgical treatment of a cerebellar tumor, using the gamma knife. This device generates a highly focused beam of radiation but also had "nicked" the IC on that side and annihilating wave V, contralateral to the ear with affected hearing (as expected neuroanatomically).[203] The wave shown in Figure 3–15 (dashed line) is the computed/estimated missing wave V, which could be derived from computations on data from the two-channel "clinical" recordings used in that patient.

Lesions in the crossover areas of the central auditory pathway also can affect ABRs on both sides. Extensive lesions overall, involving mid to upper pontine or higher lesions, also can do so from pressure or other effects (pending type of lesion, space-occupying, neural degerative, or vascular). Theoretically, lesions involving the brainstem between the ipsilesional DVCN (that is, lesion same side as the affected ear) and the IC could produce AEP responses as simulated in Figure 6–33A: delayed I–III latency on the ipsilesional side (right) and delayed III–V latency in the contralesional side (left). Therefore, thorough analysis of AEPs for both ears is paramount in differential diagnostic testing. Another example (here from an actual case, panel B), a lesion higher in the auditory brainstem can be seen to have affected only the later waves (bilaterally, but similar ABRs), as in the nail gun accident victim (again, recall Figure 3–15) . In this case, these results were for a young adult who suffered from the development of air emboli in the course of neurosurgery to remove an astrocytoma. She demonstrated a moderate, relatively flat hearing loss, as another manifes-

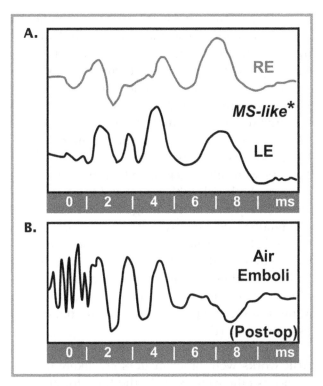

Figure 6–33. A. Quasimodeled variants of effects of sites of lesion in the pontine brainstem as can be expressed unilaterally or bilaterally differentially, such as in multiple sclerosis (inherently involving multiple lesions, thus multisite). **B.** A case of a lesion in the pons caused by air emboli having developed, unfortunately, secondary to surgery for an astrocytoma (postoperative ABR recording).

tation of her apparent central auditory processing disorder.

As intriguing are such cases, it is beyond the scope of this text to delve further into the many types and variants of retrocochlear lesions and issue of how well, versus not well, ABR testing proved useful in their diagnoses. The focus of the final discussion on its differential diagnostic applications will be brought back to the example of the acoustic tumor. Historically, demand for ABR testing for this purpose likely has exceeded that of all others, yet painfully for the audiology profession, those referrals suffered a dramatic drop into the 1990s and to this day. An NIH panel in 1991 indicated that the gold standard for tumor detection was Gd-DTPA MRI. This imaging provides identification, size, and location of intracanalicular acoustic tumors as small as 3 mm. Standard ABR measures detect acoustic tumors >1.0 cm with ~97% accuracy, smaller tumors (<1.0 cm) with 86% sensitivity, but a false negative rate from 7% to 37%.[190] Tumors by size were identified by ABRs in 100% for large tumors (>2 cm), 93% for medium tumors (1.1–2.0 cm), and 12 % for small tumors (<1.0). False positives occurred in 12% of patients.[204] Tumors were also catagorized by risk of having a tumor: high risk with a probability of 30% was based on asymmetrical hearing loss with <30% word recognition and tinnitus; intermediate risk with a 5% probability of having a tumor based on tinnitus, asymmetrical HL, plus one other symptom of a feeling of fullness, numbness of the face, double vision, or headache; low risk at 1% probability of a tumor if the symptom is tinnitus and there is no asymmetry of HL.

In fairness to the many ways the trusty click-ABR works well, other matters are likely to confound its effictiveness, as in the hunt for acoustic tumors. For example, the average population of individuals who acquire vestibular schwannomas are middle aged, namely also likely to be developing age-related hearing loss.[205] As demonstrated earlier, this often reduces ABR-wave amplitudes. The fundamental problem is that these tumors do not necessarily compress the nerve fibers for which the conventional click-ABR provides best sensitivity, given the bias of this response toward high frequencies. The overall story leading to the development of the stacked-ABR was related earlier, and the approach has been shown to be efficacious in detection acoutic tumors below a centimeter in diameter, as likely to be missed using the click.[206] Still, the method has yet to be fully developed or accepted in routine practice. Nevertheless, the concept has added to the fervor for clinical use of chirps. The issue is whether the chirp-elicited ABR can provide the same performance as the original method and thus in a more user-friendly paradigm.[133] So just how sensitive is the ABR morphology to the underlying "culprit" supposed (the naturally occuring phase dispersion of Nature's own mechanism)? Another demonstration is in order. As for the BIC "demo" (in effect; recall Figure 6–10), that a pristine model of the ABR was employed to avoid trying to see effects readily

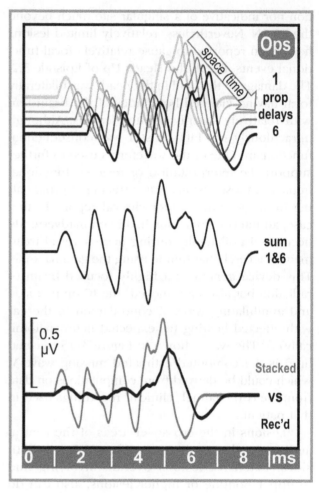

Figure 6–34. Concept recap of the "stacked ABR" and rationale of the chirp stimulus; demonstration using a computer simulation. (Ops—math operations on the model ABR; see text.)

without the distraction of the inevitable noise of actual recordings. As shown in Figure 6–34 (top), the ABR signal is delayed step-wise by 0.2 ms sequentially, as if having recorded as in practice. As such, the pickup is from a virtual test point in the ABR's far field. As was raised in discussion of what ECochG recordings "see" (recall Episode 5.2), it was shown that the cochlea itself makes the view from the outside less than optimal. Here too it "fails" too give the examiner the "best" view of the signal desired; in this case, not cochlear potentials but by not initiating the neural responses "in-sync." A net shift of ≈1 ms should certainly have some impact, although the overal response is over

5 times that in duration of the full wave complex. Glancing first just at the sum of sample delays numbers 1 and 6, already suggest potential untoward effects on wave V measurement, although this first impression is perhaps not all bad, if simply bigger is better for success. However, this is phasor math along the basilar membrane; it does not vibrate in discrete pieces. The net results are more of a sliding average over both traveling wave space and time. What more realistically is happening is represented by the bottom signal in Figure 6–34 plotted in black, effectively integrating over the ups and downs of all components over all six samples. Focusing on the IV–V complex, in the net there is still a relatively robust wave V, yet at a substantial loss of peak-to-peak amplitude versus that of the stacked ABR (gray line). Fundamentally, this is what the chirp does—"stacks the deck" preemptively to enhance the response by compensating for the phase dispersion. Validity of the chirp is supported by the earlier demonstration that the stacked-band approach could be accomplished equally using a set of ABRs sampled using Blackman-gated sinusoidal pulses over a comparable range of frequencies (thus places along the basilar membrane).[26] It is reasonable to expect that the chirp can be counted upon to improve the ABR signal recorded. As yet, chirps are still undergoing further research,[29,207] but certainly, stay tuned to future developments.

Despite recent advances in imaging, the development of sensitive ABR measures is still needed to detect small retrocochlear lesions in general. Even with imaging studies, ABRs tested in individuals suspicious of having small lesions are valuable to predict the extent of lesions and their functional impact, especially toward higher brainstem areas. Improved performance may also be sought through combined tests. For example, results of recent studies[208–210] suggest the use of a combination of acoustic and vestibular evaluations that include caloric responses, vestibular evoked myogenic responses, and results of the video head-impulse test. A recent meta-analysis compared multiple types of nonimaging measures to screen for acoustic tumors in an effort to reduce the number of individuals who need MRI evaluations.[211] Unfortunately, the conclusion was that not enough quality studies provided evidence to support using any of the tests for screening. Similarly, tests to increase sensitivity to small tumors also require the results of more comprehensive investigations. Whatever the future of research and development efforts is, one thing is not speculative, and that is the continued lack of a global standard of health and access to health care. The importance of advances in medical imaging is not in doubt, but the cost of instrumentation and personnel is a significant financial burden for many patients. The conventional click-ABR test permitted catching acoustic and other tumors before they became life threatening. The stacked-ABR, chirp, narrowband chirp, and other innovations in the differential diagnostic protocol are dedicated to the aim of improving test performance significantly. The ABR and related instrumentation is relatively inexpensive compared to other medical devices and diagnostic procedures. If the service-delivery site is difficult to staff at the specialized professional level, tele-medicine/tele-audiology is advancing with great strides—and this genre of test is well suited for such use.

HEADS UP

Differential Diagnostic Case Studies and the Challenge of Auditory Neuropathy

This edition of Heads Up provides several intriguing cases demonstrating differential diagnostics involving tests of the ABR but also looking beyond. Perhaps a subtitle might be (if a "stretch"), "Difficult to Judge a Book by Its Cover," if the audiogram is the cover, as often appears in the patient's chart (namely as one of the first pages). The cases presented will be shown to demonstrate remarkably different pathologies, yet surprisingly similar functional effects in some ways and a variety of outcomes, thus not necessarily what might have been expected from initial impressions and/or conventional audiological findings.

Case 1

A 7-month-old girl was seen in the audiology clinic with a history of having failed the **newborn hearing screening (NHS)** for the left ear. Repeated NHS testing was administered using CEOAE testing in both the newborn nursery and (subsequently) outpatient clinic at a regional hospital. The first two measurements yielded "refer" results, but the third screening result was interpreted as a "pass." This is why the patient was referred late for a more definite diagnostic hearing evaluation. Such management and the underlying rationales will be subjects of a later episode. It suffices to say here that the likelihood of obtaining "pass" results is increased when NHS is repeated due to a transient conductive condition common to newborns and that can last for some days at times. In any event, practices at the time were consistent with those of a NHS guideline,[127] thus according to the prevailing standard of care.

The patient's hearing subsequently was evaluated toward a definite diagnosis. Tympanometry using a 1000-Hz probe tone suggested normal middle-ear function at that time. Hearing thresholds were estimated via click-evoked ABR testing, and for the right ear, were taken to be at least no worse than 25 dB nHL. However, wave V was not observed upon testing the left ear, even at 90 dB nHL (Figure 6–35). In this patient's case, both transient CEOAEs and DPOAEs were measured (see panel B). Both tests demonstrated results within normal limits. The middle ear and outer hair cells both can be ruled out as the major lesion, among the possible anatomical structures capable of causing profound deafness suspected on the left. It is thus the mismatch between OAE and ABR results that strongly point to this differential diagnosis, namely a defect in neural transmission from the sound-transduction process peripheral to the CANS.

Therefore, information about the sound is not being received by the brain. By the merits of these results, the suspected site of lesion is the 8th nerve, potentially due to an auditory neuropathy—a failure of a nerve to function normally—or what is arguably more appropriately called in practice (as noted earlier), **ANSD (*auditory neuropathy/dyssynchrony disorders*)**,[189,212] in turn connoting the concept of a **spectrum** of disorders and also a matter of some controversy.[213] Nevertheless, the results summarized, thus far, do not permit definition of the actual pathology, so, and rightfully, they were followed up with further evaluation via **imaging**.

Computerized tomography or **CT scan** was ordered for the temporal bone to evaluate anatomical differences between the right and left inner ears. In this case, it proved to be the internal auditory meatus itself that was the cause. Its aperture through the left petrous pyramid was found to be severely narrowed (Figure 6–35C, white arrow pointing to the portion of the internal canal in question). Several reports in the literature have demonstrated the relationship between the width of the internal auditory meatus and hearing loss.[214-216]

At three years of age, the patient was evaluated via conventional audiometry. The results confirmed a profound hearing loss in the left ear (panel D). However, evaluation of speech recognition ability showed scores for 1-syllable words and 2-syllable words (open-set lists) and sentences in quiet of 61.1%, 70%, and 100%, respectively! The patient fortunately enjoyed normal development of speech language. Although less likely in unilateral-loss cases, such patients nevertheless should be followed up regularly with assessment of language development, especially phonological development. In general, they may require accommodation(s) in places like school to ensure favorable listening. This often includes preferential seating in the classroom, since the head casts an acoustic shadow on the side of the "good ear" for sounds coming from the side of the "dead ear." Although far less disabling than bilateral deafness, issues of unilateral hearing loss

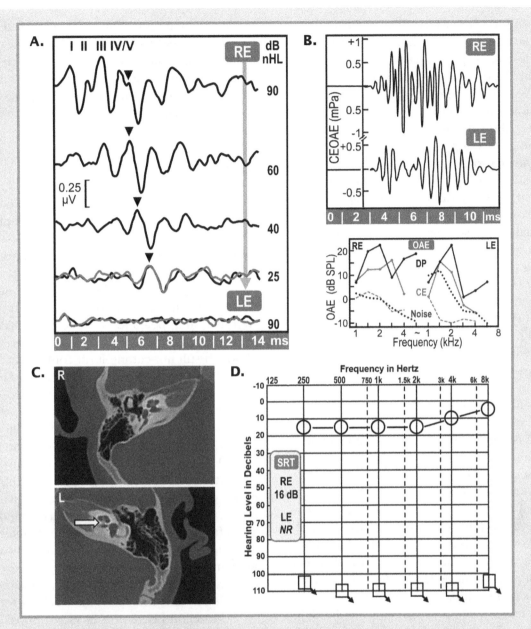

Figure 6–35. Results of differential diagnostic workup in Case 1: **A.** auditory brainstem response to clicks; **B.** transient/click-elicited (CE; half-octave band levels) and distortion-product (DP) otoacoustic emissions; **C.** computerized tomography scans; **D.** audiometric report.

have drawn appropriately increased attention. Although this child apparently was doing well, it still was important to have comprehensive evaluation of the patient and gratifying in this case to have led to a definitive diagnosis, even if untreatable medically.

Case 2

Detection of retrocochlear lesions among patients with variable, asymmetric hearing losses is always a challenge to clinicians. Interaural or interpeak latency delays are indirect evidence for retrocochlear lesions (as learned in the last episode), but their sensitivity to actual lesions is quite variable and often multifactorial.[190] Comparisons between traditional click-evoked and chirp-evoked ABR results for screening retrocochlear lesions were made in this case, the latter with the hope of further informing the diagnosis.

A 48-year-old female patient complained of left-side hearing loss with tinnitus; she also reported suffering dizziness. Although a negative history of traumatic acoustic exposure (as an initial diagnostic suspicion), her pure-tone audiogram showed a V-shape configuration of hearing loss—notch frequency at 2 kHz—on the left (Figure 6–36A). Hearing sensitivity on the right was within normal limits (thresholds ≤25 dB HL). Speech recognition scores demonstrated poor speech discrimination ability (28%) with presentation to the left ear as well.

Measurements of the ABR using the two different stimuli (click and chirp) at suprathreshold levels were analyzed for latencies (click) and amplitudes (chirp). The chirp (again) is designed to minimize high frequency dominance of the click-ABR as stimulus level increases.[133] In this patient, click-evoked ABR showed no pathological latency delays on either side, but the waveform of the chirp-evoked ABR revealed left-right amplitude differences in wave V, indicating the possibility of a retrocochlear lesion (panel B). As discussed earlier, chirp stimuli are designed to effect neural firing as if elicited simultaneously along the whole basilar membrane. Consequently, amplitude differences between ears due to some unilateral pathology are expected to be measureable more readily/reliably. Again, as AEP measurement is only a functional test, other modes of evaluation are required for a definitive diagnosis. In this case, ***magnetic resonance imaging (MRI)*** with contrast enhancement was conducted to confirm the suspected presence of retrocochlear pathology (if indeed present) and to discern its likely etiology. Results were affirmative, and the lesion proved to be a 0.6-cm vestibular schwannoma (see Figure 6–36C).

Both imaging technologies discussed here have benefited from continued research and development for decades to enhance test efficiency and resolution, and thereby to help to ease the burden on clinicians to get to the "right answers."

Reflection

How might these two cases have some common ground and/or each suggest some "deception" if not considered more deeply than a first impression? The first case has two interesting features, beyond the patient's intriguing pathology and the troubling auditory dysfunction that it can cause its victims. The left nerve dysfunction appears to be from the temporal bone "putting the squeeze" on the nerve, although still not cutting it off completely. This is attested by substantial speech recognition ability through that ear. Furthermore, close inspection of both the CEOAE and DPOAE results suggest that the hearing loss is literally sensorineural—not purely neural—as the levels of OAE in both tests are significantly lower in the left than in the right ear. This would be expected with compression of the cochlear artery, so not just the auditory nerve bundle. Therefore, the cochlear blood supply likely is compromised as well.[202] The hair cells are known to be acutely sensitive to reduction of the oxygen supply to the cochlea as is largely provided by this branch of the basilar artery.

The second case presents the opposite extreme of hearing dysfunction in the affected ear, a relatively modest loss of hearing and minimal effect on the conventional click-ABR. Indeed, in some cases of such small acoustic tumors, both can appear normal. On the other hand, the tumor compresses the nerve's subset of primary auditory neurons affected by this tumor but presumably minimally or not involving the cochlear artery. However, it took a more advanced analysis to "sniff" this one out, stacked-ABR analysis, again implemented using the chirp.

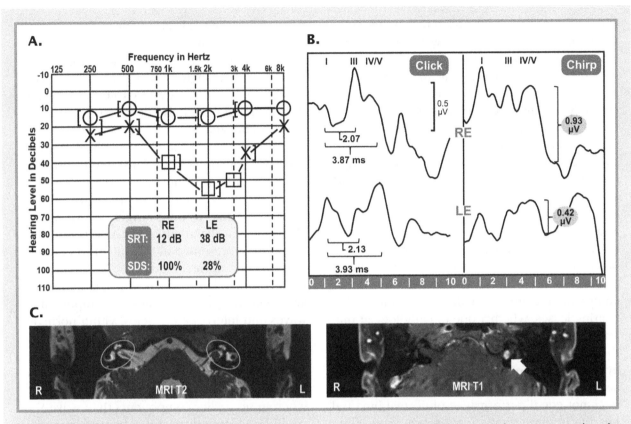

Figure 6–36. Results of workup in Case 2: **A.** audiometric report (SRT—speech reception threshold; SDS—speech discrimination score); **B.** sample ABR tracings for clicks and chirps (as indicated); **C.** magnetic resonance imaging (MRI) scans. Note: Computer processing of such images (especially when paired with the use of a contrast substance injected into the cerebral spinal fluid) permits highlighting certain tissues (like bony versus soft-tissue structures/lesions), hence the two views requested in this case. The T2 MRI (in which the authors have outlined much of the petrous portion) vividly highlights the cochlea itself and the horizontal semicircular canal. The tumor on the left side is distinguishable in this view (*a darkish mass*), but literally lights up in the T1 view.

Case 3

The final case, at a glance, may suggest similarities to Case 1, but the admonition about the frailty of book cover judgments also will resound as its intriguing details are revealed. Having contrasted in the last episode the differential effects among several types of neural disorders and of which the first two cases are exemplary, it will be instructive to take a still closer look at the disorder effectively featured here. To recap,[217,218] people with ANSD may have normal hearing or sensorineural hearing losses ranging from mild to severe, thus not precisely by any one degree or configuration of loss and which can be fluctuating losses. If a general trend, it is that of essentially flat or rising audiometric configuration. Still, the salient conventional audiometric finding is poor speech-perception ability that is not readily reconcilable with the pure-tone audiogram—speech discrimination scores poorer than expected from the audiogram. Additionally, as noted before, the contrast of the presence of OAEs (if not entirely normal) with ABRs either abnormal or not reliably demonstrated represents a diagnostically significant discordance. In general, ANSD cases present bilateral hearing losses that are more or less symmetrical. However, significant asymmetrical losses can be observed, including unilateral hearing losses. This may—or may not—be one such case, but the prospect is certainly worthy of consideration.

A 14-year-old girl presented at the second author's otolaryngology clinic. Like Case 1, she had passed the universal newborn hearing screening. She was doing well academically and socially in school. Although a lack of awareness of a hearing loss by family members, teachers, and friends, she reported a preference to listen to the phone with her left ear. She also noted problems of accurately localizing sounds and with speech discrimination in noise—a commonly recognized challenge of unilateral hearing losses, whether due to pathology at the level of the middle ear or beyond. As hinted in the review of Case 1, having one "good" ear, even if supporting reasonably good hearing sensitivity and other basic auditory functions, does not equal performance of normal binaural hearing in three-dimensional space, especially in the noisy real world.

Audiometric findings revealed, indeed, hearing within normal limits on the left, while results for the right ear demonstrated a substantial hearing loss of rising audiometric configuration (Figure 6–37A). The speech detection threshold in the right ear was quite high (80 dB HL), requiring presentation at 105 dB for optimal speech recognition, about 85%. Results of annual audiological tests since have remained consistent. Immittance testing revealed normal middle ear admittance in both ears, acoustic reflexes present stimulating the left ear, but absent on the right—a red flag for a possible retrocochlear lesion. In contrast, analyses of the DPOAEs (panel B) also demonstrated robust distortion products bilaterally, with the exception of output in the right ear at 3000 Hz. However, DPOAE magnitude at such frequencies is vulnerable to ear-canal resonance effects (for better or worse) and/or effects of inherently sharp ups and downs, again called "ripple." As noted in Episode 5.1, ripple effects are more readily demonstrated in spectral analyses using far narrower intervals along the frequency axis than typical of clinical tests and are normal effects. Therefore, this nuance does not detract from the surprisingly good DPOAE findings on the left, confirmed as well by CEOAEs robustly demonstrated bilaterally (panel B).

ECochG and ABR testing were then pursued. Results of the former (tested at 90 dB nHL, but not shown) demonstrated clearly the presence of both summating and whole-nerve action potentials bilaterally, although slightly reduced SP and AP on the right. SP/AP ratios also were not remarkable. For ABR testing, clicks were presented at 90 and 70 dB nHL (19/s repetition rate; Figure 6–37, panel C). Results for the left ear were clinically unremarkable, with robust and replicable component waves and interpeak latencies within normal limits. Results for the right ear showed a response at 90 dB, although poorer replicability, suggestive of neural dyssynchrony. This effect was clearer at 70 dB in the right ear wherein no earlier components than wave V could be identified reliably. Although not a conventional medical term, in the "back room" of the clinic, the results overall might be called a "mixed bag." In any event and especially in a still young patient, conservative management is warranted.

In conclusion, results were consistent with normal function on the left, but on the right, the results of a comprehensive evaluation of the sensorineural pathology did not permit completely ruling out a lesion of the 8th nerve. The case thus was followed up with MRI.

Before going there, another pause and reflection will be useful. A diagnostic problem may arise given only moderately abnormal ABR findings combined with essentially normal otoacoustic emissions. This effect can occur with ANSD, in principle, although the most pervasive scenario is very limited to no reliable demonstration of an ABR—not the profile here. However, this scenario can be consistent with a diagnosis of cochlear dysplasia—defined by a small, underdeveloped cochlea (namely, with formation of less than two turns). An additional curiosity of this case is the air-bone gap in

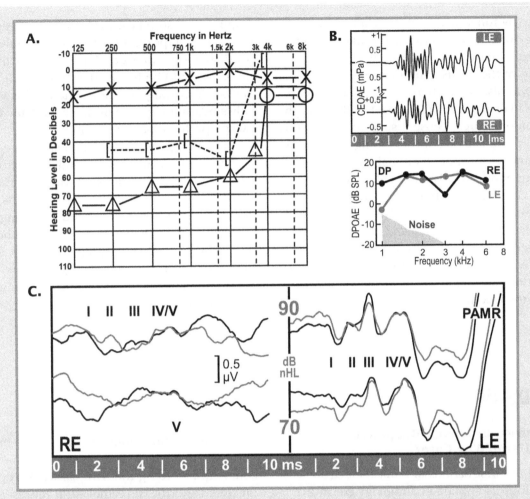

Figure 6–37. Results of workup in Case 3: **A.** Pure-tone audiogram; **B.** Otoacoustic emission analyses—click-OAEs and DP-gram; **C.** ABR test–retest tracings for stimulus levels indicated (alternating click), incidentally providing an example of the presence of a potential featured in the upcoming Heads Up—the beginning of a postauricular muscle response (PAMR). For the analysis intended, it is only a minor interference so not adversely affecting this case's ABRs and their interpretation.

the mid- to lower frequencies. A mixed loss in fact? That could account for the reflex findings, if indeed the case. Yet, that diagnosis was supported by neither the tympanometric findings nor otoscopy. An alternative mechanism is that of a virtual middle-ear defect as in the Heads Up of Episode 5.3—the case of superior semicircular canal dehiscence, thus a normal acoutico-mechanical conductive system being terminated by a hydromechanically abnormal cochlea. Another well-known pathology that had challenged diagnosticians in the past was cochlear otosclerosis, rather than the far more common variety manifested simply as a sclerosis (an abnormal bone growth) on the exterior wall of the cochlea, effectively fixating the stapes footplate in the oval window, yet without internal cochlear damage. Back to the conclusion.

The MRI findings revealed this patient to have a unilateral cochlear dysplasia, rather than pathology of the 8th nerve itself or a neuropathy, as rigorously defined. It is always problematic to define AN or any disorder entirely by functional tests. Critically assessing etiology falls in another domain (like imaging and histopathology). Interestingly, given the red flag of the acoustic reflexometry findings, there was also a "red herring" flagged (at least for the likes of an AN diagnosis) in the speech recognition scores. Those results suggested this patient to be capable of "benefiting" nearly full recruitment, given good enough audibility—not common in AN. The ECochG findings were not as compelling in this regard, but at the same time not "screaming" AN!

Nevertheless, as in Case 1, the course of management certainly was just. The outcomes of the considerable workup begged a definitive resolution, thus still more in-depth follow-up to define the true nature of the patient's disorder, helping to ensure best long-term management. It thus was important to rule out not only ANSD but any other possible etiologies that (in turn) could be health-/life-threatening or perhaps medically treatable, should this young lady's hearing impairment have continued to escape professional attention.

The foregoing cases demonstrate the great advances within and beyond clinical electrophysiology in audiology and teach the importance of thorough workup of all cases. This starts with not jumping to conclusions and not being taken in by preconceptions of "just another one of those," rather keeping an eye out for the exception(s) that might urge the need to learn more about the case before drawing conclusions.

HEADS UP

Postauricular Muscle Response—Friend/Foe/Why Care?

One of the first lessons of clinical electrophysiology as applied in audiology (recall Episode 4.1) was that of a reality check. The patient is not an electronic instrument generating a given AEP so is not capable of generating a perfectly stationary signal without significant background noise. Much attention was given and repeated in subsequent episodes to the need to recognize and minimize interference, including artifacts arising from muscle contractions (like eyeblinks). This feature is dedicated to one such possible signal that is only an "artifact" in the sense of being both myogenic—neither strictly neurogenic (as typically desired of clinical electrophysiology in audiology)—nor the generally targeted AEP—but still is a sound-evoked electrophysiological response.[219,220] This "two-faced" potential is the *postauricular muscle response (PAMR)*. As a myogenic artifact, it certainly can interfere with the most pristine recording of AEPs with which it may overlap in the time domain. This face is the one most familiar to clinicians, such as in the course of recording the ABR, as will be demonstrated shortly. Nevertheless, it represents a phenomenon worthy of purposeful pursuits. The PAMR indeed caught the attention of one of the field's greatest minds and contributors to the research and development of AEP-measurement/applications. This was the late A. Roger D. Thornton who in his youth was one of the earliest investigators of the PAMR as an auditory phenomenon.[221]

As a nuisance (that is, appearing uninvited rather than the focus of a systematic assessment of this potential), the PAMR demonstrates some seemingly erratic behavior. An example of the PAMR is provided in Figure 6–38A from recordings in an adult patient who was seen for differential diagnostic testing, namely in the recording from the right but not the left ear. The PAMR appears around 10 ms or more in latency, depending on stimulus level and/or filtering (as any other AEP). If observed, a part of its capricious

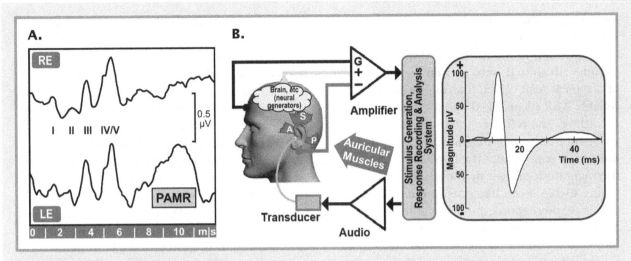

Figure 6–38. A. The first "face" of the postauricular muscle response, lurking in the ABR recording during testing of the patient's right ear (alternating-polarity clicks presented at 75 dB nHL). **B.** Partial reprint of Figure 2–16 to underscore the PAMR as an auditory evoked potential, recordable by the same approach as the ABR and other neurogenic AEPs, yet an evoked motor potential from the posterior auricular muscle (P), not the anterior (A) and/or superior (S) auricle muscles. *Gray-boxed plot*: Optimized recording for the PAMR, seen well within the latency window of the PAMR artifact in the ABR recording (*panel A*). (Based on data courtesy of Dr. K. Agung.)

behavior in the course of a test protocol is that of not being present under all conditions, by level and/or by ear. This may be more a matter of protocol and/or other extenuating circumstances than that of the PAMR simply being "unruly." It naturally is affected by stimulus level which usually is varied and/or manipulated in various sequences, pending the purpose of the examination. Appearing while testing one but not the other ear may be more about the subject becoming more or less relaxed—or conversely less or more tense/uncomfortable, respectively—as the examination progresses. For reliable measurements of the ABR, much encouragement is given to the importance of a relaxed state, wherein the patient need not be attentive during the test (indeed, can be allowed to doze off). In contrast, the PAMR tends to be augmented in the backdrop of increase in myogenic activity.[222] A common experience of examiners is that of observing some overall reduction of background noise during the test and the PAMR subsiding, if it had been present initially. In the example presented in Figure 6–38A, the hearing sensitivity was slightly better on the right and (per protocol) was the first ear tested.

That the PAMR is a ***myogenic response*** is a straightforward call; it arises from one of the three auricular muscles (per its name) that support the auricular system of the human pinna and of other mammals that can orient their ears to incoming sounds.[219,220] The source of this evolutionary holdover response is attributed in humans uniquely to the postauricular muscle (Figure 6–38, panel B). However, it has no functional value in humans, not even to wiggle the ears—a cute trick if mastered, but different muscles are involved. In other words, the PAMR's source is a vestigial muscle, yet the reflex arc has been maintained (see panel B, gray-boxed plot)—go figure. The PAMR thus is an ***acoustic-evoked motor response*** that is variable in both elicitation and manifestation. Hence, this multifactorial phenomenon is vulnerable on both sides of the stimulus-response relationship—the neurophysiological (auditory stimulus encoding) and the neuromuscular (muscle activation)—potentially including all the variables that can affect both sides of reflex arcs, in general.

Returning to the ABR recording, the samples illustrated were chosen for a balance of a typical ABR (given filtering favored for reliable ABR recordings) and a typical PAMR recording. The reflex arc involved may be vestigial, but by AEP magnitude standards, the PAMR is no wimp. It can be several times the magnitude shown by the response in Figure 6–38A, even into tens of microvolts, and is readily recorded in normal-hearing adults when recorded using both a recording montage and filter parameters that are optimal for the PAMR itself (see Figure 6–38B).[223] Fortunately, pickup of the PAMR may only be a problem for properly displaying the ABR, especially when its magnitude becomes substantially larger than the IV/V complex. If the display is set to auto-scale the waveform, a computer algorithm will scale the PAMR according to the peak-to-peak voltage of the overall epoch chosen for display, namely as the reference for full-scale display (whether a part of or full screen). With an "overbearing" PAMR, this will diminish the relative amplitude in the display of the ABR. As an incidental practical note, how the response is displayed is the user's choice and can be set to display tracings for some specific percentage of the full-screen display (N µV of signal). Alternatively, an algorithm can be switched on to check automatically what is the range of plus and minus voltages for a given record to be displayed, such that all responses displayed on the screen will have the same vertical space, regardless of how big or small is the response and/or its residual noise! Not only for the likes of a PAMR but as a general admonition, the examiner needs to stay tuned to the true magnitude of the recorded signals as displayed. Figure 6–37C (left ear) of the previous Heads Up gives another example of interference by a PAMR. Seemingly running off the allotted display area, it clearly is larger than the one in Figure 6–38A (right ear) and more on the order of the PAMR deliberately recorded in Figure 6–38B. Still, the display was manageable in the example of Figure 6–37C in favor of the ABR under examination, by way of an appropriate setting of the display scale in the first place.

Perhaps seeming counterintuitive, the treatment of a PAMR artifact is generally not one of readjusting the limits of artifact rejection, and a rather large PAMR might cause an excessive number of rejected sweeps. Also, fortunately, once the subject is settled in and fully relaxed, the PAMR presents less of a problem, if any, throughout the rest of the examination. It is even less likely to be an issue during ERA because many of the test conditions naturally will be at low sensation levels. As an auditory activated response, it too will tend to diminish with decreasing levels of stimulation (as will be demonstrated shortly).

So is the PAMR good for anything? In fact, yes! Possible practical applications of the PAMR have been explored substantially in the overall research and development of objective tests of auditory sensitivity/function.[224,225] For decades, the PAMR has drawn attention as a potential tool or adjunct to screening auditory function, including in newborns/infants.[223] Robust responses in normal hearing adults, as shown in Figure 6–39, have encouraged this line of work. The PAMR, with posturing of the neck and/or encouraging eye movements in lower mammals, provides the technical basis for obtaining reliable responses for clinical or research purposes.

The overall input-output function for the PAMR is demonstrated in Figure 6–39A; the potential systematically increases in amplitude with SPL. As demonstrated in panel B, as expected of neurogenic AEPs, effects of sensorineural hearing loss are readily evident. The recordings in this example are from an adult subject but are equally demonstrable in children. In the SNHL data set, a recruitment effect also is evident (again, a more rapid growth of amplitude per dB relative to the normal input–output function). The PAMR thus

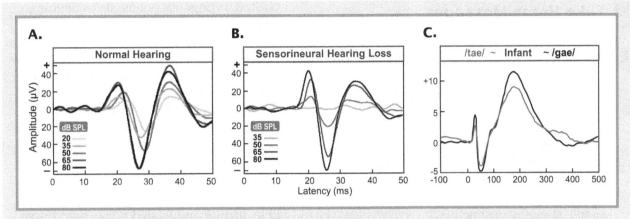

Figure 6–39. Exemplary data (grand averages) demonstrating the PAMR upon purposeful recording, showing robust responses across stimulus level, in (**A**) normal-hearing young adult, (**B**) aging adult with sensory neural loss, and (**C**) infant around 5 months of age. Stimuli: A and B—brief tone bursts; C—speech tokens, as indicated. (Based on data courtesy of Dr. K. Agung.)

appears to have plenty of "the right stuff" to be applicable to ERA. Clicks, chirps, brief tone bursts, and speech tokens[222] can be used as stimuli (panel C). Although with substantially longer latencies, the PAMR can be recorded in infants. The example in panel C is from a 5-month-old infant being stimulated with a couple of speech tokens. This paradigm is motivated by the notion that more environmentally relevant stimuli might be more effective on the assumption of being less "abstract" than sinusoidal pulses.

From the initial remarks (on the side of artifact), the PAMR naturally can be recorded via the C_Z-M or related electrode montages, but its intentional recording is improved as the distance between electrodes is decreased, for instance using C_3-M_1 and C_4-M_2 (left versus right side, respectively). Although there are some stimulus-specific effects, including the I-O function, as well as intensity-dependent latency shifts (Figure 6–39A), no adaptation effects are evident.

In routine assessment of the ABR, the PAMR also should not be discounted as a mere artifact. After all, it is the nervous system that is responding to the stimulus applied, like the acoustic/stapedius muscle reflex (the audiologist's "knee-jerk" reflex). Thus, at times, the PAMR can be a gift, even if it was not the intended metric of the evaluation. The PAMR is seen at times in too-noisy situations or uncooperative, difficult-to-test patients, such that the ABR results are equivocal/impossible to interpret. In such cases, something is much better than nothing. Certainly, it is disheartening for all concerned to have to terminate the test session empty handed.

The PAMR's story bespeaks the old adage to "never look a gift horse in the mouth." Whether the next generation of research and development finally leads to routine use of PAMR-ERA and/or other applications remains to be seen. Regardless, it seems prudent for the clinician to be well informed about the PAMR. Routinely, it is a priority for the examiner to be vigilant in identifying this potential and to endeavor to "control" it as an artifact to minimize the risk of it compromising the intended ABR evaluation. It also is a responsibility of clinicians to be vigilant for the PAMR should circumstances of the case render it informative and to be open-minded should a potentially efficacious audiological application of evoked-PAMR measurement come forth through further research and development.

■ Take Home Messages

Episode 1

1. Paramount to clinical/research applications of AEP tests is full knowledge of their "normal" nuances and nonpathological effects—from the bottom up.
2. Reliable ABR recordings depend upon thoughtful use of test parameters.
3. Few factors are as impactful on the ABR as simple stimulus parameters.
4. Particularly striking are the effects of stimulus intensity, both in magnitude and latency.
5. In practice, the ABR proves to be the AEP most influenced by issues of transducers.
6. As with OAEs, there are time-frequency interactions manifested in added complexities in the behavior of the ABR.
7. Testing via bone conduction is both feasible and a method demanding special considerations to avoid technical problems and misinterpretation.
8. A huge factor is the subject, even when perfectly neurologically normal—starting with natural individual differences and thereafter factors like early maturation.

Heads Up

10. The ABR stimulated bilaterally (same nHL and given ears equally sensitive) appears nearly double in amplitude, especially the IV/V complex, but not exactly.
11. Taking the difference between the sum of the monaural and the binaural amplitudes yields the BIC and thus reflects some aspect(s) of the binaural pathways and their signal processing.

Episode 2

1. Not only on/off, transient stimuli (at least in effect), brainstem potentials can be efficiently elicited as ongoing potentials to ongoing (state-state) stimuli.
2. The brainstem's potentials in response to an amplitude-modulated (steady) carrier follow both the stimulus's envelope and the carrier's frequency and side tones.
3. Such potentials reflect both linear and nonlinear aspects of the transduction of the stimulus, starting with the hair cells, followed by neural excitation, and yielding a form of rectification.
4. Other ongoing stimuli that elicit FFRs and EFRs include modulated noise, brief bursts of stimuli repeated over time, and vowel (speech) tokens.
5. Previous examples were all (except vowels that are not diphthongs, as well as the cat's meow) variants of amplitude modulated signals; however, frequency modulation works as well.
6. Above around nominally 80 Hz, generators of the EFRs to modulated carriers are attributed to brainstem generators, in common with the transient-elicited ABR.

Heads Up

7. Using the appropriate paradigm, the transient-ABR can be evoked readily using brief speech stimuli, providing a sort of neurological record of its brainstem-level encoding.
8. Their spectra reflect underlying components of envelop and frequency following; these speech-elicited brainstem responses have enjoyed extensive research and have promising clinical applications.

Episode 3

1. Various AEPs are potentially applicable to ERA, especially the "classical" ABR—a transient EP, used extensively; yet the ASSR provides another useful approach.
2. With inherent inefficiencies of conventional ABR-based ERA, judgments and/or applicable statistical tests profit little from relation

of response to stimulus, as is strong for 80Hz-ASSR.
3. ASSR takes advantages of spectrally based rather than temporally based analyses, including both magnitude and phase.
4. ASSR substantially addresses several problems enumerated apropos ABR-ERA, including potential efficiency enhancements of simultaneous tests over multiple frequencies and/or ears.

Episode 4

1. The ABR historically is the most broadly adopted for routine objective audiometry and uses frequency-specific stimuli—brief tone bursts and more recently narrowband chirps.
2. The strategy for searching for the VDL is important to economize on time, which also applies to sequencing of levels tested for a given frequency.
3. Effective evoked-response audiometry must be goal-driven, systematic, and involve timely practices that are different from those of behavioral audiometry.
4. Bone conduction testing can be efficacious, if respecting issues raised earlier, clinical research in the area, and a solid background in conventional audiometry with BC.
5. Effective masking levels are equally important between behavioral and objective audiometry and have been investigated, including the important parameter of interaural attenuation.
6. BC sensitivity and EMLs are not the same for adults and infants, although largely comparable been older children and adults.
7. ERA-ASSR is efficacious; a variety of stimuli have been used with roughly comparable frequency specificity, although still not equal to a pure tone.
8. BC testing using ASSR measurement has not been as extensively studied as AC-ERA, but the results are promising.
9. The concern for excessive stimulus artifact is not trivial and potentially more problematic for ASSR-ERA, requiring caution of interpretation in cases requiring high-level stimulation.
10. The M-ASSR offers possibly increased efficiency but has not been found (for instance) to be entirely proportional to the number of carrier frequencies combined.
11. SLR measurement can be applied to estimation of hearing thresholds by a variety of tools, but examiners must be familiar with and respect their limits, and still more research is needed.

Episode 5

1. General bases of interpretation of ABRs for differential diagnostics are considerably a "game" of logic.
2. Some audiometric configurations have systematic effects on ABR, others not, but that's a part of the logic too.
3. Dealing with peripheral hearing losses requires understanding and finesse.
4. Severe peripheral hearing losses, like large conductive losses, are challenging.
5. To some extent, yet not perfectly, the ABR test has keen site-of-lesion diagnostic capability.
6. Few to no AEP tests are a mountain—all powerful and/or standing alone; none are tests of the actual pathology, only functional effects suggestive of site involved.
7. Undoing what the cochlea has done with the click's spectrum may improve detectability of small lesions, at least of the 8th nerve.

Heads Up

8. The three cases featured provide interesting contrasts in similar sites of lesion, demonstrating functional tests like ABR measurement are just that but do not define etiology.
9. The 8th nerve can be "crippled" or worse by there not being enough of a channel to pass a normally functioning nerve to connect the cochlea to the brainstem.

10. The expression "sensorineural" hearing loss hedges the bet on what is not working, but Case 1's OAE versus ABR results provided demonstration of an essentially pure neural lesion.
11. The 8th nerve naturally can have the squeeze put on it by even a very small tumor, as the second case demonstrated.
12. Case 2's results nicely showed how the chirp can effect a "stacked ABR" and revealed a lesion not so readily "picked up" by the conventional-click ABR.
13. Case 3, although suspected of auditory neuropathy (as also had been Case 1), turned out to be one of malformation of the cochlea on the affected side and still hedging on "sensory/neural".
14. The tests of etiology and paths to the final truths were the imaging studies, providing incredible views inside each patient's skull.
15. The functional tests, nevertheless, helped to pave the way to appropriate management.

Heads Up

16. The PAMR is "fickle," precariously adding to the ABR waveform, although not likely directly interfering with the main wave components.
17. It still is a sign that something must be working in a patient's auditory system, hence possibly a "gift" in some cases when nothing else is going well or useful in other applications.

References

1. Jewett, D., & Williston, J. S. (1971). Auditory-evoked far fields averaged from the scalp of humans. *Brain, 94*(4), 681–696.
2. Sohmer, H., & Feinmesser, M. (1967). Cochlear action potentials recorded from the external ear in man. *Annals of Otology Rhinology and Laryngology, 76*(2), 427–435.
3. Hall, J. W. (2007). *New handbook of auditory evoked reponses*. Pearson.
4. Sininger, Y. S., & Don, M. (1989). Effects of click rate and electrode orientation on threshold detectability of the auditory brainstem response. *Journal of Speech and Hearing Research, 32*(4), 880–886.
5. Picton, T. W. (2011). *Human auditory evoked potentials*. Plural Publishing.
6. Hood, L. (1998). The normal auditory brainstem response. In L. Hood (Ed.), *Clinical applications of the auditory brainstem response* (pp. 126–144). Singular Publishing.
7. Stockard, J. J., Stockard, J. E., Westmoreland, B., & Corfits, J. (1979). Brainstem auditory-evoked responses: Normal variation as a function of stimulus and subject characteristics. *Archives of Neurology, 36*(13), 823–831.
8. Burkard, R. E., & Don, M. (2007). The auditory brainstem response. In R. E. Burkard, M. Don, J. J. Eggermont (Eds.), *Auditory evoked potentials: Basic principles and clinical application* (pp. 229–253). Lippincott Williams & Wilkins.
9. Burkard, R. F., & Sims, D. (2001). The human auditory brain-stem response to high click rates: Aging effects. *American Journal of Audiology, 11*(1), 53–61.
10. Brugge, J. F., Anderson, D. J., Hind, J. E., & Rose, J. E. (1969). Time structure of discharges in single auditory nerve fibers of the squirrel monkey in response to complex periodic sounds. *Journal of Neurophysiology, 32*(3), 386–401.
11. Zwislocki, J. J. (1975). Phase opposition between inner and outer hair cells and auditory sound analysis. *Audiology, 14*(6), 443–455.
12. Gorga, M. P., Kaminski, J. R., & Beauchaine, K. L. (1991). Effects of stimulus phase on the latency of the auditory brainstem response. *Journal of American Academy of Audiology, 2*, 1–6.
13. Fowler, C. G. (1992). Effects of signal phase on the auditory brainstem response. *Journal of Speech and Hearing Research, 35*, 167–174.
14. Coats, A. C., & Martin, J. L. (1977). Human auditory nerve action potentials and brain stem evoked responses: Effects of audiogram shape and lesion location. *Archives of Otolaryngology, 103*(10), 605–622.
15. Arnold, S. A. (2007). The auditory brainstem response. In R. J. Roeser, M. Valente, & H. Hosford-Dunn (Eds.), *Audiology. Diagnosis* (pp. 426–442). Thieme.
16. Durrant, J. D. (1986). Combined ECochG-ABR approach versus conventional ABR recordings. *Seminars in Hearing, 7*, 289–305.
17. Picton, T. W. (1990). Auditory evoked potentials. In D. D. Daly & T. A. Pedley (Eds.), *Current practice of clinical electroencelography* (2nd ed., pp. 625–678). Raven Press.

18. Yamada, O., Yagi, T., Yamane, H., & Suzuki, J. (1975). Clinical evaluation of the auditory evoked brain stem response. *Auris Nasus Larynx, 2*(2), 97–105.
19. Van Campen, L. E., Sammeth, C. A., Hall, J. W., & Peek, B. F. (1992). Comparison of Etymotic insert and TDH supra-aural earphones in auditory brainstem response measurement. *Journal of American Academy of Audiology, 3*(5), 315–323.
20. Mueller, G. (2006). Where in the world is KEMAR? *The Hearing Journal, 59*(4), 10–16.
21. Gorga, M. P., & Thornton, A. P. (1989). The choice of stimuli for ABR measurement. *Ear and Hearing, 10*(4), 217–230.
22. Durrant, J. D., & Hyre, R. (1993). Relative effective frequency response of bone versus air conduction stimulation examined via masking. *Audiology, 32*(3), 175–184.
23. Teas, D. C., Eldredge, D. H., & Davis, H. (1962). Cochlear responses to acoustic transients: An interpretation of whole-nerve action potentials. *Journal of the Acoustical Society of America, 34*(8), 1438–1459.
24. Kiang, N-YS., Watanabe, T., Thomas, E. C., & Clark, L. F. (1967). Discharge patterns of single fibers in the cat's auditory nerve. *Journal of Anatomy, 101*(Pt. 1), 176–177.
25. Don, M., & Eggermont, J. J. (1978). Analysis of the click-evoked brainstem potentials in man using high-pass noise masking. *Journal of the Acoustical Society of America, 63*(4), 1084–1092.
26. Philibert, B., Durrant, J. D., Ferber-Viart, C., Duclaux, R., Veuillet, E., & Collet, L. (2003). Stacked tone-burst-evoked auditory brain-stem response (ABR): Preliminary findings. *International Journal of Audiology, 42*(2), 71–81.
27. Gorga, M. P., Kaminski, J. R., Beauchaine, K. L., Jesteadt, W., & Neely, S. T. (1989). Auditory brainstem responses from children three months to three years of age: Normal patterns of response II. *Journal of Speech, Language and Hearing Research, 32*(2), 281–288.
28. Don, M., Kwong, B., Tanaka, C., Brackmann, D., & Nelson R. (2005). The stacked ABR: A sensitive and specific screening tool for detecting small acoustic tumors. *Audiology and Neurotology, 10*(5), 274–290.
29. Don, M., Elberling, C., & Malof, E. (2009). Input and output compensation for the cochlear traveling wave delay in wide-band ABR recordings: Implications for small acoustic tumor detection. *Journal of American Academy of Audiology, 20*(2), 99–108.
30. Cebulla, M., & Elberling, C. (2010). Auditory brain stem responses evoked by different chirps based on different delay models. *Journal of American Academy of Audiology, 21*(7), 452–460.
31. Durrant, J. D., Gerich, J. E., Mitrakou, A., Jensen, T., & Hyre, R. (1991). Changes in BAEP under hypoglycemia: Temperature related? *Electroencephalography and Clinical Neurophysiology/Evoked Potentials Section, 80*(6), 547–550.
32. Marshall, N. K., & Donchin, E. (1981). Circadian variation in the latency of brainstem responses and its relation to body temperature. *Science, 212*(4492), 356–358.
33. Durrant, J. D., Sabo, D. L., & Hyre, R. J. (1990). Gender, head size, and ABRs examined in large clinical sample. *Ear and Hearing, 11*(3), 210–214.
34. Don, M., Ponton, C. W., Eggermont, J. J., & Masuda, A. (1993). Gender differences in cochlear response time: An explanation for gender amplitude differences in the unmasked auditory brain-stem response. *Journal of the Acoustical Society of America, 94*(4), 2135–2148.
35. Don, M., Ponton, C. W., Eggermont, J. J., & Masuda, A. (1994). Auditory brainstem response (ABR) peak amplitude variability reflects individual differences in cochlear response times. *Journal of the Acoustical Society of America, 96*(6), 3476–3491.
36. Salamy, A., McKean, C. M., & Buda, F. B., (1975). Maturational changes in auditory transmission as reflected in human brain stem potentials. *Brain Research, 96,* 361–366.
37. Jacobson, J. T., Morehouse, C. R., & Johnson, J. (1982). Strategies for infant auditory brainstem response assessment. *Ear and Hearing, 3*(5), 263–270.
38. Hecox, K., & Galambos, R. (1974). Brain stem auditory evoked responses in human infants and adults. *Archives of Otorhinolaryngology, 99*(1), 30–33.
39. Kileny, P., & Niparko, J. (1994). Neurophysiologic intraoperative monitoring. In J. Jacobson (Ed.), *Principles and applications in auditory evoked potentials* (pp.447–476). Allyn & Bacon.
40. Riedel, H., & Kollmeier B. (2002). Comparison of binaural auditory brainstem responses and the binaural difference potential evoked by chirps and clicks. *Hearing Research, 169*(1–2), 85–96.
41. Zhou, J., & Durrant, J. D. (2003). Effects of interaural frequency difference on binaural fusion evidenced by electrophysiological versus psychoacoustical measures. *Journal of the Acoustical Society of America, 114*(3), 1508–1515.
42. Moore, J. K. (1987). The human auditory brain stem as a generator of auditory evoked potentials. *Hearing Research, 29*(1), 33–43.
43. Fowler, C. G., & Leonards, J. S. (1985). Frequency dependence of the binaural interaction component

of the auditory brainstem response. *Audiology, 24*(6) 420–429.

44. Fowler, C. G. (1989). The bifrequency binaural interaction component of the auditory brainstem response. *Journal of Speech, Language, and Hearing Research, 32*(4), 767–772.

45. McPherson, D. L., & Starr, A. (1995). Auditory time-intensity cues in the binaural interaction component of the auditory evoked potentials. *Hearing Research, 89*(1–2), 162–171.

46. Cone-Wesson, B., Ma, E., & Fowler, C. G. (1997). Effect of signal level and frequency on ABR and MLR binaural interaction in human neonates. *Hearing Research, 106*(1–2), 163–178.

47. He, S., Brown, C. J., & Abbas, P. J. (2010). Effects of stimulation level and electrode pairing on the binaural interaction component of the electrically evoked auditory brain stem response. *Ear and Hearing, 31*(4), 457–470.

48. Gopal, K. V., & Pierel, K. (1999). Binaural interaction component in children at risk for central auditory processing disorders. *Scandinavian Audiolology, 28*(2), 77–84.

49. Van Yper, L. N., Vermeire, K., De Vel, E. F., Beynon, A. J., & Dhooge, I. J. (2016). Age-related changes in binaural interaction at brainstem level. *Ear and Hearing, 37*(4), 434–442.

50. Gunnarson, A. D., & Finitzo, T. (1991). Conductive hearing loss during infancy: Effects on later auditory brain stem electrophysiology. *Journal of Speech, Language, and Hearing Research, 34*(5), 1207–1215.

51. Pratt, H., Polyakov, A., Aharonson, V., Korczyn, A. D., Tadmor, R., Fullerton, B. C., . . . Furst, M. (1998). Effects of localized pontine lesions on auditory brain-stem evoked potentials and binaural processing in humans. *Electroencephalography and Clinical Neurophysiology/Evoked Potentials Section, 108*(5), 511–520.

52. Levine, R. A., Gardner, J. C., Fullerton, B. C., Stufflebeam, S. M., Carlisle, E. W., Furst, M., . . . Kiang, N. Y. S. (1993). Effects of multiple sclerosis brainstem lesions on sound lateralization and brainstem auditory evoked potentials. *Hearing Research, 68*(1), 73–88.

53. Picton, T. W., John, S. M., Dimitrijevic, A., & Purcell, D. W. (2003). Human auditory steady-state responses. *International Journal of Audiology, 42*(4), 177–219.

54. Plack, C. J. (2018). *The sense of hearing* (3rd ed.). Routledge.

55. Lins, O. G., Picton, P. E., Picton, T. W., Champagne, S. C., & Durieux-Smith, A. (1995). Auditory steady-state responses to tones amplitude-modulated at 80–110 Hz. *Journal of the Acoustical Society of America, 97*(5), 3051–3063.

56. Nuttall, A. L., Ricci, A. J., Burwood, G., Harte, J. M., Stenfelt, S., Cayé-Thomasen, P., . . . Lunner, T. (2018). A mechanoelectrical mechanism for detection of sound envelopes in the hearing organ. *Nature Communications, 9*(1), 1–11.

57. Moore, B. C., & Glasberg, B. R. (1983). Suggested formulae for calculating auditory-filter bandwidths and excitation patterns. *Journal of the Acoustical Society of America, 74*(3), 750–753.

58. John, S. M., Purcell, D. W., Dimitrijevic, A., & Picton, T. W. (2002). Advantages and caveats when recording steady-state responses to multiple simultaneous stimuli. *Journal of the American Academy of Audiology, 13*(5), 246–259.

59. Purcell, D. W., John, S. M., Schneider, B. A., & Picton, T. W. (2004). Human temporal auditory acuity as assessed by envelope following responses. *Journal of the Acoustical Society of America, 116*(6), 3581–3593.

60. Tichko, P., & Skoe, E. (2017). Frequency-dependent fine structure in the frequency-following response: The byproduct of multiple generators. *Hearing Research, 348*, 1–15.

61. Kuwada, S., Anderson, J. S., Batra, R., Fitzpatrick, D. C., Teissier, N., & D'Angelo, W. R. (2002). Sources of the scalp-recorded amplitude-modulation following response. *Journal of the American Academy of Audiology, 13*(4), 188–204.

62. Coffey, E. B., Herholz, S. C., Chepesiuk, A. M., Baillet, S., & Zatorre, R. J. (2016). Cortical contributions to the auditory frequency-following response revealed by MEG. *Nature Communications, 7*(1), 1–11.

63. Joris, P., Schreiner, C. E., & Rees, A. (2004). Neural processing of amplitude-modulated sounds. *Physiological Reviews, 84*(2), 541–577.

64. Bidelman, G. M. (2018). Subcortical sources dominate the neuroelectric auditory frequency-following response to speech. *Neuroimage, 175*, 56–69.

65. Bidelman, G. M. (2015). Multichannel recordings of the human brainstem frequency-following response: Scalp topography, source generators, and distinctions from the transient ABR. *Hearing Research, 323*, 68–80.

66. Herdman, A. T., Lins, O., Van Roon, P., Stapells, D. R., Scherg, M., & Picton, T. W. (2002). Intracerebral sources of human auditory steady-state responses. *Brain Topography, 15*(2), 69–86.

67. Cohen, L. T., Rickards, F. W. & Clark, G. M. (1991). A comparison of steady-state evoked potentials to modulated tones in awake and sleeping humans.

Journal of the Acoustical Society of America, 90(5), 2467–2479.

68. White-Schwoch, T., Anderson, S., Krizman, J., Nicol, T. G., & Kraus, N. (2019). Case studies in neuroscience: Subcortical origins of the frequency-following response. *Journal of Neurophysiology, 122*(2), 844–848.

69. John, S. M., Dimitrijevic, A., & Picton, T. W. (2003). Efficient stimuli for evoking auditory steady-state responses. *Ear and Hearing, 24*(5), 406–423.

70. Herdman, A. T., Picton, T. W., & Stapells, D. R. (2002). Place specificity of multiple auditory steady-state responses. *Journal of the Acoustical Society of America, 112*(4), 1569–1582.

71. Dimitrijevic, A., Alsamri, J., John, M. S., Purcell, D., George, S., & Zeng, F. G. (2016). Human envelope following responses to amplitude modulation: Effects of aging and modulation depth. *Ear and Hearing, 37*(5), e322–35.

72. Bharadwaj, H. M., Masud, S., Mehraei, G., Verhulst, S., & Shinn-Cunningham, B. G. (2015). Individual differences reveal correlates of hidden hearing deficits. *Journal of Neuroscience, 35*(5), 2161–2172.

73. Picton, T. W., Skinner, C. R., Champagne, S. C., Kellett, A. J., & Maiste, A. C., (1987). Potentials evoked by the sinusoidal modulation of the amplitude or frequency of a tone. *Journal of the Acoustical Society of America, 82*(1), 165–178.

74. John, S. M., Dimitrijevic, A., Van Roon, P., & Picton, T. W. (2001). Multiple auditory steady-state responses to AM and FM stimuli. *Audiology and Neurotology, 6*(1), 12–27.

75. Dimitrijevic, A., John, S. M., Van Roon, P., & Picton, T. W. (2001). Human auditory steady-state responses to tones independently modulated in both frequency and amplitude. *Ear and Hearing, 22*(2), 100–111.

76. Burkard, R. F., & Shi, Y. A. (1990). A comparison of maximum length and Legendre sequences for the derivation of brainstem auditory-evoked responses at rapid rates of stimulation. *Journal of the Acoustical Society of America, 87*(4), 1656–1664.

77. Herdman, A., & Stapells, D. R. (2003). Auditory steady-state response thresholds of adults with sensorineural hearing impairments. *International Journal of Audiology, 42*(5), 237–248.

78. Stapells, D. R. (2000). Threshold estimation by the tone-evoked auditory brainstem response: A literature meta-analysis. *Journal of Speech-Language Pathology and Audiology, 24*(2), 74–83.

79. Aiken, S. J., & Picton, T. W. (2006). Envelope following responses to natural vowels. *Audiology and Neurotology, 11*(4), 213–232.

80. Skoe, E., & Kraus, N. (2010). Auditory brain stem response to complex sounds: A tutorial. *Ear and Hearing, 31*(3), 302–324.

81. Easwar, V., Banyard, A., Aiken, S. J., & Purcell, D. W. (2018). Phase-locked responses to the vowel envelope vary in scalp-recorded amplitude due to across-frequency response interactions. *European Journal of Neuroscience, 48*(10), 3126–3145.

82. Choi, J. M., Purcell, D. W., Coyne, J. A. M., & Aiken, S. J. (2013). Envelope following responses elicited by English sentences. *Ear and Hearing, 34*(5), 637–650.

83. Easwar, V., Purcell, D. W., Aiken, S. J., Parsa, V., & Scollie, S. D. (2015). Effect of stimulus level and bandwidth on speech-evoked envelope following responses in adults with normal hearing. *Ear and Hearing, 36*(6), 619–634.

84. Vanheusden, F. J., Chesnaye, M. A., Simpson, D. M., & Bell, S. L. (2019). Envelope frequency following responses are stronger for high-pass than low-pass filtered vowels. *International Journal of Audiology, 58*(6), 355–362.

85. Easwar, V., Banyard, A., Aiken, S. J., & Purcell, D. W. (2018). Phase delays between tone pairs reveal interactions in scalp-recorded envelope following responses. *Neuroscience Letters, 665*, 257–262.

86. Easwar, V., Purcell, D. W., Aiken, S. J., Parsa, V., & Scollie, S. D. (2015). Evaluation of speech-evoked envelope following responses as an objective aided outcome measure: Effect of stimulus level, bandwidth, and amplification in adults with hearing loss. *Ear and Hearing, 36*(6), 635–652.

87. Easwar, V., Scollie, S. D., & Purcell, D. W. (2019). Investigating potential interactions between envelope following responses elicited simultaneously by different vowel formants. *Hearing Research, 380*, 35–45.

88. Aiken, S. J., & Picton, T. W. (2008). Envelope and spectral frequency-following responses to vowel sounds. *Hearing Research, 245*(1–2), 35–47.

89. Easwar, V., Beamish, L., Aiken, S., Choi, J. M., Scollie, S., & Purcell, D. (2015). Sensitivity of envelope following responses to vowel polarity. *Hearing Research, 320*, 38–50.

90. Krishnan, A., Gandour, J. T., Bidelman, G. M., & Swaminathan, J. (2009). Experience dependent neural representation of dynamic pitch in the brainstem. *Neuroreport, 20*(4), 408–413.

91. Ananthakrishnan, S., Krishnan, A., & Bartlett, E. (2016). Human frequency following response: Neural representation of envelope and temporal fine structure in listeners with normal hearing and sensorineural hearing loss. *Ear and Hearing, 37*(2), e91–e103.

92. Ananthakrishnan, S., & Krishnan, A. (2018). Human frequency following responses to iterated rippled noise with positive and negative gain: Differential sensitivity to waveform envelope and temporal fine structure. *Hearing Research, 367*, 113–123.
93. Krishnan, A. (1999). Human frequency-following responses to two tone approximations of steady-state vowels. *Audiology and Neurotology, 4*(2), 95–103.
94. Krishnan, A. (2002). Human frequency-following responses: Representation of steady-state synthetic vowels. *Hearing Research, 166*(1–2), 192–201.
95. Krishnan, A., Xu, Y., Gandour, J. T., & Cariani, P. A. (2004). Human frequency-following response: Representation of pitch contours in Chinese tones. *Hearing Research, 189*(1–2), 1–12.
96. Plyler, P. N., & Ananthanarayan, A. K. (2001). Human frequency-following responses: Representation of second formant transitions in normal-hearing and hearing-impaired listeners. *Journal of the American Academy of Audiology, 12*(10), 523–533.
97. Ananthakrishnan, S., Luo, X., & Krishnan, A. (2017). Human Frequency following responses to vocoded speech. *Ear and Hearing, 38*(5), e256–e267.
98. Ananthakrishnan, S., Luo, X., & Krishnan, A. (2017). Human frequency following responses to vocoded speech. *Ear and Hearing, 38*(5), e256.
99. Galambos, R., Makeig, S., & Talmachoff, P. A. (1981). A 40-Hz auditory potential recorded from the human scalp. *Proceedings of the National Academy of Sciences, 78*(4), 2643–2647.
100. Linden, R. D., Campbell, K. B., Hamel, G. & Picton, T. W. (1985). Human auditory steady state evoked potentials during sleep. *Ear and Hearing, 6*(3), 167–174.
101. Stapells, D. R., Galambos, R., Costello, J. A., & Makeig, S. (1988). Inconsistency of auditory middle latency and steady state response in infants. *Electroencephalography and Clinical Neurophysiology/Evoked Potentials Section, 71*(4), 289–295.
102. Kuwada, S., Batra, R., & Maher, V. L. (1986). Scalp potentials in normal hearing and hearing impaired subjects in response to sinusoidally amplitude-modulated tones. *Hearing Research, 21*(2), 179–192.
103. Rickards, F. W., & Clark, G. M. (1984). Steady state evoked potentials to amplitude modulated tones. In R. H. Noda & C. Barber (Eds.), *Evoked potentials II* (pp. 163–168). Butterworth.
104. Lins, O. G., Picton, P. E., Picton, T. W., Champagne, S. C., & Durieux-Smith, A. (1995). Auditory steady-state responses to tones amplitude-modulated at 80–110 Hz. *Journal of the Acoustical Society of America, 97*(5), 3051–3063.
105. Rance, G., Rickards, F. W., Cohen, L. T., Di Vidi, S., & Clark, G. M. (1995). The automated prediction of hearing thresholds in sleeping subjects using auditory steady state potentials. *Ear and Hearing, 16*(5), 499–507.
106. Lins, O. G., & Picton, T. W. (1995). Auditory steady-state responses to multiple simultaneous stimuli. *Electroencephalography and Clinical Neurophysiology/Evoked Potentials Section, 96*(5), 420–432.
107. Lins, O. G., Picton, T. W., Boucher, B. L., Durieux-Smith, A., Champagne, S. C., Moran, L. M., . . . Savio, G. (1996). Frequency-specific audiometry using steady-state responses. *Ear and Hearing, 17*(2), 81–96.
108. Dimitrijevic, A., & Ross, B. (2008). *The auditory steady-state response: Generation, recording and clinical applications* (pp. 83–108), Plural Publishing.
109. Perez-Abalo, M. C., Savio, G., Torres, A., Martín, V., Rodríguez, E., & Galán, L. (2001). Steady state responses to multiple amplitude-modulated tones: An optimized method to test frequency-specific thresholds in hearing-impaired children and normal-hearing subjects. *Ear and Hearing, 22*(3), 200–211.
110. Dimitrijevic, A., & Cone, B. (2015). Auditory steady-state response. In J. Katz (Ed.), *Handbook of clinical audiology* (7th ed., pp. 267–291). Wolters Kluwer.
111. Tlumak, A., Durrant, J. D., & Collet, L. (2007a). 80-Hz auditory steady-state responses (ASSR) at low-conventional and high audiometric frequencies. *International Journal of Audiology, 46*, 26–30.
112. Hood, L. (2015). Auditory brainstem response: Estimation of hearing sensitivity. In J. Katz (Ed.), *Handbook of clinical audiology* (7th ed., pp. 249–266). Wolters Kluwer.
113. Kaf, W. A., Durrant, J. D., Sabo, D. L., Robert Boston, J., Taubman, L. B., & Kovacyk, K. (2006). Validity and accuracy of electric response audiometry using the auditory steady-state response: Evaluation in an empirical design. *International Journal of Audiology, 45*(4), 211–223.
114. Valdes, J. L., Perez-Abalo, M. C., Martin, V., Savio, G., Sierra, C., Rodriguez, E., & Lins, O. (1997). Comparison of statistical indicators for the automatic detection of 80 Hz auditory steady state responses. *Ear and Hearing, 18*(5), 420–429.
115. Dobie, R. A., & Wilson, M. J. (1993). Objective response detection in the frequency domain. *Electroencephalography and Clinical Neurophysiology/Evoked Potentials Section, 88*(6), 516–524.

116. Gescheider, G. A. (1997). Psychophysics: The fundamentals (3rd ed.). Psychology Press.
117. Valdes-Sosa, M. J., Bobes, M. A., Perez-Abalo, M. C., Perera, M., Carballo, J. A., & Valdes-Sosa, P. (1987). Comparison of auditory-evoked potential detection methods using signal detection theory. *Audiology, 26*(3), 166–178.
118. Elberling, C., & Don, M. (1984). Quality estimation of averaged auditory brainstem responses. *Scandinavian Audiology, 13*(3), 187–197.
119. John, M. S., & Picton, T. W. (1998). MASTER: A windows program for recording multiple auditory steady-state responses. *Computer Methods and Programs in Biomedicine, 61*(2), 125–150.
120. Pérez-Abalo, M. C., Rodríguez, E., Sánchez, M., Santos, E., & Torres-Fortuny, A. (2013). New system for neonatal hearing screening based on auditory steady state responses. *Journal of Medical Engineering & Technology, 37*(6), 368–374.
121. Picton, T. W., Dimitrijevic, A., Perez Abalo, M., & Van Roon, P. (2005). Estimating audiometric thresholds using auditory steady-state responses. *Journal of the American Academy of Audiology, 16*(3), 140–146.
122. Picton, T. W. (2011). Auditory steady state and following responses: Dancing to the rhythms. In T. W. Picton (Ed.), *Human auditory evoked potentials* (pp. 285–334). Plural Publishing.
123. Savio, G., & Perez Abalo, M. C. (2008). Auditory steady state responses and hearing screening. In G. Rance (Ed.), *The auditory steady-state response: Generation, recording and clinical applications* (pp.185–199). Plural Publishing.
124. Luts, H., Desloovere, C., Kumar, A., Vandermeersch, E., & Wouters, J. (2004). Objective assessment of frequency-specific hearing thresholds in babies. *International Journal of Pediatric Otorhinolaryngology, 68*(7), 915–926.
125. Savio, G., Cardenas, J., Perez Abalo, M., Gonzalez, A., & Valdes, J. (2001). The low and high frequency auditory steady state responses mature at different rates. *Audiology & Neurotology, 6*(5), 279–287.
126. Savio, G., Perez Abalo, M., Gaya, J., Hernandez, O., & Mijares, E. (2006). Test accuracy and prognostic validity of multiple auditory steady state responses for targeted hearing screening. *International Journal of Audiology, 45*(2), 109–120.
127. Joint Committee on Infant Hearing. (2007). Year 2007 position statement: Principles and guidelines for early hearing detection and intervention programs. *Pediatrics, 120*(4), 898–921.
128. Stapells, D. R. (2000). Frequency-specific evoked potential audiometry in infants. In R. C. Seewald (Ed.), *A sound foundation through early amplification: Proceedings of an international conference* (pp. 13–31). Phonak AG.
129. Small, S. A., & Stapells, D. R. (2003). Normal brief-tone bone-conduction behavioral thresholds using the B-71 transducer: Three occlusion conditions. *Journal of the American Academy of Audiology, 14*(10), 556–562.
130. Oates, P., & Stapells, D. R. (1997a). Frequency specificity of the human auditory brainstem and middle latency responses to brief tones. I. High pass noise masking. *Journal of the Acoustical Society of America, 102*(6), 3597–3608.
131. Oates, P., & Stapells, D. R. (1997b). Frequency specificity of the human auditory brainstem and middle latency responses to brief tones. II. Derived response analyses. *Journal of the Acoustical Society of America, 102*(6), 3609–3619.
132. Shore, S. E., & Nuttall, A. L. (1985). High-synchrony cochlear compound action potentials evoked by rising frequency-swept tone burst. *Journal of Acoustical Society of America, 78*(4), 1283–1295.
133. Elberling, C., & Don, M. (2008). Auditory brainstem responses to a chirp stimulus designed from derived-band latencies in normal-hearing subjects. *Journal of the Acoustical Society of America, 124*(5), 3022–3037.
134. Dau, T., Wegner, O., Mellert, V., & Kollmeier, B. (2000). Auditory brainstem responses with optimized chirp signals compensating basilar membrane dispersion. *Journal of the Acoustical Society of America, 107*(3), 1530–1540.
135. Cebulla, M., Lurz, H., & Shehata-Dieler, W. (2014). Evaluation of waveform, latency and amplitude values of chirp ABR in newborns. *International Journal of Pediatric Otorhinolaryngology, 78*(4), 631–636.
136. Kristensen, S. G., & Elberling, C. (2012). Auditory brainstem responses to level-specific chirps in normal-hearing adults. *Journal of the American Academy of Audiology, 23*(9), 712–721.
137. Cargnelutti, M., Cóser, P. L., & Biaggio, E. P. V. (2017). LS CE-Chirp® vs. click in the neuroaudiological diagnosis by ABR. *Brazilian Journal of Otorhinolaryngology, 83*(3), 313–317.
138. Bell, S. L., Allen, R., & Lutman, M. E. (2002). An investigation of the use of band-limited chirp to obtain the auditory brainstem response. *International Journal of Audiology, 41*(5), 271–278.
139. Wegner, O., & Dau, T. (2002). Frequency specificity of chirp-evoked auditory brainstem responses. *Journal of the Acoustical Society of America, 111*(3), 1318–1329.

140. Chaiklin, J. B. (1967). Interaural attenuation and cross-hearing in air conduction audiometry. *Journal of Auditory Research, 7*, 413–424.
141. Killion, M. C., Wilber, L. A., & Gundmundson G. I. (1985). Insert earphones for more interaural attenuation. *Hearing Instruments, 36*(2), 34–35.
142. British Columbia Early Hearing Program. (2012). Diagnostic audiology protocol [PDF document]. *Provincial Health Services Authority*. http://www.phsa.ca/Documents/bcehpaudiologyassessmentprotocol.pdf
143. Stapells, D. R., Gravel, J. A., & Martin, B. A. (1995). Thresholds for auditory brain stem responses to tones in notched noise from infants and young children with normal hearing or sensorineural hearing loss. *Ear and Hearing, 16*(4), 361–371.
144. Gorga, M. P., Neely, S. T., Hoover, B. M., Dierking, D. M., Beauchaine, K. L., & Manning, C. (2004). Determining the upper limits of stimulation for auditory steady-state response measurements. *Ear and Hearing, 25*(3), 302–307.
145. Foxe, J. J., & Stapells, D. R. (1993). Normal infant and adult auditory brainstem responses to bone conducted tones. *Audiology, 32*(2), 95–109.
146. Small, S. A., & Stapells, D. R. (2017). Threshold assessment in infants using the frequency-specific auditory brainstem response and auditory steady-state response. In A. M. Tharpe & R. Seewald (Eds.), *Comprehensive handbook of pediatric audiology* (2nd ed., pp. 505–549). Plural Publishing.
147. Clemis, J. D., Ballad, J. J., & Killion, M. C. (1986). Clinical use of an insert earphone. *Annals of Otology, Rhinology, & Laryngology, 95*(5), 520–524.
148. Wong, W., & Stapells, D. R. (2004). Brainstem and cortical mechanisms underlying the binaural masking level difference in humans: An auditory steady-state response study. *Ear and Hearing, 25*(1), 57–67.
149. Small, S. A., & Hansen, E. E. (2012). Effective masking levels for bone-conducted amplitude- and frequency-modulated tones in adults with normal hearing: A behavioural study. *International Journal of Audiology, 51*(3), 216–219.
150. Lau, R., & Small, S. A. (2020). Effective masking levels for bone-conduction auditory brainstem response stimuli in infants and adults with normal hearing. *Ear and Hearing* [ePub ahead of print].
151. Small, S. A., Hatton, J. L., & Stapells, D. R. (2007). Effects of bone oscillator coupling method, placement location, and occlusion on bone-conduction auditory steady-state responses in infants. *Ear and Hearing, 28*(1), 83–98.
152. Small, S. A., & Stapells, D. R. (2005). Multiple auditory steady-state response thresholds to bone-conduction stimuli in adults with normal hearing. *Journal of the American Academy of Audiology, 16*(3), 172–183.
153. Tlumak, A. I., Rubinstein, E., & Durrant, J. D. (2007). Meta-analysis of variables that affect accuracy of threshold estimation via measurement of the auditory steady-state response (ASSR). *International Journal of Audiology, 46*(11), 692–710.
154. van Maanen, A., & Stapells, D. R. (2005). Comparison of multiple auditory steady-state responses (80 versus 40 Hz) and slow cortical potentials for threshold estimation in hearing-impaired adults. *International Journal of Audiology, 44*(11), 613–624.
155. Attias, J., Karawani, H., Shemesh, R., & Nageris, B. (2014). Predicting hearing thresholds in occupational noise-induced hearing loss by auditory steady-state responses. *Ear and Hearing, 35*(3), 330–338.
156. Herdman, A. T., & Stapells, D. R. (2001). Thresholds determined using the monotic and dichotic multiple auditory steady-state response technique in normal-hearing subjects. *Scandinavian Audiology, 30*(1), 41–49.
157. Ishida, I. M., & Stapells, D. R. (2012). Multiple-ASSR interactions in adults with sensorineural hearing loss. *International Journal of Otolaryngology, 2012*, doi.org/10.1155/2012/802715.
158. Hatton, J. L., & Stapells, D. R. (2011). Efficiency of single- vs. multiple-stimulus auditory steady-state responses in infants. *Ear and Hearing, 32*(3), 349–357.
159. Hatton, J. L., & Stapells, D. R. (2013). Monotic versus dichotic multiple-stimulus auditory steady state responses in young children. *Ear and Hearing, 34*(5), 680–682.
160. Ishida, I. M., Cuthbert, B. P., & Stapells, D. R. (2011). Multiple-ASSR thresholds to bone conduction stimuli in adults with elevated thresholds. *Ear and Hearing, 32*(3), 373–381.
161. Small, S. A., & Stapells, D. R. (2004). Artifactual responses when recording auditory steady-state responses. *Ear and Hearing, 25*(6), 611–623.
162. Gorga, M. P., Johnson, T. A., Kaminski, J. R., Beauchaine, K. L., Garner, C. A., & Neely, S. T. (2006). Using a combination of click- and tone burst-evoked auditory brain stem response measurements to estimate pure-tone thresholds. *Ear and Hearing, 27*(1), 60–74.
163. Hatton, J. L., Rowlandson, J., Beeres, A., & Small, S.A. (2019) Telehealth-enabled auditory brainstem

response testing for infants living in rural communities: The British Columbia Early Hearing Program experience. *International Journal of Audiology, 58*(7), 381–392.

164. Kaf, W. A., Sabo, D. L., Durrant, J. D., & Rubinstein, E. (2006). Reliability of electric response audiometry using the 80-Hz auditory steady-state response: Evaluation in an empirical design. *International Journal of Audiology, 45*(8), 477–486.

165. Durrant, J. D. (1986) Combined ECochG ABR versus conventional ABR recordings. *Seminars in Hearing, 7,* 289–305.

166. Burkard, R. F., Eggermont, J. J., & Don, M. (2007). *Auditory evoked potentials: Basic principles and clinical application.* Lippincott Williams & Wilkins.

167. Oliveira, C. A., & Schuknecht, H. F. (1990). Pathology of profound sensorineural hearing loss in infancy and early childhood. *Laryngoscope, 100*(8), 902–909.

168. Suzuka, Y., & Schuknecht, H. F. (1988). Retrograde cochlear neuronal degeneration in human subjects. *Acta Oto-laryngologica, 105*(Suppl. 450), 1–20.

169. Ng, M., Srireddy, S., Horlbeck, D. M., & Niparko, J. K. (2001). Safety and patient experience with transtympanic electrocochleography. *Laryngoscope, 111*(5), 792–795.

170. Seo, Y. J., Kwak, C., Kim, S., Park, Y. A., Park, K. H., & Han, W. (2018). Update on bone-conduction auditory brainstem responses: A review. *Journal of Audiology and Otology, 22*(2), 53.

171. Hatton, J. L., Janssen, R. M., & Stapells, D. R. (2012). Auditory brainstem responses to bone-conducted brief tones in young children with conductive or sensorineural hearing loss. *International Journal of Otolaryngology, 2012,* doi.org/10.1155/2012/284864.

172. McGee, T. J., & Clemis, J. D. (1982). Effects of conductive hearing loss on auditory brainstem response. *Annals of Otology, Rhinology & Laryngology, 91*(3), 304–309.

173. Clemis, J. D. (1973). The co-existence of acoustic neuroma and otosclerosis. *Laryngoscope, 83*(12), 1959–1985.

174. Clemis, J. D., Toriumi, D. M., & Gavron, J. P. (1988). Otosclerosis masking coexistent acoustic neuroma. *American Journal of Otology, 9*(2), 117–121.

175. Fowler, C. F., & Durrant, J. D. (1994). The effects of peripheral hearing loss on the auditory brainstem response. In J. T. Jacobsen (Ed.), *Principles & applications in auditory evoked potentials* (pp. 237–250). Allyn & Bacon.

176. Gorga, M. P., Worthington, D. W., Reiland, J. K., Beauchaine, K. A., & Goldgar, D. E. (1985). Some comparisons between auditory brain stem response thresholds, latencies, and the pure-tone audiogram. *Ear and Hearing, 6*(2), 105–112.

177. Keith, W. J., & Greville, K. A. (1987). Effects of audiometric configuration on the auditory brain stem response. *Ear and Hearing, 8*(1), 49–55.

178. LePage, E. L. (1987). Frequency-dependent self-induced bias of the basilar membrane and its potential for controlling sensitivity and tuning in the mammalian cochlea. *The Journal of the Acoustical Society of America, 82*(1), 139–154.

179. Stapells, D. R., Picton, T. W., & Smith, A. D. (1982). Normal hearing thresholds for clicks. *The Journal of the Acoustical Society of America, 72*(1), 74–79.

180. Stapells, D. R., Gravel, J. S., & Martin, B. A. (2006). Thresholds for auditory brain stem responses to tones in notched noise from infants and young children with normal hearing or sensorineural hearing loss. *Foundations of Pediatric Audiology: Identification and Assessment, 16*(4), 261.

181. Fowler, C. G., & Noffsinger, D. (1983). Effects of stimulus frequency and repetition rate on the auditory brain stem responses of normal, cochlear-impaired, and retrocochlear-impaired subjects. *Journal of Speech and Hearing Research, 26*(4), 560–567.

182. Orlando, M. S., & Folsom, R. C. (1995). The effects of reversing the polarity of frequency-limited single-cycle stimuli on the human auditory brain stem response. *Ear and Hearing, 16*(3), 311–320.

183. Fowler, C. G., Bauch, C. D., & Olsen, W. O. (2002). Diagnostic implications of stimulus polarity effects on the auditory brainstem response. *Journal of the American Academy of Audiology, 13*(2), 72–82.

184. Wang, C. Y., & Dallos, P. (1972). Latency of whole-nerve action potentials: Influence of hair-cell normalcy. *The Journal of the Acoustical Society of America, 52*(6B), 1678–1686.

185. Durrant, J. D., & Fowler, C. G. (1996). ABR protocols for dealing with asymmetric hearing loss. *American Journal of Audiology, 5*(3), 5–6.

186. Fowler, C. G. & Mikami, C. M. (1992). Effects of clicks and 1000 Hz tone pips on the ABR of subjects with high frequency cochlear hearing losses. *Journal of the American Academy of Audiology, 3*(5), 324–330.

187. Telian, S. A., & Kileny, P. R. (1989). Usefulness of 1000 Hz tone-burst-evoked responses in the diagnosis of acoustic neuroma. *Otolaryngology-Head and Neck Surgery, 101*(4), 466–471.

188. Selters, W. A., & Brackmann, D. E. (1977). Acoustic tumor detection with brain stem electric response audiometry. *Archives of Otolaryngology, 103*(4), 181–187.
189. Starr, A., Sininger, Y., Nguyen, T., Michalewski, H. J., Oba, S., & Abdala, C. (2001). Cochlear receptor (microphonic and summating potentials, otoacoustic emissions) and auditory pathway (auditory brain stem potentials) activity in auditory neuropathy. *Ear and Hearing, 22*(2), 91–99.
190. Koors, P. D., Thacker, L. R., & Coelho, D. H. (2013). ABR in the diagnosis of vestibular schwannomas: A meta-analysis. *American Journal of Otolaryngology, 34*(3), 195–204.
191. Thomason, J. E. M., Smyth, V., & Murdoch, B. E. (1993). Acoustic neuroma and non-tumour retrocochlear patients: Audiological features. *Scandinavian Audiology, 22*(1), 19–23.
192. Musiek, F. E., McCormick, C. A., & Hurley, R. M. (1996). Hit and false-alarm rates of selected ABR indices in differentiating cochlear disorders from acoustic tumors. *American Journal of Audiology, 5*(1), 90–96.
193. Halliday, J., Rutherford, S. A., McCabe, M. G., & Evans, D. G. (2018). An update on the diagnosis and treatment of vestibular schwannoma. *Expert Review of Neurotherapeutics, 18*(1), 29–39.
194. Harun, A., Agrawal, Y., Tan, M., Niparko, J. K., & Francis, H. W. (2012). Sex and age associations with vestibular schwannoma size and presenting symptoms. *Otology & Neurotology, 33*(9), 1604–1610.
195. Schmidt, R. F., Boghani, Z., Choudhry, O. J., Eloy, J. A., Jyung, R. W., & Liu, J. K. (2012). Incidental vestibular schwannomas: A review of prevalence, growth rate, and management challenges. *Neurosurgical Focus, 33*(3), E4.
196. Sunami, E., Nagayama, H., Yamazaki, M., Katsumata, T., & Katayama, Y. (2006). A case of infarction in brainstem and cerebellum as a initial symptom with bilateral hearing loss. *Brain and Nerve, 58*(9), 791–795.
197. Elwany, S., & Kamel, T. (1988). Sensorineural hearing loss in sickle cell crisis. *Laryngoscope, 98*(4), 386–389.
198. Cohen, B. E., Durstenfeld, A., & Roehm, P. C. (2014). Viral causes of hearing loss: A review for hearing health professionals. *Trends in Hearing, 18*, doi.org/10.1177/2331216514541361.
199. Santarelli, R., & Arslan, E. (2002). Electrocochleography in auditory neuropathy. *Hearing Research, 170*(1–2), 32–47.
200. Furman, J. M., Durrant, J. D., & Hirsch, W. L. (1989). Eighth nerve signs in a case of multiple sclerosis. *American Journal of Otolaryngology, 10*(6), 376–381.
201. Ananthanarayan, A. K., & Durrant, J. D. (1991). On the origin of wave II of the auditory brain stem evoked response. *Ear and Hearing, 12*(3), 174–179.
202. Robinette, M. S., Cevette, M. J., & Probst, R. (2007). Otoacoustic emissions and audiometric outcomes across cochlear and retrocochlear pathology. In M. S. Robinette & T. J. Glattke (Eds.), *Otoacoustic emissions clinical applications* (3rd ed., pp. 227–272). Thieme.
203. Durrant, J. D., Martin, W. H., Hirsch, B., & Schwegler, J. (1994). 3CLT ABR analyses in a human subject with unilateral extirpation of the inferior colliculus. *Hearing Research, 72*(1–2), 99–107.
204. Bauch, C. D., Olsen, W. O., & Pool, A. F. (1996). ABR indices: Sensitivity, specificity, and tumor size. *American Journal of Audiology, 5*(1), 97–104.
205. Stangerup, S. E., & Caye-Thomasen, P. (2012). Epidemiology and natural history of vestibular schwannomas. *Journal of Neurological Surgery Part B: Skull Base, 73*(S 02), A227.
206. Don, M., Masuda, A., Nelson, R., & Brackmann, D. (1997). Successful detection of small acoustic tumors using the stacked derived-band auditory brain stem response amplitude. *American Journal of Otology, 18*(5), 608–685.
207. Cho, S. W., Han, K. H., Jang, H. K., Chang, S. O., Jung, H., & Lee, J. H. (2015). Auditory brainstem responses to CE-Chirp® stimuli for normal ears and those with sensorineural hearing loss. *International Journal of Audiology, 54*(10), 700–704.
208. Brown, C. S., Peskoe, S. B., Risoli Jr, T., Garrison, D. B., & Kaylie, D. M. (2019). Associations of video head impulse test and caloric testing among patients with vestibular schwannoma. *Otolaryngology-Head and Neck Surgery, 161*(2), 324–329.
209. Constanzo, F., de Almeida Teixeira, B. C., Sens, P., & Ramina, R. (2019). Video head impulse test in vestibular schwannoma: Relevance of size and cystic component on vestibular impairment. *Otology & Neurotology, 40*(4), 511–516.
210. Kjærsgaard, J. B., Szeremet, M., & Hougaard, D. D. (2019). Vestibular deficits correlating to dizziness handicap inventory score, hearing loss, and tumor size in a Danish cohort of vestibular schwannoma patients. *Otology & Neurotology, 40*(6), 813–819.
211. Hentschel, M., Scholte, M., Steens, S., Kunst, H., & Rovers, M. (2017). The diagnostic accuracy of non-imaging screening protocols for vestibular schwannoma in patients with asymmetrical hearing loss

and/or unilateral audiovestibular dysfunction: A diagnostic review and meta-analysis. *Clinical Otolaryngology, 42*(4), 815–823.

212. Starr, A., Picton, T. W., Sininger, Y., Hood, L. J., & Berlin, C. I. (1996). Auditory neuropathy. *Brain, 119*(3), 741–753.

213. Hayes, D., & Sininger, Y. S. (2008). Auditory neuropathy spectrum disorder (ANSD) guidelines development conference: Identification of infants and children with auditory neuropathy. Lake Como, Italy, June 19–21, 2008, http://www.thechildrenshospital.org/pdf/Guidelines%20for%20Auditory%20Neuropathy%20-%20BDCCH.pdf, (pp. 3–8).

214. Jang, J. H., Kim, J. H., Yoo, J. C., Kim, C. H., Kim, M. S., Chang, S. O., . . . Lee, J. H. (2012). Implication of bony cochlear nerve canal on hearing in patients with congenital unilateral sensorineural hearing loss. *Audiology and Neurotology, 17*(5), 282–289.

215. Lim, C. H., Lim, J. H., Kim, D., sung Choi, H., Lee, D. H., & Kim, D. K. (2018). Bony cochlear nerve canal stenosis in pediatric unilateral sensorineural hearing loss. *International Journal of Pediatric Otorhinolaryngology, 106*, 72–74.

216. Yi, J. S., Lim, H. W., Kang, B. C., Park, S. Y., Park, H. J., & Lee, K. S. (2013). Proportion of bony cochlear nerve canal anomalies in unilateral sensorineural hearing loss in children. *International Journal of Pediatric Otorhinolaryngology, 77*(4), 530–533.

217. Hood, L. J. (2015). Auditory neuropathy/dyssynchrony disorder: Diagnosis and management. *Otolaryngologic Clinics of North America, 48*(6), 1027–1040.

218. Starr, A., & Rance, G. (2015). Auditory neuropathy. In G. Celesia & G. Hickok (Eds.), *The human auditory system, Handbook of clinical neurology* (Vol. 129, pp. 495–508). Elsevier.

219. Bickford, R. G., Jacobson, J. L., & Galbraith, R. F. (1963). A new audio motor system in man. *Electroencephalography and Clinical Neurophysiology, 15*, 921–925.

220. Gibson, W. P. R. (1978). *Essentials of clinical electric response audiometry*. Churchill Livingstone.

221. Thornton, A. R. D. (1975). The use of post-auricular muscle responses. *Journal of Laryngology & Otology, 89*(10), 997–1010.

222. Agung, K., Purdy, S. C., Patuzzi, R., O'Beirne, G. A., & Newall, P. (2005). Rising-frequency chirps and earphones with an extended high frequency response enhance the post-auricular muscle response. *International Journal of Audiology, 44*(11), 631–636.

223. Purdy, S.C., Agung, K B., Hartley, D., Patuzzi, R.B., & O'Beirne, G.A. (2005). The post-auricular muscle response: An objective electrophysiological method for evaluating hearing sensitivity. *International Journal of Audiology, 44*(11), 625–630.

224. Patuzzi, R. B., & Thomson, S. M. (2000). Auditory evoked response test strategies to reduce cost and increase efficiency: The postauricular muscle response revisited. *Audiology and Neurotology, 5*(6), 322–332.

225. Agung, K., Purdy, S. C., Patuzzi, R., & O'Beirne, G. A. (2001). Objective hearing assessment using the post auricular muscle response: Stimulus and insert earphone transducer effects. *Australian and New Zealand Journal of Audiology, 23*, 67.

7

Testing Midbrain and Cortical Projection Pathways

The Writers

Episode 1: Joaquín Tomás Valderrama-Valenzuela
Episode 2: Cynthia G. Fowler and So E. Park
Episode 3: Thierry Morlet and So E. Park
Heads Up: Cynthia G. Fowler and So E. Park

■ Episode 1: Auditory Middle Latency Response and 40-Hz Auditory Steady-State Response—Signals En Route to the Cortex

This episode further explores time and space in the central auditory pathway, starting with the classical transient stimulus-response paradigm, picking up from the saga of AEP generation from the ongoing barrage of evoked electrical activity expressed in the brainstem response, yet not to be forgotten. Having refined a bit the terminology applied to the short-latency responses—distinguishing components measured using or related to electrocochleography and tests of the pontine-brainstem responses—the AEP lexicon will be enhanced a bit further. Like the ABR, the transient middle latency response (MLR) is variably named in the literature, either simply as MLR or ***auditory middle latency response (AMLR)***, as adopted henceforth. The AMLR is described commonly as comprising three voltage oscillations that appear within the first 50 or so millisecond time frame from the stimulus onset. The AMLR overall provides a basis for measurements to help the clinician evaluate the status of the central auditory pathway, indeed further up the way, through the thalamus and beyond. Its optimal stimulus-response paradigms effectively support some other advantages even in evoked response audiometry. So, onward!

The components of the AMLR are the N_0, P_0, N_a, P_a, N_b, and P_b, or N's and P's subscripted by nominal latencies, like P_{50} (alias Pb, arising at about 50 ms). The former scheme will largely be used here. It is straightforward (whether subscripted by letters or numbers), reflecting simply a progression in time. Following the convention adopted for representing the ABR graphically, positive voltage components are labeled with the letter "P," while "N" is used for the voltage-negative ones. Illustrations of the response will continue to be (as most broadly observed in audiology) by way of plotting voltage-positive peaks upwardly—for instance, C_z positive up, as in Figure 7–1 (top panel). The most robust component of the AMLR is the N_a-P_a complex. ***Amplitudes*** and ***latencies*** are measured much as described for the ABR, with characteristic values for the AMLR summarized in Table 7–1. These values are from a sample of normal-hearing adults tested monaurally and stimulated using 8 clicks per second at 70 dB nHL.[1]

Echoing essentially Figure 1–1, Figure 7–1 (bottom panel) presents a more detailed representation

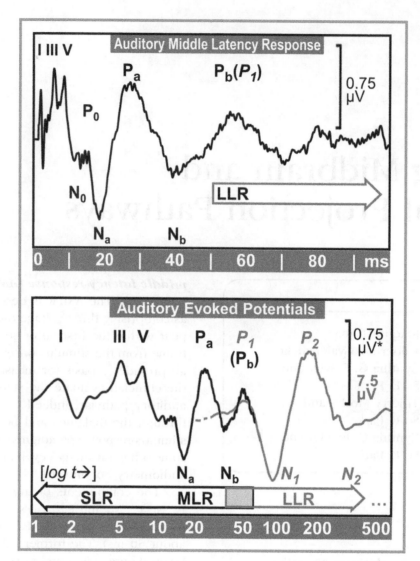

Figure 7–1. *Top panel*: Example of an auditory middle latency response (AMLR) recorded in a young adult with normal hearing. The AMLR appears in between the short-latency auditory brainstem response (ABR) and the long-latency response (LLR; a cortical auditory evoked potential). *Bottom panel*: Figure 1–1 presented a schematic diagram of the overall AEP, in deference to challenges of getting all of the component waves on the same plot, essentially requiring a logarithmic time base. Here are a couple of recordings—the SLR-MLR segment from panel A and the LLR replotted from Figure 4–12 partially overlapped naturally and are presented here on a log-time scale, underscoring the reality of the underlying time continuum of the AEPs. Substantial differences in magnitudes are also a challenge; here the two segments are simply adjusted by gain (see calibration bar).

Table 7–1. Characteristic Values of Latencies and Amplitudes of Component Potentials of the Auditory Middle-Latency Responses

	Latency (ms)		Amplitude (μV)
N_a	18.6 ± 3.1	N_a-P_a	1.27 ± 0.4
P_a	26.8 ± 2.9	N_b-P_b	0.59 ± 0.2
N_b	40.7 ± 1.7		
P_b	53.8 ± 3.0		

Table 7–2. Useful Stimulus and Recording Parameters for AMLR

Stimulus		Acquisition	
Transducer	Insert earphones	Electrode Positions	F_z, C_z referenced to as TP_9/TP_{10} (temporal-parietal, above L/R mastoids to minimize PAMR)
Type	Clicks or tone bursts	Filter	Wide: [1–2000] Hz Narrow: [1–200] Hz
Ear	Monaural or diotic	Amplification	>50,000
Polarity	Any	Analysis window	100 ms
Level	<70 dB HL	Number of responses	>1000
Rate	<10 stim/s	Sampling rate	Wide: 10 kHz Narrow: 1 kHz

of the AEPs along the ascending pathway. This figure shows that the AMLR, as its name implies, falls simply between the short- and later-latency components, as traditionally defined. This classification of AEPs[2] was motivated by the practical difficulty of representing all AEPs together in the same plot. This figure comprises a couple of edited responses. The technical challenge is the problem of optimal filtering and adequate temporal resolution among the three "time zones"; those for the best measurements for SLR components are inadequate for LLR components and vice versa. Currently, research is being devoted to explore new signal processing algorithms to overcome this technical limitation.[3,4] Meanwhile, this episode will address the nuances and parameters of stimulus and recording for the AMLR derived in deference to its different coordinates in time and space in AEPdom, as the "message" from the peripheral system continues ascending the auditory pathway. Note: For various figures thus far, computer modeling and/or other processing has been used to enhance illustrations/demonstrations of effects under discussion. This episode is no exception but also relies upon data acquired largely from the same subject (per top panel) whose responses both follow well the central tendencies of magnitudes and latencies and show all recognized components of AMLRs generally recordable in normally hearing/neurologically intact subjects. As often the rationale for modeling (for example, to have a signal that is known unequivocally, even if "burying" its awful noise), this is to minimize obscuring the effects of interest from inherent nonpathological variances among individual subjects and/or test methods, especially across studies.

An understanding of the **neural generators** of the AMLR components is key to providing a correct interpretation of the signal. The generator sources of these components are mainly the inferior colliculus, the thalamic auditory structures, and the auditory cortex.[5] However, the exact location of each is subject to some controversy. The N_a component has been associated with neural activity originating from the midbrain, thalamus, and thalamocortical radiations.[6] From a study using intracerebral electrodes (in surgical cases),[7] it was reported that the P_a component in humans was generated in the medial portion of the primary auditory cortex, N_b from the lateral section, and P_b from secondary auditory cortex. In contrast, results of other investigations suggest that the P_a originates from the mesencephalic reticular formation in children[8] and medial geniculate body.[9] Moreover, it has been documented that the P_a prevails despite bilateral lesions affecting the primary auditory cortex.[10]

Table 7–2 presents a summary of parameters recommended for an AMLR test protocol. All the parameters specified are discussed further in the following text.

Both 100-μs **clicks** and brief **tone bursts** have been shown to elicit robust AMLRs.[11] As for the ABR, tone bursts provide some degree of frequency specificity of transient stimuli. Tone bursts for measuring the AMLR today are often "built" as Blackman-windowed, four-cycle sinusoidal pulses. Recall (Episode 2.2) that the choice of number of cycles (or duration) is a compromise between frequency specificity—the more cycles, the more concentrated sound energy is along the frequency axis—and abruptness of onset—required to enhance synchronous firing of the neurons but at risk of more spectral splatter. Higher-frequency tone bursts have been reported to elicit larger-magnitude AMLRs.[11] However, it also has been found that the P_b component was easier to detect for lower-frequency (500 Hz) compared to higher-frequency (4000 Hz) tone bursts or clicks.[12] In any event, the AMLR tends to be more robustly stimulated at frequencies below 1000 Hz, than is the ABR (a matter examined further in the upcoming episode).

Figure 7–2 shows AMLR signals evoked by clicks and tone bursts at different frequencies, presented at 70 dB nHL at a rate of 8 stimuli per second in a normal-hearing, young adult subject. Consistent with the aforementioned literature, this figure shows that in this particular subject, (1) clicks evoked indeed have a larger magnitude AMLR than tone bursts; (2) the N_a-P_a-N_b complex presented a greater magnitude with the 4000-Hz tone burst compared with the 500 Hz; and (3) the P_b component was more prominent at the 500-Hz tone burst compared with the 4000-Hz tone burst. In contrast to ABR and electrocochleography (ECochG), the **polarity** of the stimulus is not critical in AMLR recordings.[13]

Similar to the binaural effect seen in the ABR, the magnitude of the AMLR is greater with **diotic** presentation of the stimulus, compared to the **monotic** (monaural) response.[14] Figure 7–3 shows AMLR signals obtained from a normal-hearing, young adult subject using clicks presented at 70 dB nHL at a rate of 8 stimuli per second delivered simultaneously to the two ears versus the left and right ears monaurally.

The AMLR components are sensitive to the stimulus **level**, as expected from effects of this stimulus parameters observed in SLRs. In general

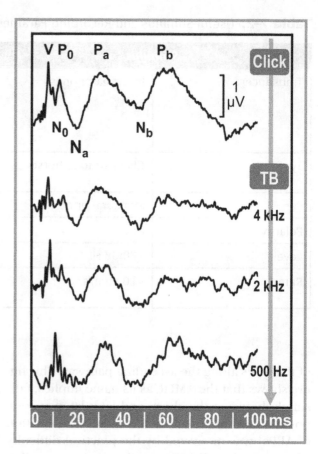

Figure 7–2. AMLRs evoked by the acoustic click and tone bursts (TB) at different frequencies, presented at 70 dB nHL with a rate of 8 stimuli per second.

terms,[15,16,17] amplitudes decrease and latencies increase as stimulus level decreases (Figures 7–4 and 7–5). However, trends for the AMLR have their own nuances (Figure 7–4A). Amplitudes gradually increase upward of 70 dB SPL but then remain nearly constant. In signals-and-systems parlance, it is as if output of the overall AMLR generator is saturating at the upper dynamic range of hearing. Figure 7–4 shows also variance (by way of measurements of standard errors of the amplitudes) for the two measurements over stimulus level, from a sample of five normal-hearing subjects.[17] Figure 7–5 shows an example AMLR obtained at different levels (normal-hearing subject as before). This figure illustrates again how amplitudes naturally decrease as level decreases, but with less evident latency-intensity shift and decreased parallel shift of longer-latency components than for the ABR (recall Figures 6–3B and 6–5).

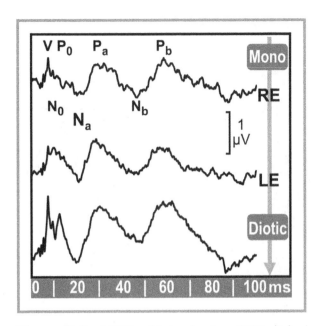

Figure 7–3. AMLRs obtained using 4000 clicks/trial presented at 70 dB nHL with a rate of 8 stimuli per second, delivered simultaneously in the two ears (diotic) versus monaurally in the left and right ears.

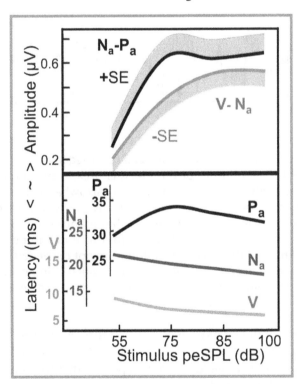

Figure 7–4. Trends of input-output functions of amplitude differences of ABR wave V to N_a versus AMLR components N_a (N_{19}) to P_a (P_{30}) at suprathreshold levels. Lighter-gray areas approximate standard errors (for simplicity plotted as + or − SEs, as indicated) about the approximate group means. (Acoustic clicks presented at levels in peak-equivalent SPLs; based on data of Fobel [2003].[17])

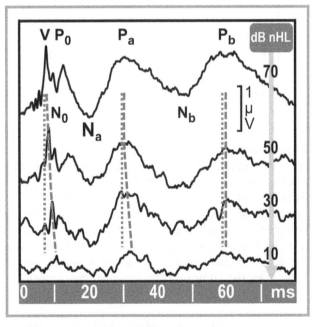

Figure 7–5. Examples of AMLRs obtained, again using acoustic clicks at several levels specified in dB nHL.

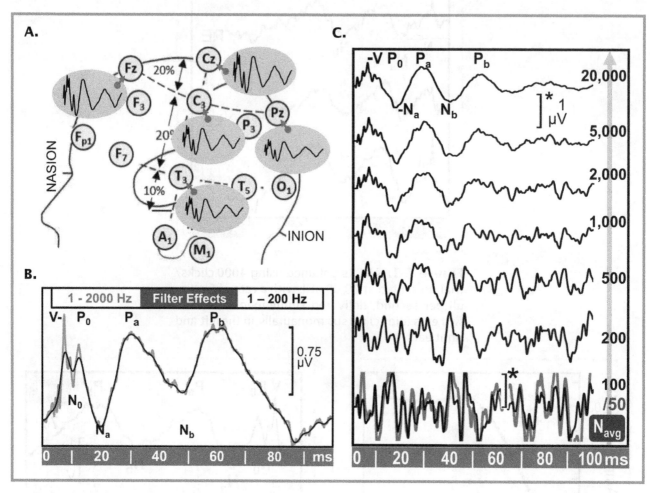

Figure 7–6. A. An AMLR recorded at C_z is taken as a model and scaled in replots as if recorded at clinically "popular" electrode positions on the scalp, showing that the magnitude of the AMLR is greater in central midline and somewhat frontal electrodes. **B.** AMLRs obtained with relatively wide- versus narrowband filters, as indicated. **C.** AMLRs at different numbers of responses averaged. Note: Averages for *Ns of 50 and 100 are overlaid to show some seemingly coherent signals yet as much noisy intervals throughout (thus not coherent) in a background of noise that (overall) exceeds the limits of the display set for this figure but did not clip any others (N ≥200). This is also to note that the limits of the A/D conversion were not exceeded in the actual recording, as that naturally is a real no-no; a limit of acceptance of a sampled epoch is imposed at least by the computer/artifact-rejection algorithm to avoid nonlinear signal averaging (recall Episode 4.1).

Since the magnitude of the AMLR is greater in midline central and frontal areas of the cortex (see Figure 7–6A), the single-channel EEG electrode montage usually consists of placing an electrode at Cz (although the hairline-forehead site, popular in ABR tests, is also efficacious); this electrode is connected to the noninverting input of the recording amplifier. The inverting input is connected conventionally to an electrode placed on ipsilateral mastoid or earlobe and the ground electrode at the nasion. Overall, the montage and polarity convention of this hookup is similar to those of recordings devoted to pontine brainstem and some cortical potentials to yield evoked responses that routinely are plotted with Cz+ potentials "up."

An amplifier gain around 75,000 is adequate for AMLR recordings. The EEG is often filtered using a wide bandwidth (for instance, 1–2000 Hz) to include the ABR components. However, narrower filter settings also can be applied (such as, 1–200 Hz), but including largely/distinctively only the AMLR components. Panel B in Figure 7–6 shows an example of the AMLR for two filter configurations. Recall that to avoid aliasing, the sampling rate must be greater than twice the value of the low-pass cutoff frequency of the filter (recall Episode 2.1, Figure 2–9). The most typical sampling rates are 10 kHz and 1 kHz for the wide and narrow filter configurations, respectively. For AMLRs, an analysis time window of 50 ms to 100 ms is typical. Also applicable to any AEPs (SLRs and beyond) is adding to the time-domain view ahead of stimulus onset—thus, a prestimulus interval as a part of the recording to better judge the recording baseline—for example, 10 ms for the AMLR (although not shown in Figure 7–6B in this rather stable recording). As with other AEP recordings, the quality of the AMLR recorded increases as the number of averaged sweeps increases. For each doubling of number sweeps (stimulus repetitions), the SNR of the AMLR is expected to increase by as much as 3 dB. This already has been demonstrated for both SLRs and LLRs (recall Episodes 4.1 and 4.2), but it is of such fundamental importance as to fill in the "MLR gap" here, namely for another seeing-is-believing demonstration. Shown in panel C of Figure 7–6 are AMLRs emerging from the noise floor, as a function of sweeps averaged. The wider band filtering (that was used for panel B) permits observing directly the ABR for comparison. This figure shows, indeed, that AMLR quality is augmented substantially with increasing numbers of sweeps averaged, but not without some cost: increased recording/test time. Consequently, the number of averaged sweeps must be determined reaching a compromise between the qualities of the response needed per application versus test efficiency. At least 500 to 1,000 sweeps are recommended to ensure a reliably detected and/or representative sample of the AMLR waveform, particularly at low stimulus levels. There is at the examiner's finger tips the same digital tools for further processing, as in ABR measurement. Going back to the earlier point of relative robustness of responses, the demonstration of panel C shows (as was hinted previously) the AMLR "emerging earlier" than the ABR (compare $N = 200$ versus 500).

The AMLR is also influenced by the stimulus *rate*. In clinical practice, it is common to use a fixed stimulus rate, recalling that the interstimulus interval (ISI) is the inverse of the stimulus rate. When using a fixed stimulus rate, it is important that the ISI is larger than the duration of the response of interest in order to avoid contamination of the AMLR by subsequent responses.[18] Since the duration of the AMLR arguably can extend to 100 ms, the maximum rate that can be used nominally is 10 stimuli per second (1/100 ms). In most studies in adults, the researchers used stimulus presentation rates around 8/s. The amplitude of the P_a component remains relatively stable from rates of 1/s to 10/s, but latencies are shorter for very slow rates (1/s or less).[19,20] In contrast, as the stimulus rate increases (ISI decreases), the latency of the P_b component increases and the amplitude decreases.[21]

AMLRs can be recorded, nevertheless, at stimulus rates faster than 10/s with the aid of **deconvolution** of the epoch, (again, a mathematical derivation that disentangles overlapping signals). In this case, it is required that the ISIs of the stimulus sequence are not fixed. The most relevant techniques that allow deconvolution of overlapping AEPs are maximum length sequences,[22] continuous loop averaging deconvolution,[23] least-squares deconvolution,[24] and iterative randomized stimulation and averaging.[1] In the classical approach, in which very long ISIs are used (>100 ms), the neurons involved are presumed to be ready to fire each time a stimulus is presented because they have had enough time to repolarize from the previous stimulus, thus leading to synchronous firing of a large number of neurons and yielding AMLR components of large amplitudes. In contrast, at fast stimulus rates, the neurons have less time to repolarize (or recover) from the previous stimulus, which leads to more neurons being in their refractory periods, thus less neurons ready to fire synchronously when a new stimulus is presented. The consequence is AMLRs of lower magnitude at faster rates; this effect is what is considered as neural adaptation (recall Episode 6.1).[25] Figure 7–7A shows examples at different stimulus rates obtained from a normal-hearing subject. Figures 7–7B and C represent changes in amplitudes and latencies as a function of stimulus rate.

A number of **artifacts** of different nature can affect the recording of the AMLR. First, **power line** noise can be induced (50/60 Hz) and is an artifact of particular concern on the EEG. Since AMLR signals usually present energy at those

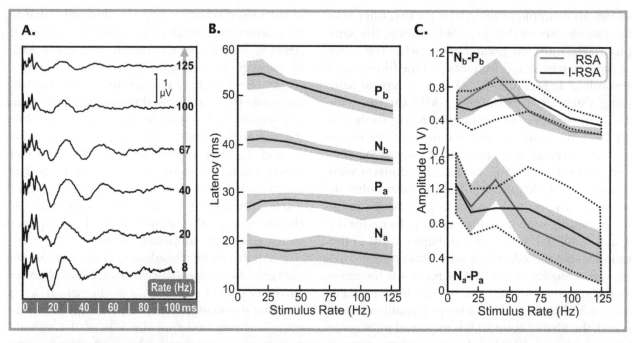

Figure 7–7. A. Example AMLRs obtained at different stimulus rates (Hz representing stimuli per second; individual subject's responses, as before). **B–C.** Mean (and +/-1 standard deviations areas) of the latencies (panel B) and amplitudes (panel C) of the AMLR components as indicated. (C: greater amplitudes in RSA [*gray*, based on averaging] at 40 Hz compared to IRSA [*black*, based on a deconvolution] indicate that averaged responses in RSA are 'contaminated' by adjacent responses, to be demonstrated in the next figure; based on data of Valderrama and colleagues, 2014).

frequencies, the use of a notch filter is not recommended. Rather, the most recommended approach is to ground properly the EEG recording system, and, if necessary, include an additional power line filter to attenuate the effect of this artifact. In addition, the transducer of the earphone again can radiate **stimulus artifact**. The most effective way to attenuate this artifact is to shield the earphones with mu-metal, connected to the same ground as the EEG recording system (if available to the examiner). However, use of tubal-insert type earphones, also successful with ABR testing, is generally effective in AMLR testing, as the transducer element itself can be positioned somewhat away from the electrodes. However, given electrodes placed in the frontal area of the head, the recording naturally can be contaminated with artifacts of **eyeblink** and **eye movement** (recall Episode 4.2). As with the ABR, the test systems artifact-rejection algorithm is useful to minimize adverse effects of these and other myogenic artifacts. For the most critical work, they can often be attenuated offline, using advanced signal processing algorithms. AMLRs are also susceptible to interference by the postauricular muscle response, highlighted in the last Heads Up (see Figure 6–38). The PAMR can be even more troubling than it is in ABR recordings, due to overlap of early AMLR/neurogenic components. The PAMR is most likely to emerge when the stimulus level is relatively high (>70 dB nHL) and when one of the active electrodes is close to the postauricular muscle (thus, just behind the ear) and/or when the neck of the test subject is tense. If suspected to be interfering significantly with the recording, effective strategies to reduce/evade the artifact are placement of the electrode further from the mastoid (like the nape of the neck), lower the stimulus level (given that this option is acceptable), and/or provide a couch or reclining chair wherein the participant can support the neck and shoulders more comfortably. The lattermost is also good practice in general for overall relaxation of the examinee.

It was mentioned earlier, that the ISI has to be greater than the duration of the targeted response's epoch (averaging window) to avoid the responses overlapping, thus contaminating their recording by possible overlapping of the individual AMLR component waves (or even those of other AEPs). However, is this necessarily a bad thing? Figure 7–8 shows the effects of using a fixed ISI higher versus lower than the duration of the averaging window, demonstrated using a model of the transient AMLR. The first row shows these model responses as if elicited at a stimulus interval of 333 ms (stimulus rate of 3 Hz). The top signal shows the instances when the stimuli were presented via a DC pulse, also used as a marker. This example shows that the responses are far from overlapping. At 8 Hz (second row, with ISI = 125 ms), the responses still do not overlap (as expected); however, at rates greater than 10 Hz (hence, ISIs lower than 100 ms), the responses do overlap. Given then fixed stimulus repetition rates, overlapping responses have substantial effects, in fact resulting in a periodic signal whose period is equal to the ISI (reciprocal of the stimulation rate = 1/frequency). As suggested previously, the "original" response is being contaminated by subsequent responses. However, something more curious is happening than expected from the likes of adaptation. Depending on the stimulus rate, this contamination can express constructive or destructive interference. This figure shows that the stimulus rate of 40 Hz produces a remarkable constructive interference, thus resulting in the model response having a greater amplitude than the original![26] This suggests that this response should be detected more readily in a background of noise. The constructive interference is a consequence of the N_a-P_a component overlapping with the N_b-P_b component of subsequent responses during stimulus repetition. The real AEP elicited by a stimulus at the rate of 40 Hz does exactly this and is known as the *40-Hz auditory steady-state response (40-Hz ASSR)*. Galambos and his coworkers[27] first recognized that these natural "time zones" of the AMLR's components

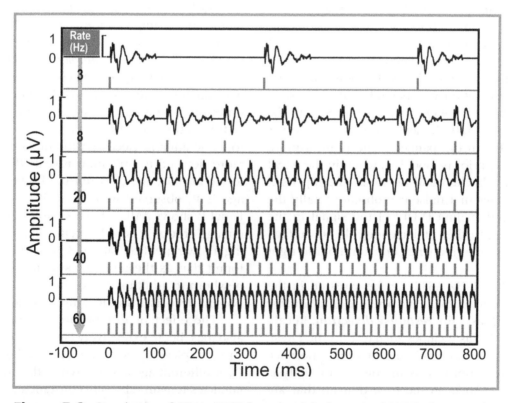

Figure 7–8. Simulation of 40-Hz ASSR from model of transient AMLR, showing the naturally recurring effects of such overlapping of the responses (see text).

should manifest as such and thus serve as the basis for an efficacious, alternative paradigm for measuring the AMLR.

The 40-Hz ASSR can be evoked by clicks, as modeled in the previous figure or by frequency-specific stimuli. To recap from Episode 6.3 dedicated to the 80-Hz ASSR, one of these options is the use a of a sinusoidal signal modulated in amplitude by another sinusoid—SAM, sinusoidal amplitude modulation (Figure 7–9A, left). A robust ASSR, indeed, can be evoked by SAM signals wherein the modulating frequency (F_M) is fixed at/near 40 Hz. As before, the carrier presents different frequencies audiometrically in order to explore the ASSR response evoked by different places (in effect) along the hearing organ. Common carrier frequencies thus are 500 Hz, 1000 Hz, and 2000 Hz. Figure 7–9A shows the representation in the time and frequency domains of these stimuli.

The panel on the top left corner of Figure 7–9B shows a segment of an ASSR evoked at 40 Hz. This ASSR is not real but, rather, a signal synthesized without noise for demonstration purposes to enable scrutiny with more precision. This figure shows that the 40-Hz ASSR indeed is a periodic signal (T = 25 ms = 1/40 Hz). So far, the model AMLRs have been analyzed in the time domain, but as learned in Episodes 6.2 and 6.3, the analysis of ASSRs is more effective in the frequency domain. Their representation via spectral analysis is seen as a series of peaks of energy in multiples of 40 Hz: 40 Hz, 80 Hz, 120 Hz, and so forth (see lower left panel B). In the panels to the right, a more realistic "scenario" is modeled, wherein the ASSR appears in a background of noise. The top right panel B shows that noise can obscure totally the visual detection limit (VDL) of the signal in the time domain, further underscoring the advantage of analysis in the frequency domain (bottom right panel B).

That the 40-Hz ASSR can be assessed in the frequency domain facilitates the use of *objective (statistical) tests for response detection*. Recalling Table 4–1, this includes such tests as the *F*-test, Hotelling T^2, and magnitude-squared coherence (MSC).[28] This approach is in contrast to analysis of transient AMLRs in the time domain that are typically scored according to the examiner's judgment when determining the VDL of the response.

As for the 80-Hz ASSR (recall Figure 6–21), these tests are applied to the ASSR's spectrum to determine whether or not a response is present by comparing the energy at the frequency in which the neural response is expected (here nominally, 40 Hz—as predetermined) and the energy of the surrounding frequencies. The latter is presumed to be noise only, hence the major source of variance in the response measurement.[29] Recent AEP test systems provide *online assessment*, as an automatic criterion for stopping averaging. This is another advantage and one that can save time.

Both the transient AMLR and 40-Hz ASSR will be taken up in the subsequent episode dedicated to objective audiometry using these responses. There are still some basic nonpathological variables (in addition to those on the more technological side), and they bring the discussion back to the transient AMLR by which so much of the foundational information was developed. This starts with the highly important aspect of *developmental changes*, to which the AMLR is highly susceptible. Maturation is indeed a substantial "game changer," firstly by potentially bringing the stimulus rate down to around 1/s in order to detect the P_a component in infants and young children.[30] Figure 7–10A shows the prevalence of the N_a and P_a components as a function of age. This figure shows overall that the percent detectability of both components increases with age following a sigmoidal function, thus demonstrating asymptoticlike growth and achievement of full maturation of the response, essentially before and after, respectively, the first decade of life. More detailed examination reveals that N_a is detected at most ages, yet not until 8 years or so of age is P_a observed in at least 50% of the cases. Panel B shows AMLRs from samples in five different age groups at two different stimulus levels, using a low repetition rate of 3.3/s. It thus has been found that as the auditory system matures from newborn to adulthood, the latency of the P_a component decreases and its amplitude increases.[20]

The effect of *advancing age* on the AMLR also has been extensively studied. Figure 7–11 shows typical latencies and amplitudes for P_a and P_b at different ages. As shown in this figure, while latencies remain relatively constant across all ages, amplitudes tend to increase as age increases.[31-33] The increase in the amplitude of the AMLR with

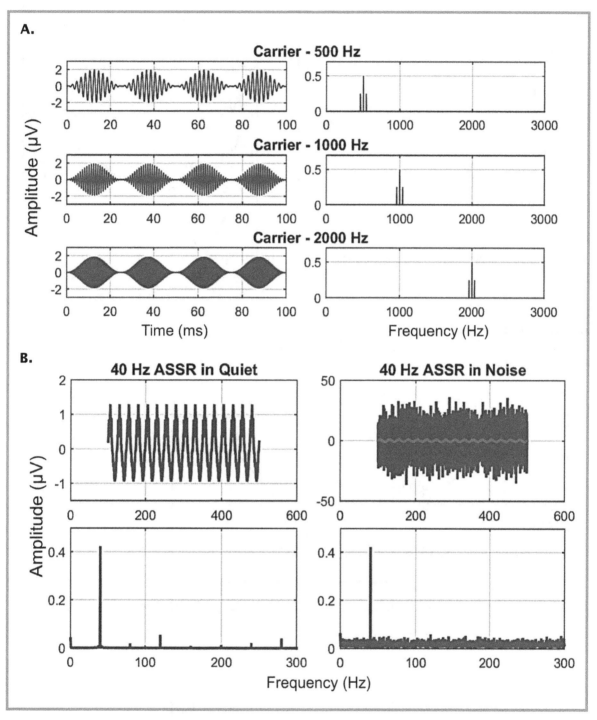

Figure 7–9. A. Sinusoidally amplitude modulated signal at different carrier frequencies represented in the time (*left*) and frequency (*right*) domains. **B**. Demonstration using a synthesized 40-Hz ASSR signal in the time (*top*) and frequency (*bottom*) domains—in quiet (*left panels*) and in noise (*right panels*). The noise is seen to totally obscure the response in the time history, whereas the presence of the response is clearly evident in the spectral view.

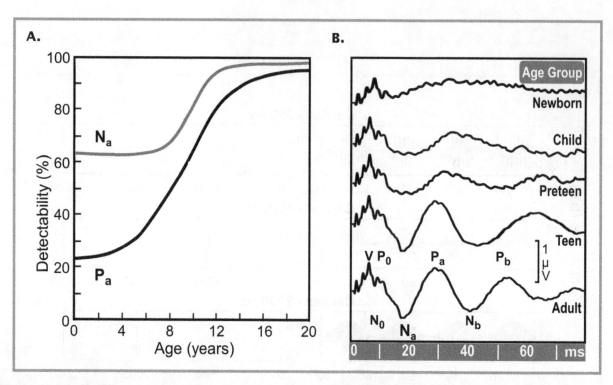

Figure 7–10. **A.** Effects of maturation on the N_a and P_a components (central tendencies, based on data of Kraus and associates [1987][30]). **B.** Quasimodeled AMLRs typical of five different age groups indicated (70 dB nHL; stimulus rate 3.3/s; based in part on data of Tucker and Ruth [1996][20]).

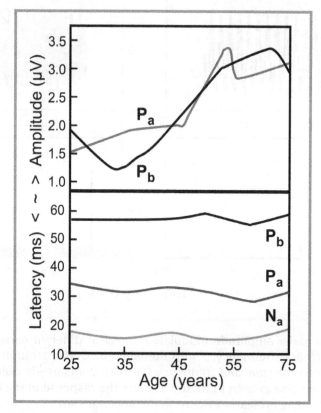

Figure 7–11. Trends of amplitude and latencies of the P_a and P_b components at different ages (based on data of Amenedo and Diaz [1998][32]).

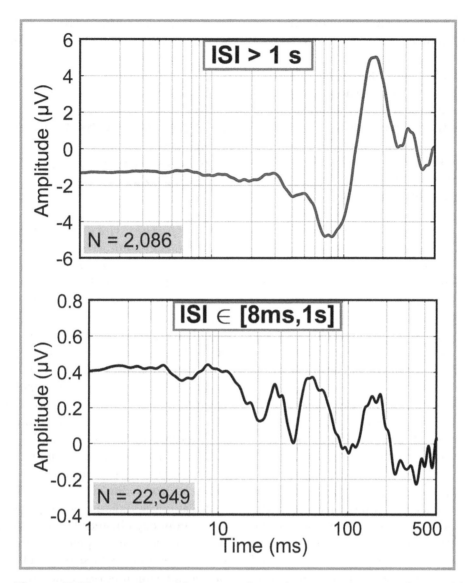

Figure 7-12. AEPs derived from recordings during presentation of natural/free-running speech; the time window of display is expanded to accommodate both MLRs and LLRs (essentially as in Figure 7-1B; note here too the use of a logarithmic time base). Results reflect changes in the makeup of the overall AEP with respect to the effective stimulus repetition rates inherent to continuous speech and their differential effects on components of the overall AEP (see text), namely effects of less (*top panel*, processed to emphasize events of ISIs > 1s) versus more neural adaptation (*bottom panel*, ISIs of 0.8 ms).

advancing age has been associated with three possible mechanisms: (1) a reduction in inhibition at subcortical levels (in particular, at the inferior colliculus and medial geniculate body); (2) a reduction in inhibition on the downward pathways from the auditory cortex to the brainstem; and/or (3) a reduction in the white matter at prefrontal regions of the cortex, which are involved in the inhibition of neural activity evoked by different sensory areas.

In general, the *sex* of the examinee is not a statistically significant factor influencing the AMLR.[34,35] There are, however, some authors who have reported apparent trends consistent with the well-documented male-female differences of ABRs—larger amplitudes and shorter latencies in females (on average). For example,[32] it has been found that, although the N_a latency was longer for male than female subjects, the latency of the remaining components—as well as the amplitude of all components—were similar between the sexes. It should also be noted that the effects of age and sex on the AMLR are interactive[36]; therefore, it is a common practice to include these two factors in data analysis to rule out their possible influence of the reported outcomes.

Moving on with a peek ahead, the analysis of adapted MLRs—obtained at fast stimulus-repetition rates—may also help to study how the auditory system responds to more *ecologically-valid stimuli*, like real free-running speech. In a recent study,[37] the researchers derived ABRs and MLRs from continuous natural speech, having the subjects listen to an audiobook. This was done by deconvolution to "unwrap" the overlapping AEPs, relative to time instants in which glottal pulses occurred (regarding voice pitch; recall Episode 6.2). The present writer and colleagues[38] have taken a similar approach and found that the morphology of the AEPs is not time invariant, rather dependent (in effect) on the interstimulus interval from the previous glottal pulse. In other words, the morphology of the elicited AEP differed whether the glottal pulse was at the onset or in the middle of a word, due to neural adaptation (lesser versus greater, respectively). This effect is presented in Figure 7–12. The top panel shows that large-magnitude MLR and LLR/cortical responses to be elicited at the onset of a sentence; this is when the ISI of the preceding glottal pulse is longer than 1 s. The bottom panel shows that in the middle of a word, when the ISI of the preceding glottal pulse is between about 0.1 s and 1 s, both MLRs and LLRs are present but with lower magnitudes due to increased neural adaptation. The methodological tools proposed in these studies may help to elucidate how the human auditory system processes speech, which can facilitate the study of cognitive processes like language and selective attention.

The objective of the present episode has been to explore the more fundamental aspects of elicitation and recording of the MLRs as well as their nonpathological variables. Now on to potential *audiological applications* of MLR measurement in the realms of ERA, differential diagnostics, and other special interests.

Episode 2: Why Evoked Response Audiometry (ERA) Using AMLR or 40-Hz ASSR Measures

The big picture: The use of AEP measures to estimate limits of auditory sensitivity traditionally has been called *evoked response audiometry (ERA)*. Yet, ERA does not imply any one AEP as the metric to get the job done. The general ERA approach—seeking the VLD of a given AEP—started with the long-latency response but clearly is applicable to all (at least in principle)—short, middle, and long latency responses. True in practice, estimation of auditory thresholds across the life span is primarily accomplished with evaluation of the auditory brainstem response, despite limitations but also in deference to its strengths. Still, ABR-ERA is not without some weakness attributed predominantly to perceptions of increased difficulty to record reliably and/or reduced accuracy of threshold estimates at lower audiometric frequencies (<1000 Hz). Low-frequency-elicited ABRs require longer rise times for adequate frequency specificity, while this potential is most robust when elicited by stimuli of shorter stimulus rise times for optimal neural synchrony. The problem will be aggravated if filtering of the recording is too aggressive and, particularly, if the high-pass frequency cutoff is set too high (recall the lesson of Figure 4–16). However, the AMLR effectively integrates energy of the sound over longer durations of sinusoidal pulses, so this potential inherently makes more efficacious use of longer-duration/rise-time stimuli. Meanwhile, as a longer latency potential, longer duration stimuli can be used without risk of interference of stimulus artifact. *AMLR-ERA* then, provides a reasonable alternative electrophysiological basis for ERA or a supplementary approach to ABR-ERA. The focus of this episode is to provide more foundational knowledge and evidence supporting audiological threshold estimates using

AMLR measurement, including nuances and practical matters of ERA, using both *transient* and *steady-state* stimulus-response paradigms.

A brief recap of the normative features of the AMLR is useful to highlight its aspects that impact threshold estimation. Recall from Figure 7–1A, P_a is the most consistent component of the AMLR. P_a occurs at 25 ms to 35 ms after stimulus onset and typically has an amplitude of 0.5 µV to 1 µV at stimulus levels of 60 dB nHL to 70 dB nHL. The P_b, which has a latency of 50 ms to 80 ms, is less consistent and even absent in some individuals with normal auditory systems. The positive peak, P_o, which precedes P_a, is smaller and variable among individuals. Because N_a and P_a are recorded reliably in older children and adults, the N_a-P_a complex has been used most often to estimate auditory thresholds. The postauricular muscle response can be an artifact. It is more apt to be recorded at high stimulus levels, given recording montage and parameters typically used for AMLR recordings, but it can be a problem for threshold estimation. With typical latencies of 12 ms to 15 ms, the PAMR can be larger than P_a, thus obscuring the true neurogenic AMLR.

Tests of the AMLR are accomplished with methods similar to ABR-ERA. The AMLR can be recorded either in isolation or simultaneously with the ABR or the auditory long latency response (ALLR). These recordings can be done with two separate channels or a single channel. With the latter approach, the simultaneous recordings of ABR and AMLR are obtained best with relatively broad band-pass filter settings to incorporate the requirements of both AEPs (for example, 10 Hz–1500 Hz). More restrictive band-pass filters (for example, 1 Hz–300 Hz) are adequate for the simultaneous recordings of AMLR and ALLR. Examples of both are illustrated in Figure 7–13. In Figure 7–13 (top panel), the ABR wave V and AMLR waves N_a-P_a-N_b-P_b are evident in an 80-ms time window; however, if the focus is only on waves V and P_a, the time window can be shortened to 50 ms. In 7–1 (bottom), the AMLR complex P_a-N_b-P_b and the LLR complex, P_1-N_1-P_2-N_2 are shown in a time window of approximately 500 ms. It should be remembered that P_b, and P_{50} (nominally middle-latency components; recall Figure 7–1, bottom) and P_1 (nominally a long-latency component) are merely different names for

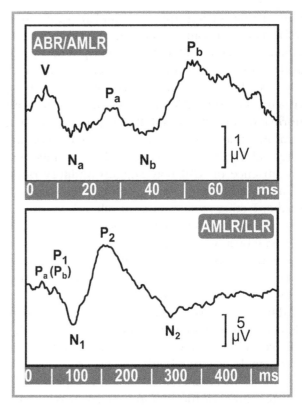

Figure 7–13. Auditory middle latency responses recorded simultaneously with either brainstem (ABR, *top panel*) or cortical (LLR, P_1-N_1-P_2 complex, *bottom panel*), responses using relatively broader bandpass filter settings and longer epochs than might be preferred respectively (typically) for each of the shorter-latency responses alone. ABR/AMLR: Band-pass of 10 Hz to 1500 Hz; epoch of 80 ms. This recording should be contrasted with that in Figure 7–1 (*top panel*) and others in the last episode; in this recording P_b is more prominent than P_a. Although less common, variability of responses is itself a variable (as noted), yet this variant would not be expected to compromise response detectability/ERA; in fact, it would be more likely to improve detection (relative to the ABR; see text). AMLR/LLR: Bandpass of 1.0 Hz to 300 Hz; epoch of 450 ms. Contrast this recording with that of Figure 7–1 (*bottom panel*); same "take-home" message, even without a log transform of the time base, given a broader filter as in this example (based on data of Park [2018][63]).

the same potential—just recorded differently (as will be discussed here shortly as well as in the subsequent chapter). In any event, simultaneous recordings of these two types of AEPs/responses (per conventional latency classifications) can be both a time-saving approach and possibly more informative in some clinical applications. In particular, the status of both the peripheral system and CANS can be evaluated more comprehensively (that is, along the central pathway) by recording concurrently the ABR and AMLR. If the ABR is abnormal or absent, the AMLR may provide information on auditory sensitivity in the same recording. Alternatively, the presence of AMLR combined with the absence of ABR may suggest auditory brainstem abnormalities, which require follow-up with further testing and/or medical referral.

There are several reasons as to how the AMLR-ERA can be advantageous over ABR-ERA. Although the ABR can be elicited below 1000 Hz (typically 500 Hz in practice), the AMLR is again fundamentally more reliable for testing below 1000 Hz. The AMLR typically is larger, so it is expected to be detected more readily than the ABR. At face value, this certainly should ensure better ability to detect signals at low stimulus levels—the "name of the game" in ERA. The AMLR can compensate for shortcomings of the high-frequency bias in ABR-based threshold estimations. These potential advantages will now be scrutinized further, as what may seem reasonable according to basic characteristics of a given AEP, tends to be more relatively than absolutely true in AEP-dom. For example, a larger potential is only more detectable if the noise floor somehow has not increased, namely relative to its underlying spectrum and practical filter settings or if the targeted potential's increase in amplitude manages to "out run" any rise in residual noise. The SNR is the bet hedger in this game of response/no response evaluation.

Stimuli for AMLR-ERA include both clicks and tone bursts, so the question arises as to the relative detectability between paradigms, hence presumably the more effective for hearing threshold estimates. An investigation dedicated to this issue compared VDLs of click-elicited responses between the ABR and AMLR in adults.[39] The results revealed that the most common responses observed near hearing threshold levels were, in descending order, the AMLR-P_a, ABR-V, and AMLR-P_b. The VDLs reported were within 10 dB of audiometric threshold. The AMLR-P_a had the advantage of being larger for all stimulus levels. In another study, the AMLR and ABR were compared directly in adults with normal hearing versus high-frequency hearing losses.[40] The two responses were recorded concurrently using a single-channel system, thus presumably common levels of residual noise. The stimuli used were clicks and 500 Hz Gaussian (windowed) tone bursts, which were presented at three levels: 70 dB nHL, 30 dB nHL, and 20 dB nHL. For the waves of interest, ABR-V and AMLR-N_a and P_a, virtually all waves were detectable at 70 dB nHL in all participants for both stimuli. In contrast, at 20 dB nHL, more than 80% of the participants had responses for Na and Pa, whereas fewer than 20% had responses for ABR-V. The conclusion here is that the AMLR is more likely to produce a response near threshold levels with a lower-frequency sinusoidal pulse. Like the Blackman-windowed tone bursts, the Gaussian window provides good frequency specificity.

The AMLR also can be recorded reliably for ERA in some individuals in whom the ABR is absent due to the degree of hearing loss. The reason for this apparent disconnect is that the synchrony of the elicitation of AMLR is less dependent on stimulus onset than the ABR and sensorineural hearing loss often compromises such synchrony. Hence, the combined ABR-AMLR strategy may be an efficient strategy to begin the evaluation, or the AMLR may be a supplementary evaluation following an initial ABR assessment, if necessary.

Figure 7–14 shows examples of the ABR/AMLRs recorded and tracked down to (essentially) VDLs (in SPLs) for a young adult with normal hearing (panel A) and an older adult with a low-frequency, sensorineural hearing loss (panel B). The responses were obtained at 500 Hz; VDLs are seen to be 40 dB SPL for ABR-V and 30 dB SPL for AMLR-P_a. The results in panel B are the same VDLs, 90 dB SPL, for both ABR and AMLR. This is likely because of the recruitmentlike effects for both potentials; if still different this might be demonstrated using 5-dB steps. Regardless, the AMLR is seen to be a more robust response. It is also interesting to note that the extent to which VDLs for both responses are close in panel A is because of the more-favorable lower-frequency cutoff per the filtering used for the AMLR, akin to the demonstration of Figure 4–16 and the "lesson" therein.

AMLR-ERA has been used in the pediatric population for decades. Because young children are prone to middle ear disorders that often in-

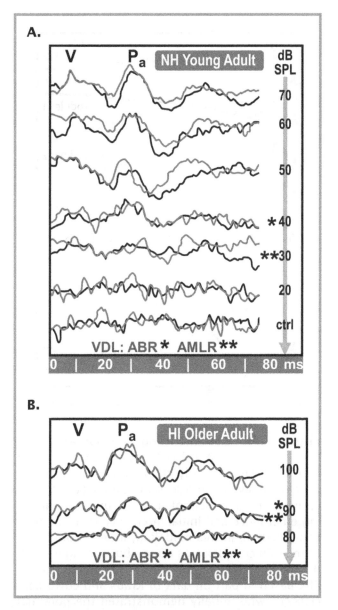

Figure 7–14. An example of ABR/AMLR recordings to 500-Hz tone bursts to estimate hearing thresholds in two subjects. **A.** Young adult with normal-hearing. **B.** Older adult with sensorineural low-frequency hearing loss. Visual detection limits as scored in each case are indicated. Test tracings (*black*) and retest tracings (*gray*) shown for both (Ctrl—control, nonstimulus trial).

clude low-frequency hearing losses, it is important not to underestimate such losses. Lower-frequency threshold estimations may help to identify the problem and/or to monitor recovery from treatment. Accurate thresholds across the audiometric frequency range are needed if a child is to be fitted adequately with a hearing aid.

There are restrictions on using the AMLR in the estimation of auditory thresholds. AMLR latencies and amplitudes are, again, substantially affected by chronological age, state of arousal (awake or asleep), and (if required) sedation level.[41,42] Fortunately, in adolescents and adults, P_a undergoes only minor changes across sleep states and during mild sedation.[43] In deep sleep, the amplitude of P_a may be marginally reduced and latency is likely to be increased. In sedation-induced sleep (for example, by administration of secobarbital), thresholds to 1000-Hz tone bursts in adults can vary by about 6 dB; for example, VDLs ranging from 15 dB SL in light sleep to nearly 22 dB SL deep sleep.[41,42] Such issues will be taken up again in a subsequent chapter (stay tuned).

However, the issue of states of arousal are pervasive and will receive recurrent attention; they have particularly clinically important impacts on the recordings of the AMLR in the younger pediatric population. The N_a wave has the most prominent peak in infants, followed by P_a. In infants and young children, the AMLR is clearly recorded in REM (rapid eye movement) sleep, waking, and light sleep (stage 1). The AMLR becomes more variable and inconsistent in sleep stage 2 and is poorly detectable or absent in the deeper sleep of stages 3 and 4.[44,45] Sleep state 4 is of particular importance in testing of infants and young children because of its negative effect impact on AMLRs. The EEG waves—that is, the un-averaged/"raw" continuous EEG recording—can be used to monitor sleep stage and to inform the clinician when the child is in sleep stages more or less conducive to acquiring reliable responses.[46] Figure 7–15 shows schematic illustrations of morphological changes in the AMLR across sleep stages in young children.

The detectability and reliability of AMLR measures during sleep state improves with age of the infant. Newborn infants spend about half of their sleep time in REM sleep for their first two weeks and accordingly the AMLR is recordable in newborn infants without sleep-stage monitoring.[47] In the first few years after birth, REM sleep decreases to about 25% and stage 4 deep sleep increases up to 46% of total sleep time, resulting in a significant decrease in the detectability of AMLR during sleep

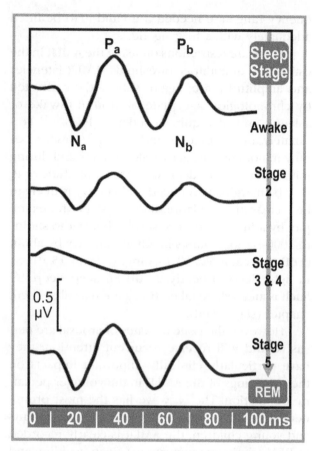

Figure 7–15. Schematic representation of changes in the morphology of AMLR that can occur due to sleep, particularly characteristics of effects of sleep stage in young children (based in part on data reported by Hall [2007][13]).

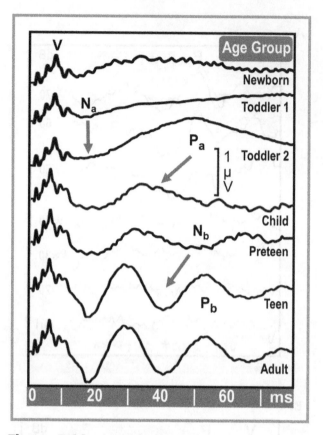

Figure 7–16. Quasimodeling of responses, in part from Figure 7–10B in the last episode, expanded a bit per trends in early childhood. (Toddler 1 and 2—essentially first and second years of age; child—early elementary-school age; *arrows*—highlighting emergence and initial latency changes in main components.) In this modeling, little manipulation of the ABR complex was done—but see Figure 6–9, devoted to changes during the first few years of life. Based in part on data of Kraus and coworkers (1987)[30] who initially demonstrated the potential value of combined ABR/AMLR recording.

in young children.[46] With maturation of generator sources for the AMLR, such as the thalamocortical pathway, the P_a wave becomes consistent and more robust during sleep.[44] The changes during preadult development are more compelling, as seen in Figure 7–16.[48] The detectability of AMLR increases with age up through the first decade of life, with a progressive decrease in latency and increase in amplitude of P_a. Ipsilaterally recorded AMLRs can be obtained from neonates and young children, but the contralateral response continues to develop over the first decade of life.

Recording parameters to optimize detectability of the AMLR are several. Stimulus rates and filter settings highly affect P_a in infants and young children, with significant interaction with the effects of chronological age.[49,50] The P_a is reliably recorded at rates in the range of 10/s to 13/s and responses become even more robust at slower rates, with a concurrent increase in the detectability.[30,50] Slower rates, however, extend the test time. As in the case of the ABR, clinical tests tend to be administered at the faster rates. Unfortunately, as stimulus rates increase, the AMLR amplitudes decrease, the latencies increase, and morphology becomes poorer. The P_a peak proves to be most resilient at these faster stimulus rates, whereas P_b

is best recorded at rates below 1.1/s. The decimal point is not misplaced here; this component requires such slower rates because the time-space frontier of LLRs is being "breached." This slower rate is consistent with P_b sitting on the conventionally defined border between the middle and long-latency AEPs, where it has characteristics that fit both AEP categories. This potential then is defined both as the latest AMLR component (P_b) and as the leading component of the complex of potentials (P_1-N_1-P_2) initiating the "late" AEPs.[51] At these slower rates, P_a is also consistent and reliably recorded in sleeping adults, while P_b is lost in stages of deep sleep (stages 3 and 4). Not all studies of the AMLR include P_b (by way of duration of the epoch recorded) because of its variability in this context. Shortly, P_b will be discussed as part of the 40-Hz ASSR and, in a subsequent episode, the same potential (a.k.a., P_1/P_{50}) will be considered in the context of long-latency AEPs.

In summary, detectability and amplitude of AMLRs in infants and young children increase with slower stimulus rates in an appropriate sleep/wakefulness state and at appropriate high-pass filter settings. As hinted along the way, filtering of the record is an issue. An optimal filter setting reduces contamination of background EEG and/or other interference with minimal distortion of the true response. AMLR waveforms in young children are likely to be contaminated by extraneous EEG activity of high-amplitude low-frequencies, namely below 20 Hz.[52] Therefore, N_a and P_a waves are recorded best with high-pass filters set to 3 Hz to 15 Hz in adults and 10 Hz to 15 Hz in infants and children.[53] In some adults, however, interference from low-frequency myogenic activity may require a compromise setting of the high-pass cutoff to as high as 30 Hz. Regardless of the high-pass filter setting (low-frequency limit of the intended bandwidth of recording), P_a is more consistently recorded using low-pass filter settings (high-frequency cutoff of band) greater than 300 Hz. The cutoff frequencies of the passband at the analog stage (front-end of the AEP test system) are not the only consideration in filtering; rate of attenuation (roll-off in dB/oct) outside the passband is important too (recall Episode 2.1). Classically, slopes of analog filters were –6 dB/octave or –12 dB/octave, although some work has been done with filters capable of roll-offs of 24 dB or 48 dB per octave. As described earlier (Episode 4.2), digital filters can be programmed readily in modern test systems for more types of filters, steeper slopes, and/or cutoff frequencies. Caution is needed as such filters can distort the AMLR waveforms unacceptably and create AMLR-like artifacts in the absence of the true AMLR.[54]

As discussed in the last episode, stimulus rates at/near 40 Hz elicits quasiperiodic steady-state oscillations in the AMLR. Peak-to-peak amplitudes can exceed 1 µV. The amplitude (+/– residual noise) is stable from cycle-to-cycle of the 40-Hz ASSR, thus not adaptive over duration of stimulation with the continuous modulated carrier.[5] This effect of repetition rate (or modulation frequency of the carrier) is indeed counterintuitive, in reference to both the foregoing discussion of the transient AMLR and in the last episode. It is being effectively facilitated by this relatively high rate of modulation given an underlying response of relatively longer latency, compared to SLRs like the ABR component potentials. Evidence that the 40-Hz ASSR actually responds to the low-frequency end of the cochlea when elicited using a lower carrier frequency (thus appropriately place specific in the cochlea) was demonstrated by the presence of the 40-Hz ASSR in individuals with high-frequency sensorineural hearing losses. The hearing loss thus prevented the high-frequency end (places) of the cochlea from contributing to the response excited explicitly toward the apex.[55] Recall Heads Up 6.2 and how ill-fated was application of FFR measurement for purposes of ERA, as such, and thus favoring the envelop following responses (40- and 80-Hz ASSR) for conducting ERA.

Consequently, the AMLR has the "right stuff" for ERA; but just how good is it? Routinely, the 40-Hz ASSR tends to be used with adults rather than infants and young children. As noted in Episode 6.3 in introducing the 80-Hz response, it is subject to sleep state, just as the AMLR, thus consistent with the derivation of the 40-Hz ASSR from the AMLR. For children, a steady-state response is produced better by a lower stimulation rate, close to 20 Hz.[52] Figure 7–17 depicts the magnitudes of AEPs potentials obtained from adults and infants at various stimulus repetition rates, including a 40-Hz stimulus-response paradigm with evaluation of responses in the frequency domain.[56] Again, the

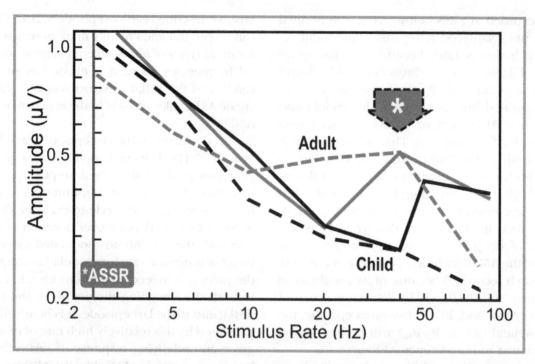

Figure 7–17. AEP amplitudes as a function of stimulus/repetition rate: dashed lines—black for primary school-aged children and gray for young adults (all normally-hearing subjects). Solid lines effectively summarize results of a meta-analysis of the literature from studies of stimulus rate effects on AEPs, carried out in development of a study of ASSRs over a broad range of rates. Both show 40-Hz responses to be considerably reduced in children, but substantially increased in adults, as expected from the first episode (based on data of Tlumak et al. [2012][56]).

80-Hz ASSR is impervious to sleep state; consequently, it is the choice for ASSR-ERA in infants and young children.

The 40-Hz ASSR, like the transient AMLR, improves response detectability in the lower audiometric frequencies as compared to the ABR. The 40-Hz ASSR-ERA thus may have an edge in approximating the true behavioral thresholds. In adults with normal hearing, the amplitudes of the 40-Hz ASSR are substantially larger compared to amplitudes of the AMLR for clicks and tone bursts; this amplitude advantage is maintained as the stimuli are decreased to near-threshold levels. Levels of 40-Hz ASSR detection average 5 dB to 30 dB above audiometric thresholds from 500 Hz to 4000 Hz, with the highest ERA-behavioral threshold differences occurring in the higher frequencies.[57]

Threshold estimates in adults with sensorineural hearing losses are typically closer to behavioral thresholds than they are in adults with normal hearing, due to neural recruitmentlike behavior. Figure 7–18A demonstrates results by way of Galambos's original method[27] in a study based primarily on time-domain analysis.[58] For demonstration purposes here, results of this study were used by the first author to effect a comparison of the 40-Hz ASSR between 500 Hz and 2000 Hz (originally 1500 Hz and 3000 Hz, but essentially the same results at the two high frequencies, justifying collapsing these data). The results are for a subject tested in whom a predominantly low-frequency hearing loss was simulated by simultaneously presenting a low-pass filtered noise with the test stimuli. The VDLs were observed to be 75 dB and 45 dB SPL, respectively, at 500 Hz and 2000 Hz. The responses recorded have been overlaid on 40-Hz sine waves approximating them in amplitude and phase. Note the phase shifts across levels. The tracings below the VDLs fail to have the sinusoidal (thus periodic) morphology as well as

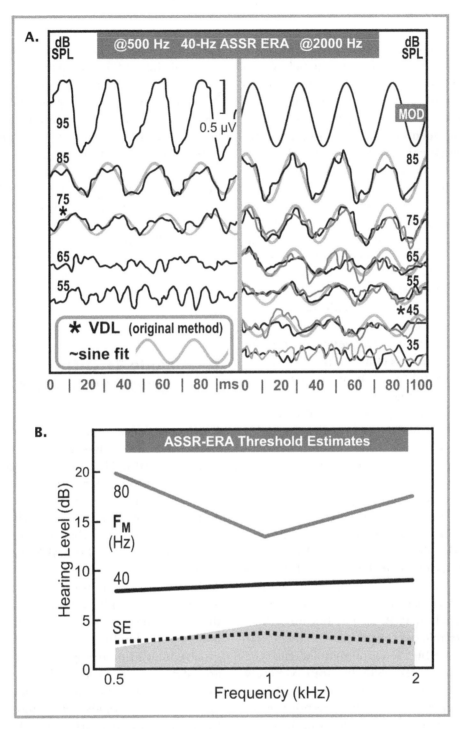

Figure 7–18. A. Virtual demonstration of determining VDLs of 40-Hz ASSRs in a case of simulated low-frequency hearing loss (see text). Here the recorded 40-Hz signal (analyzed in the time domain), traditionally via conventional ERA and overlaid with a 40-Hz sinusoid (*the MOD, modulator in gray*), is fitted to each response deemed at or above VDL for each test (carrier) frequency. **B.** Comparisons in normal-hearing subjects between 40-Hz and 80-Hz ASSRs for carrier frequencies of 500 Hz, 1000 Hz, and 2000 Hz. ASSR thresholds are closer to behavioral thresholds at 40-Hz versus 80-Hz rate at all three test frequencies (SE–standard error; based on data of Petito et al. [2005][59]).

the usual lack of test–retest cross correlation (2-kHz side). The mean differences between behavioral thresholds and the 40-Hz ASSR-ERA estimations observed were 5 dB and 9 dB, respectively. In individuals with actual low-frequency hearing loss, the 40-Hz VDLs had been found to fall overall within 19 dB of audiometric thresholds, wherein they better approximated behavior thresholds of lower than higher frequencies.

Results from a more recent study employing current ASSR methods are summarized in Figure 7–18B and permit comparisons in normal-hearing subjects of results using both 40- and 80-Hz ASSR tests for audiometric frequencies—500 Hz, 1000 Hz, and 2000 Hz.[59] Estimates from the 40-Hz ASSR tests were substantially better at all three test frequencies, with no compelling trend of substantial differences over frequency. Current instrumentation provides spectral and phase analyses and other tools useful to aid the examiner to estimate thresholds more rigorously than by visual detection (as discussed in Episodes 4.1 and 6.2).

Various underlying factors can alter the 40-Hz ASSR. Because it results from virtually overlapping transient responses, comprising both ABR and AMLR components, an absent or abnormal ABR can reduce the amplitude advantage of the 40-Hz ASSR over the AMLR. A 40-Hz ASSR is recorded reliably in adults who are awake or in light sleep. The 40-Hz ASSR diminishes and detection limits increase during deep sleep,[60] which implies that P_b is included in the overlapping responses. As discussed previously, the P_b indeed is affected by sleep state, whereas P_a is not. Because P_b in the AMLR is variable, its contribution to the 40-Hz ASSR is likely variable. Sedation may increase the threshold of the 40-Hz ASSR by approximately 15 dB.[61] In sum, changes in the 40-Hz ASSR during sleep stages may interfere with superposition of the wave components, thereby elevating hearing-threshold estimates.[62]

This episode focused on the use of the AMLRs to estimate audiometric thresholds, but the transient AMLR has other clinical applications, which are explored in the upcoming episode. Historically, AMLRs overlapped applications with the shorter latency responses, although the AMLR has not stirred up the same level of interest in research and development, nor for routine use in clinical electrophysiology. Nevertheless, the AMLR in the guise of the 40-Hz response, effectively launched a new wave of interest in AMLRs overall and fostered a family of auditory steady-state responses with a large range of repetition rates that are applicable to the assessment of brainstem through auditory cortex. Within this group, the 40-Hz ASSR stands out, literally, with its robust amplitude. New analyses since Galambos' revelation have emerged, primarily by moving analyses to the frequency domain. The related tools deserve to be in the clinician's toolbox and clinicians should remain mindful of them. Research and development continues, as is warranted, and innovative applications are expected to continue to emerge.

■ Episode 3: Differential Diagnostic Applications of AMLR

Previously, overall nuances were explored of both transient and steady-state MLRs and their applications to ERA. This final episode in the series is dedicated to exploration of the potential roles of the AMLR in differential diagnosis. On the one hand, a comprehensive review is beyond the scope of this episode, given that such a role is not yet as well defined as that of the ABR and yet the volume of literature apropos is substantial. Still, as with the ABR, there are several disorders for which AMLR testing appears to have tangible clinical value. On the other hand, the place of the AMLR in AEPdom is also considerably more expansive for possible involvement in neurological disorders. There also are interests beyond site-of-lesion-based effects on the AMLR. Such effects are related to the inherently diffuse etiologies, yet are those that can cause substantial dysfunctions for which the AMLR could assist in their evaluation.

The first point of discussion is that of the ***target population*** of the AMLR. Because the AMLR tests a specific region of the auditory system, its clinical use is warranted when clinicians suspect an issue at this level or when there is a need to evaluate the consequences of peripheral impairment at a more central level than is covered by tests of the ABR. The AMLR is used commonly in conjunction with other auditory evoked potentials (mainly the ABR) as well as other tests of auditory function, including behavioral evaluations. The AMLR components are estimated to reflect aspects of auditory processing, such as activities involved in primary (recognition, discrimination, and figure-ground) and nonprimary (selective attention, auditory sequence, auditory novelty, and audio-visual integration) listening skills.[64,65] Therefore, suspicions of decrease or impairment of such functions would justify recording/evaluating the AMLR.

Numerous studies have been devoted to investigations of the possible clinical roles of the AMLR in evaluating the thresholds of hearing in patients too young or unable to be tested behaviorally, in diagnosing hearing loss, and in evaluating central auditory processing functions. These roles are much the same as the roles of the ABR in clinical audiology; so what might be some advantages of the AMLR? First, the AMLR (again) typically has a larger amplitude than the ABR. As extraction of the target potential is playing the SNR game, a greater signal certainly should have an advantage in the objective measure of hearing sensitivity/other auditory function. This expectation was shown to be somewhat realized with the AMLR measures in the last episode despite their own limitations. This clinical application was limited, in particular, by AMLR having some dependence on state of arousal. This limitation is significant for clinical applications in newborns, infants, and other young children when natural sleep or sedation is necessary to perform the evaluation. These matters are equally applicable to use of the response for other clinical purposes, including differential diagnosis. AMLR testing, in practice, is typically reserved for individuals with relatively normal peripheral hearing sensitivity who present with deficits that suggest involvement of the CANS, especially beyond the generator sites for the ABR, as the AMLR generators are situated further long the AEP space continuum. A consistently absent or reduced AMLR combined with a normal or near-normal ABR, good hearing sensitivity by conventional audiometry, and a suggestive history are strong indicators of thalamocortical, central auditory involvement.[66]

The AMLR *generators* must be considered in any application of AMLR. Just as the interpretation of ABR results requires consideration of the relevant part of the auditory pathway, so does the AMLR. To reiterate, this AEP represents the earliest cortical responses or more, specifically, the ***thalamocortical potentials***, which have different components labeled by their voltage polarity and temporal sequence after stimulus onset (i.e., P_0, N_a, P_a, N_b, and P_b), as reviewed in Figure 7–19 and which now warrant a bit more discussion of details. The presence of the initial wave P_0 tends to be variable and vulnerable to contamination with myogenic potentials. P_0, therefore, has limited clinical application for now and (for purposes of this book) will not be treated here. The consensus has come to be that the AMLR components are mainly generated by the auditory cortex, with possible contributions of the upper brainstem and thalamus.[7] Otherwise, the N_a component (with a peak latency around 15 ms to 25 ms) originates from the posteromedial parts of Heschl's gyrus, while the posteromedial Heschl's gyrus, Heschl's sulcus, planum temporale, and the posterior superior temporal gyrus appear to all contribute to the P_a component (peak latency around 25 ms to 30 ms) with additional contributions from the mesencephalic reticular formation, at least in young children.[8] The N_b component arises from sources in the midbrain or auditory cortex. P_b emerges around 50 ms and is generated laterally in the primary area of the cortex, although its origin is still being debated and no anatomical localization of lesion can be inferred from its alteration.

Considerations of ***measures of clinical interest*** and ***recording montage*** for clinical evaluation focus commonly on conditions optimal to determine the presence or absence of the N_a and P_a components and/or their amplitudes and latencies. However, unlike the ABR, the AMLR's advantage for diagnostic utility is predominantly its amplitude, rather than its latency.[66] Because the AMLR has component potentials that originate from sources close to the surface of the scalp, they tend to show more variation with electrode position compared to the ABR. Electrodes, therefore, must be placed accurately using conventions such as the International 10-20 system (recall Figure 3–3). The electrodes should be placed over each hemisphere to evaluate the ear and electrode-location effects, which can help in the localization of a lesion. For neurological evaluation, electrodes connected to

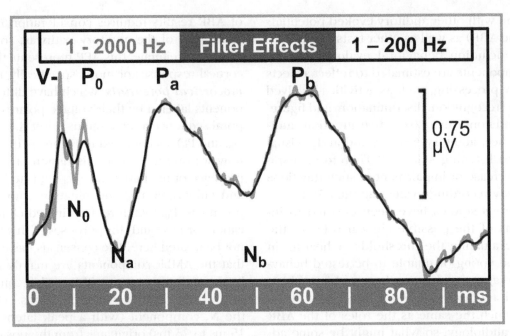

Figure 7–19. Courtesy recap of salient features of the AMLR, for two different passbands of analog filtering (replot of Figure 7–6B), as the focus now fully embraces the N_a-to-P_b components, as virtually highlighted by the 1-200-Hz "version."

the noninverting input of the preamplifier are placed at the vertex (C_z or F_z) and on the left (C_3-C_5) and right scalp (C_4-C_6) over the temporal lobes (recall Figure 7–6A). Binaural stimulation, if used, the AMLR is best recorded between C_z or F_z and at the back of the neck (at C_7). The use of multiple indices, including ear effects, electrode-location effects, delayed latencies, and/or reduced amplitudes (compared to norms) increase the sensitivity of the recorded AMLR to lesions. Using the AMLR with other diagnostic procedures, especially tests of the ABR, enhances the tool. In fact, simultaneously recording the ABR and AMLR allows for more precise site-of-lesion determination, namely to distinguish between brainstem and midbrain lesions.[67] An important question remains, however, about the degree to which an abnormal ABR related to a brainstem lesion may influence the subsequent AMLR morphology.

There is undeniably a potential value of the AMLR from the diagnostic perspective across lesion types, especially for those affecting the cortical and subcortical areas rostral to the brainstem. In fact, there are situations, such as cases of central deafness, in which AMLR is one of the few audiological alternatives that can lead to the diagnosis of this disorder. This is particularly true in patients with auditory complaints, normal cochlear function, and normal ABR but abnormal ALLR. The AMLR overall appears to be fairly sensitive to brainstem/midbrain lesions.[68] Sensitivity for group studies ranged from 0.29 to 0.89, with an average sensitivity of 0.56. Sensitivity was similar overall for neurodegenerative diseases, ranging from 0.21 to 0.73 with an average sensitivity of 0.48. Sensitivity was higher for stroke cases, with a range of about 0.52 to 0.64. In cases of head injury, sensitivity was lower overall (range: 0.38–0.55; average = 0.47). In accordance with these values from reports on relatively specific lesions and in the studies that combined lesion types, overall sensitivity was roughly 0.50. AMLR also can be used to monitor recovery from neural damage and evaluate the efficacy of rehabilitation protocols. The AMLR is an objective and noninvasive technique that can be applied at all ages, with some limitations as described in the following text.

In *differential neurodiagnosis*, the AMLR may provide information regarding the site of lesion and thereby help to support/refute a given diagnosis. Considerable evidence confirms that the AMLR is of value for evaluating lesions or dysfunctions of the central auditory nervous system and is especially sensitive to lesions of the auditory cortex and thalamocortical connections.[10,69,70] Typically, only the early components of the AMLR, N_a, and P_a are used clinically as the P_b wave is not reliably evoked by typical clinical AMLR paradigms,[68] although the detectability of P_b can be enhanced using slow repetition rates (no greater than ≈1.1/s) and is best recorded from an electrode at F_Z (connected to the noninverting preamplifier input) and an electrode for a noncephalic reference (like C_7), connected to the inverting input. Its amplitude (again) is generally greater when a relatively lower-frequency, as well as longer-duration, stimulus is used.[12]

The AMLR may be reduced or absent when recorded over the lesioned temporal lobe and interhemispheric amplitude difference for the P_a component reflects the side of the cortical lesion, regardless of which ear is stimulated. The N_a and P_a generator sites are essentially bilateral, from two dipole sources located within the temporal lobes. Consequently, patients with unilateral temporal lobe lesions present with reduced or absent P_a over the involved hemisphere, whereas this component is unchanged over the contralateral hemisphere.[10,71] Similarly, because N_a generators are separate from P_a, P_a is most affected by lesions of the posterior aspect of the superior temporal gyrus, while N_a amplitude is not affected. The decrease in the AMLR response has been linked to impaired performance in a psychoacoustic discrimination test in patients with a unilateral auditory cortex lesion, thereby reinforcing the role of AMLR in neurodiagnosis.[72] In contrast, investigators on several studies failed to find AMLR asymmetries in patients with cortical lesions that did not affect the temporal lobes, as well as in cases of unilateral anterior temporal lobectomy (a neurosurgical procedure used in treatment of epileptics with intractable seizures).[69,73]

The AMLR has been shown to have potential informational value in **neurodegenerative disorders**, starting with **multiple sclerosis (MS)**. Increased latencies of the waves P_a and P_b or an absence of waveform components occur in about 50% of patients diagnosed with MS among several studies.[68] In evaluating the efficacy of tests of ABR, AMLR, and ALLR to detect multiple sclerosis,[74] abnormalities were identified in these responses in 65%, 42.5%, and 30% of the cases sampled for these AEPs, respectively. The combined sensitivity of ABR and AMLR tests amounted to 80%, and 87.5% when all three tests were considered together. However, MS is a variable disorder (over time and location(s) of lesions), so the pattern of AEP responses affected is inevitably variable among patients.

In cases of **stroke**, AMLR latencies have been found to be related to the recovery from aphasia, as measured by the Boston Aphasia Examination.[73] In particular, the N_b peak latency recorded during the first days after stroke was related to the language score difference after 6 months. In line with this study, others showed that AMLR could be used to monitor the effectiveness of therapy, such as in stutterers.[75]

Effects of **traumatic brain injury (TBI)** have come under increasingly more scrutiny. Head trauma has a wide range of causes, including falls, sports (professional and recreational), vehicular accidents, and other accidents, including those involving explosives. The severity can range from mild to severe in all the ways that the injury occurs. As observed in an investigation of a sizable cohort (nearly 300 victims), an association was found between the severity of TBI and the extent of auditory dysfunction.[76] The amplitude of N_a and P_a decreased with increased severity, along with an increase in wave V and I–V interpeak latency of the ABR. Other studies reported indicated that the P_b/P_{50} response suggested reduced sensory gating (to be discussed shortly) in the TBI group compared to the control group, although no differences occurred among the mild, moderate, and severe subgroups of TBI.[77] However, other studies[78] have not yielded findings of significant AMLR changes in patients with head trauma, probably reflecting a difference in the sites of lesion among studies, test protocols, and/or time intervals between the brain injury and the AMLR assessment. Further studies are warranted to assess critically the clinical role of AMLR in the follow-up after injury to monitor improvement and course of improvement in TBI.

Central auditory processing disorders (CAPDs) have challenged the field of audiology to develop rigorous methods of testing and critically monitored treatment. Clinicians are confronted with teasing apart peripheral versus central processing deficits and addressing other problems that may present in this heterogeneous group where other disorders, such as language impairment and learning disabilities, frequently coexist. For some time, the AMLR has been used to evaluate children with CAPD because this electrophysiological test removes attention and memory (up to a certain degree) from the measurement process. The AMLR can detect abnormalities even when behavioral measures suggest normal function. Further, the AMLR is related less to the state of arousal and attention compared to late/cortical AEPs, which is an advantage in this particular population because attention deficits can influence testing.[44] Because the AMLR arises from the thalamocortical pathways, implying possible involvement of both subcortical and cortical auditory structures, the AMLR is a promising tool in evaluating children with listening complaints or suspected CAPD. For example, lower amplitudes of the AMLR in a CAPD group have been observed, compared to those of a control group of children.[79] Both latencies and amplitudes of the P_a and N_a components as well as the binaural interaction component of the AMLR (coming soon) have been reported to differ in children suspected of CAPD.[80] The AMLR in some children with CAPD may have delayed latencies and reduced amplitudes and can be used to identify abnormal central auditory asymmetries with implications in monitoring changes during management of the CAPD, as indicated in the following text. AMLR measures, however, do not specify particular auditory processing abilities as assessed by behavioral tests. They are, rather, indicative of presumed functional measures, like auditory discrimination, masking, or performance in the presence of degraded acoustic signals.

Another advantage of the AMLR is that it can be used to measure posttherapy improvements in central auditory function. After having several weeks of auditory training, children had AMLRs with significant changes in wave amplitude/detectability that correlated with measures of their behavioral improvement[79,81,82]. Therefore, the AMLR can serve as an objective measure of the changes that occur with auditory training.

Abnormalities in AMLR (and later AEP components) also have been reported in children with a wide range of communication disorders. Typical findings are prolonged N_a and/or P_a latency and smaller N_b amplitude in children with listening difficulties,[83] learning,[84,85] or language impairments.[86] Such results are taken to suggest slower processing and possibly more asynchronous neural firing in the auditory thalamocortical pathways that contribute to the AMLR components. Results reported from various studies have shown delayed latencies for N_a in the left hemisphere in children with learning disabilities, including reading and writing disorders. From such results, it has been hypothesized that the dysfunction of the left contralateral auditory pathway can produce difficulties in sound decoding.[87] Consequently, this dysfunction can also lead to losses in the association of linguistic components with visual components and/or induce flaws in association of auditory information with the linguistic information at primary and nonprimary cortical areas. For instance, the error in processing speed may explain the inability to read and write properly. The reticular formation, likely involved in the generation of the AMLR as stated earlier, may be involved in some of the AMLR abnormalities seen in children with learning disabilities. The reticular formation modulates overall arousal and receptiveness to sensory input, but a defective reticular formation could not carry out its brain-regulating process effectively and thereby would prevent important auditory information from being processed adequately by the cortex.

An intriguing effect (as hinted earlier), coined **sensory gating** in the psychiatry and neurology literature, features the P_{50} component at the "border" between the AMLR and the ALLR, developed originally in relation to diagnosis and treatment of schizophrenia. More recently, the effect and further refinement of the method is generating attention in relation to some auditory deficits. Sensory gating (as defined) is a preattentive, natural response of the brain to attenuate irrelevant sensory stimuli, a difficult feat for individuals with schizophrenia. The gating response is thought to be a critical underlying psychophysiological and protective mechanism of brain function, namely to prevent sensory overload and subsequent cognitive disturbances. A typical sensory gating paradigm is that of presenting stimuli in pairs that are 500-ms apart, with a 10 s interval between pairs. The first stimulus (S1) elicits an excitatory P_{50} (naturally) before an inhibitory response can develop and thus reflects the capacity of the neuronal system to respond in the absence of inhibition. The second stimulus (S2) elicits a diminished P_{50} because the inhibitory mechanism was activated by S1. Therefore, this is a test of the "strength" of the inhibitory mechanisms activated or conditioned during the first stimulus.[88] Sensory gating or P_{50} suppression is measured by the ratio of amplitudes of P_{50} responses to S1 and S2 (S2/S1). S2/S1 ratios of <0.4 in adults imply intact sensory gating.[89]

Use of the AMLR overall, and P_{50} in particular, has been explored for many years in various clinical populations. Some of the disorders that may attract auditory interest in P_{50} include Alzheimer's disease, mild cognitive impairment, traumatic brain injury, developmental disorders, and autism spectrum disorders. For example, Alzheimer's disease patients produced S2/S1 ratio of 0.89 versus S2/S1 ratio of 0.58 in healthy older adults, suggestive of reduced sensory gating, as shown in Figure 7–20.[90] In patients, increased P_{50} ratios may represent a functional disconnection to the prefrontal cortex which exerts inhibitory control over multiple subcortical and cortical regions,[91] including auditory cortical responses.[92-94] Significantly increased S2/S1 ratio or poor P_{50} suppression thus can serve as a biological marker of abnormal inhibitory processing in patients with Alzheimer's disease/other disorders.

Although testing the P_{50} is broadly promising for differential-diagnostic applications, compelling **limitations** must be considered. One is the lack of established paradigms, without which norms cannot be developed. Another factor is the large within-group variability, notwithstanding good within-subject reliability. Both latency and amplitude values are highly variable depending on stimulus and recording parameters, including specific electrode placement.[66,95] Other barriers to the clinical use of P_{50} are the current disagreements as to the specific generator sites of the components, the elusive nature of specific auditory functions, and the uncertain clinical interpretation of findings.

Effects of **early maturation** and **advanced age** were shown in Episodes 7.1 and 7.2 to be important factors in AMLR measurement and inter-

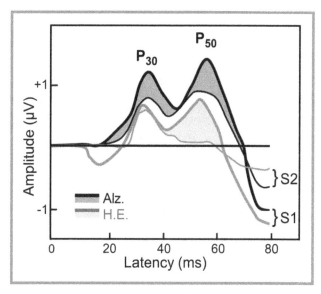

Figure 7–20. Simplified model of P_{50} waveforms recorded at the vertex and trends comparatively of results of tests of auditory sensory gating (S2/S1 ratio) in Alzheimer's (Alz.) patients and healthy elderly (H.E.) control subjects. Central tendencies for the two groups are overlaid for the two stimuli, respectively in the sensory-gating paradigm (S1 and S2; see text). Alzheimer's patients tend to have more responses to S1 for both P_{30} and P_{50} components and with a lesser amount of overall suppression per areas between the P_{50} S1 and S2 curves (*dark versus light gray*) and/or stronger/more-complete suppression of P_{50} in the control group (based on data of Thomas et al. [2010][90]).

pretation. Added to the latter is the potential confound of **age-related hearing loss**. The effects of early maturation were overviewed and shown in Figure 7–10. To both recap and further characterize trends, the AMLR undergoes changes in morphology, latency, and amplitude like the other types of AEPs as they reflect the maturation of the peripheral and central auditory systems. In infants and young children, P_a is of smaller amplitudes with longer latencies until adultlike values are reached around 8 to 10 years of age. The P_b component matures more slowly, up to around 15 years of age.[5,96] The detectability of P_a has be found to be less than 50% in sleeping children under the age of 10 years, and even only 20% of children under 1 year of age had a P_a response, while about 65% demonstrated the N_a wave.[48] However, the presence of AMLR component

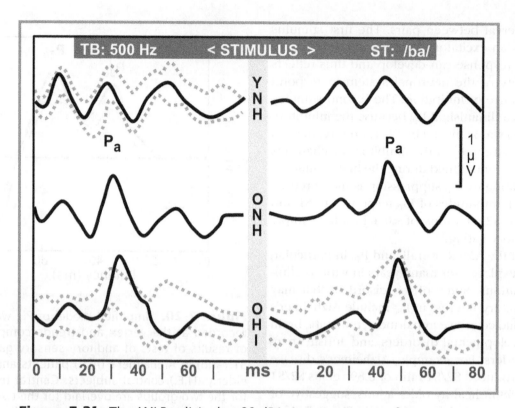

Figure 7–21. The AMLRs elicited at 90 dBA, Leq, a measure of SPL made using the A-scale frequency response of the sound level meter with time-weighted averaging. This approach was to balance the stimulus levels of the two types of stimuli used—500-Hz tone bursts (*left*) and the syllable /ba/ (*right*). Three groups of subjects were employed: young normal-hearing adults (YNH); older adults with near-normal hearing (ONH); older hearing-impaired adults (OHI). The OHI group shows the largest AMLR, followed by ONH and YNH group in descending order. TB—tone burst; ST—speech token (as indicated). Black lines are grand means (across group) averages. Dotted lines approximate pointwise ranges of individual-response tracings, similar overall, so only shown for a few averages. The exception is the OHI group tone-burst condition that had one substantial outlier, perhaps biasing the group mean slightly, yet without substantially affecting overall outcomes (based on data of Park and Fowler [2021][103]).

waves becomes close to 100% around 10 to 12 years of age. Still, others have reported observing AMLRs in all awake children from the ages of 7 years and up.[97] The AMLR can be recorded in infants and young children, given appropriate stimulus rate, filter settings, and stage of arousal. The combination of ABR and AMLR testing in infants may increase the diagnostic sensitivity of neurophysiologic assessment of the functional status of the peripheral and central auditory systems.[98]

Moving along the life span—after the AMLR achieves a period of stability in young and middle adulthood —the AMLR undergoes appreciable changes with advancing age, as was demonstrated in Figure 7–11. As hearing sensitivity tends to decrease with aging, these morphological effects warrant further scrutiny to discern peripheral from central auditory system changes. In particular and as seen in Figure 7–21, the P_a component significantly increases in amplitude with a constant or slightly prolonged latency in older adults.[31] Furthermore, age-related enhancement of P_a amplitude increases in combination with hearing loss (see OHI data). The data presented in this figure are derived from a study using both a tone burst and a speech token for stimuli. N_a-P_a and P_a-N_b (peak-to-peak) amplitudes approximately double in older adults, and baseline-peak measures of the P_a component produce an even more substantial increase, yet seemingly with little increases in variance. These changes occur consistently with both monaural and binaural stimulation. The age-related variation in the P_a component is not necessarily accompanied by changes in N_a, reflecting the fact that different neural sources may be at the respective origins of N_a and P_a. Whereas P_b amplitude increases with age, its latency shortens.[99]

The AMLR is not acutely dependent on as "sharp" an onset of the stimulus for adequate synchrony as (again) is the ABR. To recap, AMLRs may be measurable despite neural dyssynchrony disorders, such as caused by damage at the level of the 8th nerve or in the lower brainstem pathway. Therefore, the ABR and AMLR recorded together can be useful particularly to evaluate deficits from the periphery to the auditory cortex. ABR results therein are taken to be substantially indicative of lesions from the periphery through to the pontine brainstem; AMLR results can be used to evaluate more central dysfunction. This differentiation is particularly useful in older adults wherein hearing problems, indeed, may derive from a mix of peripheral and central processing problems. Consequently, the AMLR is helpful to tease apart effects of aging on the auditory system.[100]

As hearing loss and aging tend to go hand in hand (to some extent), such as teasing-out in differential diagnostics (as for the ABR, recall Episode 6.5), it is always important to account for relatively peripheral versus central dysfunction, and in that order. High-frequency sensorineural hearing loss can reduce the dynamic range of the AMLR, yet has been seen to produce a greater increase in the AMLR with increasing sound level.[101] Still, is this not simply a recruitment effect?[102] Some results are summarized in Figure 7–22 that speak to this issue.[103] Here, AMLRs were measured in young adults with normal hearing (control group, YNH1) and in a group of older subjects with hearing impairment (OHI). Test stimuli were tone bursts presented at relatively high SPLs (70 dB–100 dB, upper dynamic range of hearing) at 500 Hz and 2000 Hz. The input-output functions for the YNH1 group show nearly saturated

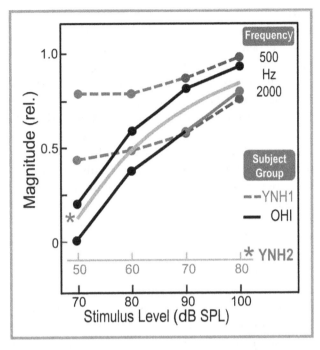

Figure 7–22. Amplitude-intensity functions of AMLR P_a for each type of stimulus (500-Hz and 2000-Hz tone bursts) with increasing sound levels. The solid lines represent older hearing-impaired (OHI) listeners and dashed lines represent young normal-hearing (YNH1) listeners. Slopes of the P_a amplitude growth functions were clearly steeper in OHI listeners, indicating faster growth rate in P_a amplitude in the aging auditory system. The solid gray line approximates input-output functions at 1000 Hz from a recent study that included 40-Hz ASSRs, effecting another group for comparisons (YNH2). In that group/study, the intensity range examined did not exceed 80 dB, hence 50-dB to 80-dB data but which coincidentally closely follows the OHI functions. At the same time, this function is showing saturation beginning at the same tests for the YNH1 group when placed on the same SPL scale (primary graphs based on data from Park and Fowler [2021][103]; added function, gray line, based on data of Tlumak and coworkers [2016][104]).

growth (outputs) at such levels. The I-O functions of the OHI group are seen to converge on the YNH1 group's functions, respectively. In an earlier study, the I-O function of the 40-Hz ASSR was examined in a similar young adult group (YNH2)—at 1000 Hz but mid- rather than upper-dynamic range levels. A similar function as that of the OHI group was reported by other researchers from results in normal-hearing subjects (see Figures 7–4[17] and 7–22, function in gray[104]). The OHI group's trends thus bespeak primarily a recruitment effect (output similar to "normal" once the hearing loss is substantially "overcome"), thus attributable primarily to hearing loss of peripheral origin.

Nevertheless and as previously stated (Episode 7.1), age-related loss of inhibitory inputs into the subcortical levels (such as the inferior colliculus and medial geniculate body) can cause an imbalance between inhibitory and excitatory functions in the CANS resulting in the enhanced amplitude of AMLR in older adults. Age-dependent enhancement of AMLR may be attributed to age-related functional reorganization. A prominent notion is that of plasticity in the CANS follows peripheral damage.[105] Similarly, enhanced amplitude with age also has been found in the visual[106,107] and somatosensory evoked potentials.[108] A possible underlying mechanism is that of an age-dependent increase in a theoretical central gain (amplification), perhaps following compensatory down regulation of GABAergic inhibition and subsequent overactive neural networks forming the central generators of sensory EPs like the AMLR. Although much of the theoretical basis for generation of AEPs naturally centers on excitatory processes, inhibition occurs broadly in the nervous system. It thus is reasonable to assume some role of inhibition in AEP generation, and thus a component of changes over the life span. By virtue of arborization within the CANS (recall Episode 3.2), enhanced central gain or whatever aging effects can be expected to occur at multiple stages, consequently, produce more pronounced increase in the amplitude of neural responses at higher levels of the auditory pathway. Such effects have been suggested at the cortical level and are likely to occur independently of hearing loss.[109] However, age-related morphological changes in AMLR have substantial intra- and intersubject variability,[110] as was seen in Figure 7–21. A variety of alterations in AMLR with advancing age may be attributable to various neural sources changing differentially as physiological processes age, again at both subcortical and cortical levels of the auditory system.[111–113]

In line with age-related enhancement of the P_a component, the P_b amplitude increases with normal aging.[114,115] Age-related increase in P_b amplitude is even larger as recorded over the left versus right hemisphere with contralateral (right ear) stimulation,[33] which may reflect right-ear advantage in older adults.[116,117]

AMLR has also been used to study binaural processing in normal-hearing and hearing-loss patients. For example, a strong correlation has been reported between the binaural masking level difference (MLD) and the P_a-N_a, binaural interaction component.[118] Moreover, they observed reduced binaural processing in subjects with symmetrical pure-tone sensitivity but asymmetrical performance on a word recognition in noise test (with and without hearing loss). However, the ever-intriguing issue of binaural interaction will be deferred now to the upcoming Heads Up, dedicated to searching beyond the ABR-BIC (featured earlier), probing for similar effects at the AMLR's level of AEP time-space and beyond.

There remain some "special interest" clinical groups worthy of consideration for AMLR testing, namely for other auditory/neurological disorders or audiological concerns for which AMLR findings might provide insights. The first are patients with *tinnitus*. Tinnitus can occur regardless of presence of hearing loss or degree of hearing impairment. Morphological alterations of the AMLR have been demonstrated in individuals reporting tinnitus. A marked enlargement of N_a and P_a amplitude of AMLR has been reported in normal hearing adults with tinnitus compared to individuals without tinnitus.[119] The enlargement occurred without correspondingly larger ABR potentials,[120] thus suggestive of changes at the level of neural generators for AMLR in individuals with tinnitus. Similarly, in individuals with hearing loss, AMLR waves were also greater with tinnitus than without tinnitus. However, AMLR waves were clearly larger in the elderly compared to hearing-matched adults with tinnitus, even though there is a large interindividual variability in AMLR waves in both the elderly and individuals with tinnitus.[120] Figure 7–23 shows a schematic illustration of AMLRs for issues of and/or interactions of normal versus hearing loss, tinnitus, and aging. Such marked differences in electrophysiological findings may be associated with altered neuronal excitability following a loss of intracortical inhibition in the functionally reorganized central auditory system. In particular,

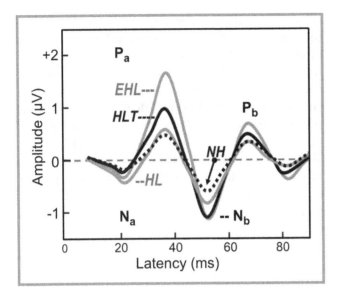

Figure 7–23. Schematic illustration of the auditory middle latency responses to 1-kHz tone bursts in normal hearing adults (NH), adults with hearing loss (HL), adults with hearing loss and tinnitus (HLT), and elderly adults with hearing loss (EHL)(based on data of Gerken and coworkers [2001][120]).

there are effects of stimulus frequency in AMLRs and 40-Hz responses that have been observed in tinnitus patients, which are attributable to tonotopic-map reorganization in tinnitus-frequency regions.[121] However, the pathophysiology of tinnitus remains unclear, and further research is needed to evaluate if the morphological alterations in the middle-latency responses can provide objective detection of tinnitus and/or other neurophysiological information apropos the origin and/or effective management of tinnitus.

Another group of interest are patients with **hearing aids**. Modern hearing aids generally are designed with nonlinear circuits, matching the reality that so is the auditory system (as noted earlier). Simply amplifying all frequencies of sounds at all sound levels linearly, thus just making sound louder, proves not to be efficacious for most patients needing amplification. Fitting nonlinear hearing aids requires information about loudness to optimize the prescriptive fit. However, obtaining loudness data (using behavioral measures) in some clinical populations is difficult, if not impossible, such as young children and individuals with cognitive and/or intellectual disabilities. Therefore,

there is an interest in using auditory evoked potentials to associate loudness judgments with corresponding objective measures over virtually the full auditory dynamic range of hearing, from soft to loud sounds. It has been suggested that ABR wave V and AMLR-P_a latencies appear to be sensitive indicators of changes in the listener's perception of loudness for brief tone-burst stimuli.[122]

In this same vein, patients with **cochlear implants** stimulated interests in all types of AEPs, a topic for a dedicated/comprehensive overview (coming soon!). Electrically elicited AMLRs (eAMLRs, stimulated via the device but otherwise recorded as in acoustic stimulation) can be recorded in patients post cochlear implantation. This test is deemed useful for an objective evaluation of auditory cortical functions and postoperative habilitation[123] in addition to the eABR. In adults, eAMLR thresholds positively correlate with acoustic thresholds obtained with the CI, therefore suggesting a role in the evaluation of infants and young children before (or when) a behavioral response cannot be obtained. Other studies, however, have not found well-defined relations between the eAMLR and speech recognition measures, which suggest that the AMLRs may not be clinically as useful in the early stages of implantation.[124] Nevertheless, CIs created a "hot bed" of research that continues; thus, further studies are warranted and, likely, eAMLR testing perhaps will turn up in the highly specialized but robust toolbox that has come to be richly supported for pre- and postimplantation management.

Notwithstanding limitations noted along the way, AMLR measurement has been a constant tool in the AEP toolbox for nearly as long as the other AEPs and certainly should be considered as part of a differential-diagnosis test battery, as long as limitations are understood in any given application. It is also important to note that several features of the AMLR response are not yet fully understood, so the results of ongoing/future research studies are needed to expand clinical applications. Among the features being investigated currently is the unlocked oscillatory EEG activity and represents a rich source of information about brain function. The assessment of these EEG oscillations has implications for P_{50} in the context of sensory gating.[125] More elaborated protocols are also being used to evaluate auditory perceptual organization with AMLR and top-down influences on brainstem activity from the thalamocortical pathways. "Central" masking evaluation is also under evaluation using contralateral masking of the AMLR.[126] The reduced dependency of the AMLR on synchrony is useful in disorders such as ANSD and other central neurological/dyssynchrony disorders. Although recent studies have focused more on ALLR responses in ANSD patients than on AMLR, these potentials may have a role to play in complex patients who present with a combination of ANSD (such as, impaired periphery) and central impairment. Lastly, the relationships between AMLR features and speech processing in different listening environments (such as, in noise) have yet to be fully explored. There clearly is plenty to do and can be done by researchers and clinicians alike "in the middle" of AEPdom. Meanwhile, in current practice of clinical electrophysiology in audiology, the middle-latency responses certainly never should be discounted out of hand, as modern AEP test instrumentation equally certainly has placed the necessary tools in clinicians' hands. Now, on to a few more parting words about MLRs and even a peek ahead.

HEADS UP

BIC Update—Whither Beyond Pontine CANS

The Heads Up of Episode 6.1 presented the **binaural interaction component (BIC)** of the ABR—its measurement and underlying rationale and interest. The classic procedure to derive the ABR-BIC can and has been applied as well to the **AMLR** and **ALLR**, including the P_1-N_1-P_2 **complex** and beyond in AEP timespace. This Heads Up is the continuing saga of the BIC, both of its relative robustness—as a **derived AEP** component/response—and further consideration of its meaning.

In Figure 7–24A (left) are recordings and derived waveforms for a relatively broadband recording and epoch to include the AMLR (thus retaining some semblance of the ABR for reference). Recapping the conditions and data processing for deriving a BIC, from top to bottom in this figure, are the right and left monaural, the binaural, and the L+R responses; finally, the BIC is computed as (R+L)-BIN.

In Figure 7–24A (right) are the same ensemble of tracings (directly recorded or derived computationally) as was used for processing the AMLR but now applied to recordings for the ALLR, essentially dominated by the P_1-N_1-P_2 complex. The substantially larger amplitudes of the N_1-P_2 components (note the different scales between potentials, by a factor of 10) are accompanied by a larger amplitude of its BIC than observed for the AMLR-BIC. At face value, the larger amplitude suggests a possible practical advantage over BICs of shorter latency responses. This assumption will be so only if, in practice, the inherently rising magnitude of the background EEG/other interference (as the high-pass cutoff of recording is lowered for optimal recording of the ALLR) does not offset the advantage per SNR. In these recordings, the advantage is realized handily, as the residual noise is well below the amplitude of the ALLR-BIC's component waves. These results answer the more basic question in the title of this Heads-Up: Yes, the likes of binaural interaction—as is true of both shorter latency responses—can be expected to remain evident in the great beyond of longer latency/cortical AEPs.

What, it may be asked, were the expectations in the first place? Purportedly, the BIC should reflect the proportion of neural resources that are devoted to binaural processing, and by the nuances of the AEPs effectively moving toward the cortex, should not only have longer latencies but also larger amplitudes. The number of neurons relative to generation of the ABR are expected both

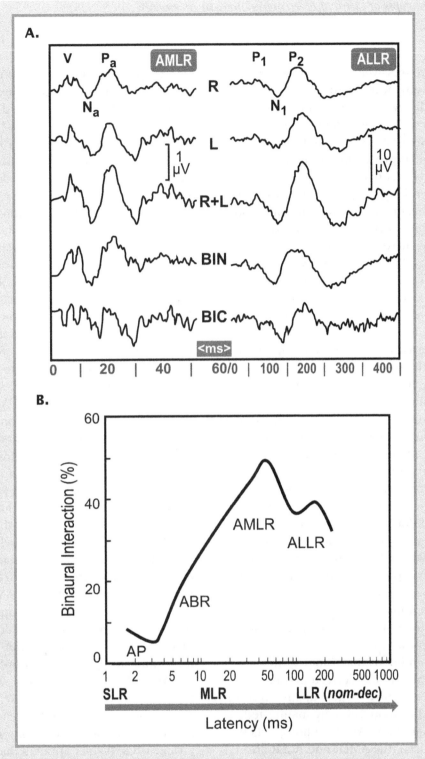

Figure 7-24. Binaural interaction occurs over the entire time domain of the AEPs. **A.** Examples here are of the derived BIC of the auditory middle (AMLR) and long latency responses (ALLR). Right (R) and left monaural (L); sum (R+L); binaural (BIN); binaural interaction component (BIC). **B.** Evolution of strength of binaural interaction (% = 100 × BIC/[L+R]) over the nominal, time-zone decades (nom-dec) of types of AEPs, thus along the primary spatial dimension of the auditory pathway (based on data of McPherson and Starr [1993])[133].

to increase progressively and to represent greater involvement in binaural processing along the auditory pathway to the cortex.[127] The cortex is well known to be greatly involved in binaural processing, built on substantial initial processing in the brainstem. Therefore, each neuroanatomical level above the pons potentially can give rise to a BIC at each level—thalamus, medial geniculate body, primary auditory cortex, if not beyond—and coincidentally, increasingly larger potentials. However, if the AEPs naturally are increasing in amplitude (as is the trend overall), then the BIC itself could simply reflect this growth. This scenario does not necessarily support the notion of greater binaural interaction. Hence, the question arises as to how to compare the BICs among the three major "time zones" in AEPs; namely, how best to "level the playing field"? The solution is one more computation, the ratio BIC/(L+R), which can be expressed readily as a percentage. Viewed accordingly, the ABR typically demonstrates a 16% to 25% reduction of the binaural responses compared to the L+R, whereas BICs of both the AMLR and ALLR show reductions of around 40%. Still, this ratio does not tell the whole story of the actual trend of the evolution of the apparent growth of binaural interaction, given the multiple components of these AEPs. This function is characterized in Figure 7–24B and seen to reflect a fairly smooth increase, yet begins to saturate, if not declining, beyond the P_1-N_1-P_2 complex.

The bottom line is that, indeed, the binaural interaction and derived potentials are not only well and alive further upstream from the ABR-BIC, but more robustly manifested by both the AMLR and ALLR. Although clicks typically are used, the AMLR and ALLR are compatible particularly with a wider selection of stimuli. The ALLR can be tested with speech tokens as well. The most commonly used tone bursts are 500 Hz and 4000 Hz, with 500 Hz producing the larger amplitudes for all the AEPs discussed here for infants[128] and adults.[129] The larger BICs for 500 Hz across the board appear to subserve stronger binaural function in the low frequencies. From this perspective, the 500 Hz should be the best choice for clinical applications. These characteristics all should bode well for the clinical measurement of the BIC based on mid-to-long latency AEPs, begging the final question—for what applications?

Several clinical applications have been suggested for clinical use of the AMLR-BICs. One is measurement of the AMLR-BIC to study the maturation of binaural processing in infants.[130] The peak amplitude of the BIC was reported from one study to occur at N_{20} for infants versus N_{40} for adults (negative components of approximately 20 ms and 40 ms, respectively). These results were interpreted to be consistent with neural development from the peripheral to more central structures. In another study, both ABR- and AMLR-BICs were derived from responses in neonates elicited using both clicks and tone bursts of 500 Hz and 4000 Hz.[128] The parent waveforms were present in an equal number of neonates regardless of the stimulus. However, fewer infants demonstrated the AMLR-BIC than the ABR-BIC, which suggests immaturity at the level of the AMLR generators. More research is needed for confirmation and follow-up in infants to determine the time course for maturation of binaural processing at the level of the AMLR.

At the higher end of the aging spectrum, in a study on young versus older males for matched hearing losses,[131] there were reported no significant differences between groups in the ABR-BIC. The AMLR-BICs were found to be normal for the young group. In contrast, the older group showed no difference between BIN and L+R waveforms, signifying undetectable or absent BICs. It thus appears that underlying binaural processing of the BIC is reduced with advanced aging.

The AMLR-BIC has been suggested to be a useful diagnostic tool for individuals suspected of having CAPD. In one such application, AMLR-BIC was compared in 60 children with suspected CAPD and 60 age-matched, healthy children. The AMLR-BIC has been reported to be significantly delayed in latency and reduced in amplitude in the children with CAPD, compared to the control group of children.[80] The investigators thus suggested that the AMLR-BIC might provide an objective measure of CAPD.

Spatial processing disorder (SPD) is a type of binaural processing dysfunction that is a possible comorbidity in children with CAPD. This combination of difficulties results in problems of sound source segregation and speech understanding difficulties in the presence of competing noise.[132] Children suspected of SPD may benefit from training that targets this deficit. In a recent study, the investigators did just that; they studied the effects of auditory lateralization training (in reference to their interaural time differences) on the AMLR-BIC.[81] There were two sizable subject samples ($N = 60$), control versus training groups of children suspected of CAPD with SPD. After the training, the "trained" group demonstrated AMLR-BICs with significantly decreased latencies and increased amplitudes that were much closer to normal. The results were in good agreement with the improvement of behavioral auditory processing observed in some CAPD tests, such as those of selective auditory attention and speech recognition ability in noise. The findings of this study suggests that that the AMLR-BIC may be a good indicator of outcomes for auditory training in children with CAPD.

Far fewer studies are published for the ALLR-BIC compared to the ABR- and AMLR-BIC, although (again) the wave amplitudes are much larger at this level. From one of the investigations, the grand-averages (responses averaged across subjects) of ALLR-BICs elicited by clicks were reported to have nominal peaks of N_{90}, P_{100}, and N_{200}, each with binaural reductions around 36%.[133] Other stimuli have been used in an effort to obtain larger BICs. BIC ratios from ABR, AMLR, and ALLR each were larger when measured using 500-Hz tone bursts, rather than clicks. Furthermore, the ratios for the ALLR-BICs were equal when measured using the speech token *ba* versus a 500-Hz tone burst.[134] Lastly, still less research has been done beyond the initial ALLR components. Study of the BIC in the "beyond" generally requires the use of more elaborate paradigms than have yet to be covered—coming soon!

As a finale to the BIC saga, it is appropriate to note a couple of studies dedicated directly to fundamental hallmarks of binaural function—sound lateralization, localization, and fusion. When two tones are presented dichotically to the two ears, but simply at equal sound levels and synchronously, the perception is of a centered, fused sound image. The question is, how much of a change in either time or level for one ear will be perceived to have changed the apparent location of the sound in the head (lateralization) or space (localization). Correspondingly, the BIC can be measured to determine electrophysiologically how much of a change will cause the BIC to be eliminated. From an investigation of the ABR, the BIC was not observed when the interaural level difference (ILD) was >30 dB to 35 dB or when the interaural time difference (ITD) was >0.8 ms to 1.2 ms.[135] The psychoacoustical (behavioral response) and electrophysiological functions for both the ILD and ITD were quite similar, suggesting the metrics used to be testing the same underlying mechanisms. In contrast, in another study, the AMLR-BIC was measured over an interaural frequency-difference range that was very limited for a percept of a singular/fused sound source.[136] However, the investigators saw no effect of interaural frequency difference on the BIC. This observation challenges the notion that the BIC necessarily reflects binaural processing, as such, and offered an alternative, neuroanatomical (rather than neurophysiological) explanation of the BIC. The monaural response arises from a majority of nerve fibers on the contralateral side of the pontine brainstem (after the initial crossover; recall Figures 3–12 and 5–8). Still, a minority of ipsilaterally ascending neurons contribute. This minority (in effect) is shared in the true binaural condition. If so, the R+L response is inevitably an overestimation of the BIN response—simply on the grounds of basic neuroanatomy of the pathways. Nevertheless, these findings and theory do not preclude the BIC being a useful biomarker for underlying neural processes. The neuroanatomy, after all, is the substrate (by definition), including possible dysfunctions/lesions of the CANS.

Take Home Messages

Episode 1

1. Understanding the neural generator of these components is key to providing a correct interpretation of the signal, but the AMLR is not an island in AEPdom.
2. Filtering, other parameters of processing, and stimuli (relative to those of SLRs), naturally differ for optimizing recordings of longer-latency responses.
3. Stimulus level has substantial effects on latency of peaks, yet minimally on waveform, especially in comparison to the ABR, even at low intensities.
4. Rate, as for the ABR, has important effects but with an unexpected "twist" that suggests an alternatively useful stimulus-response paradigm.
5. The apparent "magic" of stimulus rates near 40 Hz is the inherent near-periodic intervals among the "native" peaks, namely a period of about 25 ms: $1/0.025 = 40$ Hz.
6. The analysis in the time domain, especially given a clear target frequency determined by the stimulus rate (unlike the transient AMLR) empowers objective analyses.
7. One of the first considerations in practice—maturation—applies here too, including somewhat different effects of level of arousal on 40-Hz ASSR versus transient AMLR.
8. As with the SLRs, AMLR applications are also being pursued and are promising for examining the brain's processing of natural speech.

Episode 2

1. N_a and P_a are the most reliable components of AMLR for clinical assessments.
2. Recording considerations in AMLR depend on the patient and purpose of test.
3. Common parameters for recording AMLR include stimuli and band-pass filters specific to optimizing middle-latency components, yet also overlapping SLRs/LLRs per application.
4. Clinical application of AMLR includes frequency-specific estimation of auditory thresholds, in turn with robust responses even to lower frequencies stimuli.
5. AMLR waveforms indeed reflect developmental changes in pediatric patients, wherein parameters favoring both ABR wave V and AMLR components are particularly useful.
6. Again, state of arousal exerts clinically important influences on the AMLR to be borne in mind in practice.
7. Clinical applications of 40-Hz ASSR began with ERA (time domain); modern ASSR-ERA (frequency domain) demonstrates good threshold-estimation attributes.

Episode 3

1. By the very time-space "coordinates" of the AMLR, it is justifiably worthy of attention as a potential tool of differential diagnosis or to supplement other tests.
2. AMLR can provide information regarding the site of lesion (neurodiagnosis).
3. AMLR can help to identify/confirm central auditory processing disorders.

4. Here too parameters favoring combined ABR (V) and AMLR (Na and Pa) recording are particularly useful.
5. In addition to strong attributes for use in pediatrics, AMLR is also applicable in geriatric patents to help scrutinize/tease apart effects of dementia, hearing loss, and/or tinnitus.
6. MLR P_b (a.k.a., P_{50}) and LLR P_1 are the same and are also of research/clinical interests in the progression of AEPs, perhaps reflecting higher-level processing, like so-called sensory gating.

Heads Up

7. Binaural interaction components are indeed seen beyond time and space coordinates of the ABR and are more strongly manifested by the middle- and longer-latency components.
8. The effect appears to "top out" in the midlatency time frame.

References

1. Valderrama, J., de la Torre, A., Alvarez, I. M., Segura, J. C., Thornton, A. R. D., Sainz, M., & Vargas, J. L. (2014). Auditory brainstem and middle latency responses recorded at fast rates with randomized stimulation. *Journal of the Acoustical Society of America, 136*(6), 3233–3248.
2. Davis, H. (1976). Principles of electric response audiometry. *Annals of Otology, Rhinology, and Laryngology, 85*, 1–96.
3. de la Torre, A., Valderrama, J., Segura, J. C., & Alvarez, I. M. (2019). Matrix-based formulation of the iterative randomized stimulation and averaging method for recording evoked potentials. *Journal of the Acoustical Society of America, 146*(6), 4545–4556.
4. Kohl, M. C., Schebsdat, E., Schneider, E. N., Niehl, A., Strauss, D. J., Özdamar, Ö., & Bohorquez, J. (2019). Fast acquisition of full-range auditory event-related potentials using an interleaved deconvolution approach. *Journal of the Acoustical Society of America, 145*(1), 540–550.
5. Pratt, H. (2007). Middle-latency responses. In R. Burkard, M. Don, & J. Eggermont (Eds.), *Auditory evoked potentials: Basic principles and clinical application* (pp. 463–481). Lippincott Williams & Wilkins.
6. McGee, T., Kraus, N., Comperatore, C., & Nicol, T. (1991). Subcortical and cortical components of the MLR generating system. *Brain Research, 544*(2), 211–220.
7. Liegeois-Chauvel, C., Musolino, A., Badier, J. M., Marquis, P., & Chauvel, P. (1994). Evoked potentials recorded from the auditory cortex in man: Evaluation and topography of the middle latency components. *Electroencephalography and Clinical Neurophysiology, 92*(3), 201–214.
8. Kraus, N., McGee, T., Littman, T., & Nicol, T. (1992). Reticular formation influences on primary and nonprimary auditory pathways as reflected by the middle latency response. *Brain Research, 587*(2), 186–194.
9. McGee, T., Kraus, N., Littman, T., & Nicol, T. (1992). Contributions of medial geniculate body subdivisions to the middle latency response. *Hearing Research, 61*(1–2), 147–154.
10. Kileny, P., Paccioretti, D., & Wilson, A. F. (1987). Effects of cortical lesions on middle-latency auditory evoked responses (MLR). *Electroencephalography and Clinical Neurophysiology, 66*(2), 108–120.
11. Woods, D. L., Alain, C., Covarrubias, D., & Zaidel, O. (1995) Middle latency auditory evoked potentials to tones of different frequency. *Hearing Research, 85*(1–2), 69–75.
12. Nelson, M. D., Hall, J. W., & Jacobson, G. P. (1997). Factors affecting the recordability of auditory evoked response component Pb (P1). *Journal of the American Academy of Audiology, 8*(2), 89–99.
13. Hall, J. W. (2007). *New handbook of auditory evoked responses*. Pearson.
14. Özdamar, Ö., Kraus, N., & Grossmann, J. (1986). Binaural interaction in the auditory middle latency response of the guinea pig. *Electroencephalography and Clinical Neurophysiology, 63*(5), 224–230.
15. Madell, J. R., & Goldstein, R. (1972). Relation between loudness and the amplitude of the early components of the averaged electroencephalic response. *Journal of Speech and Hearing Research, 15*(1), 134–141.
16. Thornton, A. R. D., Mendel, M. I., & Anderson, C. (1977). Effect of stimulus frequency and intensity on the middle components of the averaged auditory electroencephalic response. *Journal of Speech and Hearing Research, 20*(1), 81–94.
17. Fobel, O. (2003). *Auditory brainstem and middle-latency responses with optimized stimuli: Experiments and models* (Doctoral dissertation, Universität Oldenburg). http://oops.uni-oldenburg.de/217/

18. Kjaer, M. (1980). Brain stem auditory and visual evoked potentials in multiple sclerosis. *Acta Neurologica Scandinavica, 62*(1), 14–19.
19. McFarland, W. H., Vivion, M. C., Wolf, K. E., & Goldstein, R. (1975). Reexamination of effects of stimulus rate and number of the middle components of the averaged electroencephalic response. *Audiology, 14*(5–6), 456–465.
20. Tucker, D. A., & Ruth, R. A. (1996). Effects of age, signal level, and signal rate on the auditory middle latency response. *Journal of the American Academy of Audiology, 7,* 83–91.
21. Onitsuka, T., Ninomiya, H., Sato, E., Yamamoto, T., & Tashiro, N. (2003). Differential characteristics of the middle latency auditory evoked magnetic responses to interstimulus intervals. *Clinical Neurophysiology, 114*(8), 1513–1520.
22. Eysholdt, U., & Schreiner, C. (1982). Maximum length sequences: A fast method for measuring brain-stem-evoked responses. *Audiology, 21*(3), 242–250.
23. Özdamar, Ö., & Bohorquez, J. (2006). Signal-to-noise ratio and frequency analysis of continuous loop averaging deconvolution (CLAD) of overlapping evoked potentials. *Journal of the Acoustical Society of America, 119*(1), 429–438.
24. Bardy, F., Dillon, H., & Van Dun, B. (2014). Least-squares deconvolution of evoked potentials and sequence optimization for multiple stimuli under low-jitter conditions. *Clinical Neurophysiology, 125*(4), 727–737.
25. Burkard, R., Shi, Y., & Hecox, K. E. (1990). A comparison of maximum length and Legendre sequences for the derivation of brain-stem auditory evoked responses at rapid rates of stimulation. *Journal of the Acoustical Society of America, 87*(4), 1656–1664.
26. Bohorquez, J., & Özdamar, Ö. (2008). Generation of the 40-Hz auditory steady-state response (ASSR) explained using convolution. *Clinical Neurophysiology, 119*(11), 2598–2607.
27. Galambos, R., Makeig, S., & Talmachoff, P. J. (1981). A 40-Hz auditory potential recorded from the human scalp. *Proceedings of the National Academy of Sciences of the United States of America, 78*(4), 2643–2647.
28. Sturzebecher, E., & Cebulla, M. (2013). Automated auditory response detection: Improvement of the statistical test strategy. *International Journal of Audiology, 52*(12), 861–864.
29. Dobie, R. A., & Wilson, M. J. (1996). A comparison of t test, F test, and coherence methods of detecting steady-state auditory-evoked potentials, distortion-product otoacoustic emissions, or other sinusoids. *Journal of the Acoustical Society of America, 100*(4), 2236–2246.
30. Kraus, N., Smith, D. I., McGee, T., Stein, L. K., & Cartée, C. S. (1987). Development of the middle latency response in an animal model and its relation to the human response. *Hearing Research, 27*(2), 165–176.
31. Woods, D. L., & Clayworth, C. C. (1986). Age-related changes in human middle latency auditory evoked potentials. *Electroencephalography and Clinical Neurophysiology, 65*(4), 297–303.
32. Amenedo, E., & Diaz, F. (1998). Effects of aging on middle-latency auditory evoked potentials: A cross-sectional study. *Biological Psychiatry, 43*(3), 210–219.
33. Yamada, T., Nakamura, A., Horibe, K., Washimi, Y., Bundo, M., Kato, T., ... Sobue, G. (2003). Asymmetrical enhancement of middle-latency auditory evoked fields with aging. *Neuroscience Letters, 337*(1), 21–24.
34. Özdamar, Ö., & Kraus, N. (1983). Auditory middle-latency responses in humans. *Audiology, 22*(1), 34–49.
35. Rodriguez-Holguin, S., Corral, M., & Cadaveira, F. (2001). Middle-latency auditory evoked potentials in children at high risk for alcoholism. *Neurophysiology Clinics, 31*(1), 40–47.
36. Cowell, P. E., Turetsky, B. I., Gur, R. C., Grossman, R. I., Shtasel, D. L., & Gur, R. E. (1994). Sex differences in aging of the human frontal and temporal lobes. *Journal of Neuroscience, 14*(8), 4748–4755.
37. Maddox, R. K., & Lee, A. K. C. (2018). Auditory brainstem responses to continuous natural speech in human listeners. *eNeuro, 5*(1), e0441–17.
38. Valderrama, J., de la Torre, A., Van Dun, B., & Segura, J. C. (2019, July). Towards the recording of brainstem and cortical evoked potentials from the fine structure of natural speech. In R. Cowan & M. Sharma (Co-Chairs), *XXVI International Evoked Response Audiometry Study Group (IERASG)*. Talk conducted at the meeting of International Evoked Response Audiometry Study Group, Sydney, Australia. http://www.ierasg.ifps.org.pl/files/IERASG_2019_abstracts.pdf.
39. Musiek, F. E., & Geurkink, N. A. (1981). Auditory brainstem and middle latency evoked response sensitivity near threshold. *Annals of Otology, Rhinology & Laryngology, 90*(3), 236–240.
40. Scherg, M., & Volk, S. A. (1983). Frequency specificity of simultaneously recorded early and middle latency auditory evoked potentials. *Electroencephalography and Clinical Neurophysiology, 56*(5), 443–452.
41. Mendel, M. I., Hosick, E. C., Windman, T. R., Davis, H., Hirsh, S. K., & Dinges, D. F. (1975). Audiometric

comparison of the middle and late components of the adult auditory evoked potentials awake and asleep. *Electroencephalography and Clinical Neurophysiology, 38*(1), 27–33.

42. Skinner, P., & Shimota, J. (1975). A comparison of the effects of sedatives on the auditory evoked cortical response. *Ear and Hearing, 1*(2), 71–78.

43. Erwin, R., & Buchwald, J. S. (1986). Midlatency auditory evoked responses: Differential effects of sleep in the human. *Electroencephalography and Clinical Neurophysiology, 65*(5), 383–392.

44. Kraus, N., McGee, T., & Comperatore, C. (1989). MLRs in children are consistently present during wakefulness, stage 1, and REM sleep. *Ear and Hearing, 10*(6), 339–345.

45. Okitsu, T. (1984). Middle components of the auditory evoked response in young children. *Scandinavian Audiology, 13*(2), 83–86.

46. McGee, T., Kraus, N., Killion, M., Rosenberg, R., & King, C. (1993). Improving the reliability of the auditory middle latency response by monitoring EEG delta activity. *Ear and Hearing, 14*(2), 76–84.

47. Roffwarg, H. P., Muzio, J. N., & Dement, W. C. (1966). Ontogenetic development of the human sleep-dream cycle. *Science, 152*, 604–619.

48. Kraus, N., Smith, D., Reed, N., Stein, L., & Cartee, C. (1985). Auditory middle latency response in children: Effects of age and diagnostic category. *Electroencehpalography and Clinical Neurophysiology, 62*(5), 343–351

49. Fifer, R. C., & Sierra-Irizarry, B. (1988). Clinical applications of the auditory middle latency response. *The American Journal of Otology, 9*, 47–56.

50. Stapells, D. R., Galambos, R., Costello, J. A., & Makeig, S. (1988). Inconsistency of auditory middle latency and steady-state responses in infants. *Electroencephalography and Clinical Neurophysiology/Evoked Potentials Section, 71*(4), 289–295.

51. Tucker, D. A., Dietrich, S., Harris, S., & Pelletier, S. (2002). Effects of stimulus rate and gender on the auditory middle latency response. *Journal of the American Academy of Audiology, 13*(3), 146–153.

52. Suzuki, T., Hirabayashi, M., & Kobayashi, K. (1983). Auditory middle responses in young children. *British Journal of Audiology, 17*(1), 5–9.

53. Kraus, N., Reed, N. D., Smith, I., Stein, L., & Cartee, C. (1987). High-pass filter settings affect the detectability of MLRs in humans. *Electroencephalography and Clinical Neurophysiology, 68*(3), 234–236.

54. Scherg, M. (1982). Distortion of the middle latency auditory response produced by analogue filtering. *Scandinavian Audiology, 11*(1), 57–69.

55. Dauman, R., Szyfter, W., Charlet de Sauvage, R., & Cazals, Y. (1984). Low frequency thresholds assessed with 40 Hz MLR in adults with impaired hearing. *Archives of Otorhinolaryngology-Head & Neck Surgery, 240*(1), 85–89.

56. Tlumak, A., Durrant, J. D., Delgado, R. E., & Boston, J. R. (2012). Steady-state analysis of auditory evoked potentials over a wide range of stimulus repetition rates: Profile in children vs. adults. *International Journal of Audiology, 51*(6), 480–490.

57. Sammeth, C., & Barry, S. (1985). The 40-Hz event-related potential as a measure of auditory sensitivity in normal. *Scandinavian Audiology, 14*(1), 51–55.

58. Fowler, C. G., & Swanson, M. R. (1989). The 40-Hz potential and SN10 as measures of low-frequency thresholds. *Scandinavian Audiology, 18*(1), 27–33.

59. Petitot, C., Collet, L., & Durrant, J. D. (2005). Auditory steady-state responses (ASSR): Effects of modulation and carrier frequencies. *International Journal of Audiology, 44*(10), 567–573.

60. Linden, R. D., Campbell, K. B., Hamel, G., & Picton, T. W. (1985). Human auditory steady state evoked potentials during sleep. *Ear and Hearing, 6*(3), 167–174.

61. Szyfter, W., Dauman, R., & de Sauvage, R. C. (1984). 40 Hz MLR to low frequency tone-pips in normally hearing adults. *Journal of Otolaryngology, 13*(5), 275–280.

62. Osterhammel, P. A., & Shallop, J. K. (1985). The effect of sleep on the auditory brainstem response (ABR) and the middle latency response (MLR). *Scandinavian Audiology, 14*(1), 47–50.

63. Park, S. E. (2018). *Auditory evoked potentials and speech-in-noise perception: Effects of aging and hearing loss* (Doctoral dissertation). Retrieved from ProQuest Dissertations & Theses Database. (10931873)

64. McPherson, D. L., Ballachanda, B. B., & Kaf, W. (2008). Middle and long latency evoked potentials. In R. J. Roeser, M. Valente, & H. H. Dunn (Eds.), *Audiology: Diagnosis* (pp. 443–477). Thieme.

65. Slabu, L., Escera, C., Grimm, S., & Costa-Faidella, J. (2010). Early change detection in humans as revealed by auditory brainstem and middle-latency evoked potentials. *European Journal of Neuroscience, 32*(5), 859–865.

66. Musiek, F., & Lee, W. (1999) Auditory middle and late potentials. In F. Musiek & W. Rintelmann (Eds.), *Contemporary perspectives on hearing assessment* (pp. 243–272). Allyn & Bacon.

67. Musiek, F. E., Geurkink, N. A., Weider, D. J., & Donnelly, K. (1984). Past, present, and future applications

of the auditory middle latency response. *Laryngoscope, 94*(12), 1545–1553.
68. Musiek, F., & Nagle, S. (2018). The middle latency response: A review of findings in various central nervous system lesions. *Journal of the American Academy of Audiology, 29*(9), 855–867.
69. Shehata-Dieler, W., Shimizu, H., Soliman, S. M., & Tusa, R. J. (1991). Middle latency auditory evoked potentials in temporal lobe disorders. *Ear and Hearing, 12*(6), 377–388.
70. Schochat, E., Rabelo, C. M., & Musiek, F. E. (2014). Electroacoustic and electrophysiological auditory measures in the assessment and management of central auditory processing disorder. In F. E. Musiek & G. D. Chermak (Eds.), *Handbook of central auditory processing disorder, Volume 1, Auditory neuroscience and diagnosis* (2nd ed., pp. 471–496). Plural Publishing.
71. Kraus, N., Özdamar, Ö., Hier, D., & Stein, L. (1982). Auditory middle latency responses (MLRs) in patients with cortical lesions. *Electroencephalography and Clinical Neurophysiology, 54*(3), 275–287.
72. Scherg, M., & von Cramon, D. (1986). Psychoacoustic and electrophysiologic correlates of central hearing disorders in man. *European Archives of Psychiatry and Neurological Sciences, 236*(1), 56–60.
73. Sosa, M. R., Martínez, M. F., Gómez, J. O., & Jáuregui-Renaud, K. (2009). Early auditory middle latency evoked potentials correlates with recovery from aphasia after stroke. *Clinical Neurophysiology, 120*(1), 136–139.
74. Japaridze, G., Shakarishvili, R., & Kevanishvili, Z. (2002). Auditory brainstem, middle-latency, and slow cortical responses in multiple sclerosis. *Acta Neurologica Scandinavica, 106*(1), 47–53
75. Angrisani, R. M. G., Matas, C. G., Neves, I. F., Sassi, F. C., & de Andrade, C. R. F. (2009). Electrophysiological auditory evaluation in stutterers pre and post treatment. *Pró-Fono Revista de Atualização Científica, 21*(2), 95–100.
76. Munjal, S. K., Panda, N. K., & Pathak, A. (2010). Relationship between severity of traumatic brain injury (TBI) and extent of auditory dysfunction. *Brain Injury, 24*(3), 525–532.
77. Arciniegas, D., Olincy, A., Topkoff, J., McRae, K., Cawthra, E., Filley, C. M., . . . Adler, L. E. (2000). Impaired auditory gating and P50 nonsuppression following traumatic brain injury. *The Journal of Neuropsychiatry and Clinical Neurosciences, 12*(1), 77–85.
78. Gaetz, M., & Weinberg, H. (2000). Electrophysiological indices of persistent post-concussion symptoms. *Brain Injury, 14*(9), 815–832.
79. Schochat, E., Musiek, F. E., Alonso, R., & Ogata, J. (2010). Effect of auditory training on the middle latency response in children with (central) auditory processing disorder. *Brazilian Journal of Medical and Biological Research, 43*(8), 777–785.
80. Abdollahi, F. Z., Lotfi, Y., Moosavi, A., & Bakhshi, E. (2019). Binaural interaction component of middle latency response in children suspected to central auditory processing disorder. *Indian Journal of Otorhinolaryngology and Head & Neck Surgery, 71*(2), 182–185.
81. Lotfi, Y., Moosavi, A., Abdollahi, F. Z., & Bakhshi, E. (2019). Auditory lateralization training effects on binaural interaction component of middle latency response in children suspected to central auditory processing disorder. *Indian Journal of Otorhinolaryngology and Head & Neck Surgery, 71*(1), 104–108.
82. Morlet, T., Berlin, C. I., Norman, M., & Ray, B. (2003). Fast ForWord™: Its scientific basis and treatment effects on the human efferent auditory system. In C. I. Berlin & T. G. Weyand (Eds.), *The brain and sensory plasticity: Language acquisition and hearing* (pp. 129–148). Delmar Learning.
83. Mattsson, T. S., Lind, O., Follestad, T., Grøndahl, K., Wilson, W., Nicholas, J., . . . Andersson, S. (2019). Electrophysiological characteristics in children with listening difficulties, with or without auditory processing disorder. *International Journal of Audiology, 58*(11), 704–716.
84. Arehole, S., Augustine, L. E., & Simhadri, R. (1995). Middle latency response in children with learning disabilities: Preliminary findings. *Journal of Communication Disorders, 28*(1), 21–38.
85. Purdy, S. C., Kelly, A. S., & Davies, M. G. (2002). Auditory brainstem response, middle latency response, and late cortical evoked potentials in children with learning disabilities. *Journal of the American Academy of Audiology, 13*(7), 367–382.
86. Miličić, D., Alçada, M. N. M. P., Clemente, L. P., Večerina-Volić, S., Jurković, J., & Clemente, M. P. (1998). A study of auditory afferent organization in children with dyslalia. *International Journal of Pediatric Otorhinolaryngology, 46*(1–2), 43–56.
87. Frizzo, A. C. (2015). Auditory evoked potential: A proposal for further evaluation in children with learning disabilities. *Frontiers in Psychology, 6*, 788.
88. Adler, L. E., Olincy, A., Cawthra, E. M., McRae, K. A., Harris, J. G., Nagamoto, H. T., . . . Ross, R. G. (2004). Varied effects of atypical neuroleptics on P50 auditory gating in schizophrenia patients. *American Journal of Psychiatry, 161*(10), 1822–1828.
89. Siegel, C., Waldo, M., Mizner, G., Adler, L.E., & Freedman, R. (1984). Deficits in sensory gating

in schizophrenic patients and their relatives: Evidence obtained with auditory evoked responses. *Archives of General Psychiatry, 41*(6), 607–612.
90. Thomas, C., Berg, I., Rupp, A., Seidl, U., Schröder, J., Roesch-Ely, D., ... Weisbrod, M. (2010). P50 gating deficit in Alzheimer dementia correlates to frontal neuropsychological function. *Neurobiology of Aging, 31*(3), 416–424.
91. Knight, R. T., Scabini, D., & Woods, D. L. (1989). Prefrontal cortex gating of auditory transmission in humans. *Brain Research, 504*(2), 338–342.
92. Weiland, B. J., Boutros, N. N., Moran, J. M., Tepley, N., & Bowyer, S. M. (2008). Evidence for a frontal cortex role in both auditory and somatosensory habituation: A MEG study. *Neuroimage, 42*(2), 827–835.
93. Mayer, A., Hanlon, F., Franco, A., Teshiba, T., Thoma, R., Clark, V., & Canive, J. (2009). The neural networks underlying auditory sensory gating. *Neuroimage, 44*(1), 182–189.
94. Golubic, S. J., Aine, C. J., Stephen, J. M., Adair, J. C., Knoefel, J. E., & Supek, S. (2014). Modulatory role of the prefrontal generator within the auditory M50 network. *NeuroImage, 92*, 120–131.
95. Picton T. W. (2011). *Human auditory evoked potentials*. Plural Publishing.
96. Ponton, C. W., Don, M., Eggermont, J. J., Waring, M. D., & Masuda, A. (1996). Maturation of human cortical auditory function: Differences between normal-hearing children and children with cochlear implants. *Ear & Hearing, 17*(5), 430–437.
97. Schochat, E., & Musiek, F. E. (2006). Maturation of outcomes of behavioral and electrophysiologic tests of central auditory function. *Journal of Communication Disorders, 39*(1), 78–92.
98. Luo, J. J., Khurana, D. S., & Kothare, S. V. (2013). Brainstem auditory evoked potentials and middle latency auditory evoked potentials in young children. *Journal of Clinical Neuroscience, 20*(3), 383–388.
99. Chambers, R. D., & Griffiths, S. K. (1991). Effects of age on the adult auditory middle latency response. *Hearing Research, 51*(1), 1–10.
100. Jerger, J., Oliver, T., & Chmiel, R. (1988). Auditory middle latency response: A perspective. *Seminars in Hearing, 9*(1), 75–86.
101. Hesse, P. A., & Gerken, G. M. (2002). Amplitude-intensity functions for auditory middle latency responses in hearing-impaired subjects. *Hearing Research, 166*(1–2), 143–149.
102. Cai, S., Ma, W. D., & Young, E. D. (2009). Encoding intensity in ventral cochlear nucleus following acoustic trauma: implications for loudness recruitment. *Journal of the Association for Research in Otolaryngology, 10*(1), 5–22.
103. Park, S., & Fowler, C. G. (2021). *Effects of presbycusis on early and middle latency auditory evoked potentials: Neural correlates of speech-in-noise perception*. Manuscript in preparation.
104. Tlumak, A. I., Durrant, J. D., & Delgado, R. E. (2016). The effect of stimulus intensity and carrier frequency on auditory middle-and long-latency evoked potentials using a steady-state-response approach. *American Journal of Audiology, 25*(1), 62–74.
105. Turrigiano, G. G. (2007). Homeostatic signaling: The positive side of negative feedback. *Current Opinion in Neurobiology, 17*(3), 318–324.
106. Dustman, R. E., & Beck, E. C. (1969). The effects of maturation and aging on the waveform of visually evoked potentials. *Electroencephalography and Clinical Neurophysiology, 26*(1), 2–11.
107. Dustman, R. E., Shearer, D. E., & Snyder, E. W. (1982). Age differences in augmenting/reducing of occipital visually evoked potentials. *Electroencephalography and Clinical Neurophysiology, 54*(2), 99–110.
108. Desmedt, J. E., & Cheron, G. (1981). Non-cephalic reference recording of early somatosensory potentials to finger stimulation in adult of aging normal man: Differentiation of widespread N18 and contralateral N20 from the prerolandic P22 and N30 components. *Electroencephalography and Clinical Neurophysiology, 52*(6), 533–570.
109. Salvi, R. J., Wang, J., & Ding, D. (2000). Auditory plasticity and hyperactivity following cochlear damage. *Hearing Research, 147*(1–2), 261–274.
110. Lenzi, A., Chiarelli, G., & Sambataro, G. (1989). Comparative study of middle-latency responses and auditory brainstem responses in elderly subjects. *Audiology, 28*(3), 144–151.
111. Deiber, M. P., Ibanez, V., Fischer, C., Perrin, F., & Mauguiere, F. (1988). Sequential mapping favours the hypothesis of distinct generators for Na and Pa middle latency auditory evoked potentials. *Electroencephalography and Clinical Neurophysiology/Evoked Potentials Section, 71*(3), 187–197.
112. Gerken, G. M. (1996). Central tinnitus and lateral inhibition: An auditory brainstem model. *Hearing Research, 97*(1–2), 75–83.
113. Jacobson, G. P., Kraus, N., & McGee, T. J. (1997). Hearing as reflected by middle and long latency event-related potentials. In B. R. Alford, J. Jerger, & H. A. Jenkins (Eds.), *Electrophysiologic evaluation in otolaryngology. Advances in otorhinolaryngology* (Vol. 53, pp. 46–84). Karger.

114. Amenedo, E., & Diaz, F. (1999). Ageing-related changes in the processing of attended and unattended standard stimuli. *Neuroreport, 10*(11), 2383.
115. Golob, E. J., Irimajiri, R., & Starr, A. (2007). Auditory cortical activity in amnestic mild cognitive impairment: relationship to subtype and conversion to dementia. *Brain, 130*(3), 740–752.
116. Jerger, J., Chmiel, R., Allen, J., & Wilson, A. (1994). Effects of age and gender on dichotic sentence identification. *Ear & Hearing, 15*(4), 274–286.
117. Roup, C. M. (2011). Dichotic word recognition in noise and the right-ear advantage. *Journal of Speech, Language and Hearing Research, 54*(1), 292–297.
118. Leigh-Paffenroth, E. D., Roup, C. M., & Noe, C. M. (2011). Behavioral and electrophysiologic binaural processing in persons with symmetric hearing loss. *Journal of the American Academy of Audiology, 22*(3), 181–193.
119. Singh, S., Munjal, S. K., & Panda, N. K. (2011). Comparison of auditory electrophysiological responses in normal-hearing patients with and without tinnitus. *Journal of Laryngology & Otology, 125*(7), 668–672.
120. Gerken, G. M., Hesse, P. S., & Wiorkowski, J. J. (2001). Auditory evoked responses in control subjects and in patients with problem-tinnitus. *Hearing Research, 157*(1–2), 52–64.
121. Wienbruch, C., Paul, I., Weisz, N., Elbert, T., & Roberts, L. E. (2006). Frequency organization of the 40-Hz auditory steady-state response in normal hearing and in tinnitus. *Neuroimage, 33*(1), 180–194.
122. Korczak, P. A., Sherlock, L. P., Hawley, M. L., & Formby, C. (2017). Relations among auditory brainstem and middle latency response measures, categorical loudness judgments, and their associated physical intensities. *Seminars in Hearing, 38*(1), 94–114.
123. Wang, B., Cao, K., Wei, C., Gao, Z., & Li, H. (2019). Evaluating auditory pathway by electrical auditory middle latency response and postoperative hearing rehabilitation. *Journal of Investigative Surgery, 32*(6), 542–551.
124. Gordon, K. A., Papsin, B. C., & Harrison, R. V. (2005). Effects of cochlear implant use on the electrically evoked middle latency response in children. *Hearing Research, 204*(1–2), 78–89.
125. Smucny, J., Olincy, A., Eichman, L. C., Lyons, E., & Tregellas, J. R. (2013). Early sensory processing deficits predict sensitivity to distraction in schizophrenia. *Schizophrenia Research, 147*(1), 196–200.
126. Özdamar, Ö., & Bohórquez, J. (2008). Suppression of the Pb (P1) component of the auditory middle latency response with contralateral masking. *Clinical Neurophysiology, 119*(8), 1870–1880.
127. Debruyne, F. (1984). Binaural interaction in early, middle, and late auditory and late auditory evoked responses. *Scandinavian Audiology, 13*(4), 293–296.
128. Cone-Wesson, B., Ma, E., & Fowler, C. G. (1997). Effect of signal level and frequency on ABR and MLR binaural interaction in human neonates. *Hearing Research, 106*(1–2), 163–178.
129. Fowler, C. G., & Horn, J. (2012). Effects of stimulus frequency on binaural interaction in the auditory brainstem and auditory middle latency evoked potentials. *American Journal of Audiology, 21*, 90–98.
130. McPherson, D. L., Tures, C., & Starr, A. (1989). Binaural interaction of the auditory brain-stem potentials and middle latency auditory evoked potentials in infants and adults. *Electroencephalography and Clinical Neurophysiology/Evoked Potentials Section, 74*(2), 124–130.
131. Kelly-Ballweber, D., & Dobie, R. A. (1984). Binaural interaction measured behaviorally and electrophysiologically in young and older adults. *Audiology, 23*(2), 181–194.
132. Camerson, S., Glyde, H., & Dillon, H. (2012). Efficacy of the LiSN & learn auditory training software: Randomized blinded controlled study. *Audiology Research, 2*(1), 15
133. McPherson, D. L., & Starr, A. (1993). Binaural interaction in auditory evoked potentials: Brainstem, middle-and long-latency components. *Hearing Research, 66*(1), 91–98.
134. Fowler, C. G., Heller, A., & Herskovitz, J. (2018, October). Binaural interaction components: Early to late auditory evoked potentials. In D. W. Swanepoel (Chair), *World Congress of Audiology*. Talk conducted at the World Congress of Audiology, Cape Town, South Africa.
135. Furst, M., Levine, R. A., & McGaffigan, P. M. (1985). Click lateralization is related to the β component of the dichotic brainstem auditory evoked potentials of human subjects. *Journal of the Acoustical Society of America, 78*(5), 1644–1651.
136. Zhou, J., & Durrant, J. D. (2003). Effects of interaural frequency difference on binaural fusion evidenced by electrophysiological versus psychoacoustical measures. *Journal of the Acoustical Society of America, 114*(3), 1508–1515.

Cortical Level Testing

The Writers

Episode 1: Barbara K. Cone
Episode 2: Linda J. Hood, Rafael E. Delgado, and Abreena I. Tlumak
Heads Up: John D. Durrant and Martin Walger
Episode 3: Mridula Sharma
Heads Up: Ronny K. Ibrahim and Mridula Sharma
Heads Up: Fabrice Bardy

Episode 1: Call Them Late, But They Were the First AEPs for Practical ERA—LLRs

Curiously, auditory evoked potentials have been classified by their latencies—short, middle, long (alternatively, early, middle, and late)—as that does little to explain their generator sources. Given that the use of auditory evoked potentials (AEPs) in audiology is tied intimately to site-of-lesion determination, the naming of these electrophysiological indices has importance when communicating findings. The short and middle latency responses were refined by more specific naming in previous episodes. In this episode, the term "*cortical auditory evoked potential*" (***CAEP***) is used to refer to the auditory *long latency response* (***LLR***), which this episode formally introduces. More specifically, this episode provides an overview of the CAEP *onset response*, known as the P_1-N_1-P_2 *complex*. The P_1-N_1-P_2 is considered an *obligatory* response of the brain, as opposed to a *cognitive response*, although it certainly is an *event-related potential* (***ERP***). This complex is often classified as an *exogenous* ERP, meaning that its latency and amplitude are primarily determined by stimulus parameters. This classification is opposed to *endogenous* ERPs for which perceptual and cognitive mechanisms heavily influence latency and amplitude; endogenous ERPs are discussed in a subsequent episode.

Historical perspectives again will serve as a point of departure as they often establish the rationale for measurement of a given AEP and its clinical interest. For this obligatory response the history is obligatory as the source of all that developed into viable clinical methods, both for ERA and differential diagnostic applications. Pauline Davis was the first to describe the CAEP.[1] Concerning the translation of research findings to the clinic, Ann Barnett and Isabelle Rapin also must be recognized. Barnett was among the first to use CAEP measurement for the detection of hearing loss in the pediatric population[2] and to describe the development of the CAEP in humans.[3] Rapin's seminal publication[4] set the stage for the next half century of use of CAEPs not only in audiology but also in diagnosing developmental language disorders. Mention of the "day of yore" in ERA begs a tad more of the history—simple but enormously important, Pauline Davis' husband, Hallowell, championed her findings, built upon them, and involved himself extensively in both psychoacoustical and neurophysiological research. By the 1960s, Hallowell Davis was developing the foundational method of evaluating the visual limit of detection of the CAEP, which is used to this day in ERA. Davis's efforts also led to production of the first commercially available AEP-test system. It is beyond the scope here to survey thoroughly the multidecade history of research and development of applications of CAEP measurement. As an example, by the 1980s in Canada, workers seeking compensation for employment-related loss of hearing came to be compelled to have confirmation of their pure-tone audiogram via ALLR-ERA.[5] The ERA area of application of this CAEP will be taken up in the upcoming episode.

The purpose of this episode is to provide the groundwork for understanding the CAEP and potential clinical interests. The neural generators and stimulus-response characteristics of the transient elicited P_1-N_1-P_2 will be the AEP at center stage and thus first reviewed. Included are the developmental dependencies and other subject-related factors that can affect the presence, latency, and amplitude of this response.

The neural generators of the P_1-N_1-P_2 complex have been described well since the 1970s,[6] although ever-improving methodologies such as invasive methods in experimental animals, dipole-source localization algorithms, and brain-mapping technologies have refined the "view." Each component of the P_1-N_1-P_2 complex has both distinct and overlapping sources. In general, the P_1-N_1-P_2 is generated bilaterally by the primary auditory cortex on the superior aspect of the temporal lobe, also involving the parabelt regions (also known as association cortices). There can be involvement of the premotor cortex and the thalamocortical radiation, which in turn can include some reticular formation input.

The ***P1 component***, occurring at 50 ms to 70 ms following stimulus onset, may have contributions from the hippocampus, planum temporale, and lateral temporal cortex, depending on the complexity of the stimuli—speech tokens versus tone or noise bursts. Another factor is that the test paradigm controls for attention switching as may take place on an involuntary basis. Many investigators have considered P_1 of the CAEP and ***Pb*** of the auditory middle latency response (AMLR)—more specifically, the ***thalamocortical response***—to be the same component. Given that the AMLR is usually obtained with brief, noncomplex stimuli presented at much faster rates and with different EEG filter settings than typical for recording P_1, it is no surprise that some differences in the generator sites can be found, depending on the stimulus and recording parameters.

The ***N1 component***, occurring at 90 ms to 120 ms following stimulus onset, has multiple generators in primary and secondary auditory cortices, and three subcomponents have been defined.[7] There is an ***N_1b*** component that is largest when recorded from the vertex and is described as "frontocentral negativity" from ERP topographical maps (as sketched roughly in Figure 7–6A). Its generator source is localized to the superior portion of the temporal lobe. A positive-going "T-complex" is another aspect of the N_1 and is discerned in the recordings made from midtemporal scalp regions. Whereas the N_1b has vertically oriented dipoles, the T-complex has a radial source in the secondary auditory cortices. The third subcomponent of N_1 has a latency of 100 ms and is observed when the interstimulus intervals are >1/s; this N_1 is an indicator that the cortex has been activated by a stimulus. Specific neural generators among the primary and secondary cortices have not been determined. Clinically, CAEPs are recorded with an electrode at the vertex connected to the noninverting amplifier input, which provides a view of N_1 as a unitary component. Obtaining the subcomponents of N_1 or the T-complex requires the use of a multielectrode array (recall Figure 3–2B).

The P_2 has generators from multiple areas of primary and secondary auditory cortices and occurs at 180 ms to 200 ms following stimulus onset. Heschl's gyrus is involved in the generation of P_2 and also subcortical contributions from the mesencephalic activating system have been described. The generators of P_2 are influenced by the type of stimulus paradigm used, particularly with respect to controls for attention and stimulus salience as well as the age and cognitive status of the listener.

Figure 8–1 provides both a recap of the typical approach to measuring amplitudes of transient-elicited AEPs and illustration specifically of the wave morphology of the P_1-N_1-P_2 complex. Indi-

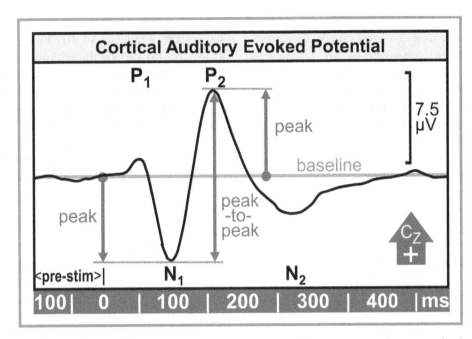

Figure 8–1. Recap of conventional measures of transient, auditory evoked potentials, applied here to the typical P_1-N_1-P_2 complex, an obligatory response of the brain. This example is typical of responses elicited in the midfrequencies and at moderate hearing levels of the audiogram. In addition to the highlights discussed (*in gray text*), plotting the response to show a segment of the interstimulus interval immediately before stimulus onset can be useful for the most critical assessment of quality of the recording.

cated are the definition of baseline and peak versus peak-to-peak measurements. As with earlier AEPs, latencies usually are measured at the most positive or negative maxima within a circumscribed time window of the component/complex targeted (that is, rather than endeavoring to determine reliably response onset in reference to baseline of a given component potential). The illustration expresses overall nuances typical of the CAEP in normal-hearing, neurologically intact adults, using stimuli presented at moderate (conversational) sound levels. The nature of effects on the obligatory CAEP of a variety of factors now will be considered.

Like the earlier AEPs, ***stimulus-response dependencies*** are substantial for the CAEP. However, an advantage of the CAEP over the more ubiquitous target for AEP testing clinically—the auditory brainstem response (ABR)—is the greater variety of stimulus types that can be used in a clinical evaluation with considerably less concern for stimulus artifact and with greater efficacy of substantially longer stimuli. These include clicks, tone bursts, pure tones, consonants, vowels, consonant-vowel, consonant-vowel-consonant, vowel-consonant-vowel tokens, and words. These stimuli can be presented in quiet or noise (with ipsilateral or bilateral maskers) and are delivered with insert, supraaural, or circumaural phones or in a sound field. Considering this variety of stimulus options and presentation modes, the CAEP is very much at home in the audiology clinic.

In any audiological test (as emphasized in Episode 2.3 on calibration and others since, in effect), the interpretation of the recorded AEP cannot be fully realized in the absence of knowledge of the acoustic path of the stimulus (namely, multiple transfer functions along the way). Accordingly and a priori, anything—as strongly hinted earlier—about the effective stimulus reaching the hearing organ must be considered. The good news is that their effects are relatively straightforward, namely well understood as stimulus-level effects. Contrasting issues that were controversial for some time in applying bone conduction to ABR-ERA (recall Episodes 6.1 and 6.4 with more coming soon), any special issues for BC-CAEP-ERA are much the same as in conventional audiometry.

These signals are not foreign to audiologists, and such knowledge can be applied to understanding stimulus-response variables required to interpret CAEP findings. The P_1-N_1-P_2 complex often can be detected down to 10-dB or less sensation level (Figure 8–2A). As with other AEPs, the accuracy of visual detection level (VDL) rests upon the SNR of the CAEP (regarding background EEG noise levels), so optimizing the response-to-noise level is paramount. Sensorineural hearing loss affects the relationship between the stimulus level and the VDL, such that the CAEP response threshold may be found, indeed, at or merely a few dB above the behavioral threshold. CAEP input-output functions are approximately linear in semilogarithmic plots initially (for instance, voltage versus dB SPL) but then follow more of a saturating-nonlinear function starting between 40 dB SPL to 70 dB SPL (Figure 8–2B, top right).[8] Results of a recent study of the N_1-P_2 I-O function in the mid-dynamic range suggest growth of response more reflective overall of a power function, such as is characteristic of perceived loudness versus dB SPL (a log-log plot, given dB being a log transform).[9]

Stimulus level also affects CAEP latency (Figures 8–2A and B). Overall, latencies decrease inversely with stimulus level, although there are differences in the latency-level functions for the individual response components (P_1, N_1, and P_2), with P_2 exhibiting longer latency delays at lower levels than the other components (panel B). Latencies shifts are (20 ms–40 ms) within 10 dB to 20 dB of the behavioral threshold with just under 1 ms/dB from 20 dB nHL to 80 dB nHL.[10]

The amplitude of the CAEP is also determined by stimulus frequency. Given the equivalence of all other stimulus parameters, CAEP amplitudes decrease as stimulus frequency is increased. The differences in amplitude as a function of frequency

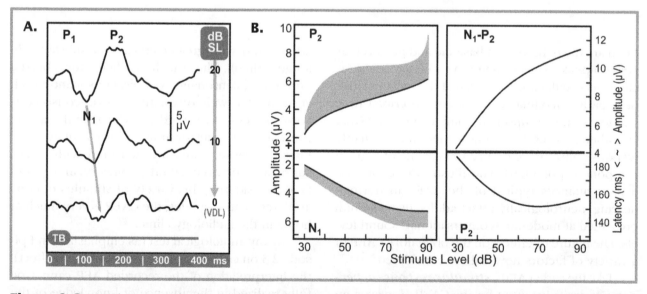

Figure 8–2. **A.** The N1 tracked to limit of visual detection (regarding sensation level) in a normal-hearing adult, with the gray line highlighting a concomitant latency shift; for the CAEP, this is more readily seen approaching its VDL. **B.** Overall trends of growth and variance (roughly mean and + or − 1 standard deviation) for N_1 and P_2 components, seen to be somewhat different for the two components. CAEP amplitude is often measured peak-to-peak as "N_1-P_2." Latency dependence of N_1 demonstrated (*left panel*) is largely paralleled by that of P_2 (*right panel*) again expressed most dramatically at lower sound/sensation levels (based in part on data of Adler and Adler [1991][8]).

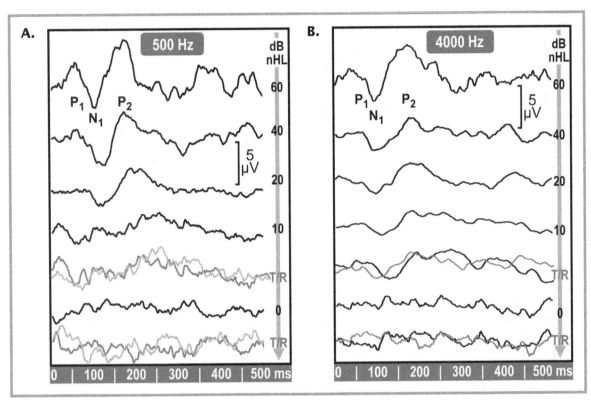

Figure 8–3 A–B. Overall trends of recordings expected of the CAEP, tested at 500 Hz and 4000 Hz in adults given hearing thresholds within normal limits at both frequencies tested, in terms of both input-output and latency-intensity characteristics. Both averaged and individual test/retest (T/R) recordings are shown at the lower levels.

are thought to be due to the tonotopic mapping of the cochlear response areas at the level of the cortex, and the location of these cortical areas with respect to the scalp topography of the CAEP. For CAEP recordings made from vertex (Cz) or fronto-vertex (Fz) positions, the CAEPs tend to have larger amplitudes for lower frequency stimuli. There are also systematic latency differences as a function of frequency, with latencies decreasing with increasing frequency. These nuances are illustrated in Figure 8–3, recordings typical overall of those observed in young adults with normal hearing.

The rate of stimulation has a profound effect on CAEP amplitude. In adults, the CAEP amplitude increases dramatically as stimulus rate decreases; there is a 50% change in amplitude when the stimulus rate is increased from 0.1 Hz (a 10 s ISI, not practical for clinical use) to 1.0 Hz.[11] For more clinically applicable rates, the overall change in amplitude has been reported to be 1.4 µV/Hz for a rate change of 0.5 Hz to 2.0 Hz,[12] as shown in Figure 8–4A. These trends are also apparent from research applying a steady-state stimulus-response approach to obtaining the CAEP, permitting an objective measure of relative magnitude (panel B) at stimulus rates much higher than those conventionally used for obtaining the CAEP transient response.[13] Again, it can be seen that the magnitude increases dramatically as stimulus rate decreases.

Similar effects of rate are seen in children; however, the nuances are remarkably different during infancy and early childhood. The maturational differences from younger children are centered on the immaturity of the N1 component. N1 is not evident in CAEP recordings made (from vertex), unless the interstimulus interval exceeds 2 s to 3 s (0.5 Hz–0.3 Hz). Because most published CAEP studies over the past quarter-century employed rates of 1.0/s or higher, N1 was often reported in

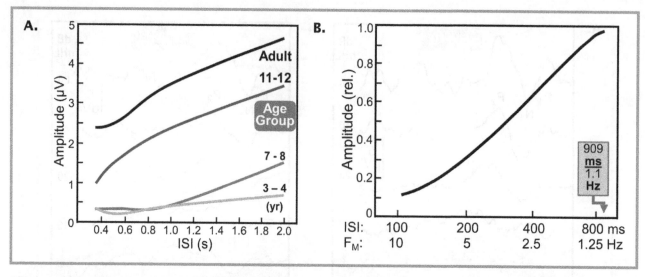

Figure 8–4. A. Amplitude of the CAEP as a function of stimulus rate, thus interstimulus interval (ISI, here in seconds) in the adult and in children per years of maturation (based on data of Gilley and associates [2005][12]). **B.** Trends of change in overall magnitude of the CAEP over a range starting with repetition rates more typical of AMLR measurement down to a modulation frequency (F_M) of 1.1 Hz—thus an interstimulus interval of 1/1.1 = 909-ms ISI—falling in the range most popular in practical CAEP testing (modeled from data of Tlumak and coworkers [2011][13] of measurements of steady-state equivalent responses; technical details of paradigm to be presented in the upcoming episode).

the literature as not being apparent until the age of 10 to 11 years.[10] The sensitivity of the CAEP to rate effects during development are evident in the graphs of CAEP amplitude as a function of stimulus rate in Figure 8–4A, with subject age as the parameter.

Other stimulus parameters that can affect the latency and amplitude of the CAEP are stimulus envelope rise-time and its spectro-temporal complexity. Rise-times longer than 30 ms can reduce response amplitudes compared to those evoked by stimuli that have shorter rise times. There can also be latency effects commensurate with the delay in reaching the peak stimulus level. Thus, in order to estimate pure-tone thresholds for tonal stimuli, stimulus rise-time, duration, and rate should be constant across frequency.

Stimuli like speech are used readily to evoke the CAEP, but their spectro-temporal complexity also affects latency and amplitude. These effects are observed for speech features, such as consonant-vowel (CV) tokens depending, for instance, on whether the consonant is voiced or unvoiced. The effect of voice onset time can be observed in the latency and morphology of the CAEP.[14,15] Similarly, vowel tokens with higher frequency components, such as /i/, should result in lower amplitude responses than /u/, based upon the frequency dependencies of the CAEP. Similarly, /ʃi/ evokes a larger response than /si/ because of the spectral complexity of frication compared to sibilance.

In summary, as with any AEP test used as an audiological tool, it is necessary to maintain an exacting consideration of stimulus parameters and the way they affect the response and interact with the status of the underlying auditory system. Attention is now turned to the *listener-related variables* that will affect the response.

The first variable is maturation; its effects on the CAEP are substantial both in infancy and throughout much of childhood, as was shown by Figure 8–4A. Nevertheless, CAEPs are evident during fetal development and have been recorded remotely from across the maternal abdominal wall in fetuses from 32 to 38 weeks gestational age.[16] Furthermore, CAEPs have be recorded in prematurely born infants, at 24 weeks gestational age.[17] The morphology of CAEPs obtained from premature infants is negative across the scalp, and neuromagnetic recordings also demonstrate this negativity[18] yet are consistent with a dipole source in the auditory cortex. Between 36 to 40 weeks, the CAEP polarities from central versus lateral scalp positions appear to change and can be of different polarities, although by term, the CAEP obtained from vertex electrodes is a positive-going potential. These changes in scalp topography and morphology reflect the ongoing maturation of the subcortical and cortical auditory pathways and their dipole orientations.

During early infancy, the most prominent component of the CAEP is a positive going peak with a latency of 200 ms to 250 ms. The presence and morphology of the CAEP are, however, highly dependent upon the rate of stimulation during infancy and early childhood. In most of the research on development, clicks, tone bursts, or speech tokens (CV) have been used, presented at rates of 1/s or higher. A P_1 response is evident with latencies between 100 ms to 200 ms during the first year of life, even when stimulus rates are at 1 to 2/s. It is possible to discern a N_1 peak during the first year of life if the stimulus rate is in the range of 0.25 to 0.5/s (rates well below any typically used in conventional testing). Stimulus rates on the order of 0.25 Hz permitted investigators to discern N_1 in typically developing infants and children ranging in age from newborns to 6 years.[19] Similarly, the author has provided norms for CAEPs evoked by tonal and speech tokens obtained from infants under one year of age.[20] In that study, for a stimulus rate of 0.5 Hz, CAEP component P_2 was evident in 70% of infants tested at levels as low as 20 dBA SPL, and N_1 components were present in 85% to 100% of infants for levels at 30 to 60 dBA SPL. The latencies of the P_1-N_1-P_2 components (for stimuli at 60 dBA SPL) were 132 ms, 216 ms, and 333 ms, respectively. The latency and amplitude maturation of these components showed a latency decrease for all components over the first 6 years of life. When stimulus rates are at or above 1 Hz, adultlike latencies are not apparent until 10 to 12 years of age[21] and are also influenced by the electrode montage used to obtain the CAEP.

In summary, CAEPs can be obtained from as early as 24 weeks gestational age; the latencies, amplitudes, and scalp topographies undergo substantial maturational development during the first 12 years of life. Still, CAEPs are reliably recorded for near-threshold stimuli even in infants under the age of 12 months. Illustrated in Figure 8–5 are the effects of maturation on the CAEP. The most significant change in latency takes place during the first 2 years of life for the P1 component. Substantial variability in stimulus and recording parameters used over the past five decades of research makes the characterization of maturational trends for the N_1 and P2 components difficult. Because P_1 and N_1 latencies are highly correlated, the shape of the N1 latency development curve should be close to that of P_1 when stimulus rates are optimized for obtaining N_1 in the very young. Developmental latency data for click-evoked CAEPs obtained in sleeping infants and toddlers (see inset panel of Figure 8–5) were published by Barnet and coworkers more than three decades earlier,[22] reflecting essentially the same time course of early maturation of P_1.

The next important factor, the "flip-side" of early maturation, is that the CAEP changes during aging. Specifically, some changes in the CAEP occur

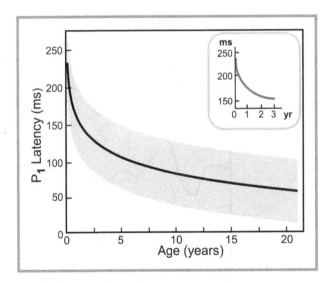

Figure 8–5. Trend of maturation of the P_1 component. Based on data and equation of Ponton and coworkers (2002).[21] Overall ranges of values about the approximate mean are represented here simply applying the same function at values defining limits that accounted for nearly all scatter in the data. Inset: Trend from data reported earlier by Barnet and associates (1975) over the first few years of development.[22]

that appear to be independent of age-related hearing loss. A common finding is that CAEP amplitudes are increased relative to those found in younger adults. In animal models of auditory system aging, these large amplitudes are attributed to decreased neural inhibition throughout the auditory system.[23] The N_1 and P_2 latencies also have been noted to be prolonged in older normal-hearing adults compared to young normal-hearing adults. These findings suggest that reduced neural synchrony as well as reduced central inhibitory processes may be responsible. Another finding was revealed using research paradigms designed to investigate perceptual and electrophysiological aspects of temporal processing, such as (from psychoacoustics) studies of **binaural masking level differences** and **interaural timing differences**. Results reflected diminished capacities among older adults (>60 years) relative to younger listeners, regardless of hearing status.[24,25] These perceptual and electrophysiological differences are correlated with diminished speech perception abilities, particularly in noise. Recordings in Figure 8–6 are illustrative of responses overall of the effects of stimulus rate on the CAEP for younger (nominally, in the 20s) versus older adults (in the 60s+) with normal hearing.

As implied from discussions of the earlier AEPs, there is always a concern for potential effects—good, bad, or at least different—of the level of arousal of the patient. The examiner must know and understand the effects of the sleep stage and level of consciousness for any evoked potential test; this knowledge is fundamental to interpreting the results. Listeners in studies employing a variety of P_1-N_1-P_2 test paradigms exhibit robust responses when passively alert with their eyes open. The effect of sleep, whether natural or sedated, is more complicated but, in any event, can dramatically alter CAEP amplitude and thus

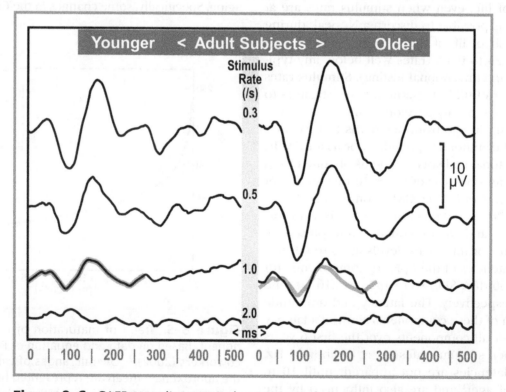

Figure 8–6. CAEP recordings typical comparatively in younger adults and their elders, which are particularly evident at the lower stimulus repetition rates. Nevertheless, as shown by the light-gray-highlighted tracing of the younger subject's response at the 1/s rate (again, more typical of that used in practice), the differences of amplitudes and/or peak latencies are still discernable.

affect detectability. Latencies are also affected. These effects also change systematically with different sleep stages and yet can limit the replicability of the response. Both the P_1-N_1-P_2 complex and the background noise (physiological and EEG) are particularly challenging to tease apart with time-domain analyses of transient AEPs. As sleep state could change during the CAEP test, stationarity of both the signal (response) and noise cannot be assumed, and this potentially reduces the effectiveness of signal averaging. These complexities of sleep-related changes are one reason why CAEPs were abandoned for ERA in infants and children, who typically were tested during sedated sleep. At the same time, there were considerable advances in ERA when it was shown that the ABR was stable during even sedated sleep. As now known, it is possible to obtain robust CAEPs for suprathreshold stimuli in awake infants.[20,26]

The level of arousal and attention can also affect the CAEP. With increased attention or listening effort, the amplitude of the P_2 and subsequent N_2 components increase, or that of P_2 decreases while N_2 is increased. These changes may be absent in those with mild cognitive impairment,[27] and thus be a harbinger of a neurocognitive deficit.

The effects of sensorineural hearing loss have been of considerable interest for CAEP-measurement efforts. Because the CAEP can be evoked by tones or speech tokens that better approximate those used in pure-tone and speech audiometry (given greater duration/spectral complexity), effects of hearing loss on the CAEP are expected to manifest similarly to results of conventional audiometry. At least, results of CAEP-ERA can be counted upon for accurate representation of any configuration of loss. There are still other applications for the clinical use of CAEPs, indeed including speech audiometry.

It is well documented[28] that, upon eliciting CAEPs using speech tokens, the latencies for N_1 and P_2 increase with the severity of hearing loss. At the same time, the amplitude variability of CAEP components is increased for those with hearing loss compared to those with normal sensitivity. The presence of N_1 and P_2 components diminishes with the severity of hearing loss, although P_1 and N_1 may be present within 5 dB of the psychophysical threshold, for which recruitment mechanisms appear to play a key role. N_2 latencies demonstrate a high correlation (r >0.70) with pure-tone thresholds in the range of 2.0 kHz to 4.0 kHz, but here N_2 was measured in an active listening paradigm. In general, the presence of the N_1 component indicates that the stimulus was sufficient to evoke a synchronized neural response at the level of the cortex. Therefore, in the neurologically and cognitively intact person, the CAEP response is highly correlated with psychophysically measured detection thresholds.

In summary of the functional and clinical significance of the CAEP, the P_1-N_1-P_2 complex is sensitive to several stimulus parameters and is also dependent upon the integrity of the peripheral auditory system as well as its cortical generators. The presence of the CAEP indicates that the cortex has responded to sound in a way that provides enough neural synchrony to obtain a time-locked (coherent) evoked potential. Obtaining this response can be especially relevant in those with auditory neuropathy,[29] who do not have acoustic reflexes or ABRs, or those who are too young or cognitively impaired to participate in behavioral tests. Additionally, the latency of the P_1 has been used as a "biomarker" of auditory system development in deaf infants and children who have received a cochlear implant.[30]

Table 8–1 provides a summary of recommended stimulus and recording parameters in the clinical context. The P_1-N_1-P_2 complex can be obtained handily, particularly for the passively alert infant, child, or adult. Pure-tone stimuli can be used to evoke this CAEP, and thus thresholds can be estimated from the lowest level at which the response is present. Its use for cases of malingering has a robust evidence base[5,31,32] (coming soon!). CAEP evaluation also has been used in hearing aid verification in infants.[33] Computerized detection algorithms have been implemented and are undergoing further research and development.[13,34] The incorporation of CAEP tests in an EHDI program has been shown to lower the age of hearing aid fitting on a population basis.[35] CAEPs can be obtained using acoustic or electric stimuli, as transduced by a cochlear implant (mentioned along the way and discussed in-depth in the next chapter). Further information about the P_1-N_1-P_2 complex as an index of stimulus change will be forthcoming as well as CAEPs/other LLRs obtained in special populations, such as those with dyslexia, central

Table 8–1. Useful Stimulus and Recording Parameters for Testing CAEP Onset-Response

Stimulus types: click, tone burst, and speech
Rise-fall time: 10 ms–20 ms
Plateau: 20 ms–200 ms
Carrier frequency: 125 Hz–8000 Hz
Speech token: natural or synthesized

Examples:
    Vowel: /a/
    Consonant: /m/
    CV: /ba/
    CVC: /dad/

Stimulus rate (transient-elicited): 0.3 Hz–1.1 Hz
Calibration of stimulus level: dB SPL, HL, nHL, or SL

Recording parameters:
    Epoch duration: 500 ms–1000 ms
    Prestimulus: 10% of poststimulus time
    Sampling rate: 250 Hz–500 Hz
    EEG filter: 1 Hz–30 Hz
    Amplification: 50,000 to 100,000 (or recommended by equipment manufacturer)

Electrode Montage:
    Cz (noninverting)
    Mastoid or ear lode ipsi or contra to the stimulus ear or jumpered together to inverting input (pending channel and interests)
    Ground: nasion or mastoid or earlobe (contra to stimulus ear; pending for single channel)

auditory processing disorders, or other developmental disabilities.

Consequently, results of tests of the cortical AEPs can be used clinically and broadly to document the integrity of the auditory nervous system to the level of the cortex. Even with some level of success with conventional behavioral test methods, CAEP evaluation is particularly useful in patients for whom reliable perceptual responses are challenging to obtain. A significant advantage of CAEPs is that stimuli of considerable spectro-temporal complexity, again including speech tokens, may be used, and the latency and amplitude of the response are sensitive to the acoustic features of such stimuli. CAEPs may be present, even in those with neural dyssynchrony disorders, wherein ABRs or AMLRs are absent/abnormal. Using test protocols that tap binaural and temporal processing also may be used as an objective indicator of complex central auditory function or disorder. All the relevant methods and technologies thereto may be found in the audiologist's toolbox thanks to modern AEP-test instrumentation. However, there also is a still broader foundation to "pour" herein, both on the side of ERA-knowhow (up next) and further exploration of AEP time-space, the "late-late show" (stay tuned!).

■ Episode 2: Why ERA Using Cortical Response Measurement

Evaluation of auditory function includes assessment of the ability to both detect sounds and discriminate among sounds. Comprehensive evaluation of auditory function with both behavioral and physiologic responses provides important cross-checks in clinical decision making.[36] Inclusion of CAEPs provides evaluation of the auditory pathway from the ear to the cortex. In current clinical practice, objective assessment of detection of sound, related to threshold sensitivity, focuses on responses generated in subcortical regions, as noted in earlier discussions of the transient and steady-state brainstem responses. These early or short-latency responses dominate clinical applications of electrophysiological testing to newborn hearing screening and pediatric audiological assessment. As noted in previous chapters, the subcortical responses are less-to-negligibly influenced by effects of sleep and sedation and mature earlier than responses from cortical areas of the auditory pathway. However, there also are limitations of measures using brainstem responses that include lower-amplitudes, low SNRs, and (the downside of the advantages just recapped) the inability to characterize more than a relatively limited portion of the auditory pathway. Some patients, such as those with an auditory neuropathy or an auditory synaptopathy, simply do not have reliable subcortical responses which reduces utility of auditory electrophysiology for this critical population, if the evaluation of AEPs is limited to merely testing the subcortical potentials. The last episode, rather, demonstrated the CAEP to be a robust electrophysiological marker that can be applied to characterize various aspects of auditory function and hinted strongly that it could be altered by the same issues of both stimuli and preexisting lesions of the peripheral and/or lower-central auditory pathways. This episode focuses on application of the CAEP to detection of sound in the context of evoked response audiometry (ERA) including characteristics, advantages, and considerations and further probing of the upper pathways for still other signs of the patient's complete auditory status. Hence, more to come for this season, as AEPdom extends vastly in space and time.

The point of departure once more, nevertheless, must be a bit more of the history of discovery of AEPs. This, in particular, is the work of Hallowell Davis and his research group that focused on obtaining the first recordings of cortical electric responses to sound, namely to augment the story presented earlier. Its seminal importance warrants added consideration specifically in relation to the ERA method. Figure 8–7 provides a look back in time to Dr. Davis working at a desk with the first commercially available evoked response audiometer (developed in the 1960s), based extensively on his work at the Central Institute for the Deaf in St. Louis, Missouri. His earliest work grew out of collaboration with wife Pauline[1]; however, the technology available early on permitted cortical responses to sound to be recorded from the surface of the head only in subjects with robust responses and low background noise. Yet, this critical work provided the basis for technological breakthroughs, though only realized for practical clinical use decades later. With the machine seen in Figure 8–7, extraction of far smaller signals from the brainstem remained out of reach for a while longer. Nevertheless, two critical matters are reflected in this figure—insight and subsequent demonstration of signal averaging that allowed acquisition of repeatable records of event-related potentials. This approach led to powerful methods of efficacious ERA that are widely applicable to clinical electrophysiology in audiology to this day.

History suggests a variety of choices of AEPs to measure, including the CAEP for purposes of estimating hearing thresholds. So, a key question is: Why apply CAEP measurement to ERA, in particular?

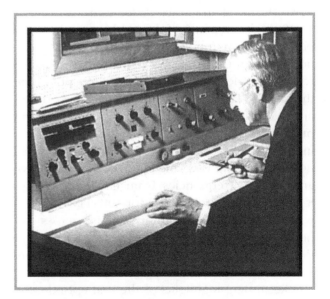

Figure 8–7. Hallowell Davis at the console of the first commercially available electric response audiometer (courtesy of Dr. S. Nittrouer).

The N1-P2 components of the CAEP are an auditory evoked potential of choice when testing older children and adults where a nonbehavioral, frequency-specific response is needed.[37] Multiple characteristics of CAEPs support their value as an assay of detection of sound; primary among these is again the close agreement between CAEP and behavioral thresholds.

A "gold standard" for threshold comparisons is generally held to be thresholds for pure tones that are obtained using a controlled behavioral paradigm (like the Carhart-Jerger modified Hughson-Westlake method[38]—a.k.a. conventional pure-tone audiometry). Consequently, comparisons between this classical benchmark of hearing sensitivity and any candidate method of evoked-potential detection needs to be made, starting with consideration of the influence of the stimulus intensity step size used. Audiometric procedures typically use initial steps of 10 dB with refinement near threshold with 5-dB steps. Due to time constraints, AEP tests typically begin with 20-dB steps and are completed/refined using 10-dB steps to define the response threshold estimate. Thus, direct comparison between behavioral and physiological thresholds is impacted by the stimulus levels used to estimate threshold. An interpolation method, wherein the AEP amplitude has met a specified criterion, has been suggested to provide a closer approximation when this is taken into consideration.[39]

Studies comparing thresholds obtained by behavioral pure-tone audiometry and visual detection levels of CAEPs report that responses can be recorded at levels close to behavioral pure-tone thresholds. The majority of studies report differences of about 10 dB between CAEP-VDLs and pure-tone behavioral thresholds.[34,39-43] These include comparisons among subjects with normal hearing, hearing loss, and simulated hearing loss, and include frequencies from 0.5 kHz through 8 kHz. Findings are similar for subjects with and without hearing loss and are similar across frequency—the other principal parameter of conventional audiometry. Additional information from some of these studies now will be considered.

Recapping highlights of the first episode, the N_1-P_2 complex (a.k.a. the vertex potential) is the waveform typically used for threshold estimation in older children and adults, while P_1 is a focus in infants and young children based upon its prominence. The P_1 component provides information about level of arousal, sensory gating (suppression), and decreases with age. N_1 reflects basic stimulus characteristics, initial selection for later pattern recognition, and increases with age. Lastly, P_2 can also provide information about selective attention, stimulus change, feature detection, and short-term memory. Thus, the limit of detection of sound is a valuable aspect where these components can be applied to ERA; however, detection is not the sole function represented.

Specific information/informational values related to latency and amplitude characteristics of the components P_1, N_1, and P_2 have been described in the last episode, as well, so will not be repeated here. In the context of measuring a VDL (to recap "method 101"), responses are obtained at varying intensities from well above response "threshold" to near, if not below, response threshold. Latency and amplitude characteristics naturally change across intensity (Figure 8–8). CAEP amplitude decreases fairly consistently with intensity changes from high to low stimulus levels. CAEP latency typically shows little to no change for a broad range of higher suprathreshold stimulus levels, again with greater latency shifts as stimulus level decreases and the VDL is approached.

A general truism applies here that's worth repeating: Achieving an acceptable SNR is critical in the application of all AEPs to ERA. A key value of CAEPs in particular in ERA is the higher amplitude of cortical responses over subcortical evoked potentials and that this increase in amplitude also manages to stay above an inherently increasing background EEG, as lowering of the low-frequency cutoff is needed for an optimal response. The result is a signal-to-noise advantage, namely more so than the AMLR versus the ABR (recall Episode 7.2). With higher amplitude responses and quiet subjects, fewer sweeps are needed in an averaged response to achieve an acceptable SNR, although the longer-latency response must be evaluated at lower repetition rates. Therefore, there is not necessarily time saved, for example, ALLR-ERA versus ABR-ERA in practice, but this also should not be the motivation of choice of test. It rather should be a more comprehensive evaluation of the auditory pathway without substantial loss of efficiency

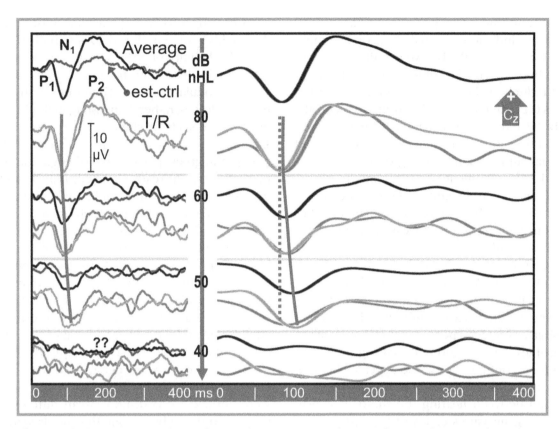

Figure 8–8. Partial replots of data from Figures 4–12 and 4–17 (extracted transient response), tone-burst elicited CAEPs, followed down to the VDL in the "Game of Waves;" before (analog filtering only, *left panel*) and after digital filtering (*right panel*), respectively. The latter, in its original presentation, thus provided a second look at the data by way of further computer processing. Here, an added feature to the post-processing is time-expanded views of the tracings for further scrutiny. A latency-intensity shift is evident in both views/panels, although slight in the initial view (*left panel*). It is more readily seen in the expanded view (*right*). Incidentally, all manipulations demonstrated herein are available at the clinician's fingertips using modern AEP test systems. The underlying latency-intensity function (*outlined in gray line with a dotted line for a no-shift reference*) might seem to "point" toward a slight negative depression in amplitude of N_1 at 40 dB—thus perhaps a real response. However, both the poor reproducibility and level of residual noise suggests otherwise. This adult patient with a mild-moderate-sloping, high-frequency sensorineural loss demonstrated, in fact, a pure-tone threshold of 40 dB HL at the test frequency of 1 kHz. The VDL and predicted hearing threshold thus would be stated as 50 dB (given no other levels tested); though slightly overestimated, the results still would be informative of this subject's hearing status at the test frequency. T/R: test/retest tracings (from split buffers) overlapped; est-ctrl: estimated residual noise computed as (T-R)/2.

of testing. This perspective will be pursued in more detail shortly. Nevertheless, the test protocol can change substantially with age of the patient. Infants' responses may be lower in amplitude and/or noisier than those obtained from adults. Infants may be active (wiggly) and cannot be instructed to remain quiet, as can be done in testing older children and adults. Choices in stimulus type, presentation, filtering, and so forth varies depending on the patient being tested and the goal of testing. Filter settings, particularly the high-pass (HP) setting (again the low-frequency cutoff), affects response amplitude. Comparisons of various HP filter settings indicates minimal effect on P2 amplitude with a setting of 0.1 Hz. An HP filter setting of 1.0 Hz, often used in clinical testing, results in significant reductions in response amplitude. For the low-pass (LP) filter setting (high-frequency cutoff), a 30-Hz LP filter is fairly standard for the CAEP testing with minimal distortion of the response and substantial suppression of background noise.

As the development of efficacious measurement of the CAEP, in effect, seeded the development of ERA, there have been many studies comparing hearing-threshold estimations across AEPs. The overall trend indicates variability among response types, yet generally closer agreement between VDLs of CAEPs and behavioral thresholds than with subcortical responses. These differences have been studied across audiometric frequencies using frequency specific stimuli and among hearing-status groups (normal hearing and varying degrees, configurations, and types of hearing loss). In the following discussion, relationships are considered between hearing thresholds and estimates among measures of CAEP (P_1-N_1-P_2), ABR, ASSR with 40-Hz modulation, and ASSR with 80-Hz modulation.

ABR measurement remains the most frequently used clinical tool for hearing-threshold estimation and (as demonstrated earlier) there is a strong evidence base supporting its use. The relationships between VDLs for ABR elicited by brief tone bursts and behavioral thresholds are well established; threshold differences in subjects with normal hearing are typically 20 dB to 30 dB in the lower frequencies and 10 dB to 15 dB in the higher frequencies.[44,45] Slightly better agreement is observed in patients with hearing loss than for those with normal hearing.[45,46] The threshold differences constitute "correction factors" that can be applied clinically to obtain estimated hearing levels (eHL), can be used in relating results to the audiogram, and are useful in planning management when hearing loss is present.

Measurement of auditory steady-state responses (ASSR) was demonstrated earlier (recall Episode 6.3) to provide another useful approach and reliable metric for ERA. This discussion will start with a corresponding brainstem response—the 80-Hz ASSR. In a study[41] described in Episode 6.4, simulated hearing loss (using masking noise to elevate thresholds) was employed to test both the validity and reliability of ASSR-ERA threshold estimates using multiple carrier frequencies and 80-Hz to 100-Hz modulation rates. The justifications for this research design, rather than testing multiple hearing-impaired subjects or clinical cohorts, were several: systematic control of the hearing loss including multiple degrees; particular/challenging audiometric configurations readily created; and all conditions tested in the same sample of brains.[47] The last issue addresses concern for adverse effects of permanent, organic hearing loss on the CANS and the possibility of related bias. In addition to the ASSR testing, the researchers recorded CAEPs for tones centered at 2 kHz and compared threshold estimations among the three modes of testing thresholds. The hearing loss configuration in question was a substantial 2000-Hz notch (somewhat like that of Case 2 in the case studies in Heads Up of Episode 6.5; Figure 6–36A). VDLs were determined for ALLR-ERA and automated scoring based on statistical criteria were applied to ASSR-ERA. Mean differences between CAEP and behavioral thresholds were about 10 dB, consistent with other studies, and ASSR and behavioral threshold differences were only slightly smaller. Differences between behavioral and CAEP and ASSR thresholds were constant across degrees of simulated sensorineural hearing loss. Comparison among the three tests administered (behavioral, CAEP, ASSR) for normal hearing and simulated hearing losses from 50 dB to 80 dB HL are illustrated in Figure 8–9. CAEP and ASSR demonstrated similar and reliable threshold estimations with correlations of AEP threshold via visual detection to behavior thresholds over 0.90 with nearly identical R^2 values: CAEP—0.84 and ASSR—0.86. (R^2 reflects the proportion of variance attributable to covariance.)

In another study,[43] results of ERA were compared between the CAEP and 40-Hz ASSR in adults with normal hearing and in two groups of patients with either mild-moderate hearing loss or severe-profound hearing loss. Test stimuli were centered at 0.5 kHz and 4 kHz. For subjects with normal hearing, CAEP-behavioral threshold differences were 10.3 dB at 0.5 kHz and 11.5 dB at 4 kHz, consistent with the 10 dB difference reported earlier across a number of studies. At 0.5 kHz, the 40-Hz ASSR thresholds were slightly poorer than

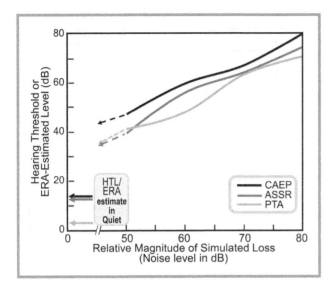

Figure 8–9. Comparisons among ERA estimates of hearing thresholds (transient-elicited CAEP and ASSR, 80 Hz) and behavioral threshold (PTA) at 2000 Hz as a function of hearing loss simulated in normal-hearing subjects by a simultaneous masking (tone-in noise) paradigm. Average unmasked behavioral thresholds as indicated (central tendencies modeled; based on data of Kaf and coworkers [2006][41]).

CAEP thresholds in subjects with normal hearing and similar across the hearing loss groups. In contrast, at 4 kHz, differences between behavioral and 40-Hz ASSR were larger for all groups. These findings were consistent with those of an earlier report of an 11-dB difference for CAEP thresholds at 1 kHz, 2 kHz, and 3 kHz in adults compared to a 19-dB difference when using a 40-Hz test paradigm.[40] Results of the more recent study[43] also provided comparisons across frequencies and subject groups, indicating that CAEP response thresholds at 0.5 kHz averaged 3 dB lower than those obtained to 4-kHz stimuli. These results were consistent with the conclusion from yet another earlier study[48] that low-frequency stimuli tend to elicit greater amplitude CAEPs than higher-frequency stimuli.

An investigation[49] comparing ERA results among tests of the CAEP, 40-Hz ASSR, and 80-Hz ASSR evaluated thresholds at 0.5 kHz, 1 kHz, and 2 kHz in adults, with most subjects having sensorineural hearing losses. The results showed that all three methods predict the degree and configuration reasonably accurately. CAEPs were comparable to ASSR though in some patients CAEP thresholds showed larger differences. Differences between behavioral and AEP thresholds, averaged across the three test frequencies available for all response types, were 20.8 for CAEP, 17.1 for 80-Hz ASSR, and 12.1 dB for 40-Hz ASSR. Thresholds for the 40-Hz ASSR method were significantly closer to behavioral thresholds though the authors of the report noted that the CAEP and 40-Hz ASSR audiogram estimates were obtained more quickly than when measuring the 80-Hz ASSR.

While the focus has been the use of tone bursts in the context of seeking detection limits of sound, CAEP testing readily accommodates more complex stimuli—including more environmentally relevant stimuli, such as speech, and also stimuli of longer duration than the tokens discussed in earlier episodes. In relation to complexity of nonspeech stimuli, comparisons have been made among pure tones, multitones, and narrow-band noise stimuli.[50] Multitones were found to yield the highest amplitude responses for stimuli centered above 0.5 kHz, supporting the benefit of complex stimuli and demonstrating that bandwidth is not driving improved response amplitude with nontonal signals. In other words, the use of such stimuli in eliciting the CAEP is reflecting more activity of the CANS' processing of sound than merely more/less energy of the stimulus (assuming appropriate sound calibration among the less-versus-more complex sounds). Since higher amplitude responses yield better SNRs, these stimuli also potentially lead to shorter test times. Continued exploration of complex stimuli, particularly while retaining frequency specificity, is thus warranted.

A common practice in AEP threshold testing is to follow latency and amplitude changes with sound level (again, Figure 8–8). Experienced testers will consider response reproducibility—per amplitude and/or latency changes for a given test–retest— in making determinations of response presence.[41] The variability and complexity of these factors in real-world testing add to the desire to have objective methods for response determination, as will be discussed shortly for the CAEP. First, some more nonpathological variables are discussed, as considered previously for both the short- and middle-latency responses.

As demonstrated in the last episode, cortical responses are affected substantially by maturation of the neural pathways; this effect reflects maturational changes in structures comprising the hemispheres of the brain, including the considerable connections between the hemispheres. Neuromaturation continues through 12 years of age.[51] Nevertheless, CAEPs can be recorded at all ages, again including in term and preterm infants,[19,20,52] although morphology of cortical evoked responses can differ in ways that affect identification/interpretation of primary components, their respective latencies and amplitudes, and distribution of these potentials across the scalp. These differences dictate the need to modify test parameters to best suit the age of the individual being tested, whether the goal is response threshold detection or studies related to perception. The key message, to reiterate, is that CAEPs can be used at all ages, including very young infants.

Measurement of the CAEP, in principle and certainly in the general and neurologically intact adult population, is best accomplished in subjects who are alert and attentive to the stimuli. While response amplitudes are less robust when patients are not attentive or (worse) not awake, they still can be recorded and produce reasonably reliable/informative results in varying circumstances. This has been discussed previously, yet bears re-emphasis. A particularly important point to recap and elaborate is the effect and importance of presentation rate, well-known to affect response amplitude substantially and to interact strongly with both subject age (recall Figure 8–4) and level of arousal. Figure 8–10 effectively "stitches together" trends of AEP amplitude plotted as a function of stimulus rate (ranging from 0.75 to 80 stimuli per second) in adults (both awake and lightly dozing) and children (6 to 9 years of age, awake).[13,53,54] These results provide an example of the interactions among factors influencing CAEPs and the need to account for such characteristics when implementing test protocols and interpreting test results.

This characteristic is intriguing, in that watching the CAEP is watching the brain literally mature into the teen years. Yet for the clinician wishing to use ERA, academic interest may hold less importance than implementation and value in the clinic, begging again the question, why the CAEP for ERA? As has been stated, it is all about turf in AEP-dom. Long latency, cortically based responses

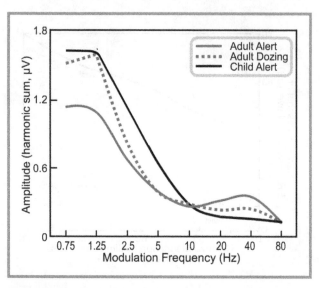

Figure 8–10. Effects of stimulus repetition on AEPs overall. Parameters are adult (mature-young subjects; awake/alert), adult dozing (lightly sleeping), and child (children 6–9 years; alert, watching a favored video on a small screen to minimize eyeblink/gaze artifacts). Magnitudes of overall responses derived from measurements in the frequency domain via a steady-state stimulus-response approach, carrier frequency of 1 kHz (based on data of Tlumak and associates [2012][53]).

provide several advantages in clinical evaluation and research settings. As suggested previously, cortical testing approaches typically demonstrate responses well approximating behavioral thresholds. Even if only "breaking even" (that is, at least as close estimates to behavioral thresholds as results of subcortical-AEP-based ERA), the inclusion of more of the auditory pathway is a strong argument of such approaches. Despite this, clinical applications of cortical responses remain very limited which may be related to factors such as minimal emphasis in training programs and lack of comfort of clinicians in response to identification and interpretation. The following discussion expands considerations of the stimulus-response characteristics that support the value of CAEPs in hearing-threshold estimation.

Cortical auditory evoked potentials literally provide a broader view of functional integrity of the auditory pathway than earlier AEPs, especially those generated subcortically. Picking up from this contention made at the outset of this episode, the presence of a cortical response demonstrates that signals have reached the primary auditory cortex and beyond, thus providing greater validity. Furthermore, CAEPs are generated at least closer (than subcortical measures) to parts of the CANS underlying true tests of the sensation called hearing, as commonly accorded to the pure-tone, behaviorally evaluated audiogram. While CAEPs used for detection testing (P1-N1-P2) in a single stimulus paradigm may not fully evaluate hearing as such, the presence of responses does provide evidence of processing across significant portions of the pathway supporting capability that underlies comprehension and communication.

Valuable considerations related to the test stimuli include greater frequency specificity, made possible with longer duration stimuli and the ability to utilize various types of stimuli such as tones, syllables, words, and so forth. Complex stimuli may have broader bandwidth which reduces frequency specificity; however, this provides opportunities to evaluate processing of speech directly and processes that underlie language. Furthermore, longer duration stimuli facilitate applications in hearing aid and cochlear implant testing and reduced susceptibility to electrical artifacts.

Use of subjective, visual detection methods to determine response thresholds (again) has been a challenge throughout AEP-ERA history. Criteria used among clinicians and researchers vary and this is a major contributor to variability in findings across both research studies and clinical sites. Automated template detection methods and application of statistical methods have moved toward desired objective analysis. Importantly, these methods should serve to make CAEP testing more accessible to clinicians by removing uncertainty in judging response presence. Furthermore, automated, algorithm-based methods improve efficiency of testing by providing objective guidance about when a sufficient number of averages has been obtained.

A CAEP test system developed at the National Acoustic Laboratories in Australia utilizes natural speech stimuli with primary energy distributed across low-, mid-, and high-frequency ranges[55] and automated detection of response presence. This system incorporates a response detection procedure where data are averaged across 101 ms to 500 ms and then divided into nine 50 ms time periods of the response. A statistical method (Hotelling's T^2) is used to calculate the presence of a response across these time bins with response presence defined as significantly different from zero which allows consideration of positive as well as negative peaks. Application of this statistical approach for detection of CAEP waveforms has been validated in adults[56] and infants.[57,58] Results demonstrated that response detection was as least as accurate as subjective identification by visual detection of the response's presence.

In further study of automated response detection,[59] the CAEP-detection algorithm "considered" residual noise levels as well as response detectability. Residual noise is estimated based on epoch to epoch variation in a latency region of interest, and the Hotelling's T^2 statistic is applied to response detection (in the study summarized earlier[50]). The investigators' results provide data related to detection sensitivity, false positive rate, and recording time. This procedure should have application to identification of suprathreshold responses, detection of response presence near threshold, and can be applied to various types of evoked potentials. Few methods have been applied in consideration of both residual noise level and response detection. One such method is Fsp,[60] long available and originally developed for/applied to the ABR, for example as an objective basis for setting a "stopping rule"—the number of repetitions of the stimulus over which to determine reliably of the coherent average (recall Table 4–1).

Another approach suggests use of the growth/I-O function, fitted across intensity as a method to objectively estimate hearing thresholds.[61] The innovators compared several metrics in adults with normal hearing that included peak-to-peak amplitude, root-mean-square amplitude (in effect power), and peak phase-locking value (PLV) features. Estimates based on PLV were found to provide the closest estimates of behavioral thresholds (namely, within an average of 2.7 dB).

The methods summarized in the foregoing have been fundamentally time-domain based. A substantially different approach and currently in research and development is a method that incorporates ASSR principles with measurement of the CAEP[62]—thus frequency-domain based and adding the advantages of the ASSR stimulus-response approach toward truly objective CAEP measurement and ERA.[13,53,54] In this paradigm, the response currently has been coined, "long-latency auditory steady-state response" (LLASSR) (Figure 8–11). Consequently, a statistically based estimation of SNR is applied and response identification can be both strictly objective and automated using rule-based decisions. The aim is to benefit in CAEP testing the use of the key "virtue" of ASSR measurement. This is that of the signal recorded being specified deterministically by the stimulus. The response can then be evaluated according to its harmonic fine structure in reference to the stimulus rate—in short, by knowing precisely (in effect) where to look in the spectrum for a significant response. In applying an ASSR approach to the CAEP, there admittedly is added complexity in comparison to that of SLR- and MLR-ASSRs, both of which can be used reliably (as surveyed in the last two chapters) by testing primarily at the fundamental frequency dictated simply by stimulus repetition rate (a.k.a., modulation frequency). The LLASSR spectrum is more complex, may not necessarily be strongest at the "fundamental," and is not as resilient to stimulus rates that overlap/convolve the responses at higher than the nominal rates optimal for the corresponding/classical transient responses. At the same time and at rates of most practical value for ERA in particular (around 1/s), the classical transient response still can be extracted in the LLASSR paradigm, the analysis of which is

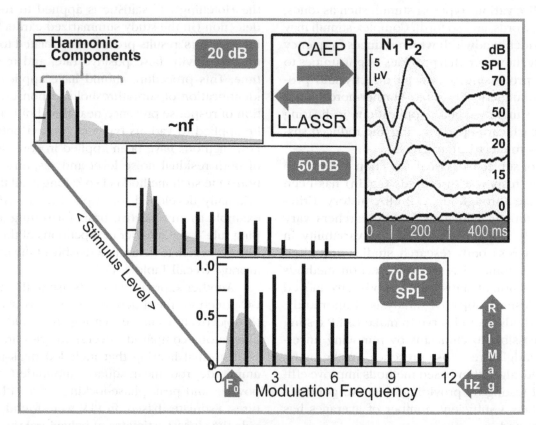

Figure 8–11. Spectra of ALLRs from a steady-state stimulus-response paradigm. While considerably more complex than the spectra of 80-Hz/40-Hz ASSRs, LLASSRs' spectra are still readily measurable and reliable for ERA/other clinical applications[62]. At low stimulation rates like 0.75/s (f_0 for the data here), the "machine" can be given rules to fully objectively evaluate true responses. At the same time, the conventional, transient-evoked response can be extracted (*seen inset/right-most panel*). Idealized/line spectra modeled from grand averages from young normal-hearing adults. Overall noise floor (nf) indicated by gray areas.

illustrated in Figure 8–11 (see Figure 8–8, demonstrating the basic stimulus-response paradigm, for reference; however, the subject for the inset-panel of the current figure had normal hearing). The clinical strength of this technique thus is the ability to measure cortical responses objectively, including near behavioral thresholds, while minimizing confounds of interference and/or subject state typically associated with traditional CAEP assessment. As the latter potentially/likely will affect both signal and noise spectra, both must be analyzed, as inherent to this method. Therefore, this and other objective methods have potential to expand and generalize the use of LLRs in clinical audiology and to help overcome issues faced by clinicians involving the interpretation of responses, indeed with changing patient state and/or maturation.

In work to date, the LLASSR method has been scrutinized in adults with normal hearing, subjects with simulated conductive hearing loss, and in patients with sensorineural hearing loss.[63,64] ERA estimates of thresholds obtained using the LLASSR approach have been compared to those of other ALLR methods and behavioral thresholds. Results indicate that LLASSR measures are within 5 dB to 10 dB of behavioral responses for frequency-specific stimuli in the 0.5 kHz to 4 kHz range. An automated response detection approach uses a harmonic sum from the signal's spectrum and noise estimates around the harmonics (similar to an approach well developed earlier in the measurement of distortion-product OAEs). The long-term goal is to further refine parameters of method of response detection, taking full advantage of the characteristics of ASSRs—again fundamentally a deterministic approach. Data collection and analysis are ongoing in infants and additional patient populations, with the goal of developing an objective method of characterizing cortical function and threshold detection that is applicable in patients of all ages from newborn infants through older adults and by a method that readily can be placed in clinicians' hands. Use of the method is intended practically to complement what the user already knows of clinical electrophysiology in audiology and enhancing information garnered from the test. Its design thus is intended neither to require of the user substantial relearning nor giving up the opportunity to scrutinize the conventional/time-domain CAEP.

Testing CAEPs to evaluate performance of patients with hearing aids and cochlear implants also offers additional merits. While evaluation of amplification with ABR is not recommended due to the need for brief stimuli,[65] longer duration stimuli can be used with ALLRs, which allows evaluation of responses with stimuli that are appropriate for processing through a hearing aid or cochlear implant.[30,66,67] Interestingly, Rapin and Graziani[68] were among the first to use CAEP measurement in the assessment of effectiveness of amplification. From a series of 5- to 24-month-old children, they reported responses to be present in the majority of children with severe-profound hearing loss, believed to reflect improvement in audibility provided by a hearing aid. This was not observed in all children, leaving the possibility of influence of specific characteristics of the hearing loss, as well as signal processing functions of the device.[69] Extensive discussion of procedures and issues, particularly as they relate to CI, is provided in the chapter to follow.

CAEPs have particular value in differential diagnosis, in patients who have no recordable subcortical neural responses, and in situations where stimulus characteristics need to be compatible with processing of signals through hearing aids and cochlear implants. Cortical responses also are valuable in differential diagnosis where a test battery includes AEPs from cortical and subcortical areas. Patients with cortical deafness can display age-normal patterns of peripheral and subcortical responses, otoacoustic emissions, and middle-ear muscle reflexes while cortical responses are absent or highly abnormal.[70]

In contrast, patients with an AN or an SD are diagnosed based on absent or highly abnormal subcortical neural responses, specifically the ABR.[71,72] The presence of cortical responses in many patients with AN/SD presents particular promise in threshold assessment in infants and children. While the usual method of establishing threshold sensitivity in infants and young children is with ABR or 80-Hz ASSR, patients either with or at risk for AN/SD do not have reliable brainstem responses. This dilemma leaves clinicians without a method of determining hearing status until a child is old enough to obtain reliable behavioral thresholds, which is typically at least 5 to 6 months of age or even longer in preterm infants and children with developmental delays. Many patients with ANSD of all ages have present cortical responses and, in these cases, CAEP measurement has been used as an approach for establishing threshold sensitivity.[66] Furthermore, relationships between presence of cortical responses and speech perception ability have been established in patients with AN/SD, providing an alternative method of gaining insight into auditory function in this patient population.[29,73]

The goal of this episode was to demonstrate the value of CAEPs in threshold-determination applications, demonstrating for clinical and research applications alike that CAEPs are viable and reliably recorded responses and that ALLR-ERA is a valid method to apply their measurement to the estimation of hearing thresholds. Findings in cooperative, awake, and mature adults have demonstrated excellent approximations of ALLR-ERA estimations to behavioral thresholds. Much more is known today and being revealed in further research and development of CAEP recording/measurement to deal with all levels of maturation and with inattentive or even sleeping subjects. There are specific advantages of CAEP measurement/ALLR-ERA over other approaches, especially if limited to use of low-amplitude responses from the brainstem and, in turn, their limitations in the types of stimuli applicable. Indeed, at this point in history, the clinician may find it more difficult to justify not including cortical responses in initial testing than rationalizing the need to follow up with such testing.

Tests of CAEPs can and thus should be implemented in both clinical and research laboratories. Much progress has been made in optimizing acquisition systems to improve data analyses and provide reliable, objective detection algorithms. Collection of data from patients in clinical settings will serve to help researchers, clinicians, and developers evaluate new systems and algorithms broadly across populations to understand the full potential of applications. This may be particularly true for those groups where behavioral testing is not possible or objective testing is needed to fully understand an individual's auditory ability, as noted here and in other chapters. While there still is some challenge(s) in testing immature systems, CAEPs can be recorded reliably in these individuals with the consideration that response characteristics differ. The case has been made for evaluating AEPs from both subcortical and cortical regions, giving clinicians a wide range of resources with an established evidence base to guide them in providing comprehensive and accurate evaluation of patients and subjects of all ages and across various auditory disorders.

HEADS UP

A Case Spared Operative Treatment Thanks To Testing of Both Brainstem and Cortical AEPs

Long-latency AEP measurement paved the road for ERA research and development but was quickly cast aside in routine practice in favor of the ABR-ERA, per its unique advantages (discussed earlier). Overlapping research and development of clinical applications of evoked response measurements was that of an imagination-catching concept and revolutionary new otological treatment—part surgical, part electronic device—and with the vision to provide some hearing ability in profoundly deaf patients. This was the birth of the "practical" *cochlear implant (CI)*. This featured story is largely a retrospective, yet one of insights and lessons for today and tomorrow. It also is a prequel to a more comprehensive coverage of the wholesome AEP and CI relationship, coming soon.

The earliest days after pioneering proof-of-concept efforts represented some commercial battles for viable and marketable CIs, timely profession-sanctioned clinical trials, and ultimately approval of agencies like the U.S. Food and Drug Administration. The path to an approval for clinical use of CIs was appropriately conservative, initially granted only for limited use in adult patients but finally in children by the late 1980s. Clinics providing the technology were sparse in number, typically based at major/regional health-care centers. Strict protocols were observed for determining candidacy for CIs. Degrees of hearing losses (sensorineural) of patients treated were severe to profound at all audiometric frequencies. Interested patients had to be counseled to have realistic expectations; if they had any success using hearing aids, they would likely be better off just sticking with that treatment. The CI thus was far from a cure-all; there naturally were surgical risks involved. At that time, a sufficient level of success functionally, such as to provide communication ability on the telephone, was realized only in a minority of cases. Imaging was not at the very high level of today, but greatly progressing and a standard part of the protocol for determining candidacy. Results needed to suggest at least a patent internal auditory canal (unlike Case 1 in the Heads Up 6.5 on case studies) and a fluid-filled cochlea for electrode insertion.

The clinical workup thus required confirmation of level of impairment. Some programs included in their workup two electrophysiological methods. One was ABR testing to corroborate objectively conventional audiometric findings of profound deafness. The other was (recall Episode 5.4) that of applying an electrical stimulus via a transtympanic electrode—TT ECochG in reverse (in effect).[74,75] This, like conventional audiometry, is a subjective test of response to the stimulus applied. During the "promontory test," the patient is instructed in some manner to indicate any sensation. The underlying rationale of this approach is that if a bioelectric signal can get to the promontory from the 8th nerve, applying electrical signals to the promontory should reach any residual nerve fibers via the same electro-anatomical pathway. This clinic's stimulus paradigm was, once the transtympanic needle electrode was seated on the promontory (placed by an otologist using an operating microscope), they were presented a series of electrical pulses. The objective was not only to confirm (possibly) any auditory sensation to electrical simulation (versus merely a tactile, if not painful, sensation) but also to evaluate the ability of the patient to detect a gap between pairs of pulses presented. The latter serves as a rudimentary discrimination test. Today it is known that just around 60% of successfully implanted CI candidates demonstrate some hearing sensation via preoperative promontory stimulation, yet this "good news" carries a high false-negative rate. There also is generally some level of discomfort caused by the procedure and/or stimulation. For these reasons, the test came to be removed from this clinic's routine CI-candidate workups. Nevertheless, there has been continued interest in transtympanic promontory stimulation.[75,76] Whether a given test proves to not seem warranted for routine usage, there always is at least some chance that in certain populations that it still could provide further insights and/or other perceived benefits of its outcome(s). In any event, the case presented here was well on her way to have the promontory test in the course of her workup.

Potential CI candidates, as with any specialty, can be and often are referred from other facilities that are not directly involved in CI treatment. This was the case for this female patient in her mid-70s, referred from an outlying hospital's otolaryngology department to be evaluated for CI candidacy at the metropolitan medical center. Although hearing status was confirmed locally—namely a profound sensorineural loss bilaterally—it is customary at the CI program's site to reconfirm hearing status. The routine was to meet with the patient and a family member/significant other, communicate considerations for candidacy, proceed to conventional audiological evaluation, and immediately be followed up with clinical electrophysiology—all before seeing the CI program's chief otologist and audiology staff involved to come to a final recommendation to the patient. Profound loss of hearing clearly is substantially debilitating and especially so when incurred acutely and/or late in life, as was the client's history. Sudden onset hearing losses of this degree are not unprecedented, but fortunately are not common either. The team thus had to be cautious to ensure the patient's hearing status, namely to have unequivocal evidence of meeting the CI program's qualifications for candidacy and a truly organic condition, in particular.

The ABR thus was evaluated, but the results were both surprising and hardly gratifying clinically, per expectations and objectives of the patient's visit. They indeed were unnerving given that only minutes later the patient was slated to be seen in the otology clinic to receive the promontory test to further support (hopefully) her candidacy to receive the miraculous treatment of a CI. The ABR results are summarized in Figure 8–12A.

Advanced age is well-known to be accompanied often by hearing losses and that such losses tend to be progressive, but not by way of sudden onset. As learned in Episode 6.5, a substantial hearing loss can obscure the interpretation of the ABR for differential diagnostic purposes. Still, with luck, there should be some ability to elicit an ABR pending degree and etiology of the loss. Presbycusis is characterized by progressive loss of hearing in the high frequencies. Stimulating at 90 dB nHL can be expected to show something of a response, even with a severe high-frequency sensorineural loss. Beyond that, with more and more involvement of the low frequencies as well, it will be difficult to record anything but background noise. Therefore, this patient was presumed to have little chance for demonstrating any ABR; yet there they were, "plain as day" and for both ears. Not only robust ABRs at 90 dB but also still impressively strong responses at 70 and suggestive responses at 40 dB nHL. Could these results also suggest the presence of some degree of hearing loss? Possibly, but nothing much more than a mild loss in the upper frequency range and certainly not the sort of degree of loss typical of candidacy for cochlear implantation at the time. Hence the question,

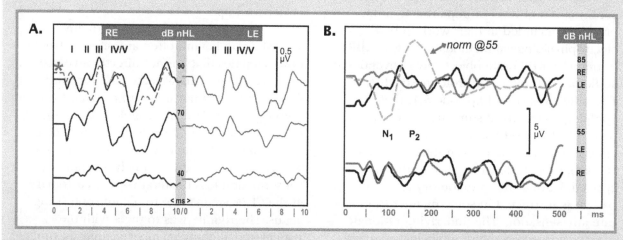

Figure 8–12. A. Results of ABR (transient-SLR) testing in a case presenting with profound deafness, as a candidate for a cochlear implant. Right (*RE, black*) tracings and left (*LE, gray-line*) tracings of responses. *LE response replotted in the RE panel (*dashed gray line*) for direct comparison and demonstration of essentially equivalent responses bilaterally. Click stimulus at 17.1 Hz repetition rate; nHLs as indicated. **B.** CAEP results, overlaying RE and LE responses at indicated nHLs. Tone burst at 500 Hz; 1.1 Hz repetition. Both tests: recording between vertex and respective mastoids; ipsilateral montage for ABR; contralateral montage for CAEP. Normative (norm) grand-average response at 55 dB nHL (*dashed gray line*) for comparison, indicating no N1-P2 evident, even at the higher test level. Yet, some coherent waves occurred, possibly actual responses, but if so, more likely of subcortical origin(s).

might the patient be feigning profound deafness for some reason?

Back to the patient's history. The patient in fact had suffered a stroke some months before—severe, but with good recovery of general health. Question: Which came first—hearing loss or stroke? Somehow, nobody quite knew that answer that day, and it certainly was difficult to resolve confidently on the spur of the moment. Meanwhile, the otology chief was wondering where the patient was, while the audiologist also was wondering, what to do?

First, think. Taking the profound deafness at face value for the moment (compelling by anecdotal information and how the patient was perceived by the staff), the ABR results compellingly argued against the presumptive auditory status. To recap, there was no worse hearing sensitivity than reasonably expected per age (regarding population statistics). Yet, no inkling either that the patient actually perceived the presence of sound. Decision: check the cortex before discharging the patient from the evoked potential lab—test her CAEP. The results are summarized in Figure 8–12B. To best ensure whether or not there were any coherent signals in the patient's recording, right- and left-ear tracings are overlaid (test–retest responses having already been averaged) for the same objective—improving chances to "see" a true response, if present. Arguably there are "bumps" in the tracings (perhaps AMLR components?) but not a N_1-P_2 waveform, whether at 55 dB (where likely she would have "reliable ABRs") or at 85 dB nHL (just below where she demonstrated robust ABRs). To iterate, no sign of a reproducible N_1-P_2 complex, in reference to the AEP lab's normative data at 55 dB and typical response from a young adult, normal-hearing subject plotted in the figure for reference. Even in the face of any clinically significant hearing loss consistent with the ABR findings, failure at the higher stimulus levels of the CAEP test could only indicate bilateral cortical deafness.

The promontory test was cancelled. Cortical deafness is not common, even in stroke victims. Thinking of the auditory space continuum, it is increasingly difficult going "north" along the pathway to shut down sound detection totally, even by a substantially disordered auditory pathway. Just too many side paths and/or crossovers along the way whereby some signal should reach the cortex, at least for merely detecting the presence of sound. Of course, the outcome was disappointing to all concerned. Here was a patient nearly in line for a CI, prepared mentally to accept surgery, and having a glimmer of hope for better days than had befallen her in the golden years by an untoward cerebrovascular event and subsequent neurological sequelae.

Failing catching the case at the candidacy confirmation stage, stimulating a true auditory response electrically surely would have failed anyway. However, failing that test would not have been a deal-breaker for moving forward with an implant, if all other criteria were met and the patient was still well motivated. There had been reasonably successful cases in the face of failing to stimulate the candidate via promontory electrical stimulation (that is, in deference to proportion of false negatives possible).

What is the teaching point here? If CAEP testing was not done, no problem; it was a moot point anyway? Certainly not! Quite the contrary. The case demonstrates that the clinical electrophysiological component of the protocol must be administered by an examiner(s) who is both competent and comfortable to pursue whatever evoked response is best indicated by any clinical questions as they arise. Need to know is the imperative. If the given clinical protocol gets sidestepped by some unforeseen variable, there must be readiness to see it through, whether in the same appointment or via rescheduling. Here, the viable ABRs put the brakes on moving forward according to the typical protocol, at least until any new question(s) could be resolved. Today, audiologists have all the wonderful tools of electrophysiological measures to evaluate the complete auditory system, if and when necessary—from the 8th nerve to the cortex. The protocol is established according to reasonable expectations based on the particular clinical population that has been shown to be well served by a given diagnosis and treatment. However, the protocol is to help ensure proper steps by best practices, as supported by its evidence base. It is not intended to be so rigid as to put blinders on the clinician.

Back to the story: Would it have been good enough simply to give the patient understanding of her not being, in fact, an appropriate candidate? That too—certainly not. The electrophysiology lab of the clinic in this case actively used longer-latency responses, not just tests of ABR alone. This was hardly the first case in which—regardless of the test "ordered"—merits of events in the actual appointment suggested another test protocol to be needed, namely the one to best get to what became the real question to be answered by results of AEP testing. Some clinicians may have adequate experience and comfort levels only for the most routine tests, admittedly favoring the brainstem responses in practice. Nevertheless, that is not enough for full competency in clinical electrophysiology in audiology.

Of course, the patient was disappointed by the outcome, yet appeased by an understanding of her real hearing problem. This lady, a widow, was still young at heart; she had recently found the new love of her life. It was actually the boyfriend who had gotten wind of the growing success of cochlear implantation. It thus was more his idea and motivation than her own. Still, they both could deal with the outcome better and be content with, at least, having pursued cochlear implantation and having benefited appropriate management.

■ Episode 3: Late-Late Shows in AEPdom—Beyond Obligatory Potentials: When Just Turning On the Same Stimulus Is Not Enough

This episode is about even later cortical responses than presented thus far, namely associated with higher-order auditory processing. The perception of a sound involves cortical-level function initiated by neural processes that elicit an **obligatory** AEP—the P_1-N_1-P_2 complex[6] in older children and adults or immature variants in young children. But wait, there is more! As presented earlier, the classical approach to measuring the CAEP is that of a straight forward, stimulus-response paradigm. A single stimulus or event (click, tone burst, or speech token) occurs in the subject's test ear; if the auditory system is nominally functional, there is a good chance that some facsimile of the CAEP will be registered by the AEP test system. In other words, given adequate sensitivity of the peripheral system, enough of an intact ascending pathway, and thus populations of neurons firing adequately synchronously to this repeated singular stimulus, the cortex has to respond, and the response readily detected, especially by modern instrumentation. Another paradigm is to have additional (two or more) stimuli that occur UNexpectedly—referred to as (targeted) **deviants, infrequent or rare stimuli**—embedded in a train of stimuli commonly referred to as **standards** or **frequent stimuli** (Figure 8–13A). The auditory cortex still actively detects but also discriminates between these types of stimuli. Consequently, the obligatory response will be elicited by the standard stimulus within the train; the deviants will elicit separately **discrimination potentials**[77,78,79] (Figure 8–13B).

The components of the CAEP were seen to operate in a time zone delimited by latencies of approximately 50 ms to (rarely much over) 200 ms in otoneurologically intact adults. Recall that the P_b falls on the nominal MLR-LLR boundary in AEPdom and identified in the context of LLRs as P_1. It, N_1, and P_2 also can be referred to as P_{50}, N_{100}, and P_{200}, respectively. The focus here, for the most

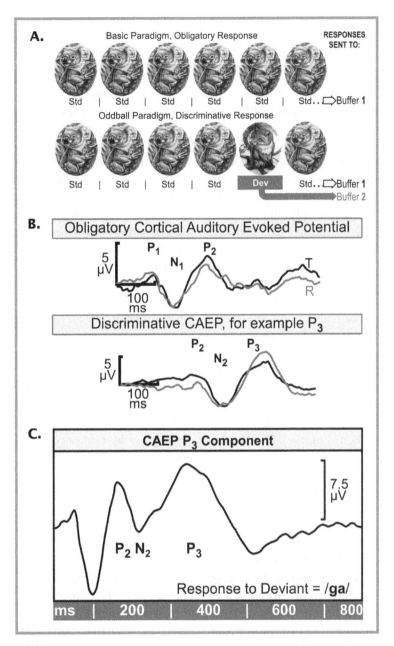

Figure 8–13. A. Visual representation of paradigms for simply eliciting an obligatory response (in effect, comprising only "standard" stimuli) versus trains of standards interspersed randomly with a "deviant" stimulus—the oddball paradigm. Here the standard (Std) stimulus is represented by the koala bear with the fox serving as the deviant (Dev), in turn with far less proportion of occurrences in the overall train of stimuli presented. Coherent averaging of data for the two events are derived from separate buffers in computer memory. (Images courtesy of Mr. M. A. Durrant.) **B.** Averaged potentials, obligatory versus discriminative responses, to the stimuli when presented in an oddball paradigm. In this example, tone bursts were used (a standard of 1000 Hz and deviant of 2000 Hz). The potentials of the P_1-N_1-P_2 complex are characteristic obligatory responses while P_3 (P_{300}) is characteristic of discriminative responses. **C.** Example of a P_3 elicited using contrasting speech tokens (/ga/ versus the standard /da/) presented in an oddball paradigm.

part, will be "the beyond"—not only for just another AEP wave but another way of teasing out fundamentally more information from AEP measurement and at another approximately 100 ms later (Figure 8–13C). Traditionally, P_{300} or simply P_3 has been referred to as an **endogenous response**. This implies that it is impacted by the cognitive context within which the stimulus occurs and that its behavior is only partially related to the physical properties of the stimulus.[80] In contrast, **obligatory cortical responses** again are regarded as **exogenous**; they are strongly dependent on the physical properties of the stimulus.[81] There are two problems with the application of these terms when defining any AEP with a cortical generator. First, all cortical responses (obligatory and discriminatory) have multiple generators that include auditory and cognitive sources that are difficult to disentangle. Second, these responses are affected by **attention** and **meaning** as much as the physical properties of the stimulus.[10] Therefore, application of these terms is inadequate and is not applied here in further discussion.

The current episode features primarily one particular discrimination potential, the P_{300}/P_3 and with emphasis specifically on the P_3b component—a large, broad, positive peak that occurs around 300 ms following the perceptible onset of an improbable or deviant stimulus[82] (Figure 8–13C). In other words, the subject must attend to the change of the stimulus that results in elicitation of this response.[83,84] The response has a centro-parietal distribution with the response observed most prominently on the scalp at midline, namely at sites suggesting a neural source in the parietal-temporal region of the cortex.[6,82,83] The P_3b has been demonstrated using visual, somatosensory, and auditory stimuli,[85] but in this overview, only the auditory stimulation is considered in detail.

Depending on the type of paradigm and the deviant stimulus, there may be another broad, positive and smaller component wave or of shorter latency than $P_{300}b$—$P_{300}a$ or simply P_3a. This component is typically observed at about 250 ms to 300 ms with fronto-central distribution and midline sites displaying the biggest response.[84] The P_3a occurs when a subject involuntarily orients or switches attention to a distinct stimulus that is not a target and, therefore, is unexpected and does not require a button-press response,[86] as frequently required of participants in P_{300} studies to help the examiner assess level of attention. This response underscores further aspects of this type of AEP that differs distinctly from obligatory AEPs with respect to both response generation and test paradigm. The P_{300} "show" still provides objective measures of the response.

The stimuli employed in P_3 complex measurement can range from novel and unrecognizable to "not-so-novel" but easily discriminable.[87] The P_3a is relatively less well understood compared to the (later) P3b, but it appears to be a consequence of a nontargeted deviant stimulus (no button pressing) or an unexpected deviant in contrast to a targeted deviant stimulus that elicits P3b and requires the subject to press the button. The difference between target and nontarget deviants is in the level of **expectation**. For instance, a target deviant occurs when participants are informed to "look out" for a deviant or press the button when a certain deviant occurs, whereas a nontarget deviant is unexpected.[77]

P_3a and P_3b responses also are characterized by their respective amplitudes (Figure 8–14A). Amplitude is often dependent on the stimulus magnitude.[77] Here, the greater the deviance between presentations of standard and deviant stimuli, the larger the amplitude of the P_3 complex (a and b components of the response) will be. The amplitude of the P_3 complex is also inversely related to probability; the lower the probability of certain stimuli occurring (rare stimulus presentations), the larger P_3a and P_3b are. The implication is that these responses must be elicited after cognitive evaluation and categorization of the stimuli.[88] At the same time, the P_3a and P_3b peak latencies differ, which is attributed to the fact that the P3a component can occur because of changes in either attentive, or nonattentive, stimuli (panel A). The P_3b peak is only elicited in response to attended stimuli[89] (panel B), and that is what makes the P_3 complex "so cool"! Overall, what makes the P_3 "show" different from testing of obligatory responses is that it is largely one of greater cooperation (subject is at least quiet and alert), if not one of "audience participation" (actively attending to a target stimulus or more, like mentally counting occurrences of a deviant stimulus or button pressing).

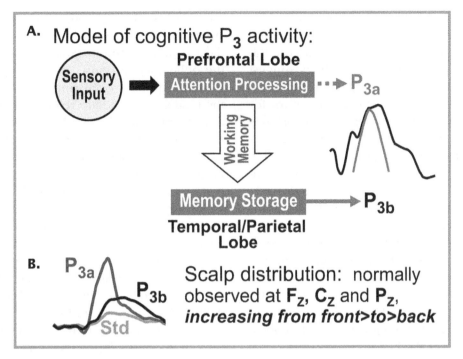

Figure 8–14. **A.** The cortical systems involved in eliciting the P_3 response. Waveform models: excerpts centered around 300 ms; gray line—underlying P_3a component. **B.** Model P_{3a} and P_{3b} responses and their individual morphology and relative amplitudes and latencies (with *underlying standard/obligatory response in light gray*).

Consequently, the difference between P_3a and P_3b, indeed, must reflect further processing by the cortex (again, Figure 8–14A). This is another example of "no free lunches" since it takes more time for such processing—thus longer latency of response. The P_3b component is produced after a decision is made about the presented stimuli (detection of changed stimuli), but what P_3b presence represents is not clear.[84] Two theories have been proposed to explain the elicitation of P_3b. One theory suggests that P_3b is the consequence of updating expectancy when an anticipated event occurs.[90] The second possibility is that P_3b is a result of "context-updating" when an unexpected event occurs.[91] Working memory is the central, executive function proposed to be associated with such updating.[84] Long-term memory, however, provides cognitive reorganization and requires conscious awareness of novel information for P_3b to be elicited —hence the different "time-space coordinates" of the auditory pathway involved in its generation.

In a more recent research report, a *late-novelty P_3 or nP_3* arising at about 400 ms and a *slow wave (SW)* following the nP_3 component have been identified.[92] Using *principal component analysis* (a statistical tool), the investigators identified the sources in the frontal and parietal lobes. The response has only been considered in a limited number of studies and is not discussed in more detail here. Still, the issue is certainly noteworthy.

The P_3a and P_3b peaks have different cortical sources (again, Figure 8–14A), suggesting different underlying neural processes. The two responses differ because of varying allocations of top-down processing resources, such as working memory and attention.[84] The P_3a occurs as a result of involuntary orienting of attention associated with a frontal source position, whereas the P_3b is representative of processes that include *working memory* and attention. P_3b is more readily observed with recordings from a more parietal location (see Figure 8–14B).[82,84,93]

Lesion studies have determined that a P_3a alone can be diminished in the frontal lobe and by focal, hippocampal lesions,[94,95] whereas the P_3b peak remains unaffected. These findings suggest different areas of neurophysiological involvement of each component with distinct generators for P_3a and P_3b components. For instance, recordings with needle electrodes from depths of the cortex (possible in some neurosurgical cases) identified generators for P_3a that included the anterior cingulate and fronto-parietal cortex. Generators for P_3b, however, included superior-temporal, posterior-parietal, hippocampal, cingulate, and frontal structures.[86,96] Similar generators were located in a low-resolution electromagnetic tomography.[97] This study identified an anterior distribution with generators in the cingulate, frontal, and right-parietal areas for P_3a, and sources in bilateral-frontal, parietal, limbic, cingulate, and temporo-occipital regions for P_3b.[97,98]

The P_3b is most commonly elicited through an oddball paradigm (see Table 8–2 for common parameters and again Figure 8–13A for illustration). To recap: An oddball paradigm consists of stimuli of high versus low probability. Stimuli that occur more frequently (70%–80% of the total number of stimuli presented) are referred to as frequent/standard/common stimuli. Such presentations elicit the obligatory response components (P_1, N_1, and P_2). Infrequently occurring stimuli are ≤30% of the total stimuli and are referred to as infrequent/deviant/rare/novel stimuli; these stimuli evoke responses that require perceptual ability to distinguish the two types of stimuli, which results in eliciting the P_3 complex. The amplitude is measured by the difference between the baseline and the response peak. The largest excursion from baseline occurs typically at ≥250 ms for P_3a and 300 ms for P_3b[84] (again see Figure 8–14). Stimuli of 1000 Hz for frequent/nontarget presentations and 1500 Hz as the rare/target stimuli provide high interclass correlations of test–retest reliability r = 0.86 and 0.89 for P_3 amplitude and latency, respectively.[99]

The amplitude of the P_3 response overall (Figure 8–15) is dependent on multiple factors, such as the type of stimuli, the probability of the stimuli occurring, and the difficulty of the task—with greater difficulty of the task resulting in more reduced amplitudes.[100] In particular, the amplitude of the P_3 is dependent on the probability of the

Table 8–2. Useful Settings for Recording P_3s

Parameter	Setup
Stimulus type	Tone burst (10-30-10 ms) or speech stimuli
Frequent stimulus	1000 Hz or speech stimuli
Infrequent stimulus	2000 Hz or can be any stimuli
Stimulus polarity	Alternating
Intensity	75 dB nHL
Presentation rate	1.1/s (interstimulus interval at least twice stimulus duration)
Time window	500 ms (is influenced by the duration of the stimuli and interstimulus interval)
Filter bands	1 Hz–30 Hz
Electrode montage	Fz—A1/A2 and Pz—A1/A2
Number of channels	2
Number of sweeps	500 ≈ number of standards/frequents to ensure adequate number of deviants/infrequents ≈ 150
Probability of infrequent	20% (although 10% is better)

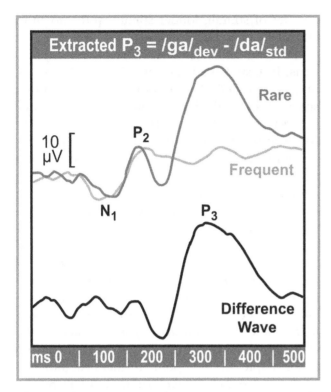

Figure 8–15. Averaged P_3 response to speech-token standard and deviant stimuli (/da/-/ga/ contrast) in a young, normal-hearing adult. The "extracted" waveform—indicated as "difference wave—is computed as "rare" minus "frequent" buffered data/signals in posttest/additional processing of the recorded potentials.

deviant stimulus. Large P_3b amplitudes are elicited with less probable stimuli; in other words, the less likelihood of the deviant stimulus occurring, the more robust the P_3b response.[82]

P_3 (a or b) latency is measured from the onset of the target stimuli and is representative of cognitive efficiency—effortful processing of the mental task or speed of allocation of attention and memory.[97,100] However, this is not the same, indeed independent, of what commonly is called "reaction time."[97,100,101] The more confident and cognitively efficient the listener is—when discriminating novel (infrequent) stimulus presentations from the frequent stimuli— the earlier the latency is.[102]

The P_3 can be elicited by a variety of stimulus changes (see parameters, Table 8–2), such as alterations in the frequency of tone bursts,[103,104] intensity,[103] duration,[103] or spatial location.[105] Researchers have been investigating how different the deviant (rare) a target needs to be from the standard stimulus presentations to elicit a P_3 complex reliably.

In summary, as the differences increase between the target and frequent stimuli and the target becomes more easily discriminated, the component latency decreases and the amplitude increases.[102] Table 8–2 also provides a summary of the most basic parameters for successfully eliciting P_3, although a variety of paradigms can be effective. Thereto, a number of effects must be considered that further can affect the P_3s, as overviewed in the paragraphs to follow.

Arousal effects: While it is accepted that P_3b is influenced by cognitive processes, state of arousal is equally relevant. Arousal has been defined as a broad-based concept that refers to a trait or state of readiness/alertness, as stated by the authors of an extensive review of the literature.[106] Their objective was to identify the influences of natural and biological factors, such as body temperature, sleep quality, exercise, food intake, common drugs, caffeine, nicotine, and alcohol that impact an individual's state of arousal and, in turn, impact on P_3b morphology. The effect of these biological factors is varied and are observed as shifts in latency and/or amplitude.

Attention effects: Generally speaking, passively ignoring stimuli results in longer P_3 latencies and smaller amplitudes, relative to when participants have actively listened to the stimuli.[107] Individual amplitude variations can occur as a result of arousal state, which affects both attention and information processing abilities such that individuals with a lower or decreased state of alertness present with lower amplitude responses and longer latencies.[84] Eyes open or closed during a stimulus paradigm was not found to cause any differences in P_3b response, as long as participants were engaged in the task and stimulus presentations.[107]

Maturation and aging effects: Results of a relatively recent systematic review of 75 studies have been reported wherein P_3b latency and amplitude had been examined (in effect) across subjects from 6 to 87 years of age.[108] In general, the P_3b latency decreased during the first years of life until they reached a minimum, from which they then were observed to increase in older adults.[109,110] The determined rate of change for P_3b latency was approximately 0.5 ms–2.0 ms/year, with a minimum latency noted to emerge at about 15 years of age.[81] Similarly, P_3b amplitude increases during childhood, whereas in older adults it decreases, possibly due to a general slowing of brain processes.[102,108] Age-related changes in P_3b amplitude tended to peak at about 20 years of age and then gradually decline.[81,108]

P_3b latency and amplitude reach their maximum (lowest latency and highest amplitude) at different ages (Figure 8–16), interpreted as reflecting different aspects of brain maturation.[108] Latency was proposed to index neural speed, dependent on myelination, whereas amplitude was theoretically reflective of cognitive resources. Consequently, in advancing age, as the speed of cognitive processing decreases due to degeneration of white matter fiber tracts, P_3b latency starts to increase and an amplitude decrease occurs.[111]

The combined systematic review and meta-analysis of P_3b latency and amplitude providing much of the information on maturation/aging that was detailed previously also revealed that there were no significant *sex effects*.[108] The latency and amplitude trajectories for males and females were found to be similar. Additionally, it was noted that differences in paradigm parameters did not significantly impact P_3b latency. However, P_3b amplitude was more likely to be affected with a higher number of stimuli; louder stimuli were shown to effectively decrease amplitude.

Moving on to clinical interests and applications, P_3 tests have been investigated extensively in a variety of clinical populations including schizophrenia, alcoholism, autism, cognitive disorders (such as Alzheimer's), and **attention deficit hyperactive disorder (ADHD)** among others.[100]

With advancing age, a frontalization of brain responses seems to occur as part of age-related, compensatory neural effects. This concept (in essence) is that more primitive structures (prefrontal cortex) come to play an increased role in governing behavior. This finding has been discussed within the **compensation-related utilization of neural circuits hypothesis (CRUNCH)** as well as in the anterior-posterior shift in aging models.[108,112] These models are based on the theory that additional neural activity is recruited as the task difficulty increases. However, this relationship is not simple. At some point, further task difficulty cannot be cognitively well-supported and performance drops. Older adults allocate more resources at relatively lower difficulty levels and this compensatory mechanism is localized in the prefrontal cortices where P_3a is elicited. Older adults with more frontal activity that require additional resources also exhibit poorer performance on neuropsychological tests of executive functions.[108,113] In sum, the association between increased frontal activity (frontalization), aging, and cognitive performance are currently not well understood. How the frontalization influences the P_3 complex requires further investigation.[112]

Schizophrenia is a mental disorder that significantly impacts cognition and has multiple other symptoms. Despite the variation in the presentation and symptomology of the disorder, the consensus is that for individuals with schizophrenia, auditory stimuli elicit longer latencies and lower amplitudes of P_3b compared to normative values.[114] P_3b latency and amplitude were reported to be impacted similarly in adults presenting with either high-functioning or low-functioning schizophrenia forms. In other words, the degree of the disorder and its impact on life did not correlate with the P_3 response findings.[115] The question remains—precisely, why are P_3b latencies and amplitudes impacted in individuals with schizophrenia?

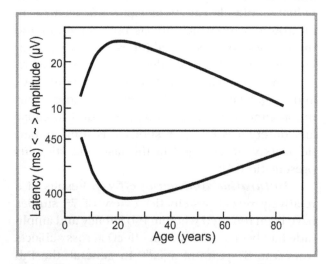

Figure 8–16. Overall trends of variation of latency and amplitude of P_{3b} as they change with age. (Central tendencies modeled, based on data reported by van Dinteren and associates [2014].[108])

The P$_3$b response was shown to be impacted in first-episode adults diagnosed with schizophrenia[116] and in their first-degree relatives.[117] This linkage may suggest a genetic predisposition to schizophrenia. However, another study found that P$_3$b amplitude (and not latency) was affected in the first-episode patients and was unaffected in healthy siblings.[118] Another possibility is that poor P$_3$b latency and amplitude in the schizophrenia population may be due to an inability to maintain attention to the task. Longer P$_3$b latencies and reduced amplitudes were present despite attention not required as a task condition.[119] Another study suggested that schizophrenia changes the allocation of attention, which consequently impacts P$_3$b latency and amplitude despite the straightforward oddball task.[120] In a more recent paper, reaction time and ability to inhibit/stop responding to task stimuli were reported to be impacted in adults with schizophrenia.[121] The authors suggested that the deficit lies in "slower initiation of the inhibitory system." In consideration of all the evidence, it appears that executive control of attention in schizophrenia is likely linked to the poor P$_3$b response findings.

Alzheimer's dementia is a progressive, degenerative disease that is one of the most common types of dementia. Although Alzheimer disease is not a disease of youth, it should not be considered as disease uniquely of elders. The disease results in anatomical changes in the brain, especially hippocampal volume. In addition, naturally occurring protein (a peptide, amyloid beta 42) in excess clumps together to form plaques in between neurons, which impacts cell function.[122] Results of a recent review of 20 studies found a smaller amplitude of P$_3$b to be a hallmark of Alzheimer's disease, relative to their magnitude observed in control groups (normal adults).[123] From another study, it was reported that the frontal response associated with P$_3$a had a prolonged latency in cases of Alzheimer's disease.[124] Therefore, if both P$_3$a and P$_3$b were measured, the ability to differentiate Alzheimer's from other cognitive disorders/diseases and from normal controls would be improved.[124] The literature review noted previously[123] also highlighted the fact that the impact of this disease was observed equally with visual and auditory stimuli. The association between Alzheimer's disease and the ranging severity of its presentation still is not explained well. It remains an area requiring further exploration.

Mild cognitive impairment (MCI) defines another clinical population of increasing interest in AEP research. This clinical entity may be a part of the "expected" aging process or a precursor to more serious cognitive decline, namely, ***aging dementia***.[125] MCI can also be associated with mild head injury. On average, populations with MCI show poor P$_3$b latencies and amplitudes. However, there is much overlap of P$_3$ latency and amplitude across the groups studied. From results of another investigation, prolonged P$_3$b latency was found to be correlated with age.[126] Hence, the question remains—are atypical P$_3$b latencies due to MCI, or do they reflect anatomical and functional aging factors associated with so-called normal aging?

In contrast, ***ADHD*** is relatively common in youth, affecting 3% to 18% of children.[127] The most prominent theoretical model suggests that individuals with ADHD have poorer/slower inhibitory control and are impacted in the anterior cingulate gyrus.[128,129] Previous studies reported that the amplitudes of the frontally generated component (P$_3$a) is reduced in children with ADHD compared to those of age-matched, normal controls.[129–131] P$_3$a has also been used to evaluate the effects of methylphenidate in this clinical population.[129] Adults with ADHD across six studies also showed a reduced P$_3$ response.[132] However, this appraisal was limited by the modest number of studies included for consideration and the small sample sizes for each study comprising the review. Another issue was that P$_3$a and P$_3$b responses to auditory and visual stimuli were collated rather than segregated into two stimulus groups. Regardless, the review provided meta-analysis encompassing results from approximately 150 adults. Other evidence has shown that populations with ADHD have reduced P$_3$ amplitude, possibly due to poorer inhibitory control in both auditory and visual modalities.[82]

Autism is a neurological, developmental disorder that is complex and multifaceted, manifesting itself within the first 3 years of life. P$_3$b amplitudes are noted to be reduced in this population with two possible explanations proposed. The first is that P$_3$b is reflective of an inability to allocate attention resources to the task, which may be an underlying rationale for why children with ADHD produce a small amplitude P_3b response.[133] The second explanation is that the reduced P_3b is more reflective of difficulty attaching meaning to novel (deviant) stimuli.[133] In a review, 32 papers were evaluated to find that P_3b amplitudes were significantly reduced in children with autism compared to control group.[134]

Adults with postlingual *hearing loss* comprise one of the few clinical populations in whom P_3b has been evaluated at the individual level.[135] Although past work was devoted to the notion of testing P_3 complex for purposes of ERA, this method is not well suited for that task.[136] P_3b amplitude is robust in cases with cochlear implants who demonstrate high performance on many auditory tasks.[135] In other words, if individuals with cochlear implants are able to perceive stimulus changes, P_3b amplitude is commensurate with normal-hearing controls.[137,138] In pediatric-CI cases in whom stimulus discrimination is poor, P_3b latency was reported to be significantly longer than age-matched controls.[139,140]

P_3a, in contrast to P_3b, was reported to be present in both good and poor adult CI users, but not in controls with normal hearing.[141] P_3a is linked to inhibitory control and orienting response and the investigators wondered if the response reflected orientation to sound, which implies that the participants were aware of the stimuli. The presence of the MMN (another discriminative potential preceding P_3, to be discussed shortly) in only good CI users also supported this suggestion. It is also possible that the presence of P_3a only in CI users (not normal hearing) indicates presence of compensatory neural activity that is normally observed in the older population to cope with a difficult task (as per the CRUNCH model).[108]

In at least one study, P_3b response was mapped across sensorineural hearing loss ranging from mild to severe/profound degree based on averaged 1000-Hz and 2000-Hz thresholds.[28] Results showed that for stimuli presented at 65 dB SPL, even mild hearing losses resulted in longer latencies for P_3b. P_3b amplitude was not impacted for mild losses but at moderate losses, amplitudes were reduced and latencies were prolonged. The same study showed that for stimuli delivered at higher levels (80 dB SPL), mild losses were associated with P_3b responses least impacted. For moderate losses, however, the 80 dB SPL presentation level resulted in longer latencies and smaller amplitudes compared to normal-hearing controls. Most adults with severe-to-profound losses showed no measurable P_3b response.

There are still other populations in which P_3 has been studied broadly. These include groups with alcoholism, mood disorders, Parkinson disease, and brain injuries as well as groups with other childhood disorders, including *auditory processing disorders*. Regarding the lattermost, a clear interpretation of the findings remains difficult. This difficulty is likely due to the high level of variability within the cohorts studied and the still ill-defined underlying mechanisms of both the disorders and P_3 responses. It has been suggested that P_3b is a measure of auditory-cognitive function, rather than a biomarker for any one particular disorder.[142]

Auditory training has attracted considerable interest in auditory neuroscience, especially regarding objective ways to determine the effect of auditory training on the CANS. In at least some populations, P_3b measures have been successfully applied. For instance, 14 adults with mild to moderate hearing loss and hearing aids were divided into two groups. Half of the group received 8 hours of auditory training and the control group received no training. Afterward, both groups were tested with P_3b. The experimental group had significantly shorter P_3b latencies compared to P_3b in the control group.[143] In an earlier study, children with auditory processing disorders who underwent auditory training had decreased P_3b latencies, whereas P_3b latency did not change in the control group.[144] In yet another study, P_3b and other AEPs were used to determine the benefits of music training in children. Two groups of children of 6 to 7 years of age were trained on music and sports, respectively, but a third group received no training. While at the baseline there were no differences between the groups, 2 years later, children in the music training group showed a greater P_3b amplitude compared to that of the children in the other two groups.[145] These are just a few examples that display how P_3b can be used to evaluate the effects of training in children and adults with and without hearing loss, readily evaluated in both clinical and typical populations.

There are several limitations as to why P_3a and P_3b have not been applied more broadly clinically.[81] Considering some 12,000 P_3 publications over nearly a half century, it has been surmised that the problem is that of it having not been possible to link this AEP to a specific cognitive process.[108] The barriers to *translational research* include the following: (1) variability even in normal populations resulting in overlap between the performance of controls versus patients of interest; (2) at present, many studies are investigating effects/impacts at group level, including (presumably) homogeneous groups of disorders—with more research needed toward determining the replicability of P_3a and P_3b responses within the normal and clinical populations of interest—thereby characterizing responses at an individual level; (3) due to the multiple processes and sources involved in the elicitation of P_3a and P_3b response, it is difficult to determine what an absence or variation in response implies for the considered disorder/disease; (4) specificity and sensitivity of the P_3a and P_3b response is low—with Alzheimer's disease, ADHD, and Autism disorders all displaying small P_3b amplitudes and therefore, differential diagnosis maybe problematic; and (5) the association between the comorbid disease processes, functional disability, the neural response behaviors and P_3a and P_3b remains unclear.

There clearly remains plenty of research potential and the need for further advancement of this AEP technology and clinical applications. Although data have come forth to elucidate the maturation of P_3b across the human life span,[108] more work is needed to characterize the P_3a equally. Test–retest reliability of the P_3a and P_3b responses must be fully assessed before sound clinical judgment can be applied to the results. While P_3b measurement does not appear efficacious for differential diagnosis at this time, it may be used to determine preserved or anomalous information processing. The current literature also demonstrates that assessing the P_3b component can be applied in the evaluation of auditory training paradigms and to monitor the effects of therapy and/or medication. Finally, the type of stimuli used to elicit both P_3 component responses and conduct their assessment requires additional research to better understand the effect of stimuli on certain clinical populations. For example, do children with reading disorders have poorer discrimination of both tonal and speech stimuli, and if there are indeed any differences, what are the implications of these stimulus effects? Moreover, if response differences to stimulus type(s) exist or findings suggest that a particular population is more sensitive to one type of discrimination (tonal or speech), this discovery may be useful in gaining further insight into underlying neural and central mechanisms.

Meanwhile, several other discriminatory potentials have received a great amount of attention in the literature and have/had considerable promise for routine clinical use. Still more research tools have become established broadly in audiology clinics. To wrap up this episode, the following is a brief overview, starting with a discrimination potential that actually precedes P_3a (as hinted earlier), this time a component of opposite polarity and that is intriguing for its particular nuances.

The *mismatch negativity (MMN)* occurs at 100 ms to 250 ms after the onset of a perceived change in a presented stimulus[146,147] (Figure 5–17, main panel) and has maximum activation in the frontal and temporal regions of the brain.[148] It is recorded at the fronto-central scalp positions (Fz/Cz).[149] The MMN is elicited when a perceived stimulus change occurs in simple tones, complex chords, or speech sounds. Stimulus changes may comprise frequency, intensity, duration, or localization variations[82,146,147] (Figure 8–17, "demo" panel). The MMN has also been observed with visual and somatosensory stimuli.[146]

Similar to the P_3b response, the MMN is a cortical auditory evoked potential that is elicited in response to change within an oddball paradigm; however, unlike the P_3b, the MMN arises as an automatic detection of change in absence of active, task attention.[148] The MMN is elicited even when the participant is actively doing another task (such as reading a book or watching a silent movie). The presence of the P_3a (which has longer latencies and occurs after the MMN) implies that the participant switched attention to the test task.[148] Lastly, the MMN, similar to the P_3b, is a result of a detected change in the stimulus and this change may be an irregularity within an expected pattern. In other words, the "standard" in an oddball paradigm may

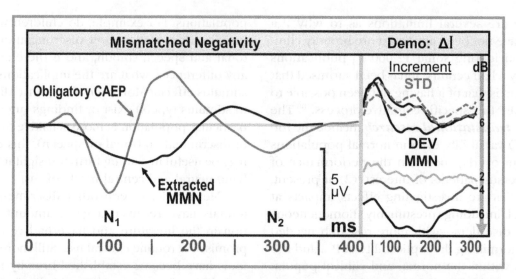

Figure 8–17. Characteristic mismatched negativity (*MMN, black line*) for young adults with normal hearing, with a typical obligatory CAEP in the background. Based on responses elicited by tone bursts of 1500 Hz for the deviant and 1100 Hz for the standard, both presented at 55 dB SPL. The response illustrated is "tapping" cortical processing of frequency discrimination by the CANS. Inset: For further demonstration (Demo) purposes, the MMN is tracked here in an intensity-discrimination paradigm, wherein the standard is held at a constant 55 dB SPL but with an increment (in dB as indicated) applied to the deviant, akin to the classical psychoacoustic test of the difference limen for sound intensity (ΔI). In the stimulus paradigm used, the rate was increased to 2.4/s which considerably adapts/reduces N_1 while leaving the MMN substantially intact, emerging robustly at decibel differences that indeed are readily audible to normally hearing listeners (based on data courtesy of Drs. B. Philibert and J. D. Durrant; stimulus paradigm, courtesy of Dr. N. Kraus).

be a single sound or a rhythm and the "deviant" being any change from the expected pattern.[149,150]

Two hypotheses have been proposed to explain why the MMN is elicited[151]—model adjustment and adaptation—which reflect differing concepts of the underlying auditory processing and neural generators. It also is unclear whether the response is an extension of N1, with generators in the temporal and/or frontal cortex.

The MMN quickly commanded the attention of researchers and clinicians alike, with a ground swell of research in the late 1990s and into the new century. Results obtained portended substantial clinical utility. The MMN was elicited without requiring active attention from the patients. It was observed in infants, children, and adults.[152,153] Patient groups tested included sleeping babies,[154] comatose patients,[155] and children with reading disorders who were tested while watching silent videos.[156] Similar to P_3b, MMN has been investigated in cognitive disorders as well as childhood disorders, with MMN being absent, smaller, or later occurring, depending on the population.[82]

Since the discovery of the MMN in the late 1970s[146] and its study across various populations, several limitations of the studies have become evident. A primary issue with most studies has been using MMN at the group level, rather than at the individual level. To date, this necessity has precluded it from use clinically. The MMN is a rather small amplitude response[79] (often less than 1 μV, similar to the ABR and some AMLR components (again see Figure 8–17) and therefore, it is often noted to be absent even in typical populations of interest.[147] Still, MMN measurement remains worthy as a research tool, and there also remains the possibility (per the history of AEPdom) that the tool simply has yet to be sufficiently developed and/or simply to find "its place" in clinical science. At this writing for instance, researchers from various laboratories are investigating how to evaluate and measure the MMN in young infants to have a measure of their auditory discrimination at the individual-subject level.

The time continuum of the AEP also has been explored beyond P_{300} for possible research/clinical applications. These "late-late" AEPs include **N_{400} (negativity that peaks at 400 ms), ELAN (early left anterior negativity), and P_{600} (positivity that peaks at 600 ms),** which can be useful in evaluating language comprehension.[157] The AEPs discussed thus far are often elicited using tones, syllables, or (single) words, but words also permit investigation of the effects of linguistic complexity of stimuli. As well demonstrated in the foregoing, cortically evoked potentials provide information about the perception of sound and/or auditory discrimination. In order to understand and evaluate the way context within sentences can influence cortical responses, "late-late" AEPs can be elicited in responses to scrutinize changes in terms of **grammar** and **meaning**.[157]

The N_{400} peaks at about 400 ms after the onset of sentence-based stimuli, with the largest peak amplitudes occurring in response to a semantic incongruency.[82] For instance,

Semantically congruent sentence: "Grandma dressed for the party."
Semantically incongruent sentence: "Grandma dressed for the table."

Collectively, all the words in both sentences would elicit an N_{400}.[158] However, the semantically incongruent sentence would elicit the larger negativity[157] (Figure 8–18A). This cortical response has been shown to generate a scalp distribution of activation that is broad and maximal for the midline plane and is recordable at the central-parietal electrodes.[159]

The ELAN and P_{600} responses consist of a negative peak (arising at approximately 150 ms–250 ms) and a positive peak (emerging at about 600 ms) respectively, and both responses occur after the onset of stimuli consisting of sentences. The ELAN is a response to identification of syntactically appropriate structure and is about "detection," whereas the P_{600} is a response to syntactic violation[157] (Figure 8–18B). An example of syntactically appropriate sentence structure is, "The professor and students involved with the discussion board had a lively debate." An example of syntactic violation is, "The professor and students had a lively in debate on the discussion board involved." Given the sentence with a syntactic violation, a robust ELAN is initially evoked indicating detection of the syntactic error, whereas P_{600} is evoked at the obvious syntactic violation. The ELAN would be generated by frontal, left sites, whereas the P_{600} would be associated with centro-parietal positivity. These violations can be combined as syntactic-semantic violation, for example, "Professor and cats had a lively in debate on the discussion board involved." In this double-violation scenario, ELAN and P_{600} will be elicited but not N_{400}.[160] The pattern of responses implies that syntactic structure precedes semantic structure and that the syntactic-semantic structure is different.[158] Because sentence processing is complex, several cortical regions are involved in semantic and syntactic processing,[160] including the anterior and posterior temporal regions as well as the inferior frontal gyrus.[157]

The "late-late" AEPs have been used to evaluate populations with neurological pathologies, such as aphasia[161], brain injury[162], Alzheimer disease[163], and Parkinson's disease.[164] The N_{400}-P_{600} responses are somewhat less explored AEPs, particularly in the hearing-loss population.[158] Despite this limitation, there is an interest in these resources, especially for investigating speech processing in a more real-world or ecologically valid approach.

The LLRs span the time-space dimensions of AEPs with intriguing nuances among them and involve widespread functional cortical areas. Although testing the later potentials extends beyond the more fundamental aspects of routine clinical utility, the more exotic responses in the realm of AEPdom may make the clinical tools more intriguing, if requiring more elaborate

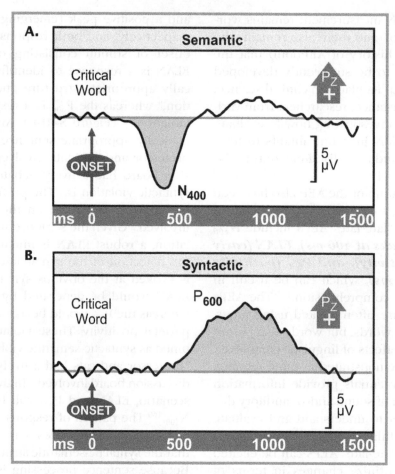

Figure 8–18. Averaged N_{400} (**A**) and P_{600} responses (**B**) to semantic versus syntactic incongruences of the sentences presented (see text). (Responses recorded in a young adult subject.)

paradigms by which to administer them. The foundational information presented early in the book was intended to support a broader understanding of AEPs even beyond those that are currently in clinical use. The upcoming chapter returns to "more basic" AEPs and the more fundamental methodologies by which they are measured, yet expands on clinical approaches that are driven by the need for suitable tests—especially for patients more difficult to test. The lower auditory pathway will again become the focus, although not exclusively. LLRs are becoming more and more efficacious in (for example) very young patients, who effectively were ignored not that long ago in most such cases. Who knows then what might be possible in the seemingly impossible cases with further research and development. As postulated before, given the history of the field, significant advances can be anticipated. With AEPdom now having been explored to the limits, there is no need to fear the new—like "fear of the dark"—as building upon the foundation given herein shall be the opportunity—the "light"—with the reward of approaching the new or a test/protocol simply beyond the routine, namely with interest and a sense of being prepared to give that "next generation" approach a fair chance. However, before leaving "the big(ger) picture" AEPdom, it will be useful to take a peek at what has been perceived as the "enemy" in endeavoring to measure AEPs, the ever-present background in their time histories. Hence, just one more thing.

HEADS UP

Peek at EEG Analyses Via Advanced Signal Processing

From the outset and now well-known by the reader in the "language" of the art and science of measuring AEPs, recording an evoke potential/response is one of data averaging. Looking to detect a response or even to measure as precisely as possible peak amplitudes and latencies of a given potential has been a task of extracting its signal from a background activity presumably behaving like a stationary, random broadband noise. This conceptual framework was to provide a reasonably valid and reliable tool to extract AEPs, indeed of numerous types of signals, yet full well recognizing that in that background lurks the "resting" EEG—brain waves! Here, now approaching the end of the "series" of the many episodes presenting the full range of AEPs, methods of testing them, and various additional "maneuvers" beyond basic coherent averaging, the question is raised on behalf of the often maligned EEG, and as the old song goes, "Is that all there is, my friends, is that all there is?"

Historically, it was the studious observation of the running EEG (tediously following lengthy recordings, literally traced out by electromechanically driven ink pens on reams of paper) that gave a clue that, indeed, there is organized brain wave activity that is reasonably assumed to be stimulus evoked—in particular, that known as the "K complex."[165,166] Researchers in the 1930s, at the dawn of EEG measurement and analysis, and into the 2000s continued to pursue the real nature of this EEG component.[166] From nearly the get-go, it was reckoned to have to do with stages of sleep and/or level of arousal. Origins were attributed to both the thalamus and frontal cortex, also implicated in the generation of some components of MLRs and LLRs, yet activity of huge magnitudes and longer latencies were only evident during sleep. In the thick of the research to examine systematically effects of sound stimulation was none other than Hallowell and Pauline Davis (recall history discussed in Episodes 8.1 and 8.2).[167] It certainly was germinal work both within their highly productive research group and with collaborators working in a state-of-the-science sleep laboratory of the era, effectively launching H. Davis' lifelong devotion and research and development, ultimately wherein signal averaging was applied to EEG analysis to reveal AEPs. These early workers, really had to "know their EEG." However, might endeavoring to treat the K-complex more like an "evoked potential"[168] have led workers of the future and today to overlook what the spontaneous EEG itself might have to offer? In fact, can more be derived from ongoing EEG and thereby more learned about activity underlying the evoked responses commonly measured, in other words, rather than "turning a blind eye"? This question begs an even more basic one: Is EEG (in effect) merely "noise," as treated in conventional AEP testing, when it comes to saying how sensory signal processing and the subsequent encoded signal headed to the cortex affect brain waves overall?

When evaluating an AEP, only activity that is time/phase *locked* to the stimulus accumulates on average; what is left is effectively deemed "noise" (random variance) and thus is discarded. Turns out that what was discarded also holds *unlocked* or "induced" activity within the overall EEG. This induced activity relates to events/stimuli and/or modulations by underlying sensory, cognitive, or linguistic processes.[169] The induced activity is rhythmic or oscillatory and therefore represents frequency-dependent changes in the EEG. However, depending on the "event," the magnitude and phase of EEG oscillations/rhythms at specific frequencies may vary from trial to trial. It is important to appreciate that the "evoked" and "induced" activities (as defined here), despite different neurophysiologic origins, are not completely independent of each other. The induced and evoked activities are linked processes in response to an event and progress in time with different, as well as overlapping, frequency components.[170] Time-frequency analyses can extract and inform from the EEG which frequencies are more robust versus which have less power at a given time. The following text is an overview of such analyses which comprise several steps.

Frequency analysis: In trying to piece together facts on how to view the signal from a different perspective, there are many different signal processing methods which can be "borrowed" to do this. Neural firing patterns have been found by previous studies to be associated with specific functions in the brain.[171] These neural firings are often periodic in nature within a certain short period of time; hence, periodic signals are often characterized by their frequency.

One of the more typical frequency analyzing tools used is (again) the Fourier transform. Recall that the Fourier transform is a complex mathematical equation to determine which frequencies are present within the signal. To better illustrate this, the Fourier transform can be represented as a prism. A prism will take a white light and split this into different colors; similarly, a Fourier transform will take a signal and split it into frequency components (Figure 8–19A). To recap, the output of a Fourier transform will generate three output parameters which includes the following:

1) Frequency: determines which frequencies are present in the signal
2) Magnitude: determines the strength of the frequency component
3) Phase: determines how the frequency components are aligned in time with each other.

There have been a number of studies that report that these frequencies are linked to a broad variety of perceptual, sensorimotor, and cognitive functions.[172–175] Hence, these frequencies are commonly grouped into frequency bands according to their functionalities (Figure 8–19B). These "EEG bands" are as follows:

1) Delta (frequencies from 0.5 Hz–3.5 Hz)
2) Theta (frequencies from 4 Hz–8 Hz)
3) Alpha (frequencies from 8 Hz–12 Hz)
4) Beta (frequencies from 13 Hz–30 Hz)
5) Gamma (frequencies from 30 and above)

The delta band has been associated with sleep and quality of sleep,[176] while the theta band has been found to be associated with control of working memory.[177] The alpha band has been found to be associated with attention and higher executive functions,[174,175] while the beta band (frequencies between 12 Hz–30 Hz) has been associated with motoric functions.[178–181] The gamma band has been found to be associated with behavior and decision making.[182]

Time-frequency analysis: Feeding the whole signal into frequency analyses shows a number of frequencies but ignores the (overall) time aspect. This motivates the introduction of time-frequency analysis. The time-frequency analysis uses the frequency analysis concept but instead of feeding the signal as a whole, the signal is divided into smaller temporal segments and each of these segments are then fed into the frequency analyzer (a.k.a., the prism). As a result, each of these segments has information on their frequency contents which, when appended together, presents how these frequency components evolve over time (Figure 8–19C). Since spectrum analysis (of each segment) already requires two-dimensions, then plotting the results of time-frequency analysis requires three-dimensions, as shown.

Normalizing time-frequency analysis: In EEG signals, the higher-frequency magnitudes are significantly lower when compared to the lower-frequency magnitudes. This would then create an issue when analyzing the frequency components as the higher-frequency components would be perceived to be negligible all the time. In trying to resolve this, the

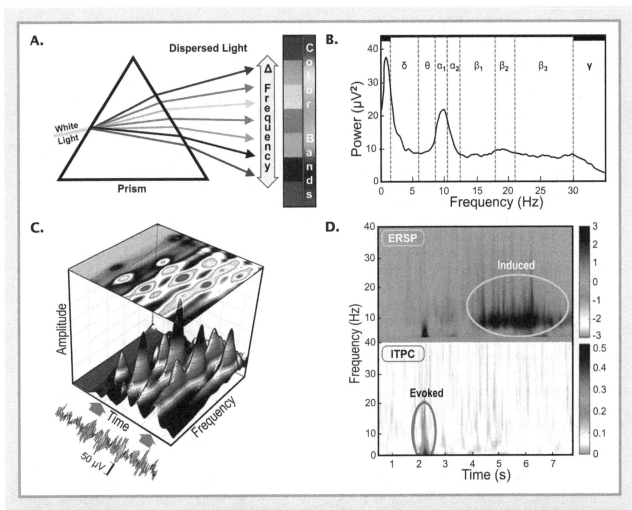

Figure 8–19. A. The prism disperses white light into different colors, just as the Fourier analysis "disperses" the signal into its component frequencies. As the frequency of a sound and its wavelength are directly related, so is this the case for light. To enhance the display of results of complex signal analyses, color-coding can be employed but here simply *represented in levels of gray with R (red), G (green), and B (blue)* to demark the three primary colors. **B.** The EEG signals are commonly grouped into specific frequencies which have specific functional significance. **C.** The time-frequency analysis divides the incoming EEG into smaller chunks and passes these smaller segments onto the "prism." **D.** Combined results of ITPC and ERSP analyses (see text) showing respectively both evoked and induced EEG activities.

frequency components are represented by magnitude changes instead of absolute values of magnitudes. In doing so, a "baseline period" is often selected to be the "reference" to which the other magnitudes are compared. The normalization process is performed for every frequency/frequency window and often called the ***event-related spectral perturbation (ERSP)***. The normalization process can be performed in essentially two ways:

1) Representing the changes in magnitude as "gains"
2) Representing the changes in magnitude as "additive"

The selection of the normalization process would highly depend upon the assumption of the physiological phenomenon. These magnitude changes are often called ***event-related synchronization (ERS)*** and ***event-related*** *desynchronization (ERD)*. ERS is for when there is a positive change (an increase of magnitude); ERD is when there is a negative change (a reduction of magnitude) compared to baseline.

Intertrial phase coherence (ITPC): As recalled from previous chapters, the amplitude of auditory evoked potentials is highly dependent on how aligned are the averaged trials. This alignment information is stored within the phase information. The more similar they (the phases) are, the higher the intertrial phase coherence value and vice versa. The intertrial phase coherence can be used to determine whether a frequency band is associated with time- and phase-locked processes ("evoked") or whether is it associated with non-time-locked processes ("induced"). One advantage of using the ITPC over (for instance) just looking at the ERP amplitude is that the ITPC can be used to determine frequency-specific bands of activity.

So, here practically is the upshot of what has been presented thus far. Were the sentence, "Mark buys three nice flowers" heard by a subject while their EEG data is being recorded, the acquired EEG data analyzed in time and frequency would appear as in Figure 8–19D. "Normalizing" this time-frequency response using the period of EEG activity prior to the sentence (a.k.a., "baseline") would yield an ERSP, also shown therein. From the ERSP, if wishing to further determine activities that are evoked and/or induced, the ITPC then can be utilized to highlight the evoked responses, specifically, that are phase locked. In panel D, it can be seen that the first increase of activity in the lower frequencies (at 2 s–2.5 s) is the evoked (phase locked) response while the later increase of activity is induced (non-phase locked activity).

After learning about all these fancy signal processing methods, "how to put them into practice?" might be asked? Recently, induced activities have been explored while measuring auditory potentials to glean as much information possible from the recorded EEG in both children and adults, including various clinical populations. For instance, in a recent study the investigators endeavored to determine if musical expertise was associated with enhanced attention skills.[183] To address this issue, the neural oscillatory activities across frequency bands, specifically the alpha band (again, frequencies between 8 Hz and 12 Hz), were extracted using the "prism," and musicians and nonmusicians were presented the speech token /da/ in quiet and in different levels of noise. Results showed that only in the most difficult listening condition, musicians showed significantly decreased energy in the alpha power (shown through the ERSP). Children with reported listening difficulties were assessed using the same paradigm. The results showed that children with listening deficits have poor auditory processing encoding.[184] Latency shifts were observed in the beta and gamma bands. There are still other studies investigating the induced activities as well as evoked responses to better understand auditory discrimination, language processing, and even reading. As Captain Barbossa (*Pirates of the Caribbean*) might say, "Waste not! There is more to EEG than meets the eye!"

HEADS UP

The Change Potential—Sometimes What's Later Tells More

Anticipating the inevitable return to the brainstem in the upcoming episode, this feature will head the reader back down the pathway, yet remain at the cortical level. It introduces another objective measure of ***auditory discrimination***, called the ***acoustic change complex*** (**ACC**), but part of the group of ALLRs covered earlier. Auditory discrimination, again, is described as the ability to recognize differences between two sounds. Of broad importance, discrimination ability is a prerequisite for distinguishing among phonemes in words and thus essential to developing spoken language.[185] The obligatory N_1-P_2 complex was characterized as a response predominantly to the onset of a sound, but it turns out that it also can be elicited by a change within an ongoing sound. The latter response—coined the ACC—can be recorded based on methods of either electroencephalography (EEG) or magnetoencephalography (MEG, coming soon) and without the subject actively attending the targeted stimulus. The response also is around 2.5 times larger than the MMN when elicited using the same stimuli. The ACC is simply interpreted as a change-detection response arising from a variation in the activation and deactivation of neural populations within the auditory cortex.[186-188]

The ACC can be elicited by a wide range of stimulus changes. This includes changes in frequency or intensity of tone bursts[189] or interaural timing differences (ITDs) in sustained stimuli.[190] The ACC also is responsive to iterated ripple noise (IRN) or change in speechlike stimuli. Correspondingly, it provides objective measures related to place and temporal pitch, loudness, binaural sound localization, and speech discrimination. Figure 8–20 shows another stimulus paradigm effective for measuring the ACC, namely involving changes in the phase of a spectral ripple noise (SRN). This approach provides an objective neural measure representing limits of spectral resolution.[191]

The robustness of the ACC and its excellent test–retest reliability suggest that it could be used clinically to determine objectively if there is discrimination integrity for a subject at

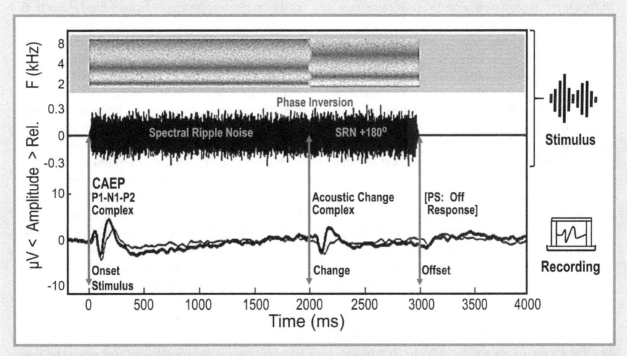

Figure 8–20. Spectrogram (*top graph*) and time history (*middle graph*) of the spectral ripple noise (SRN) stimulus used in this demonstration to record an acoustic change complex (ACC). Recorded signal below: The ACC here was elicited by a phase change in this spectrally complex stimulus (see text) occurring 2,000 ms after stimulus onset. The CAEP's onset response and the ACC response show similar morphology, but the ACC is of lower amplitude. PS: This is not "postscript" literally but is to demark an off-response that can often be seen in recordings of AEPs when elicited by tone busts/other stimuli of long enough duration, so as to not be obscured by the much larger on-response. (Recording from an adult subject.)

the cortical level.[187,192,193] The literature indicates a significant positive correlation between ACC measures and discrimination ability in adults—subjects whose speech recognition ability can be tested reliably. In fact, several researchers have concluded that the presence and magnitude of ACC can be taken as an index of perceptual discrimination.[186,193,194] The morphology of the ACC has been likened to that of the onset of the P_1-N_1-P_2 complex and observed in the majority of cases, though with a slightly longer latency and smaller amplitude (see Figure 8–20). Finally, the ACCs can be objectively interpreted by statistical algorithm, such as the Hotelling T^2 for automated detection purposes.[56] The statistical algorithm has been demonstrated to provide easy and accurate interpretation of outcomes consistent with those of experienced examiners.

The ACC, nevertheless, is considered an ***obligatory response*** arising from the primary auditory cortex, which means that it (again) does not require attention of the listener to the sound for it to be generated by the brain. This characteristic is especially important when testing young children or infants. During testing, infants are placed typically on the parent's/guardian's lap and only need to be entertained or distracted using silent toys. It thus is neither required that their attention be focused on any particular stimulus, nor be involved in the test paradigm in any way behaviorally (for instance, as required in some applications of the P_3, like pressing a button upon detection of the oddball stimulus). Further, the infant does not require administration of a sedative to remain adequately quiet for successful test completion.

It also has been demonstrated several times that the ACC can be elicited in people wearing hearing aids[195] or cochlear implants.[194,196,197] The feasibility to record the ACC in free field has been confirmed in normal-hearing adults wearing hearing amplification and tested with naturally produced speech tokens.[195] It also has been shown that it is possible to record ACCs in adult CI users directly stimulated by their indwelling electrodes, namely by alternating stimulated electrodes.[197] Larger ACCs were recorded when increasing separation between electrodes to which the stimuli were applied. However, a careful interpretation of the ACC waveform when recorded with CI users is needed because of the presence of CI artifacts. Lastly, similarly to onset CAEP, the ACC can also be elicited in adults and children with an auditory synaptopathy/neuropathy[198,199] but showing delayed latencies and smaller amplitude compared to that of a normal/control group.

The use of objective auditory discrimination measures such as the ACC is promising in evaluating young children who cannot be tested using conventional/behavioral measures. Even though hearing aids amplify sounds for them to be detected, the damaged auditory system may have limited capacity for extracting acoustic cues from speech. Discrimination ability interacts with spoken language input to influence the development of spoken language skills. If children do not progress from sound detection to discrimination, they will experience great difficulties in developing spoken language, and thereafter in developing good speech intelligibility. There thus is much emphasis on early intervention in children with hearing aids or CIs. The decision to implant children currently is made almost exclusively on the basis of hearing thresholds. By being able to determine early-life speech discrimination ability with amplification, it could be possible to make more informed management decisions. Children who have poor speech discrimination, even when aided with the best of what current hearing-aid technology has to offer, likely could benefit more from a CI, so stay tuned.

To summarize, the presence of an ACC suggests that the subject perceived and processed the sound transition at the primary auditory cortex. The implications for clinical applications with specific reference to the use of objective auditory discrimination measures to guide clinical referral for pediatric auditory habilitation/rehabilitation is to be defined further, and more research is needed to document the complex relationship between objective measures of discrimination and speech perception/language development.

Take Home Messages

Episode 1

1. The trip through AEP space and time continues with the CAEP—bigger and hugely important in the expansion of utilities of clinical neurophysiology in audiology.
2. Also known as the slow vertex potential, still other sites than C_z can be useful.
3. As with earlier multipeaked waveforms, measurement of magnitude has conventions/issues particular to the longer latency potentials.
4. Component waves (as with earlier responses) demonstrate nuances of input-output functions as well as LI shifts.
5. CAEP obtained at/near behavioral thresholds in awake, alert, and passive adults and children are particularly "friendly" to testing using tone bursts.
6. One of the singularly most influential stimulus parameters is the ISI (a.k.a,. the inverse of repetition rate), in turn, interacting with effects of maturation.
7. Maturation, especially the earlier years, is a substantial factor for cortical AEPs.
8. On the other end of the life span, CAEPs can become more robust with aging, especially upon reducing the stimulus rate.
9. Cortical-AEP measurements offer a powerful extension to that of testing earlier responses, incorporating still more of the auditory pathway and metrics of auditory function.

Episode 2

1. Although ABR/ASSR-ERA would win out over ERA based on either ALLR or ECochG, ALLR-ERA came first and upon which principles of ERA were founded.
2. As ERA is an effort to predict hearing, then why not test most of the auditory pathway?
3. Opening the door in space to the cortical level also opens the time window of stimuli, yet minimizes risk of stimulus-electrical interference.
4. The L-I effect is still "manifested" in the ALLR and potentially useful in ERA to help define its VDL.
5. Reliability of ERA is relatively high using the ALLR (among AEPs).
6. Computer-assisted response detection/analyses, including a steady-state approach, are in research and development with promising results.
7. The general attributions of the steady-state approach apply, including possibly enhancing profiling of effects of stimulus rate.

Heads Up

8. Regardless of practical considerations for purposes of ERA, the entire pathway must be considered, as the "merits" of the case and/or circumstances present.

Episode 3

1. Evoking discriminative cortical potentials requires more complex paradigms than obligatory EPs.
2. P_3 (a.k.a., P_{300} and cognitive potential) is a positive discrimination potential after the deviant (change) is presented via the oddball paradigm, readily elicited by tone bursts and speech.
3. Additional processing beyond the obligatory response proves to be more complex than a singular "entity," hence components P_{3a} and P_{3b} with their own nuances/importance.
4. Though a variety of paradigms are possible, general/fundamental nuances prevail to distinguish tests of obligatory versus discriminatory AEPs.
5. The basic oddball paradigm works well; still, more elaborate paradigms permit more sophisticated tests and/or better reliability.
6. There are both methodological considerations and numerous other factors that can impact results of the oddball paradigm, but maturation/life span issues are prominent.
7. There remain challenges for various AEP tests for "prime-time" clinical testing, hence still work to be done.

8. Other discriminatory AEPs are several, permitting testing of function from precognition—such as the MMN—to progressively higher levels of cognition—like N_{400} and P_{600}.

Heads Up

9. The point of departure to AEPdom was (in effect) the classical EEG, and research and development has greatly progressed in scope of interests in EEG.
10. Modern analyses permit a distinction between evoked—synchronized—and induced activity—both synchronized and desynchronized; so, not just "noise" after all!

Heads Up

11. The ACC is an obligatory response from the auditory cortex sensitive to a change in an ongoing sound, whether in loudness, spectral content, or phase, or to insertion of temporal gaps.
12. The approach lends itself potentially to a broad range of clinical applications (even treatment with amplification/implants) and over the life span (even young infants).

References

1. Davis, P. A. (1939). Effects of acoustic stimuli on the waking human brain. *Journal of Neurophysiology, 2*(6), 494–499.
2. Barnet, A. B., & Lodge, A. (1966). Diagnosis of deafness in infants with the use of computer-averaged electroencephalographic responses to sound. *The Journal of Pediatrics, 69*(5), 753–758.
3. Barnet, A. B. (1971). EEG audiometry in children under three years of age. *Acta Oto-laryngologica, 72*(1–6), 1–13.
4. Rapin, I. (1964). Evoked responses to clicks in a group of children with communication disorders. *Annals of the New York Academy of Sciences, 112*, 182–203.
5. Alberti, P. W., Hyde, M. L., & Riko, K. (1987). Exaggerated hearing loss in compensation claimants. *The Journal of Otolaryngology, 16*(6), 362–366.
6. Vaughan, H. G., Jr., & Ritter, W. (1970). The sources of auditory evoked responses recorded from the human scalp. *Electroencephalography and Clinical Neurophysiology, 28*(4), 360–367.
7. Näätänen, R., & Picton, T. W. (1987). The N1 wave of the human electric and magnetic response to sound: A review and an analysis of the component structure. *Psychophysiology, 24*(4), 375–425.
8. Addler, G., & Adler, J. (1991). Auditory stimulus processing at different stimulus intensities as reflected by auditory evoked potentials. *Biological Psychiatry, 29*(4), 347–356.
9. Tlumak, A. I., Durrant, J. D., & Delgado, R. E. (2016). The effect of stimulus intensity and carrier frequency on auditory middle-and long-latency evoked potentials using a steady-state-response approach. *American Journal of Audiology, 25*(1), 62–74.
10. Picton, T. W. (2011). *Human auditory evoked potentials*. Plural Publishing.
11. Hall, J. W., III (1992). *Handbook of auditory evoked responses*. Allyn and Bacon.
12. Gilley, P. M., Sharma, A., Dorman, M., & Martin, K. (2005). Developmental changes in refractoriness of the cortical auditory evoked potential. *Clinical Neurophysiology, 116*(3), 648–657.
13. Tlumak, A. I., Durrant, J. D., Delgado, R. E., & Boston, J. R. (2011). Steady-state analysis of auditory evoked potentials over a wide range of stimulus repetition rates: Profile in adults. *International Journal of Audiology, 50*(7), 448–458.
14. Novak, G. P., Kurtzberg, D., Kreuzer, J. A., & Vaughan, H. G., Jr. (1989). Cortical responses to speech sounds and their formants in normal infants: Maturational sequence and spatiotemporal analysis. *Electroencephalography and Clinical Neurophysiology, 73*(4), 295–305.
15. Sharma, A., & Dorman, M. F. (1999). Cortical auditory evoked potential correlates of categorical perception of voice-onset time. *The Journal of the Acoustical Society of America, 106*(2), 1078–1083.
16. Sakabe, N., Arayama, T., & Suzuki, T. (1969). Human fetal evoked response to acoustic stimulation. *Audiology Japan, 12*(4), 458–468.
17. Weitzman, E. D., & Graziani, L. J. (1968). Maturation and topography of the auditory evoked response of the prematurely born infant. *Developmental Psychobiology: The Journal of the International Society for Developmental Psychobiology, 1*(2), 79–89.
18. Lengle, J. M., Chen, M., & Wakai, R. T. (2001). Improved neuromagnetic detection of fetal and neonatal auditory evoked responses. *Clinical Neurophysiology, 112*(5), 785–792.

19. Wunderlich, J. L., Cone-Wesson, B. K., & Shepherd, R. (2006). Maturation of the cortical auditory evoked potential in infants and young children. *Hearing Research, 212*(1–2), 185–202.
20. Cone, B., & Whitaker, R. (2013). Dynamics of infant cortical auditory evoked potentials (CAEPs) for tone and speech tokens. *International Journal of Pediatric Otorhinolaryngology, 77*(7), 1162–1173.
21. Ponton, C., Eggermont, J. J., Khosla, D., Kwong, B., & Don, M. (2002). Maturation of human central auditory system activity: Separating auditory evoked potentials by dipole source modeling. *Clinical Neurophysiology, 113*(3), 407–420.
22. Barnet, A. B., Ohlrich, E. S., Weiss, I. P., & Shanks, B. (1975). Auditory evoked potentials during sleep in normal children from ten days to three years of age. *Electroencephalography and Clinical Neurophysiology, 39*(1), 29–41.
23. Caspary, D. M., Ling, L., Turner, J. G., & Hughes, L. F. (2008). Inhibitory neurotransmission, plasticity and aging in the mammalian central auditory system. *Journal of Experimental Biology, 211*(11), 1781–1791.
24. Eddins, A. C., & Eddins, D. A. (2017). Cortical correlates of binaural temporal processing deficits in older adults. *Ear and Hearing, 39*(3), 594–604.
25. Pichora-Fuller, M. K., & Schneider, B. A. (1991). Masking level differences in the elderly: A comparison of antiphasic and time-delay dichotic conditions. *Journal of Speech and Hearing Research, 34*(6), 1410–1422.
26. Cone, B. K. (2015). Infant cortical electrophysiology and perception of vowel contrasts. *International Journal of Psychophysiology, 95*(2), 65–76.
27. Irimajiri, R., Golob, E. J., & Starr, A. (2005). Auditory brain-stem, middle-and long-latency evoked potentials in mild cognitive impairment. *Clinical Neurophysiology, 116*(8), 1918–1929.
28. Oates, P. A., Kurtzberg, D., & Stapells, D. R. (2002). Effects of sensorineural hearing loss on cortical event-related potential and behavioral measures of speech-sound processing. *Ear and Hearing, 23*(5), 399–415.
29. Rance, G., Cone-Wesson, B., Wunderlich, J., & Dowell, R. C. (2002). Speech perception and cortical event related potentials in children with auditory neuropathy. *Ear and Hearing, 23*(3), 239–253.
30. Sharma, A., Martin, K., Roland, P., Bauer, P., Sweeney, M. H., Gilley, P., & Dorman, M. (2005). P1 latency as a biomarker for central auditory development in children with hearing impairment. *Journal of the American Academy of Audiology, 16*(8), 564–573.
31. Lightfoot, G. (2016). Summary of the N1-P2 cortical auditory evoke potential to estimate the auditory threshold in adults. *Seminars in Hearing, 37*(1), 1–8.
32. Tsui, B., Wong, L. L., & Wong, E. C. (2002). Accuracy of cortical evoked response audiometry in the identification of non-organic hearing loss. *International Journal of Audiology, 41*(6), 330–333.
33. Punch, S., Van Dun, B., King, A., Carter, L., & Pearce, W. (2016). Clinical experience of using cortical auditory evoked potentials in the treatment of infant hearing loss in Australia. *Seminars in Hearing, 37*(1), 36.
34. Van Dun, B., Dillon, H., & Seeto, M. (2015). Estimating hearing thresholds in hearing-impaired adults through objective detection of cortical auditory evoked potentials. *Journal of the American Academy of Audiology, 26*(4), 370–383.
35. Mehta, K., Watkin, P., Baldwin, M., Marriage, J., Mahon, M., & Vickers, D. (2017). Role of cortical auditory evoked potentials in reducing the age at hearing aid fitting in children with hearing loss identified by newborn hearing screening. *Trends in Hearing, 21*, 1–16.
36. Jerger, J. F., & Hayes, D. (1976). The cross-check principle in pediatric audiometry. *Archives of Otolaryngology, 102*(10), 614–620.
37. Hyde, M. (1997). The N1 response and its applications. *Audiology and Neurotology, 2*(5), 281–307.
38. Carhart, R., & Jerger, J. F. (1959). A preferred methods for clinical determination of pure-tone thresholds. *Journal of Speech and Hearing Disorders 24*(4), 330–345.
39. Lightfoot, G., & Kennedy, V. (2006). Cortical electric response audiometry hearing threshold estimation: Accuracy, speed, and the effects of stimulus presentation features. *Ear and Hearing, 27*(5), 443–456.
40. Dejonckere, P. H., & Coryn, C. P. (2000). A comparison between middle latency responses and late auditory evoked potentials for approximating frequency-specific hearing levels in medicolegal patients with occupational hearing loss. *International Tinnitus Journal, 6*(2), 175–181.
41. Kaf, W., Sabo, D. L., Durrant, J. L., & Rubinstein, E. (2006). Reliability of electric response audiometry using 80 Hz auditory steady-state responses. *International Journal of Audiology, 45*(8), 477–486.
42. Prasher, D., Mula, M., & Luxon, L. (1993). Cortical evoked potential criteria in the objective assessment of auditory threshold: A comparison of noise induced hearing loss with Ménière's disease. *Journal of Laryngology & Otology, 107*(9), 780–786.

43. Tomlin, D., Rance, G., Graydon, K., & Tsialios, I. (2006). A comparison of 40 Hz auditory steady-state response (ASSR) and cortical auditory evoked potential (CAEP) thresholds in awake adult subjects. *International Journal of Audiology, 45*(10), 580–588.
44. Gorga, M. P., Kaminski, J. R., Beauchaine, K. A., & Jesteadt, W. (1988). Auditory brainstem responses to tone bursts in normally hearing subjects. *Journal of Speech, Language, and Hearing Research, 31*(1), 87–97.
45. Stapells, D. R. (2000). Threshold estimation by the tone-evoked auditory brainstem response: A literature meta-analysis. *Journal of Speech-Language Pathology and Audiology, 24*(2), 74–83.
46. McCreery, R. W., Kaminski, J., Beauchaine, K., Lenzen, N., Simms, K., & Gorga, M. P. (2015). The impact of degree of hearing loss on auditory brainstem response predictions of behavioral thresholds. *Ear and Hearing, 36*(3), 309–319.
47. Durrant, J. D. (2004). Simulated hearing loss via masking: Research and heuristic applications. *Seminars in Hearing, 25*(1), 25–37.
48. Wunderlich, J. L., & Cone-Wesson, B. K. (2001). Effects of stimulus frequency and complexity on the mismatch negativity and other components of the cortical auditory-evoked potential. *The Journal of the Acoustical Society of America, 109*(4), 1526–1537.
49. Van Maanen, A., & Stapells, D. R. (2005). Comparison of multiple auditory steady-state responses (80 versus 40 Hz) and slow cortical potentials for threshold estimation in hearing-impaired adults. *International Journal of Audiology, 44*(11), 613–624.
50. Bardy, F., Van Dun, B., & Dillon, H. (2015). Bigger is better: Increasing cortical auditory response amplitude via stimulus spectral complexity. *Ear and Hearing, 36*(6), 677–687.
51. Moore, J. K. (2002). Maturation of human auditory cortex: Implications for speech perception. *Annals of Otology, Rhinology & Laryngology, 111*, 7–10.
52. Key, A. P., Lambert, E. W., Aschner, J. L., & Maitre, N. L. (2012). Influence of gestational age and postnatal age on speech sound processing in NICU infants. *Psychophysiology, 49*(5), 720–731.
53. Tlumak, A. I., Durrant, J. D., Delgado, R. E., & Boston, J. R. (2012). Steady-state analysis of auditory evoked potentials over a wide range of stimulus repetition rates: Profile in children vs. adults. *International Journal of Audiology, 51*(6), 480–490.
54. Tlumak, A. I., Durrant, J. D., Delgado, R. E., & Robert Boston, J. (2012). Steady-state analysis of auditory evoked potentials over a wide range of stimulus repetition rates in awake vs. natural sleep. *International Journal of Audiology, 51*(5), 418–423.
55. Purdy, S. C., Katsch, R., Dillon, H., Storey, L., Sharma, M., & Agung, K. (2004). Aided cortical auditory evoked potentials for hearing instrument evaluation in infants. In R. C. Seewald (Ed.), *A sound foundation through early amplification: Proceedings of 3rd pediatric conference* (Vol. 8, pp. 115–127). Phonak AG.
56. Golding, M., Dillon, H., Seymour, J., & Carter, L. (2009). The detection of adult cortical auditory evoked potentials (CAEPs) using an automated statistic and visual detection. *International Journal of Audiology, 48*, 833–842.
57. Carter, L., Golding, M., Dillon, H., & Seymour, J. (2010). The detection of infant cortical auditory evoked potentials (CAEPs) using statistical and visual detection techniques. *Journal of the American Academy of Audiology, 21*(5), 347–356.
58. Munro, K. J., Purdy, S. C., Uus, K., Visram, A., Ward, R., Bruce, I. A., . . . Van Dun, B. (2020). Recording obligatory cortical auditory evoked potentials in infants: Quantitative information on feasibility and parent acceptability. *Ear and Hearing, 41*(3), 630–639.
59. Bardy, F., Van Dun, B., Seeto, M., & Dillon, H. (2020). Automated cortical auditory response detection strategy. *International Journal of Audiology, 59*(11), 835–842.
60. Don, M., Elberling, C., & Waring, M. (1984). Objective detection of averaged auditory brainstem responses. *Scandinavian Audiology, 13*(4), 219–228.
61. Mao, D., Innes-Brown, H., Petoe, M. A., Wong, Y. T., & McKay, C. M. (2018). Cortical auditory evoked potential time-frequency growth functions for fully objective hearing threshold estimation. *Hearing Research, 370*, 74–83.
62. Durrant, J. D., Tlumak, A. I., Delgado, R. E., & Boston, J. R. (2017). *Steady state measurement and analysis approach to profiling auditory evoked potentials from short-latency to long latency. U.S. Patent No. 9,662,035.* U.S. Patent and Trademark Office.
63. Hood, L. J., Delgado, R. E., Durrant, J. D., Roberts, L., Racca, J., Ferguson, M., & Agboola, E. (2018, October). *Towards clinical implementation of a late latency auditory steady state response paradigm.* In D. W. Swanepoel (Chair), World Congress of Audiology. Oral presentation conducted at the meeting of the World Congress of Audiology, Cape Town, South Africa.

64. Hood, L. J., Delgado, R. E., & Durrant, J. D. (2020, January). *Application of an auditory steady state response paradigm to cortical evoked potentials.* Presented at the Midwinter Meeting of the Association for Research in Otolaryngology, San Jose, CA.
65. Gorga, M. P., Beauchaine, K. A., & Reiland, J. K. (1987). Comparison of onset and steady-state responses of hearing aids: Implications for use of the auditory brainstem response in the selection of hearing aids. *Journal of Speech, Language, and Hearing Research, 30*(1), 130–136.
66. He, S., Teagle, H. F., Roush, P., Grose, J. H., & Buchman, C. A. (2013). Objective hearing threshold estimation in children with auditory neuropathy spectrum disorder. *Laryngoscope, 123*(11), 2859–2861.
67. Gardner-Berry, K., Purdy, S. C., Ching, T. Y., & Dillon, H. (2015). The audiological journey and early outcomes of twelve infants with auditory neuropathy spectrum disorder from birth to two years of age. *International Journal of Audiology, 54*(8), 524–535.
68. Rapin, I., & Graziani, L. J. (1967). Auditory-evoked responses in normal, brain-damaged, and deaf infants. *Neurology, 17*(9), 881–881.
69. Billings, C. (2013). Uses and limitation of electrophysiology with hearing aids. *Seminars in Hearing, 34*(4), 257–269.
70. Hood, L. J., Berlin, C. I., & Allen, P. (1994). Cortical deafness: A longitudinal study. *Journal of the American Academy of Audiology, 5*, 330–342.
71. Berlin, C. I., Hood, L. J., Cecola, R. P., Jackson, D. F., & Szabo, P. (1993). Does type I afferent neuron dysfunction reveal itself through lack of efferent suppression? *Hearing Research, 65*(1–2), 40–50.
72. Starr, A., Picton, T. W., Sininger, Y., Hood, L. J., & Berlin, C. I. (1996). Auditory neuropathy. *Brain, 119*(3), 741–753.
73. Narne, V. K., & Vanaja, C. (2008). Speech identification and cortical potentials in individuals with auditory neuropathy. *Behavioral and Brain Functions, 4*(1), 15.
74. Lee, J. C., Yoo, M. H., Ahn, J. H., & Lee, K. S. (2007). Value of the promontory stimulation test in predicting speech perception after cochlear implantation. *Laryngoscope, 117*(11), 1988–1992.
75. Kuo, S. C., & Gibson, W. P. (2002). The role of the promontory stimulation test in cochlear implantation. *Cochlear Implants International, 3*(1), 19–28.
76. Alfelasi, M., Piron, J. P., Mathiolon, C., Lenel, N., Mondain, M., Uziel, A., & Venail, F. (2013). The transtympanic promontory stimulation test in patients with auditory deprivation: Correlations with electrical dynamics of cochlear implant and speech perception. *European Archives of Oto-Rhino-Laryngology, 270*(6), 1809–1815.
77. Courchesne, E., Hillyard, S. A., & Courchesne, R. Y. (1977). P3 waves to the discrimination of targets in homogeneous and heterogeneous stimulus sequences. *Psychophysiology, 14*(6), 590–597.
78. Hillyard, S. A., & Anllo-Vento, L. (1998). Event-related brain potentials in the study of visual selective attention. *Proceedings of the National Academy of Sciences, 95*(3), 781–787.
79. Picton, T. E., Bentin, S., Berg, P., Donchin, E., Hillyard, S. A., Johnson, R., Jr., . . . Taylor, M. J. (2000). Guidelines for using human event-related potentials to study cognition: Recording standards and publication criteria. *Psychophysiology, 37*(2), 127–152.
80. Donchin, E., Ritter, W., & McCallum, W. C. (1978). Cognitive psychophysiology: The endogenous components of the ERP. *Event-Related Brain Potentials in Man, 349*, 411.
81. Picton, T. W. (2010). Human auditory evoked potentials (1st ed.). Plural Publishing.
82. Duncan, C. C., Barry, R. J., Connolly, J. F., Fischer, C., Michie, P. T., Näätänen, R., . . . Van Petten, C. (2009). Event-related potentials in clinical research: Guidelines for eliciting, recording, and quantifying mismatch negativity, P300, and N400. *Clinical Neurophysiology, 120*(11), 1883–1908.
83. Hillyard, S. A. (1985). Electrophysiology of human selective attention. *Trends in Neurosciences, 8*, 400–405.
84. Polich, J. (2007). Updating P300: An integrative theory of P3a and P3b. *Clinical Neurophysiology, 118*(10), 2128–2148.
85. Snyder, E., Hillyard, S. A., & Galambos, R. (1980). Similarities and differences among the P3 waves to detected signals in three modalities. *Psychophysiology, 17*(2), 112–122.
86. Halgren, E., Marinkovic, K., & Chauvel, P. (1998). Generators of the late cognitive potentials in auditory and visual oddball tasks. *Electroencephalography and Clinical Neurophysiology, 106*(2), 156–164.
87. Katayama, J. I., & Polich, J. (1998). Stimulus context determines P3a and P3b. *Psychophysiology, 35*(1), 23–33.
88. Verleger, R., Jaśkowski, P., & Wascher, E. (2005). Evidence for an integrative role of P3b in linking reaction to perception. *Journal of Psychophysiology, 19*(3), 165–181.
89. Sussman, E., Winkler, I., & Schröger, E. (2003). Top-down control over involuntary attention switching

in the auditory modality. *Psychonomic Bulletin & Review, 10*(3), 630–637.
90. Verleger, R. (1988). Event-related potentials and cognition: A critique of the context updating hypothesis and an alternative interpretation of P3. *Behavioral and Brain Sciences, 11*(3), 343–356.
91. Donchin, E., & Coles, M. G. (1988). Is the P300 component a manifestation of context updating? *Behavioral and Brain Sciences, 11*(3), 357–374.
92. Barry, R. J., Steiner, G. Z., De Blasio, F. M., Fogarty, J. S., Karamacoska, D., & MacDonald, B. (2020). Components in the P300: Don't forget the novelty P3! *Psychophysiology, 57*(7), e13371.
93. Escera, C., & Corral, M. J. (2007). Role of mismatch negativity and novelty-P3 in involuntary auditory attention. *Journal of Psychophysiology, 21*(3–4), 251–264.
94. Knight, R. T. (1984). Decreased response to novel stimuli after prefrontal lesions in man. *Electroencephalography and Clinical Neurophysiology/Evoked Potentials Section, 59*(1), 9–20.
95. Knight, R. T. (1996). Contribution of human hippocampal region to novelty detection. *Nature, 383*(6597), 256–259.
96. Halgren, E., Baudena, P., Clarke, J. M., Heit, G., Marinkovic, K., Devaux, B., . . . Biraben, A. (1995). Intracerebral potentials to rare target and distractor auditory and visual stimuli. II. Medial, lateral and posterior temporal lobe. *Electroencephalography and Clinical Neurophysiology, 94*(4), 229–250.
97. Volpe, U., Mucci, A., Bucci, P., Merlotti, E., Galderisi, S., & Maj, M. (2007). The cortical generators of P3a and P3b: A LORETA study. *Brain Research Bulletin, 73*(4–6), 220–230.
98. Wronka, E., Kaiser, J., & Coenen, A. M. (2012). Neural generators of the auditory evoked potential components P3a and P3b. *Acta Neurobiologiae Experimentalis, 72*(1), 51–64.
99. Hall, M. H., Schulze, K., Rijsdijk, F., Picchioni, M., Ettinger, U., Bramon, E., . . . Sham, P. (2006). Heritability and reliability of P300, P50 and duration mismatch negativity. *Behavior Genetics, 36*(6), 845.
100. Polich, J., & Criado, J. R. (2006). Neuropsychology and neuropharmacology of P3a and P3b. *International Journal of Psychophysiology, 60*(2), 172–185.
101. Pritchard, W. S. (1981). Psychophysiology of P300. *Psychological Bulletin, 89*(3), 506.
102. Atcherson, S. R., & Stoody, T. M. (2012). *Auditory electrophysiology: A clinical guide.* Thieme Medical Publishers.
103. Polich, J. (1989). Frequency, intensity, and duration as determinants of P300 from auditory stimuli. *Journal of Clinical Neurophysiology, 6*(3), 277–286.
104. Vesco, K. K., Bone, R. C., Ryan, J. C., & Polich, J. (1993). P300 in young and elderly subjects: Auditory frequency and intensity effects. *Electroencephalography and Clinical Neurophysiology/Evoked Potentials Section, 88*(4), 302–308.
105. Teder-Sälejärvi, W. A., Pierce, K. L., Courchesne, E., & Hillyard, S. A. (2005). Auditory spatial localization and attention deficits in autistic adults. *Cognitive Brain Research, 23*(2–3), 221–234.
106. Polich, J., & Kok, A. (1995). Cognitive and biological determinants of P300: An integrative review. *Biological Psychology, 41*(2), 103–146.
107. Polich, J. (1986). Attention, probability, and task demands as determinants of P300 latency from auditory stimuli. *Electroencephalography and Clinical Neurophysiology, 63*(3), 251–259.
108. van Dinteren, R., Arns, M., Jongsma, M. L., & Kessels, R. P. (2014). P300 development across the lifespan: A systematic review and meta-analysis. *PloS One, 9*(2), e87347.
109. Sangal, R. B., Sangal, J. M., & Belisle, C. (1998). P300 latency and age: A quadratic regression explains their relationship from age 5 to 85. *Clinical Electroencephalography, 29*(1), 1–6.
110. Walhovd, K. B., Rosquist, H., & Fjell, A. M. (2008). P300 amplitude age reductions are not caused by latency jitter. *Psychophysiology, 45*(4), 545–553.
111. Brickman, A. M., Meier, I. B., Korgaonkar, M. S., Provenzano, F. A., Grieve, S. M., Siedlecki, K. L., . . . Zimmerman, M. E. (2012). Testing the white matter retrogenesis hypothesis of cognitive aging. *Neurobiology of Aging, 33*(8), 1699–1715.
112. Porcaro, C., Balsters, J. H., Mantini, D., Robertson, I. H., & Wenderoth, N. (2019). P3b amplitude as a signature of cognitive decline in the older population: An EEG study enhanced by Functional Source Separation. *Neuroimage, 184*, 535–546.
113. West, R., Schwarb, H., & Johnson, B. N. (2010). The influence of age and individual differences in executive function on stimulus processing in the oddball task. *Cortex, 46*(4), 550–563.
114. Bramon, E., Rabe-Hesketh, S., Sham, P., Murray, R. M., & Frangou, S. (2004). Meta-analysis of the P300 and P50 waveforms in schizophrenia. *Schizophrenia Research, 70*(2–3), 315–329.
115. Hamilton, H. K., Perez, V. B., Ford, J. M., Roach, B. J., Jaeger, J., & Mathalon, D. H. (2018). Mismatch negativity but not P300 is associated with functional disability in schizophrenia. *Schizophrenia Bulletin, 44*(3), 492–504.

116. Wang, J., Tang, Y., Li, C., Mecklinger, A., Xiao, Z., Zhang, M., . . . Li, H. (2010). Decreased P300 current source density in drug-naive first episode schizophrenics revealed by high density recording. *International Journal of Psychophysiology*, *75*(3), 249–257.
117. Bramon, E., McDonald, C., Croft, R. J., Landau, S., Filbey, F., Gruzelier, J. H., . . . Murray, R. M. (2005). Is the P300 wave an endophenotype for schizophrenia? A meta-analysis and a family study. *Neuroimage*, *27*(4), 960–968.
118. De Wilde, O. M., Bour, L. J., Dingemans, P. M., Koelman, J. H. T. M., Boerée, T., & Linszen, D. H. (2008). P300 deficits are present in young first-episode patients with schizophrenia and not in their healthy young siblings. *Clinical Neurophysiology*, *119*(12), 2721–2726.
119. Baribeau-Braun, J., Picton, T. W., & Gosselin, J. Y. (1983). Schizophrenia: A neurophysiological evaluation of abnormal information processing. *Science*, *219*(4586), 874–876.
120. Jeon, Y. W., & Polich, J. (2003). Meta-analysis of P300 and schizophrenia: Patients, paradigms, and practical implications. *Psychophysiology*, *40*(5), 684–701.
121. Matzke, D., Hughes, M., Badcock, J. C., Michie, P., & Heathcote, A. (2017). Failures of cognitive control or attention? The case of stop-signal deficits in schizophrenia. *Attention, Perception, & Psychophysics*, *79*(4), 1078–1086.
122. Butterfield, D. A., Drake, J., Pocernich, C., & Castegna, A. (2001). Evidence of oxidative damage in Alzheimer's disease brain: Central role for amyloid β-peptide. *Trends in Molecular Medicine*, *7*(12), 548–554.
123. Hedges, D., Janis, R., Mickelson, S., Keith, C., Bennett, D., & Brown, B. L. (2016). P300 amplitude in Alzheimer's disease: A meta-analysis and meta-regression. *Clinical EEG and Neuroscience*, *47*(1), 48–55.
124. Juckel, G., Clotz, F., Frodl, T., Kawohl, W., Hampel, H., Pogarell, O., & Hegerl, U. (2008). Diagnostic usefulness of cognitive auditory event-related P300 subcomponents in patients with Alzheimers disease? *Journal of Clinical Neurophysiology*, *25*(3), 147–152.
125. Medvidovic, S., Titlic, M., & Maras-Simunic, M. (2013). P300 evoked potential in patients with mild cognitive impairment. *Acta Informatica Medica*, *21*(2), 89.
126. Papaliagkas, V. T., Kimiskidis, V. K., Tsolaki, M. N., & Anogianakis, G. (2011). Cognitive event-related potentials: Longitudinal changes in mild cognitive impairment. *Clinical Neurophysiology*, *122*(7), 1322–1326.
127. Scahill, L., & Schwab-Stone, M. (2000). Epidemiology of ADHD in school-age children. *Child and Adolescent Psychiatric Clinics of North America*, *9*(3), 541–555.
128. Barkley, R. A., Koplowitz, S., Anderson, T., & McMurray, M. B. (1997). Sense of time in children with ADHD: Effects of duration, distraction, and stimulant medication. *Journal of the International Neuropsychological Society*, *3*(4), 359–369.
129. Paul-Jordanov, I., Bechtold, M., & Gawrilow, C. (2010). Methylphenidate and if-then plans are comparable in modulating the P300 and increasing response inhibition in children with ADHD. *ADHD Attention Deficit and Hyperactivity Disorders*, *2*(3), 115–126.
130. Liotti, M., Pliszka, S. R., Perez, R., Kothmann, D., & Woldorff, M. G. (2005). Abnormal brain activity related to performance monitoring and error detection in children with ADHD. *Cortex*, *41*(3), 377–388.
131. Wild-Wall, N., Oades, R. D., Schmidt-Wessels, M., Christiansen, H., & Falkenstein, M. (2009). Neural activity associated with executive functions in adolescents with attention-deficit/hyperactivity disorder (ADHD). *International Journal of Psychophysiology*, *74*(1), 19–27.
132. Szuromi, B., Czobor, P., Komlósi, S., & Bitter, I. (2011). P300 deficits in adults with attention deficit hyperactivity disorder: A meta-analysis. *Psychological Medicine*, *41*(7), 1529–1538.
133. Bomba, M. D., & Pang, E. W. (2004). Cortical auditory evoked potentials in autism: A review. *International Journal of Psychophysiology*, *53*(3), 161–169.
134. Cui, T., Wang, P. P., Liu, S., & Zhang, X. (2017). P300 amplitude and latency in autism spectrum disorder: A meta-analysis. *European Child & Adolescent Psychiatry*, *26*(2), 177–190.
135. Soshi, T., Hisanaga, S., Kodama, N., Kanekama, Y., Samejima, Y., Yumoto, E., & Sekiyama, K. (2014). Event-related potentials for better speech perception in noise by cochlear implant users. *Hearing Research*, *316*, 110–121.
136. Wall, L. G., Davidson, S. A., & Dalebout, S. D. (1991). Determining latency and amplitude for multiple peaked P300 waveforms. *Journal of the American Academy of Audiology*, *2*(3), 189–194.
137. Micco, A. G., Kraus, N., Koch, D. B., McGee, T. J., Carrell, T. D., Sharma, A., . . . Wiet, R. J. (1995). Speech-evoked cognitive P300 potentials in cochlear implant recipients. *American Journal of Otology*, *16*(4), 514–520.

138. Legris, E., Gomot, M., Charpentier, J., Aoustin, J. M., Aussedat, C., & Bakhos, D. (2018). Assessment of auditory discrimination in hearing-impaired patients. *European Annals of Otorhinolaryngology, Head and Neck Diseases, 135*(5), 335–339.
139. Kileny, P. R., Boerst, A., & Zwolan, T. (1997). Cognitive evoked potentials to speech and tonal stimuli in children with implants. *Otolaryngology-Head and Neck Surgery, 117*(3), 161–169.
140. Grasel, S., Greters, M., Goffi-Gomez, M. V. S., Bittar, R., Weber, R., Oiticica, J., & Bento, R. F. (2018). P3 cognitive potential in cochlear implant users. *International Archives of Otorhinolaryngology, 22*(4), 408–414.
141. Kelly, A. S., Purdy, S. C., & Thorne, P. R. (2005). Electrophysiological and speech perception measures of auditory processing in experienced adult cochlear implant users. *Clinical Neurophysiology, 116*(6), 1235–1246.
142. Picton, T. W. (1988). The endogenous event-related potentials. In E. Başar (Ed.), *Dynamics of sensory and cognitive processing by the brain. Springer series in brain dynamics* (Vol. 1, pp. 258–265). Springer.
143. Gil, D., & Iorio, M. C. M. (2010). Formal auditory training in adult hearing aid users. *Clinics, 65*(2), 165–174.
144. Jirsa, R. E. (1992). The clinical utility of the P3 AERP in children with auditory processing disorders. *Journal of Speech, Language, and Hearing Research, 35*(4), 903–912.
145. Habibi, A., Cahn, B. R., Damasio, A., & Damasio, H. (2016). Neural correlates of accelerated auditory processing in children engaged in music training. *Developmental Cognitive Neuroscience, 21*, 1–14.
146. Näätänen, R., & Alho, K. (1995). Mismatch negativity—A unique measure of sensory processing in audition. *International Journal of Neuroscience, 80*(1–4), 317–337.
147. Sharma, M., Purdy, S. C., Newall, P., Wheldall, K., Beaman, R., & Dillon, H. (2004). Effects of identification technique, extraction method, and stimulus type on mismatch negativity in adults and children. *Journal of the American Academy of Audiology, 15*(9), 616–632.
148. Paavilainen, P. (2013). The mismatch-negativity (MMN) component of the auditory event-related potential to violations of abstract regularities: A review. *International Journal of Psychophysiology, 88*(2), 109–123.
149. Picton, T., Alain, C., Otten, L., Ritter, W., & Achim, A. (2000). Mismatch negativity: Different water in the same river. *Audiology and Neurotology, 5*(3–4), 111–139.
150. Winkler, I. (2007). Interpreting the mismatch negativity. *Journal of Psychophysiology, 21*(3–4), 147–163.
151. Garrido, M. I., Kilner, J. M., Stephan, K. E., & Friston, K. J. (2009). The mismatch negativity: A review of underlying mechanisms. *Clinical Neurophysiology, 120*(3), 453–463.
152. Pang, E. W., Edmonds, G. E., Desjardins, R., Khan, S. C., Trainor, L. J., & Taylor, M. J. (1998). Mismatch negativity to speech stimuli in 8-month-old infants and adults. *International Journal of Psychophysiology, 29*(2), 227–236.
153. Schröger, E. (2005). The mismatch negativity as a tool to study auditory processing. *Acta Acustica United with Acustica, 91*(3), 490–501.
154. Uhler, K. M., Hunter, S. K., Tierney, E., & Gilley, P. M. (2018). The relationship between mismatch response and the acoustic change complex in normal hearing infants. *Clinical Neurophysiology, 129*(6), 1148–1160.
155. Kane, N. M., Butler, S. R., & Simpson, T. (2000). Coma outcome prediction using event-related potentials: P3 and mismatch negativity. *Audiology and Neurotology, 5*(3–4), 186–191.
156. Sharma, M., Purdy, S. C., Newall, P., Wheldall, K., Beaman, R., & Dillon, H. (2006). Electrophysiological and behavioral evidence of auditory processing deficits in children with reading disorder. *Clinical Neurophysiology, 117*(5), 1130–1144.
157. Friederici, A. D., Steinhauer, K., & Pfeifer, E. (2002). Brain signatures of artificial language processing: Evidence challenging the critical period hypothesis. *Proceedings of the National Academy of Sciences, 99*(1), 529–534.
158. Stapells, D. R. (2002). Cortical event-related potentials to auditory stimuli. In J. Katz (Ed.), *Handbook of clinical audiology* (Vol. 5, pp. 378–406). Lippincott Williams & Wilkins.
159. Kutas, M., & Federmeier, K. D. (2009). N400. *Scholarpedia, 4*(10), 7790.
160. Friederici, A. D., & Kotz, S. A. (2003). The brain basis of syntactic processes: Functional imaging and lesion studies. *Neuroimage, 20*, S8–S17.
161. Khachatryan, E., De Letter, M., Vanhoof, G., Goeleven, A., & Van Hulle, M. M. (2017). Sentence context prevails over word association in aphasia patients with spared comprehension: Evidence from N400 event-related potential. *Frontiers in Human Neuroscience, 10*, 684.
162. Kotz, S. A., Rothermich, K., & Schmidt-Kassow, M. (2012). Sentence comprehension in healthy and

brain-damaged populations. In M. Faust (Ed.), *The handbook of the neuropsychology of language* (pp. 760–777). Blackwell Publishing.
163. Olichney, J. M., Yang, J. C., Taylor, J., & Kutas, M. (2011). Cognitive event-related potentials: Biomarkers of synaptic dysfunction across the stages of Alzheimer's disease. *Journal of Alzheimer's Disease, 26*(s3), 215–228.
164. Angwin, A. J., Dissanayaka, N. N., McMahon, K. L., Silburn, P. A., & Copland, D. A. (2017). Lexical ambiguity resolution during sentence processing in Parkinson's disease: An event-related potential study. *PloS One, 12*(5), e0176281.
165. Loomis, A. L., Harvey, E. N., & Hobart III, G. A. (1938). Distribution of disturbance-patterns in the human electroencephalogram, with special reference to sleep. *Journal of Neurophysiology, 1*(5), 413–430.
166. Colrain, I. M. (2005). The K-complex: A 7-decade history. *Sleep 28*(2), 255–273.
167. Davis, H., Davis, P. A., Loomis, A. L., Harvey, E. N., & Hobart, G. (1939). Electrical reactions of the human brain to auditory stimulation during sleep. *Journal of Neurophysiology, 2*(6), 500–514.
168. Bastien, C., & Campbell, K. (1992). The evoked K-complex: All-or-none phenomenon? *Sleep, 15*(3), 236–245.
169. Makeig, S., Debener, S., Onton, J., & Delorme, A. (2004). Mining event-related brain dynamics. *Trends in Cognitive Sciences, 8*(5), 204–210.
170. Yordanova, J., Kolev, V., & Polich, J. (2001). P300 and alpha event-related desynchronization (ERD). *Psychophysiology, 38*(1), 143–152.
171. Shinomoto, S., Kim, H., Shimokawa, T., Matsuno, N., Funahashi, S., Shima, K., . . . Inaba, N. (2009). Relating neuronal firing patterns to functional differentiation of cerebral cortex. *PLoS Computational Biology, 5*(7), e1000433.
172. Başar, E., Başar-Eroğlu, C., Karakaş, S., & Schürmann, M. (2000). Brain oscillations in perception and memory. *International Journal of Psychophysiology, 35*(2-3), 95–124.
173. Aoki, F., Fetz, E. E., Shupe, L., Lettich, E., & Ojemann, G. A. (1999). Increased gamma-range activity in human sensorimotor cortex during performance of visuomotor tasks. *Clinical Neurophysiology, 110*(3), 524–537.
174. Klimesch, W. (1999). EEG alpha and theta oscillations reflect cognitive and memory performance: A review and analysis. *Brain Research Reviews, 29*(2-3), 169–195.
175. Palva, S., & Palva, J. M. (2011). Functional roles of alpha-band phase synchronization in local and large-scale cortical networks. *Frontiers in Psychology, 2*, 204.
176. Delvey, C., Pin-Chun, C., & Mednick, S. (2018, November). *Central autonomic couplings during sleep can predict sleep-induced working memory improvement.* Poster conducted at Southern California Conferences for Undergraduate Research, California State University, San Bernardino, CA.
177. Sauseng, P., Griesmayr, B., Freunberger, R., & Klimesch, W. (2010). Control mechanisms in working memory: A possible function of EEG theta oscillations. *Neuroscience & Biobehavioral Reviews, 34*(7), 1015–1022.
178. Baker, S. N. (2007). Oscillatory interactions between sensorimotor cortex and the periphery. *Current Opinion in Neurobiology, 17*(6), 649–655.
179. Lalo, E., Gilbertson, T., Doyle, L., Di Lazzaro, V., Cioni, B., & Brown, P. (2007). Phasic increases in cortical beta activity are associated with alterations in sensory processing in the human. *Experimental Brain Research, 177*(1), 137–145.
180. Zhang, Y., Chen, Y., Bressler, S. L., & Ding, M. (2008). Response preparation and inhibition: The role of the cortical sensorimotor beta rhythm. *Neuroscience, 156*(1), 238–246.
181. Pogosyan, A., Gaynor, L. D., Eusebio, A., & Brown, P. (2009). Boosting cortical activity at beta-band frequencies slows movement in humans. *Current Biology, 19*(19), 1637–1641.
182. Castelhano, J., Duarte, I. C., Wibral, M., Rodriguez, E., & Castelo-Branco, M. (2014). The dual facet of gamma oscillations: Separate visual and decision making circuits as revealed by simultaneous EEG/fMRI. *Human Brain Mapping, 35*(10), 5219–5235.
183. Meha-Bettison, K., Sharma, M., Ibrahim, R. K., & Mandikal Vasuki, P. R. (2018). Enhanced speech perception in noise and cortical auditory evoked potentials in professional musicians. *International Journal of Audiology, 57*(1), 40–52.
184. Gilley, P. M., Sharma, M., & Purdy, S. C. (2016). Oscillatory decoupling differentiates auditory encoding deficits in children with listening problems. *Clinical Neurophysiology, 127*(2), 1618–1628.
185. Martin, B. A., & Boothroyd, A. (1999). Cortical, auditory, event-related potentials in response to periodic and aperiodic stimuli with the same spectral envelope. *Ear and Hearing, 20*(1), 33–44.
186. Martin, B. A., & Boothroyd, A. (2000). Cortical, auditory, evoked potentials in response to changes of spectrum and amplitude. *Journal of the Acoustical Society of America, 107*(4), 2155–2161.
187. Tremblay, K. L., Friesen, L., Martin, B. A., & Wright, R. (2003). Test-retest reliability of cortical evoked

potentials using naturally produced speech sounds. *Ear and Hearing, 24*(3), 225–232.
188. Martin, B. A., Boothroyd, A., Ali, D., & Leach-Berth, T. (2010). Stimulus presentation strategies for eliciting the acoustic change complex: Increasing efficiency. *Ear and Hearing, 31*(3), 356.
189. Dimitrijevic, A., Michalewski, H. J., Zeng, F. G., Pratt, H., & Starr, A. (2008). Frequency changes in a continuous tone: Auditory cortical potentials. *Clinical Neurophysiology, 119*(9), 2111–2124.
190. Ross, B., Fujioka, T., Tremblay, K. L., & Picton, T. W. (2007). Aging in binaural hearing begins in mid-life: Evidence from cortical auditory-evoked responses to changes in interaural phase. *Journal of Neuroscience, 27*(42), 11172–11178.
191. Won, J. H., Clinard, C. G., Kwon, S., Dasika, V. K., Nie, K., Drennan, W. R., . . . Rubinstein, J. T. (2011). Relationship between behavioral and physiological spectral-ripple discrimination. *Journal of the Association for Research in Otolaryngology, 12*(3), 375–393.
192. Friesen, L. M., & Tremblay, K. L. (2006). Acoustic change complexes recorded in adult cochlear implant listeners. *Ear and Hearing, 27*(6), 678–685.
193. He, S., Grose, J. H., & Buchman, C. A. (2012). Auditory discrimination: The relationship between psychophysical and electrophysiological measures. *International Journal of Audiology, 51*(10), 771–782.
194. Martin, B. A., Tremblay, K. L., & Stapells, D. R. (2007). Principles and applications of cortical auditory evoked potentials. In R. F. Burkard, J. J. Eggermont, & M. Don (Eds.), *Auditory evoked potentials: Basic principles and clinical application* (pp. 482–507). Lippincott Williams & Wilkins.
195. Tremblay, K. L., Billings, C. J., Friesen, L. M., & Souza, P. E. (2006). Neural representation of amplified speech sounds. *Ear and Hearing, 27*(2), 93–103.
196. He, S., Grose, J. H., Teagle, H. F., & Buchman, C. A. (2014). Objective measures of electrode discrimination with electrically-evoked auditory change complex and speech perception abilities in children with auditory neuropathy spectrum disorder. *Ear and Hearing, 35*(3), e63–74.
197. Brown, C. J., Etler, C., He, S., O'Brien, S., Erenberg, S., Kim, J. R., . . . Abbas, P. J. (2008). The electrically evoked auditory change complex: Preliminary results from nucleus cochlear implant users. *Ear and Hearing, 29*(5), 704–717.
198. Dimitrijevic, A., Starr, A., Bhatt, S., Michalewski, H. J., Zeng, F. G., & Pratt, H. (2011). Auditory cortical N100 in pre-and post-synaptic auditory neuropathy to frequency or intensity changes of continuous tones. *Clinical Neurophysiology, 122*(3), 594–604.
199. He, S., Grose, J. H., Teagle, H. F., Woodard, J., Park, L. R., Hatch, D. R., . . . Buchman, C. A. (2015). Acoustically-evoked auditory change complex in children with auditory neuropathy spectrum disorder: A potential objective tool for identifying cochlear implant candidates. *Ear and Hearing, 36*(3), 289–301.

9

Difficult-to-Test Patients—General Methods and Newborn Screening

The Writers	
Episode 1:	Monica J. Chapchap and Patricia C. Mancini
Episode 2:	Susan A. Small
Episode 3:	Diane L. Sabo
Heads Up:	John D. Durrant and Cynthia G. Fowler
Episode 4:	Andy J. Beynon

■ Episode 1: Screening Hearing Responses Versus Threshold Estimation and Estimating Audiometric Configuration

Hearing *screening* is an approach to identifying individuals in the general population who may have been born with or acquired impairment of their hearing. It initially was performed only on a limited scale and with limited methods, testing behaviorally. Hearing screening relatively early in life was confined to school-aged children, screened using portable audiometers. This often proved to be too little too late and with too few at-risk children being identified. Justification of screening for a health issue falls on two parameters—need and ability to follow up; a successful screening program requires still other considerations. This chapter is substantially dedicated to pediatric audiology, wherein *evoked response audiometry (ERA)* has played a highly important role. The objectives of *newborn hearing screening (NHS)*, however, are substantially different from those of ERA. NHS is a strategy used to identify the possible presence of congenital hearing loss in neonates. Particularly early in maturation, hearing disorders generally will be without evident signs or symptoms. Still, hearing loss is one of the most frequent disorders presented at birth and interferes significantly with normal development of speech, language, cognition, and socialization.

In the first year of life, good quality of sound exposure, other sensorial experiences, and social interactions are fundamental for nourishing the brain's maturation in the future speaker. Delayed development of speech and language is detected by parents "with luck" at around 12 months of age but not until around 2 years for the vast majority of children.[1] *Universal* newborn hearing screening *(UNHS)* is specifically a strategy to identify hearing problems as early as possible. UNHS is essential because a targeted hearing screening program—such as testing only a high-risk population like babies from a *newborn intensive care unit (NICU)*—will miss half of the hearing-impaired infants.[2] In general, hearing screening is only the first step of a hearing health-care program and must be followed by diagnostic and intervention phases of patient management (Figure 9–1).

The ages of *identification* and initiation of adequate *intervention*, respectively, are critical in the language development of hearing-impaired infants. Both linguistic performance (expressive

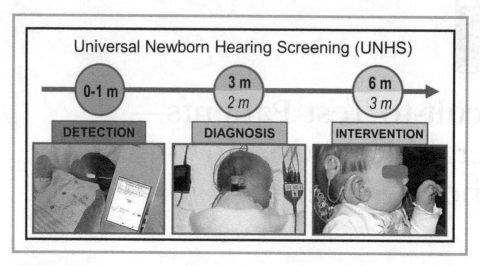

Figure 9–1. Currently recommended milestones of universal newborn hearing screening.

and comprehensive) and social development of hearing-impaired infants in whom intervention was initiated by age 6 months have been shown to be far superior to that of children identified at later ages. Indeed, the early-intervention children's performance/development has proven to be comparable to that of their normal-hearing peers (that is, age-matched). Therefore, the defining factor for success has been shown to be the age of the initiation of intervention.[3] To achieve an intervention as early as 6 months of age, it is imperative to perform the first hearing screening at the newborn nursery before discharge, and subsequently to have a ***diagnosis*** for the at-risk infant by the age of 3 months (see Figure 9–1). In some countries in which birthing of children is often in the home, the initial screen may only be available in a community center, but this could exacerbate both meeting the standard of universal NHS and doing so in an adequately timely manner.[4]

In multiple reports since the early 1990s,[5–11] UNHS has been endorsed with the recommendation—to underscore—that all babies identified should have a diagnosis by the age of 3 months and follow up with appropriate intervention by the age of 6 months. Most recently (2019), the Joint Commission on Infant Hearing (JCIH)[4] has recommended UNHS programs to have reached certain quality indicators toward meeting follow-up "milestones" of 1-3-6 months, respectively. Examples of these indicators are percentage of all newborn infants who complete screening by 1 month of age; the recommended benchmark is >95% (with age correction for preterm infants). Another is the percentage who completed a comprehensive audiological evaluation by 3 months of age; the recommended benchmark is 90%. However, the JCIH also has recommended that programs endeavor to implement the more ambitious milestones of 1-2-3 months, respectively, in other words, intervention by 3 months of age.

The principle of UNHS is applied toward identification of patients at risk for hearing loss using predetermined pass-fail criteria, in turn different from the objective and approach of ERA (estimating hearing thresholds to evaluate hearing function and/or impairment). Another aspect that differs from conventional ERA is that in the process, parents/caregivers are presented with the benefits of early identification of hearing disorders, even though they may have had no suspicion of hearing problems. The success of the treatment subsequently depends on the timeliness of the first professional contact and an understanding that UNHS is a program with the stages of detection, diagnosis, and intervention. Parent/caregivers must be convinced that minimizing potential sensory deprivation is particularly crucial in infants.

In general, the most common methods of NHS are tests of the *otoacoustic emission (OAE)* and/or the *auditory brainstem response (ABR)*. In order to minimize errors of interpretation of results and improve NHS quality among screeners and screening programs, the protocols are standardized. Both the performance and analyses of the tests are automated (to diminish testing time), applying the test at a single stimulus level and rate and evaluating the recordings for statistical significance of responses via a computer algorithm. These features are specific to UNHS and indeed differ from the same test methods as used at the diagnostic phase, in deference to the needs and requirements of their respective clinical applications.

In practice, *cost/benefit* considerations must also be made to ascertain which procedure best meets the NHS programmatic needs. There are several publications about NHS test performance showing good specificity and sensitivity (metrics to be discussed further, shortly). There are no ideal performance levels, but both OAE and ABR measurement have proven to be appropriate and efficacious for NHS.[12,13]

UNHS embraces still other considerations for implementation in a timely and rigorous manner. In many countries, UNHS broadly has become mandatory, justified, and deemed beneficial—therefore, effective in practice. Justifications for UNHS are summarized in Table 9–1. As a primary goal of UNHS is the detection of all types of hearing losses; whatever the extenuating circumstances, different methodologies among different populations may be recommended. For example, OAE testing often is recommended for the low-risk population of infants from *well-baby nurseries (WBNs)*, wherein sensory hearing loss is more common. ABR testing is often recommended for the high-risk population of "NICU graduates" in which neural hearing losses are more prevalent.

ABR-ERA offers the ability to identify hearing loss type, degree, and configuration in infants of 3 months of age using air and bone conduction testing with frequency-specific stimuli, namely at several frequencies bilaterally. These requirements are predicated on the goal to initiate efficacious hearing-aid intervention (if indicated) by 6 months of age. The 3-month diagnostic timeline is based on the difficulty in obtaining high-quality ABR results beyond this age when natural sleep becomes more limited. Results of studies have demonstrated that around 60% of hearing-impaired infants have a complete diagnostic evaluation by 3 months, and 72% of the total by the age of 1 year.[14] There is ample evidence that diagnostic delays (when they occur) are due to professionals' inability to complete a comprehensive hearing evaluation and (subsequently) come to a definitive diagnosis.[15] The

Table 9–1. Universal Newborn Hearing Screening (UNHS)—Justifications

The prevalence of congenital hearing loss in infants is high and may vary from 1 to 3 in 1,000 births at general low-risk population toward 2% to 4% at high-risk population.
Hearing loss is the most frequent affliction when compared to other routinely screened neonatal pathologies, such as phenylketonuria.
In most of the cases, hearing loss is invisible and may not be perceived unless an objective hearing screening is performed, which would identify only 50% of the hearing impaired cases.
NHS must be universal because of the risk indicators.
Healthy neonates mostly benefit from UNHS because the identification of hearing loss is typically later than in high-risk neonates.
Early identification of hearing loss and adequate intervention (hearing aids, cochlear implants), namely by 6 months, enables normal speech and language development—comparable to normal hearing pairs.
UNHS promotes timelines that permit the completion of diagnostic and intervention stages earlier than those realized without a UNHS program in place.

responsibilities of a UNHS program are great in the mandate of follow-up, especially by virtue of the tight timelines that must be observed.

In practice, this means diagnosis/decisions are based largely, indeed, upon electrophysiological tests. Behavioral evaluation will take on increased importance during follow-up as well but also with age. In any event, follow-up requires extensive cooperation beyond the audiology clinic, including with the ear, nose, and throat clinic, other medical and/or social services, and certainly the family.

In summary, a successful UNHS program requires clear purpose and the capacity for appropriate follow-up. Significant **family history, prenatal history**, and/or history of **neonatal intensive care** justify screening, without question. However, in UNHS, the interest of a more comprehensive screening program and objectives of early hearing evaluation and intervention are the justifications. Before the advent of UNHS initiatives, efforts were focused only upon and limited to risk indicators; screening efforts then served largely only the population of infants from NICUs. Still, these cases are at increased risk for hearing disorders per their general and/or neurological health issues. This, in turn, is another explanation and justification of the overall predominance of electrophysiological tests, rather than that of OAE tests, in this patient group.

In 2007, the JCIH[8] had described the risk indicators associated with permanent congenital, delayed-onset, or progressive hearing loss in childhood (Table 9–2). The identification of risk indicators is important for proper follow-up and management of newborns at risk. The details of

Table 9–2. Joint Committee on Infant Hearing (JCIH)

Risk Indicators Associated with Permanent Congenital, Delayed-Onset, or Progressive Hearing Loss in Childhood (JCIH, 2007[8])
Risk indicators that are marked with a "§" are of greater concern for delayed-onset hearing loss.
Caregiver concern§ regarding hearing, speech, language, or developmental delay.
Family history§ of permanent childhood hearing loss.
Neonatal intensive care of more than 5 days or any of the following regardless of length of stay: extra corporeal membrane oxygenation (ECMO)§, assisted ventilation, exposure to ototoxic medications (gentamicin and tobramycin) or loop diuretics (furosemide/Lasix), and hyperbilirubinemia that requires exchange transfusion.
In utero infections, such as cytomegalovirus (CMV)§, herpes, rubella, syphilis, and toxoplasmosis.
Craniofacial anomalies, including those that involve the pinna, ear canal, ear tags, ear pits, and temporal bone anomalies.
Physical findings, such as white forelock, that are associated with a syndrome known to include a sensorineural or permanent conductive hearing loss.
Syndromes associated with hearing loss or progressive or late-onset hearing loss§, such as neurofibromatosis, osteopetrosis, and Usher syndrome; other frequently identified syndromes including Waardenburg, Alport, Pendred, and Jervell and Lange-Nielson.
Neurodegenerative disorders§, such as Hunter syndrome, or sensory-motor neuropathies, such as Friedreich ataxia and Charcot-Marie-Tooth syndrome.
Culture-positive postnatal infections associated with sensorineural hearing loss§, including confirmed bacterial and viral infections (especially herpes viruses and varicella meningitis).
Head trauma, especially basal skull/temporal bone fracture§ that requires hospitalizations.
Chemotherapy.§

the follow-up can differ depending on the risk indicators identified.

The tools adopted in NHS are a matter of approach, and the technological evolution/revolution is intertwined with that of NHS. Indeed, the development of OAE technology[16] was a door-opener to screen for hearing loss in **WBNs**. The challenge in earlier stages of development of NHS was that of branching out into the WBNs to find the (proportionally) far fewer newborns who truly were at risk for hearing losses postdischarge. For all the importance of UNHS, as just overviewed and thus identifying babies at risk, results of large-scale ("population") studies have shown that in the general population the risk for congenital hearing loss is low (1 in 1,000 births).[17] The analogy of the needle in the haystack comes to mind, while the potential cost to the individual and society of not finding that baby at risk is high. Coming through the 1970s and 1980s, ABR and then *automated* ABR (*AABR*)[18] testing were the prevailing opinions but were greatly hampered by costs and test time to effectively implement. Subsequently emerging OAE tests appeared more efficient at the time and an excellent candidate for administering a screen in the most economical and timely manner,[19] namely to do so predischarge and without unnecessarily extending hospital stays.

Shown in Figure 9–2A are samples of *click-evoked otoacoustic emissions* evaluated in a nursery; results on top (nominally labeled right ear) are characteristic of recordings obtained in most normal hearing ears. In contrast, the left-ear results (panel A, bottom) demonstrate minimal/absent responses, typical of cases of hearing thresholds beyond the range of clinically normal hearing. These results for the CEOAE screen are considered thus a pass for the right versus a fail for the left ear. One caveat in using OAE testing is that it is sensitive to temporary outer and middle ear issues, potentially more so than results of *automated* screening of the *auditory brainstem response, AABR), samples of which appear in panels C and D*. This leads to a higher false positive rate than using an AABR screen.[20] This situation relates to the middle ear. Since the newborn is left with a fluid-filled ear but now having to hear in an air-filled environment (a temporary impedance mismatch), it can take a bit of time over the first few days following birth for the fluid to clear. A conductive lesion (even if small and temporary) tends to present a sort of double jeopardy for the recording of the emission—attenuating the sound into and the emission coming out from the cochlea. It often is recommended to use AABR screening as a complementary tool for neonates who fail the OAE screen and before discharge from the nursery to reduce significantly false-fail rates of the screening program. This is also useful to decrease parental anxiety in awaiting a retest postdischarge, thus ideally within 30 days. The good news is that around 70% of the neonates who fail the OAE-first screening pass AABR screening when administered the same day.[21] Such testing equally could be done the following day or so, as generally there is a short stay in the hospital even for well babies. The JCIH recommends this protocol, namely given any OAE-screen failures. However, simply rerunning the OAE screen before discharging the baby (when practical) also can substantially reduce net fail rates. The professional or professionally supervised personnel are critical to reducing OAE false-alarm rates to a reasonable level for UNHS. A typical failure rate of an OAE-based UNHS program is 1.8%.[22]

Practical UNHS programs can have significantly different needs with respect to test modality(ies), affordability, available personnel, and relative numbers of well-baby births versus births by which babies are referred to NICU. In 2019, JCIH suggested using either OAE or AABR testing of babies not of higher risks (by history/NICU graduates). As noted before, the general tendency is that of screening programs find in the WBNs predominantly cases of sensory losses, so a good match for use of the OAE "tool." Still, there is the concern of missing a case of a neural loss, particularly that of auditory neuropathy spectrum disorder (ANSD), as likely would occur in an OAE-only screening program. At the same time, an ANSD is of lower prevalence, although recently becoming recognized to be of higher prevalence than assumed initially.[23] Practically then, the goal would be to use AABR in screening at least in NICU/other at-risk babies. Nevertheless, this is also an issue of health-care economics, wherein trying to avoid missing any case of ANSD at birth simply might not be within means.

More than one technology is available for both modalities discussed. Figure 9–2 also includes

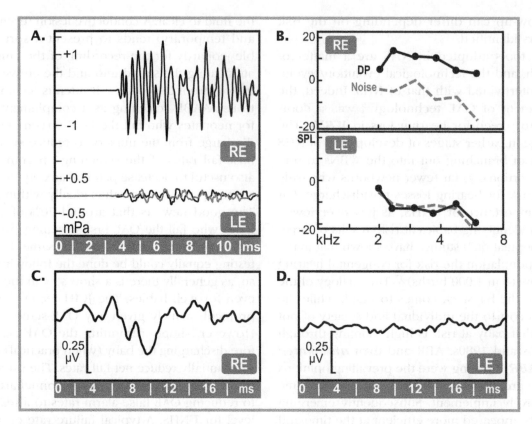

Figure 9–2. Comparison among results from screening tests of click-evoked otoacoustic emissions (**A**), distortion product OAEs (**B**), and auditory brainstem responses obtained using an automated screener (**C**, right ear and **D**, left ear). Examples of cases/ears wherein the baby passed (*top graphs in panels **A** and **B** and panel **C**, RE*) versus failed the screen (*bottom graphs in panels **A** and **B** and panel **D**, LE*). Test levels for the DPOAE were 65 dB SPL/55 dB SPL, tacked across test frequencies as well; levels fell well within +/−1 dB throughout frequency sweeps for both.

examples of **distortion product** OAEs by way of **DPOAE-grams**. These are examples of pass (right ear) versus fail results (left ear, as indicated). Going farther up the auditory pathway, both ABR and **auditory steady-state response (ASSR)** screens have inherent strengths for purposes of NHS, although the latter has yet to become mainstream in this context. ABR measurement in the role of a screening test is most broadly implemented via AABR measurement, again to detect a statistically significant response via a computer algorithm for responses elicited by a singular stimulus level and rate. There are newer generations of equipment that are hybrids, such as diagnostic units packaged compactly for ease of portability and "loaded" with flexible software to handle a variety of protocols, including automated screening. Again, examples of AABR recordings in cases of a pass versus fail are shown in Figure 9–2, panels C and D for the two cases/ears respectively. As a screening test, just one stimulus thus is used but also is presented at a somewhat elevated rate than in the adult, especially for purposes of differential diagnostic testing (typically around 20/s or less). Generally clicks are used at a rate of around 35/s for screening to expedite acquisition, and they are presented at about 45 dB nHL.

In practice, CEOAE, DPOAE, and AABR have shown comparable results in the detection of midfrequency responses (that is, the geometric-/octave-based center of the frequency range of hearing, as routinely represented by the pure-tone audiogram). Tests of these evoked responses are similarly efficacious for NHS purposes.[12] As important for any test, ***pass/fail criteria*** must be set with an understanding of ***statistical decision making***—relevant ***probability functions*** and cost/benefits of criteria set. Some of the relevant terminology already has been used/defined in earlier chapters, but a bit more detailed discussion will be worthwhile.

Any test can prove to have good or less-so effective performance, which can be evaluated quantitatively. Here the focus has been on instruments that can be trusted to identify individuals more likely than the unscreened population to have a certain condition—like hearing loss. Just how trustworthy and what are useful metrics to say so? There are at least two measures that are commonly used to evaluate test performance—***sensitivity and specificity***.[24,25] The sensitivity is a metric that reflects the probability that the screening test will be positive (that is, the patient having failed the screen) among those who truly have the targeted condition (like a disease or dysfunction). In contrast, the specificity reflects the probability that the screening test will be negative (passed the screen) among those who do not have the condition. Clinically, these concepts are important for confirming or excluding disease/dysfunction. Ideally, a screening test should provide both a high sensitivity and specificity. Calculation of sensitivity and specificity requires construction of a ***2 × 2 table*** (Figure 9–3A, upper panel)—two columns (one for "impaired" and another for "unimpaired") and two rows (one for "fail" and another for "pass"). These rows and columns create four boxes for outcomes, as follows: ***true positives*** (cell A, impaired and failed the test), ***false positives*** (cell B, unimpaired but still failed the test), ***false negatives*** (cell C, impaired yet passed the test), and ***true negatives*** (cell D, unimpaired and passed the test). Sensitivity and specificity are the most commonly reported findings of studies of the accuracy of diagnostic tools. When sensitivity is high, a negative test result is likely to rule out the condition. Still, high

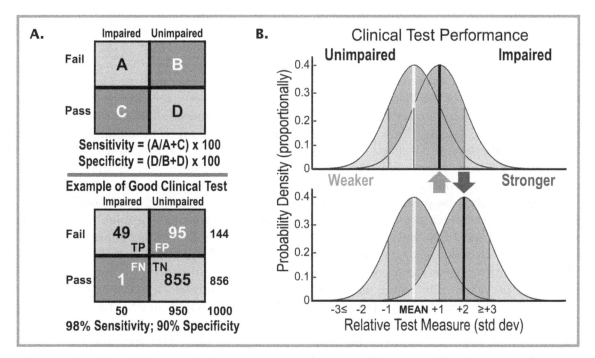

Figure 9–3. Bases of evaluating test sensitivity and specificity: **A**—2 × 2 tables; **B**—probability density functions (see text). Regarding the latter for a given test, the abscissa typically would be scaled in units of measure of that test, deemed to be of diagnostic value (such as interaural latency differences in differential diagnostic application of the ABR; recall Episode 6.5). Here, it is simply scaled in intervals of the standard deviation of the measure, as it is the respective variances of the results in the impaired versus unimpaired population that characterizes the challenges of setting test criteria. (Based in part on illustrations courtesy of Dr. D. Sabo.)

sensitivity alone/"unchecked" also would likely yield unacceptably high false positives. Specificity is the metric that provides a sort of "checkmate". When specificity is high, a positive test result is likely to rule in the condition. Consequently, a good screening test must both identify persons with the disease/dysfunction (high sensitivity) and rule out persons without the disease/dysfunction (high specificity).

For example (panel A, lower 2 × 2 table), if 1,000 people are screened for a specific disorder that has a 5% prevalence in the general population, a good clinical test must identify correctly all 50 patients with the disease and rule out all the 950 people without the disease. However, this level of performance would imply a perfect screen, something not achieved readily in the real world. Since "all tests" implies inclusion of those cases whose results were inaccurate and/or misinterpreted, such cases also must be accounted for in the analysis, thus counting false negatives and false positives. The most important characteristics of any screening test depend on the implications of an error. Sadly, mistakes or other exigencies can happen, thus making observation of both sensitivity and specificity equal to 100% unlikely. More realistic numbers might be 98% sensitivity and 90% specificity. In this case, for the same cohort, the screen will have identified correctly 49 persons with the condition and 1 case with a false negative. Additionally, the screen will have ruled out the condition in 855 truly "normal" people, while having only sent 95 people unnecessarily for follow-up evaluations (namely, false positives). Note that in this example describing a test offering good performance, 144 of the 1,000 patients failed the screen, yet only 49 of those (34%) had the condition. This apparent incongruity is a consequence of the low (5%) prevalence. Excluding temporary conductive losses, the prevalence of permanent childhood hearing loss is nearer to 1%. Whether this is good enough will come down to the cost-benefits analysis, for instance apropos costs of follow-up test(s) and the "cost" placed on missing cases of hearing loss.

Statistical variability in the presentation of a given condition in the population of interest is taken to be distributed (ideally) along the measurement value in a **bell-shaped curve**—technically, the *probability density function* (see Figure 9–3B). In a poor screening test, there is a quite high proportion of false negatives and false positives relative to true positives and true negatives (panel B, upper curves), hence great overlapping of the unpaired (nominally normal) versus impaired cohorts. In strong screening tests, much less overlap occurs (lower curves). A perfect test would have nonoverlapping distributions of results. The most important characteristics of any screening test depends on the chance for errors. In all cases, it is important to understand the performance characteristics of a test to appropriately interpret results and their implications.

Effectiveness of screens again must take into consideration cost/benefits. Many screening tests have potential adverse effects (costs) that need to be considered and weighed against the potential benefits. In addition, there are pragmatic issues of the test methods themselves to be considered, such as their availability, staff time and training, discomfort that they may cause the patient, and so forth. These too are costs. Evaluations of OAE and ABR have good test performance in detecting hearing loss greater than 35 dB HL. More restricted pass-fail criteria will yield more false-positives and consequently cause more incidents of unwarranted parental concern, in addition to the more obvious costs of more follow-up tests. Benefits in this "arena" are taken to be implied by the considerations early on in this episode—the need to have an effective, efficient UNHS program toward early identification of children with hearing losses.

It cannot be emphasized enough: NHS must be applied in a systematic manner to ensure effectiveness and benefit. Various approaches to effective screening of newborns in WBNs have been tried with successful outcomes. Figure 9–4 shows an "overview" model—a decision **flowchart** adaptable to both WBNs and NICUs. The "flow" also is shown in reference to desired timelines.

Reports from NHS programs have shown variable levels of success, from inception.[26] Still, good experiences in this area have been published.[27] Success depends on the availability of and adherence to detailed technical guidance/documentation, involvement of a team of screeners with a coordinator to achieve excellence, and measurement defined by quality indicators. Besides the

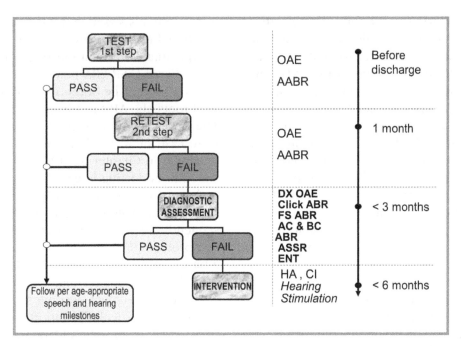

Figure 9–4. Flow chart of universal newborn screening and follow-up management.

Table 9–3. UNHS—Recommendations

National Institutes of Health, Early identification of hearing impairment in infants and young children, 1993[5]
Joint Committee on Infant Hearing, Principles and guidelines for early hearing detection and intervention programs, 2019[4],1994[6], 2000[7], 2007[8]
European Consensus, Statement on Neonatal Hearing Screening, 1998[9]
American Academy of Pediatrics, Task Force on Newborn and Infant Hearing, 1999[10]
British Society of Audiology, Guidelines for the early audiological assessment and management of babies referred from the Newborn Hearing, 2013[11]

human-resource commitments, specific characteristics such as kindness and empathy in handling neonates and their families, professional conduct, technically competent/responsible service, and highly efficient performance are very important. Given the many complexities and demands and having needed a considerable enhancement of computing and electronic instrumentation for efficacious UNHS programs, it is a tribute to the workers in this area to have succeeded overall globally and in a relatively short amount of time, including well-developed guidelines as summarized in Table 9–3.

The effects of evolving technology have an impact for the program's maintenance and success by way of technology promising a fast, standardized, and noninvasive test methodology for a specific population. However, this is not yet a "level playing field" globally. Levels of success in countries of relatively high-level/broadly accessible health-care systems are usually higher than in so-called developing countries. Great emphasis was placed on the importance of principles presented previously: early detection, reliable diagnosis, and timely intervention to improve chances of hearing-impaired infants developing skills competitive with their normally hearing peers. Unfortunately, there still are many challenges for developing countries to implement and maintain effective NHS programs.

Although the need for successful UNHS programs cannot be denied,[28] the legislative support, technology, and expertise needed to implement such programs on a national level only recently have come to be realized in more and more developing countries. Screening programs need to be part of the government health service provision in the country and with ensured funding. There also are continuing needs for staff training, maintenance of equipment, and establishment of links with education, social, and other support agencies nationally and internationally. Therefore, many challenges remain to achieve truly global UNHS. Finding the resources to implement solutions for the detection and treatment of newborns is also a major problem. Most developing countries have a high birth rate with dense populations.[29] Rates of hearing-impairment prevalence in newborns are estimated to be higher in developing countries, considering the relatively higher rate of exposure to risk factors.[30,31]

Standardizing screening and intervention programs remains an important goal to establish quality NHS programs in developing countries. Additionally, there needs to be consideration of the local culture and local resource strengths and limitations. The burden of hearing loss falls disproportionately on disadvantaged groups, mainly because they are unable to afford the preventive and routine care necessary to avoid hearing impairment or afford hearing aids (including supplies and maintenance) or other devices to treat or make their/their child's condition manageable. Fortunately, the World Health Organization has long embraced initiatives to promote and empower NHS programs.

Moving beyond NHS, clinical electrophysiology is an essential tool for follow-up to NHS, starting with ERA toward the objective of timely follow-up to the newborn screen. The focus then shifts from identification to audiological evaluation of the nature, type, and degree of the hearing loss and ultimately acquiring information needed to initiate intervention. The approach depends on the child's ability to cooperate, even for visual reinforcement or play audiometry. In early follow-up and/or for some multiply handicapped children, behavioral tests will not be feasible. Objective functional tests thus are the only practical choice for quantitative estimation of the hearing threshold. ABR- or ASSR-ERA plays the major role herein.

It also must be borne in mind that, by its classical roots, the ABR test is a neuro-diagnostic tool. The earlier mention of concern for missing a possible case of ANSD is a case in point. As demonstrated in Chapter 6, ABR measurement is well suited to evaluating integrity of the initial auditory pathway. Here the emphasis practically is again on the transient ABR, elicited typically by clicks. Consequently, a special benefit of ABR-ERA is that the test protocol, if time permits, could be expanded a bit to permit adding stimuli and/or levels for differential diagnostic testing, should indeed a retrocochlear involvement become suspected.

This is particularly important for differentiation between sensory and neural hearing disorders, indeed as management of the AN case teaches (recall Episode 6.5 and its accompanying casestudies Heads Up). If the auditory system is damaged and particularly if neurons cannot fire synchronously or suffer disruptions (from faulty synapses with the organ of Corti or within the central auditory nervous system), there may be no identifiable ABR waveform or a partial absence of waves, even though the cochlea may be functioning normally. Distinguishing pre- from postsynaptic auditory neuropathy or other dysfunctions centrally will affect choice of intervention and outcomes. As an audiological test, some assumptions are made about the patient's neurologic status; conversely, as a neurologic test, some assumptions must be made concerning the hearing status/effects (recall the rationale of interpretation of the ABR in differential diagnostic testing, again Episode 6.5). If the testing conditions are good and the recording appears technically adequate (particularly with an acceptably low level of background noise) yet no ABR is observed confidently at any stimulus level, then it is not possible to use that finding in isolation, let alone to distinguish between a neurologic and sensory losses. Hence the importance of other information and/or testing, such as OAE and/or tests of other/longer-latency AEPs.

However, the immature auditory system again can "cause" apparent abnormalities of the ABR/other AEPs which are, in fact, entirely normal for

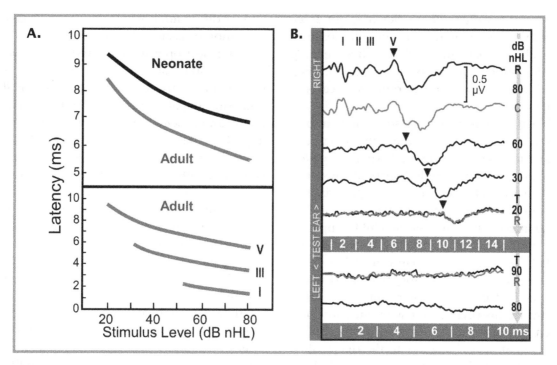

Figure 9–5. A. *Top*: Comparison of latency-intensity functions between infants and young adults (based on data of Gorga and associates, 1987[32]). *Bottom*: Trends for all three major components of the ABR, as a recap/other reminders (see text). **B.** Examples of click-elicited brainstem test results typical of follow-up testing corresponding to screening results represented in Figure 9–2 (respective test ears as indicated).

the gestational age of the child (recall Episode 6.1). So critical are these maturational effects on the ABR waveform and interpretation of test results that they warrant additional demonstration. As shown in Figure 9–5, salient effects include substantially longer latencies for neonates when compared to those of adults, as seen in panel A (top subpanel). Functions in the bottom subpanel recap overall latency-intensity functions for the three main ABR components. Recall also the lesson of Figure 6–9; for the premature and full-term newborn and infant through the first couple of years, their waveform and/or peak latencies (relative to the adult) are involved in maturation, thus affecting both absolute and interpeak intervals. The results of conventional ABR testing (click stimulus) in Figure 9–5B exemplify recordings as might be seen in cases presenting the screening results presented earlier apropos pass/fail criteria (see Figure 9–2C and D). Responses in the upper part of panel B show the sort of maturational delay portrayed in panel A.

The analysis of the ABR thus requires normal references for different age ranges. By the age of 2 years however, the latencies of waves I, III, and V generally reach the same values as those found in adults.[32] Any deviation from age-appropriate latencies should lead to follow-up investigations and appropriate management of the child. Nonetheless, since both hearing loss and neurologic disease can affect ABR latencies, distinguishing these categories of pathology can be problematic to disentangle, in the same manner discussed in Episode 6.5. Pending results/interpretation, medical referral may be in order.

For ERA, frequency-specific tests of the ABR or ASSR are essential to best overall estimations of hearing thresholds (again, to define both degree and configuration of hearing losses; recall Episode 6.4). Acceptable agreement for many purposes can be realized between behavioral thresholds and ***visual detection levels (VDLs)*** of the ABR or the statistically significant levels of the 80-Hz ASSR.

Still, there are instances where they may not agree and/or may not provide reliable-enough measures for clinical purposes intended, as when seeking information supporting intervention with hearing-aids, cochlear implants, and/or other medical/surgical treatment.

Subjective hearing tests also remain important for the management of the patient—where, when, and to what extent possible (per the child's stage of development). Audiologists always seek to have behavioral test results as appropriate to the patient's capability, starting with the history, including anecdotal reports of the child's apparent level of auditory functioning. The history is fundamentally one of the clinician's most important tools. In the case of contradictory findings between subjective- and objective-test results, the differences can be instructive and wherein care must be taken in interpretation of the results. Taking example again of ANSD, a key to the diagnosis is often the "disjoint" between subjective and objective findings, in turn dependent on differential-diagnostic objective findings that start indeed with both OAE and ABR assessments.[33] This "package" of information may reveal an apparently working hair cell system in the face of sending a poor signal or no apparent signal up to the CANS. In pediatric ANSD patients old enough to participate in some behavioral testing, other disjoints likely will be manifest, such as disagreement of the audiogram with the DP-gram and/or poor speech recognition not readily attributable to the presumed degree/configuration of hearing loss. In any event, the observation of little/no ABR cannot be taken as evidence of a full disconnect of the peripheral to the central system. This has encouraged clinicians to look beyond the pontine brainstem, thus beyond the ABR. Consequently, it is important to comprehensively determine what further management is warranted, especially toward better understanding of the patient's functional limitations/status. Much of these same considerations must be applied in any case—regardless of site of lesion beyond the auditory receptor cells—in the interests of "due diligence" and avoiding being blindsided by perceived "gold-standards" of conventional audiologic evaluation and ABR/ASSR testing. Chapters 7 and 8 included substantial coverage of applications of both middle- and long-latency responses to ERA and/or differential diagnostics, with detailed consideration of issues of maturation.

The electrophysiological test findings are often more important at very young ages in the decision making about the management of the child with a hearing impairment, by default. Older children often can participate in some adaptation of audiological evaluations, if not conventional behavioral audiometry. For them, diagnostic/treatment decisions and other follow-up are made depending more on behavioral audiological findings. At the same time, because the electrophysiological and behavioral tests provide information on different aspects of the child's auditory function, their results indeed are complimentary.

Electrophysiological testing of frequency-specific, transient ABRs has been considered for nearly a half-century to be the most reliable technique for estimating hearing thresholds. In subjects who cannot cooperate to be quiet enough for reliable recordings, they potentially will require sedation—an issue to be taken up in more detail in an upcoming episode. The use of ABR measurement remains a sort of gold standard for any other approach (as hinted previously), namely to equal or surpass ABR tests' performance and match this AEP's breadth of clinical-population applicability, including being virtually impervious to level of arousal. Skilled usage can provide reasonably accurate estimation of hearing thresholds and hearing-loss configuration, especially from 1000 Hz to 4000 Hz and in cases of mild to moderately severe hearing losses, other than of steeply sloping ("ski-slope") configurations.

For more than two decades, however, there has been increasing interest in and evidence to support the role of ASSR measurement for ERA (recall Episodes 6.3 and 6.4). Further information on clinical applications and practical considerations are pursued in the upcoming episode. One of the most important advantages of ASSR measurement is the possibility to assess several frequencies simultaneously while presenting them to both ears at the same time, thus potentially decreasing test time, if compared to the same assessment using ABR with tone-burst stimuli. Rather than depending on VDLs and latency of transient ABRs (to reiterate), ASSRs are assessed using spectral analysis and statistical tests of response components predictable from the stimulus (for example ≥80 Hz.)[34] This removes the examiner's subjective judgment of the limit of detection of the electrophysiological response. The ASSR also permits estimation of hearing thresholds across the same range with comparable accuracy to ABR-ERA.

Some ills of the classical ABR-ERA potentially (as noted earlier) may be addressed more readily/reliably with measurement of longer-latency AEPs (recall Episode 7.2), such as testing the transient-elicited AMLR (auditory middle latency response) below 1000 Hz using tone bursts. The 40-Hz steady-state "version" is another candidate, although having some limitation for testing sleeping patients. However, ERA application of transient-elicited ALLRs (the cortical auditory evoked potentials, P_1-N_1-P_2 complex) most readily permits dealing with any issue of frequency specificity (recall Episodes 8.1 and 8.2). Yet their use also requires consideration of the effects of subject state and maturation that are more complicated than in the testing of the earlier responses. This point is a reminder that ERA overall was seeded by the early work on the CAEP. More recently, it has become of greater interest and with greater success to test CAEPs in children, even infants.[35] The results promise more efficacious test methods and reliability, even in the youngest pediatric patients, in particular without requiring their attention to the stimuli and/or their being fully awake.

Until recently, there was the issue of not having a steady-state approach to measurement of the CAEP (in particular the N1-P2 complex, frequently the focus of response measurements for ALLR-ERA); such a method is now in research and development, as noted in Episode 8.2.[36] This advance offers the same advantages to cortical response testing as 40- or 80-Hz ASSR but while also extracting the conventional/transient response. Additionally, the approach permits a straightforward evaluation of effects of a parameter of testing broadly which is well known and was demonstrated earlier (recall Figures 8–4B and 8–10)—the effects of stimulus rate. Decreasing the stimulus rate below 10/s is seen to remarkably change the AEP observed. Simply measuring an overall response magnitude can be advantageous, rather than that of the traditional picking of some peak(s) and making measurements relatively interpretively. A stimulus rate profile thus can be determined without subjective wave/response identification. Rate effects indeed have been observed/reported for decades across the major latency groups of AEPs, including tests of responses beyond "time zones" of those arising from 8th-nerve and/or brainstem generators. The overall effect is expected to be reflective of overall levels of generators of the CANS, per the overall S-M-L latency ranges. Maturational changes are also significant in all three major "time zones." Hence the thought that once perfected, rate-profile assessment could provide valuable information about more of the auditory pathway than conventionally is being assessed and using purely objective methods that also could be automated.

Such work and still others continue to refine/add to the audiologist's electrophysiological toolbox and are the outgrowths of efforts to ensure the transfer of scientific results from the research laboratory to the clinic, and therein to the development of evidence-based practice of revolutionary tests. This well is reflective of the entire history of ERA and related applications, such as NHS/UNHS, even if seemingly "operating" on more of an evolutionary than revolutionary timescale. Still, phenomenal progress has been realized over the last half-century, but science is inherently and justifiably conservative to minimize the risk of "dead-ends" or worse—malpractice. The progress to date truly is revolutionary, considering that predigital electronics were literally the "dark ages" of electrophysiology. There thus is every reason to be confident that further innovations and advances will follow.

Episode 2: Bone Conduction Testing—A Special Challenge, Yet Efficacious With Understanding

As witnessed in Episode 6.4, the ABR and ASSRs are readily evoked by a bone-conducted (BC) stimulus.[37] With appropriate calibration (force rather than sound pressure level used for air conducted, AC stimuli), a BC stimulus has similar effectiveness to an AC stimulus for the estimation of hearing thresholds. Bone-conduction evoked response testing in infants has been used for more than 30 years to differentiate between types of hearing loss in the clinic: sensorineural, mixed, or conductive. **Bone-conduction ABRs** are a standard component of infant hearing assessments in many countries; **BC ASSRs** are not used as widely but are preferred in some countries where ASSRs are used (for instance in Cuba). Establishment of type of hearing loss early is critical to avoid delays in appropriate intervention for infants. Identification of a transient conductive loss due to fluid in the middle-ear space leads to a very different intervention path for a family compared to confirmation of a permanent sensorineural hearing loss.

Bone-conduction hearing sensitivity in infants differs significantly from that of adults. This **maturational difference** in BC hearing was first noted in the development of BC ABR testing methods. BC ABR studies showed that infants with normal hearing (or normal BC hearing) tended to have better low-frequency thresholds compared to higher frequencies but with some variability across studies due to age tested, frequencies selected, and likely methodology. Mean BC ABR thresholds for 500 Hz range from −11 dB nHL to 15 dB nHL and the lowest thresholds tend to be for neonates.[38–40] BC-ABR thresholds for 2000 Hz range from 4 dB nHL to 17 dB nHL (4 dB–22 dB poorer than 500 Hz). Only two studies have reported BC ABR thresholds for 1000 and 4000 Hz (one frequency each); they found similar mean thresholds of 5 dB nHL to 7 dB nHL.[39,41] Infant BC ABR thresholds also tend to be better than those estimated for adults, particularly at 500 Hz.[42]

Studies of **bone-conduction ASSRs** have provided a comprehensive view of infant-adult differences in BC sensitivity across a broad range of frequencies, in part due to the possibility of presenting **multiple BC stimuli** simultaneously (likely to one cochlea at threshold levels). Trends of findings from data reported from a series of BC-ASSR studies conducted with normal-hearing infants are summarized in Figure 9–6, reflecting that mean BC thresholds in infants age 0 to 18 months range from 11 dB HL to 18 dB HL, 5 dB HL to 10 dB HL, 20 dB HL to 26 dB HL, and 9 dB HL to 28 dB HL at 500 Hz, 1000 Hz, 2000 Hz, and 4000 Hz, respectively. As infants mature, the low-frequency thresholds tend to worsen. For

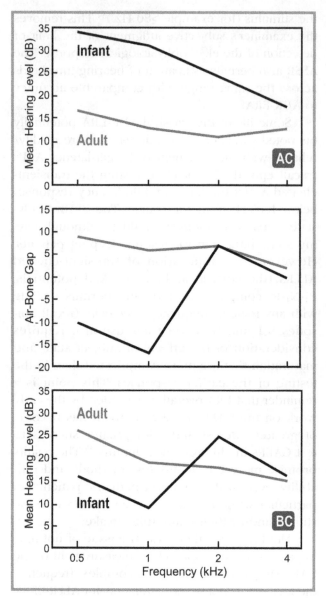

Figure 9–6. Trends of findings from data reported from a series of BC-ASSR studies conducted with normal-hearing infants (see text). Panels for AC and BC results, as indicated; mean estimate air-bone gap shown in the middle panel to further emphasize the adult-infant differences, essentially, a turnaround in the influence of test frequency on this measure. (Note: Adult plot, adaptation of Figure 6–26; see Episode 6.4.)

example, mean BC-ASSR thresholds for 10 to 24 month-old infants are 22 nHL, 13 nHL to 17 nHL, 26 nHL to 27 nHL, and 13 nHL to 19 nHL at 500 Hz, 1000 Hz, 2000 Hz, and 4000 Hz, respectively.[43] Premature infants (32–43 weeks postconception) have BC-ASSR thresholds of 16 dB HL, 16 dB HL to 17 dB HL, 35 dB HL to 37 dB HL, and 33 dB HL at 500 Hz, 1000 Hz, 2000 Hz, and 4000 Hz, respectively. These threshold estimates for premature infants reflect both maturational differences in sensitivity compared to older infants and some degree of threshold elevation due to the presence of equipment-related background noise in the nursery, as ears were not occluded.[44,45]

In sum, comparison to the younger infant group (excluding premature infants), adults have poorer BC-ASSR thresholds for 500 Hz and 1000 Hz, slightly better thresholds at 2000 Hz, and similar thresholds at 4000 Hz.[43] The mechanisms that explain these infant-adult differences in BC-ABR and ASSR sensitivity will be discussed later.

Very few BC-ASSR studies have been published to date for infants with hearing loss. In one study,[46] test results were acquired both in infants with normal hearing and with mild conductive losses at 500 Hz. For the infants with normal hearing (confirmed by ABR testing), AC- and BC-ASSRs fell within normal levels proposed.[47] For infants with mild conductive losses, not all **AC-ASSR thresholds** were elevated, so there would be some overlap of infants with normal hearing and mild conductive loss. However, as predicted, BC-ASSR thresholds did not differ for the infants who had either normal hearing versus conductive hearing loss. In another study,[48] hearing sensitivity in a group of children was assessed before and after the insertion of ventilating tubes; the findings showed that the **ASSR air-bone gap** decreased by 10 dB to 25 dB posttreatment. Nevertheless, more data still are needed—from different research groups and from infants with a range of hearing loss—to develop this technique fully.

Recent research and development has been devoted to optimizing stimuli, particularly **chirps**, begging the question—are chirps really better? Optimization of threshold estimation in infants using ABR testing methods continues to be a focus of pediatric research. One stimulus in particular is the frequency-specific **narrow-band chirp**. This stimulus has been under investigation recently because of the ability to elicit larger brainstem responses compared to those elicited by more traditional stimuli. Improvement of the signal-to-noise ratio by enhancing brainstem response itself should allow the responses to be detected more quickly and accurately, thus resulting in more efficient testing. This goal is important for reaching the objective of completing the test conditions in one appointment to avoid having to reschedule the remainder upon the infant waking. The database for AC narrowband chirp stimuli has been growing in the past several years and a few studies investigating infant thresholds to BC narrowband-chirp stimuli have emerged. ABRs to AC, narrowband CE-Chirp in neonates have shown larger amplitudes compared to brief tonal stimuli at 500 Hz, 1000 Hz, 2000 Hz, and 4000 Hz for levels ≤40 dB nHL to 60 dB nHL.[49,50]

Unfortunately, the amplitude advantage of the narrowband CE-Chirp is not consistently present for 500 Hz at low-to-moderate levels and is not present at 60 dB nHL for either 500 Hz or 4000 Hz.[50,51] For still higher levels (80 dB nHL), there is no amplitude advantage at any frequency; amplitudes are actually smaller at 500 Hz compared to traditional brief tonal stimuli.[51] The research findings in this area are a reminder that the "trick" of the chirp—to virtually eliminate adverse phase dispersion of the traveling wave for the optimal neurophysiological response—is not straightforward. The underlying, major reality is that of hair cell function being substantially nonlinear (recall Episodes 5.1 and 5.2). Hence, there have been efforts more recently to develop "level-specific" broad- and narrowband (NB) chirp stimuli (AC & BC) designed to optimize response amplitudes across presentation levels—the CE-Chirp LS.[52,53] Data from infants with normal hearing and hearing loss are needed for AC and BC NB chirps compared to brief tone bursts, as have been used and studied more extensively. Still, the utility of NB CE-Chirp LS stimuli is a priority as these stimuli are potentially the most applicable for the identification of hearing loss across frequency and for fitting of hearing aids and other devices in infants. It is also necessary to determine if potentially larger ABRs to NB chirps are either due to improved synchronization and/or simply to stimulation of wider cochlear regions that result in less place-specific responses.

Potential elicitation of **vestibular responses,** rather than auditory responses per se, to intense AC and BC stimuli is another important issue (recall

Episode 6.4). ABR tests can occasionally elicit a response at approximately 3 ms that actually arises from the vestibular system. Clinically, this response is not difficult to identify because it occurs earlier in the waveform than wave V. However, the possibility of eliciting a vestibular response is more problematic for ASSRs because responses are analyzed in the frequency domain, making it difficult to distinguish between auditory and vestibular responses. Spurious signals also have been recorded as low as 30 dB HL for BC ASSRs in individuals with profound hearing loss.[54,55] Further research and development is needed to improve analyses and/or filtering to minimize such artifacts.

The foregoing discussions/considerations raise several pragmatic questions that are addressed in the following text. First, how can what is now known about *infant BC sensitivity* be *applied in the clinic*? Electrophysiological assessment protocols for infants are designed to establish AC and BC thresholds for each ear as efficiently as possible, similar to standard pure-tone behavioral testing for cooperative adults. To achieve this goal, clinicians need infant-specific, frequency-specific, normal levels for BC-ABRs in dB nHL and BC-ASSRs in dB HL to establish whether hearing levels are within normal limits or elevated. It should be noted that ASSR stimuli are often calibrated in "adult" dB HL stimulus levels. It is not appropriate to interpret these findings without applying age-specific correction factors because, otherwise, these values do not reflect maturational differences in either AC- or BC-hearing thresholds. *Estimated Hearing Level (eHL) correction factors* to convert infant ABR and ASSR results to predicted behavioral results in dB HL are needed. An example of well-established normal levels and eHL correction factors for BC-ABR used for infant hearing assessment (using insert type earphones) are shown in Table 9–4. Suggested normal levels for BC-ASSRs are also shown for comparison. More BC-ASSR data are needed for infants with hearing loss before this technique can be implemented with confidence in the clinic.

A second question is, how is BC testing incorporated into the test protocol? Clinical protocols for assessing infants vary in different parts of the world; however, only one well-established approach used to conduct BC-ABR testing will be discussed here to illustrate how testing protocols are adapted for infants. This is the protocol recommended by the *British Columbia Early Hear-*

Table 9–4. Example of "Normal" Levels in dB "eHL" Correction Factors for Infant Tone-Burst ABR and Multiple ASSR per Methods Used by a Well-Established Early Hearing Detection and Intervention Program[56]

		500 Hz		1000 Hz		2000 Hz		4000 Hz	
		AC	BC	AC	BC	AC	BC	AC	BC
ABR	Normal (dB nHL)	35	20	32	na	30	30	25	na
	eHL correction in dB	10*	–5	10	na	5	5	0	na
ASSR	Normal (dB HL)	40–50	30	40–45	40	40	40	40	30
	eHL correction in dB†	10–20	--	10–15	--	10–15	--	5–15	--

Note.
Normal: level at which majority of normal-hearing infants have responses present.

eHL correction: ABR (dB nHL) or ASSR (dB HL) threshold minus eHL correction = estimated behavioral hearing threshold in dB HL.

*British Columbia Early Hearing Program (BCEHP) adopted a 10-dB correction factor for AC ABRs at 500 Hz in 2015.

na: not available.

--symbol: not available.

†Normal AC ASSR level and eHL correction factors—preliminary and conservative (corrections for BC-ASSR stimuli not yet available).

ing Program (BCEHP)[56]. The infant generally is tested under natural sleep, an aspect of patient management and testing considered in-depth in the upcoming episode. Initiation of the protocol starts with ABR testing using AC stimuli at normal-hearing levels in infants (2000 Hz at 30 dB nHL first in each ear), then switches to BC-ABR testing if responses are not clearly present at these levels. Stimuli are not usually presented below the normal levels—that is, no worse than 25 dB eHL for each frequency—to save testing time. When responses are found to be elevated above normal levels, AC threshold searches are then conducted across frequencies (500 Hz, 1000 Hz, 2000 Hz, and 4000 Hz), as time allows in the first appointment. The idea is to determine whether or not the AC threshold elevation, when present, is conductive (transient type is initially inferred but of course permanent conductive loss is possible) versus a primarily sensory loss. The management of these potential outcomes could be very different. The rationale for determining hearing-loss type before thresholds are established is that infant sleep time is unpredictable. If only elevated AC thresholds are obtained before the infant wakes up, management cannot begin and the parent/guardian does not know if the hearing elevation is permanent or temporary. Even if tympanometry reveals fluid in the middle-ear space, the true degree and type of hearing loss is not known.

For example, consider an infant with Down syndrome who has AC-ABR thresholds of 55 dB nHL to 65 dB nHL and flat tympanograms, but BC-ABR testing was not conducted. This is a real-case scenario from past clinical experience. Question: At that juncture, could a conductive hearing loss be assumed? The audiologist involved essentially assumed that the AC elevation resulted solely from the fluid; an otolaryngologist subsequently surgically inserted ventilating tubes. The infant was reassessed with ventilating tubes in place; unfortunately, AC thresholds did not improve. BC testing was then conducted and found to match the AC thresholds, confirming that this child, in fact, had a permanent moderate-sensorineural hearing loss. This example stresses the importance of having BC information early in the assessment process to avoid misidentifying the type of hearing loss and potentially leading to delays in appropriate intervention (hearing aids in this case) and/or perhaps averting unnecessary procedures.

The next question is, what are some *infant-friendly adaptions for conducting BC testing*? Adaptations to standard BC behavioral audiometric methods are needed for testing BC ABRs, as indeed some infant-specific issues arise. More testing time is required to conduct BC-ABR and ASSR threshold estimation in sleeping infants compared to assessing an adult using behavioral methods. This leads to potential discomfort due to the bone vibrator pressing on the skin for an extended period of time. Two methods can be used successfully to keep the bone vibrator in place for testing—*elastic headband* with sufficient tension applied or securing it *hand-held* with sufficient force—namely either instead of attempting to use a conventional bone-vibrator headband).[45] Some audiologists have reported that the handheld method is preferred to avoid waking the infant. Ideally, the vibrator is held by an assistant to optimize the ergonomics for the audiologist operating the ABR system. In any event, the parent/caregiver should never be asked to hold the bone vibrator.

Another issue, also related to infant comfort to optimize sleep time, is whether or not to remove earphones when switching between AC and BC testing, as needed for the testing protocol. Of course, covering the ears brings up the issue of the *occlusion effect,* which is taken into account when establishing adult thresholds. Interestingly, maturational differences in the occlusion effect have been noted. Despite greater increases in sound pressure level in the occluded ear canal in infants 0 to 10 months of age compared to adults, occluded BC threshold in young infants do not differ significantly from nonoccluded thresholds.[17] As a result, it is appropriate to leave earphones in place throughout testing in young infants which greatly reduces the chance of disturbing and waking the infant before testing has been completed. For older infants, it is recommended that earphones be removed (as for testing older children and adults) because the occlusion effect emerges toward the end of the first year of life.[57]

Another difference from standard pure-tone BC audiometry in adults is the selection of *position on the head*. For adults, calibration standards for BC stimuli are presented across frequency for

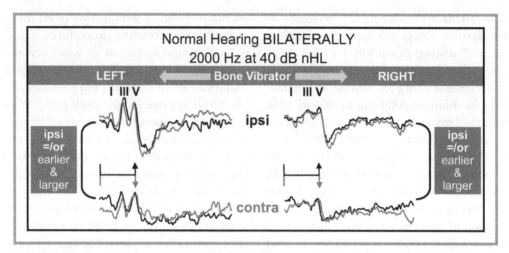

Figure 9–7. BC-ABR results typical of infants with normal hearing bilaterally: two-channel recordings with bone-conducted stimuli delivered to the left and right mastoid as indicated. Ipsilateral/contralateral (ipsi/contra) asymmetries reveal the expected pattern for normal cochleae in infants 1 to 2 years of age or conductive hearing loss (such as aural atresia). Response amplitudes are smaller and latencies are equal or later in the recording channel contralateral to the test cochlea.

two positions, the middle of the forehead and the mastoid. Infant threshold estimations via BC-ASSR-ERA have been examined across frequency as a function of different positions of the bone vibrator to determine optimal positioning on the smaller infant skull.[45] Compared were results of placements high (slightly superior and posterior to the top of the pinna) and low on the temporal bone (low mastoid) versus forehead. It was found that the positions that resulted in the largest range of usable stimulus levels (recalling inherent limits of BC versus AC audiometry) were the high temporal bone and mastoid placements. Practically speaking, it is easier to maintain a constant pressure on the flatter, high temporal bone and is preferred by clinicians. The forehead is attractive for firm vibrator placement too. However, the sensitivity is much less than that observed with vibrator placements on the high temporal bone or mastoid, in fact, by 12 dB to 18 dB on average. From these findings, forehead placement is not recommended.

Bone-conduction testing in infants reveals a curious yet quite useful *asymmetry of crossover stimulation*, as illustrated in Figure 9–7. It is well known from standard behavioral audiometry techniques used to assess adults that there is substantial crossover for BC stimulation due to minimal transcranial or *interaural attenuation (IA)*. IA in adults has traditionally been reported to be approximately 0 dB to 10 dB.[58] However, adult IA estimates were recently updated as follows: 0 dB to 10 dB at 500 Hz to 2000 Hz and 10 dB to 17 dB for frequencies greater than 3000 Hz.[59,60] For bone conduction in adults, clinical masking of the cochlea contralateral to the test ear is often required to isolate the cochlea under scrutiny in BC testing because of these low IA values. Although clinical masking is still required in some infants, isolation of the test ear without masking can often be achieved by comparing the pattern of results for two-channel BC recordings (discussed in the following text). However, clinical use of similar principles for BC-ASSRs is not as common because this has not been thoroughly investigated in infants with hearing loss.

The pattern for BC-ABR testing in question for normal-hearing infants or infants with normal BC-sensorineural hearing (for instance, in a case of aural atresia) results in wave V amplitudes and latencies that are equal to or earlier and/or larger in the response ipsilateral to the BC stimuli (the nominal "test cochlea"), compared to the response recorded contralateral to the bone vibrator (the "nontest cochlea"). As seen in Figure 9–7, when the

BC stimulus is delivered to the left mastoid, wave V is smaller (and could also be later) in the response recorded by the contralateral channel. This pattern reversed when the BC stimulus is delivered to the right mastoid in the bilaterally normal-hearing case. These predictable ipsilateral/contralateral asymmetries between sides for two-channel BC-ABR recordings determine which cochlea is actually responding to the stimulus.[61,62]

When the opposite pattern is observed (contralateral ABR greater and/or earlier compared to ipsilateral ABR), as in Figure 9–8, then the nontest cochlea is contributing more to the response than the test cochlea and a sensory loss is inferred.[63,64] Masking of the nontest ear is then necessary to establish the test-ear ABR threshold. Masking is also appropriate if the ipsi-contra waveform comparison is equivocal. Although reasonably well tested in infants with conductive loss,[38,64] the ipsilateral/contralateral comparison technique has not been as extensively investigated in infants with sensory or mixed loss. Nevertheless, this methodology is used routinely in large infant EDHI programs with reasonable group results.[65] As an aside, infant ABR wave V ipsilateral/contralateral asymmetries are also useful for recording responses to high-level air-conduction stimuli when a significant difference in the degree of hearing loss between ears is suspected. Use of ipsilateral/contralateral asymmetries to predict which cochlea is responding is quite efficient compared to masking procedures, which are more time consuming. For testing sleeping infants, efficient testing methods are paramount due to limited and somewhat unpredictable testing time available. As discussed later in this episode, there are circumstances that dictate the use of masking noise to isolate the test cochlea in infants; however, unlike adult behavioral masking procedures, infant masking procedures suitable for auditory brainstem testing are still under development.

As mentioned earlier, ipsilateral/contralateral asymmetries and their potential clinical application have not been studied as extensively for BC-ASSRs. However, a few studies have shown that two-channel EEG recordings of infant brainstem

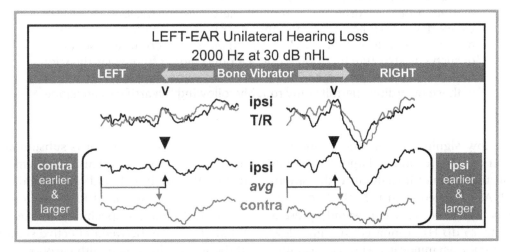

Figure 9–8. Results from an infant with unilateral, sensorineural hearing loss: two-channel EEG recordings for a BC stimulus delivered to the left and right mastoid as indicated (for simplicity, replications shown only for ipsilateral responses to characterize the stability of the recordings overall). Ipsilateral/contralateral (ipsi/contra) asymmetries reveal the expected pattern (see text) for a normal cochlea when the vibrator was positioned on the right mastoid. However, when the bone vibrator was on the left mastoid in this case, wave V is larger and earlier in the contralateral channel. This infant had normal hearing in the right ear but a profound loss in the left ear. Therefore, this is also an example in which the nominally left-ear results were attributable entirely to crossover and demonstrate the importance of effective masking in the comprehensive ABR evaluation.

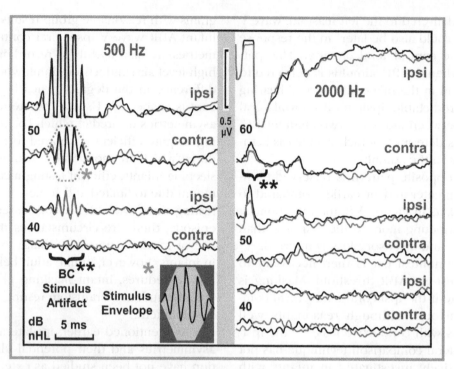

Figure 9–9. BC-ABR in an infant demonstrating elevated visual detection levels at 500 Hz and 2000 Hz, as well as the substantial stimulus artifacts,** especially at the higher stimulus levels (namely, approaching the output limits of the bone vibrator itself). Inset: Time history* of the artifact plotted in the backdrop (*gray area*) of the stimulus envelope at 500 Hz, where details can be see seen in the recordings at 40 dB nHL and 50 dB nHL. Temporal resolution of the recording does not permit representation of such fine structure for 2000 Hz. At a 4 times higher frequency, the stimulus is that much shorter, and the resolution for the sampling rate reused in these recordings permits only roughly following the artifact's envelope.

ASSRs also show significant ipsilateral/contralateral asymmetries, with responses larger and earlier in latency in the channel ipsilateral to the stimulated ear.[43,66] As expected from BC ABR findings,[64] ASSR asymmetries were most consistently present at 20 dB HL to 25 dB HL compared to higher levels. For BC-ASSRs, asymmetries were consistently present only at 500 Hz and 4000 Hz but not at 1000 Hz and 2000 Hz.[28] In contrast, published ABR findings show consistent asymmetries at 500 Hz and 2000 Hz.[66] Further research is needed in infants with asymmetrical or unilateral hearing loss to determine how well ipsilateral and contralateral BC-ASSR recordings determine the cochlea that is responding to the BC stimulus.

It was demonstrated in Figure 6–7B that the stimulus artifact (due to electromagnetic radiation) from a bone vibrator is substantially greater than that of earphones. This may seem like a scary technical issue but should not intimidate the clinician for BC testing of ABRs. First, tone bursts of sufficient frequency specificity are routinely used. While less delay between effective stimulus arrival at the test cochlea than with earphones (especially the tubal insert type), at least the overall delay of the combined electromechanical and cochlear and neural transmission times can be expected to allow measurement of the IV/V complex, namely with little risk of contamination by stimulus artifact. This is even more so the case in young infants, thanks to maturational delays, as illustrated in Figure 9–9. If hearing loss is not too severe, the artifact often is barely evident at lower stimulus levels tested. Furthermore, the artifact pickup by the contralateral recording channel is far less; the electrode on the opposite mastoid from the placement of the bone vibrator is at a greater distance. Artifact also can be scary to sort through while recording ABRs due to possible added effects of nonlinearities that come to play on the net average. Shown in the inset is the envelope of the stimulus (recall Figure 2–12). A sample of the artifact under the 500-Hz condition is overlaid, illustrating that the electrical pickup indeed is mimicking the input stimulus to the bone vibrator. However, the net average shows distortion attributable in part to nonlinear circuit components of the amplifier which is being driven to saturation; hence, it is not averaged out even if using alternating stimulus polarity. The time resolution in these recordings is less capable to represent the fine-structure of the 2000 Hz (compared to 500 Hz), but still registers the nonlinear component (comparable to envelop following; recall Episode 6.2). The inflation of the stimulus artifact overall going from AC to BC also is about the substantially larger (by about 40 dB) input signal to drive the bone vibrator rather than an earphone at the same dB nHL. Lastly, all electromechanical transducers have limits, becoming progressively nonlinear themselves when pushed to their limits (as reflected by the different audiometric limits of AC and BC calibrations on the audiometer's HL dial).

Multiple factors contribute to asymmetry effects and greater infant sensitivity. **Infants have unique characteristics** that examiners can use to evaluate their BC hearing using brainstem auditory evoked potentials. One characteristic is the structure of the skull and overlying tissues. The infant skull comprises multiple bony plates that are joined by fibrous joints or sutures to ensure even, symmetrical growth until the plates are fused together by ossification in early adulthood.[67,68] The softer connective tissue of the sutures of the infant skull results in the temporal bone oscillating in a more isolated manner compared to adults who have a fully fused skull. The soft issue in the infant skulls reduces the dissipation of BC energy to the other bony plates. As a consequence, a more intense signal is delivered to the ipsilateral cochlea.[38,69–72] As infants mature, the thickness and density of collagen and elastin increase[73] and the infant skull also increases in circumference. In addition to the obvious anatomical and structural differences in the skull and overlying tissues, systematic changes result in differences in the mechanical impedance of the immature skull from early infancy to 7 years of age. This likely contributes to the infant-adult differences in sensitivity to BC stimuli,[74] bearing in mind that the artificial mastoid used to calibrate bone vibrators was modeled and built via research and development based on the adult skull and auditory system.

These factors not only potentially contribute to infant-adult differences in BC sensitivity but also likely explain the greater IA values for infants, which have been estimated, using indirect measures, to be approximately 10 dB to 35 dB in the first year of life, as shown in Table 9–5. The greatest IAs are reported for neonates[75] and infants 0 to 6 months of age.[72] The fontanelles are also a source of dissipated sound energy, leading to an

Table 9–5. Indirect Measures of Interaural Attenuation (dB) for Bone-Conducted Stimuli for Infants (in Bold Print) and Adults Using ABR and ASSR Measures.

Study	Method	Indirect Measure	Age	Interaural Attenuation (dB)
Yang and associates (1987)[75]	ABR—clicks	Wave V Latency	Adult **Neonate** **12 months**	0–10 **25–35** **15–25**
Small and Stapells (2008)[72]	ASSR—AM/FM; 500–1000 Hz F_c	Ipsi/contra asymmetries	Adult **0–6 months**	0–10 **10–30**
Hansen and Small (2012)[80]	ASSR—AM/FM; 1000 Hz F_c	Effective masking levels (binaural AC)	Adult **0–7 months**	0 **10–15**

observable increase in IA when compared to adults.[76] Another factor which is also believed to contribute to infant-adult differences in two-channel ABR recordings is the developmental changes in the auditory brainstem, including the dipole orientation of the neurogenerators of the ABR.[61,77,78] Estimation of BC IA using sound pressure in the ear canal in infants and adults, rather than direct estimation in individuals with profound unilateral hearing loss, has been proposed as an easier way to estimate IA. However, the results are not as promising as expected. First, significant differences occurred at 500 Hz, 750 Hz, 2000 Hz, and 3000 Hz for sound pressure estimates compared to direct measures in profound cases of unilateral hearing loss.[60] Second, for young children (0–2 years), IA was greater compared to adults but less than expected compared to other indirect estimates.[74] Taken together, these findings support the conclusion that accurate estimates of BC IA still are needed for infants, similar to the foundational research for adults, by direct estimation in individuals with unilateral profound hearing loss or potentially a different method ultimately proven to yield as accurate results.

The perspective from classical pure-tone audiometry suggests another important question: Are **clinical masking procedures in infants** the same as in older children and adults? When significant asymmetries in BC thresholds exist between ears in infants, or when ipsilateral/contralateral asymmetries in the ABR are inconclusive, clinical masking of the nontest cochlea is needed to accurately determine BC thresholds specific to each cochlea. Some examples of inconclusive ipsilateral/contralateral ABR comparisons that would require masking are as follows: (i) wave V latencies and amplitudes are too similar between channels so that the cochlea responding cannot be determined with certainty; (ii) AC-ABR thresholds may be within normal limits but the contralateral ear has better thresholds, so the contralateral wave V is larger than the ipsilateral response and the BC thresholds for the test cochlea are not clear; and (iii) alternatively, BC-ABR thresholds are significantly elevated in both ears so the test cochlea is difficult to identify as the stimulus is crossing over and stimulating both cochleae.

Appropriate BC masking levels for auditory brainstem response testing methods have been formally investigated recently given that **effective masking levels (EMLs)** for conventional behavioral pure-tone audiometry are well established and have been in use for approximately 60 years.[79] Comparisons of EMLs for BC stimuli measured directly in infants were initially investigated using BC-ASSRs[47,80] then BC-ABRs.[81] Direct measures of EMLs in infants are critical for the development of efficient masking procedures appropriate for clinical use.

Estimation of EMLs for BC ASSRs (single AM/FM stimuli) and ABRs in normal-hearing infants and adults first required binaural masking noise to ensure that responses from both the test and nontest ear were eliminated. With binaural narrowband noise presented using insert earphones, EMLs for BC-ASSRs elicited by 500-Hz to 4000-Hz stimuli at 35 dB HL, were as follows: (i) infants: 81 dB, 68 dB, 59 dB, and 45 dB SPL; (ii) adults: 66 dB, 63 dB, 59 dB, and 55 dB SPL. Maturational differences in BC-EMLs are evident. Higher masking levels are required for infants compared to adults for low frequencies; 15 dB and 5 dB more masking for infants at 500 Hz and 1000 Hz, respectively. As frequency increases, the pattern changes; infants require the same amount of masking at 2000 Hz as adults but actually need 10 dB less masking at 4000 Hz.[47,80] It should be noted that it may be difficult to completely and safely mask responses from both cochleae using binaural masking at 500 Hz for stimuli that exceed 35 dB HL due to the much greater masker levels needed at this frequency compared to higher frequencies.

The EMLs for BC-ABR testing that have become available recently were determined with white-noise masking to simulate what would be typically available in clinical ABR systems. The masking pattern for BC-ABRs is similar to previously reported BC-ASSR EMLs. For infants, BC-ABRs elicited by 500-Hz and 2000-Hz stimuli presented at normal levels, 20 dB and 30 dB nHL, respectively; EMLs (binaural masking) are 82 dB and 72 dB SPL, respectively. In contrast, for the same stimulus levels in adults, EMLs are 72 dB SPL at both frequencies. In summary, for BC-ABRs, a comparison of infant and adult results shows that 10 dB more masking is required for 500 Hz for infants but the same amount of masking is needed in both age groups for 2000 Hz. It is important to note that it is also not possible to mask out BC-ABRs using a maximum binaural masking level of 80 dB SPL at 500 Hz for infants. Again, this sound level limits effective masking of BC-ASSRs to relatively low stimulus levels.[81]

Based on these findings and assuming a minimum amount of BC IA of 10 dB for the stimulus presented to the infant test ear, monaural masking levels for the nontest ear can be determined. The following monaural white-noise masking levels are recommended clinically for BC-ABR testing (B71 bone vibrator): 72 dB and 82 dB for 500 Hz at 20 dB and 30 dB nHL, respectively; 62 dB, 72 dB, and 82 dB SPL for 2000 Hz at 30 dB, 40 dB nHL, and 50 dB nHL, respectively.[81] It is also worth reminding that a BC vibrator has a much more limited range of possible stimulus levels due to distortion resulting from nonlinearity of the output compared to air-conduction transducers. For stimuli, the maximum testing levels are 51 dB for 500 Hz and 63 dB nHL for 2000 Hz. For BC-ASSRs, the following narrowband noise masker levels are recommended: 71 dB and 81 dB SPL for 500 Hz at 35 dB and 45 dB HL, respectively; 58 dB, 68 dB, and 78 dB SPL for 35 dB, 45 dB, and 55 dB HL at 1000 Hz, respectively; 49 dB, 59 dB, 69 dB, and 79 dB SPL for 35 dB, 45 dB, 55 dB, and 65 dB HL at 2000 Hz, respectively; 45 dB, 55 dB, 65 dB, and 75 dB SPL for 35 dB, 45 dB, 55 dB, and 65 dB HL at 4000 Hz, respectively.[47,80] The maximum testing levels are 60 dB HL for 500 Hz to 4000 Hz for single BC-ASSRs and 50 dB HL for multiple BC-ASSRs to avoid nonlinearity in the signal. Further research is needed to confirm accuracy of isolating the test ear in infants with hearing loss before applying these recommended EMLs clinically.

Recall Episode 6.3 for improving test efficiency via ASSR testing; a natural query arises: Are **multiple ASSRs** in fact more efficient than single-ASSR tests? As noted and certainly with strong face validity, this question is an important procedural factor, especially for assessing infants when the amount of testing time is never guaranteed. Results of ASSR studies in adults showed that ASSR amplitudes are not significantly reduced when multiple versus single stimuli are presented until presentation levels exceed 60 dB SPL[82,83] or when carrier frequencies are at least one octave apart for either adults with normal hearing or hearing loss.[84] In principle then, less testing time is needed compared to a single-stimulus presentation. In contrast, infants show interactions, demonstrated by amplitude reductions, at 60 dB SPL for the multiple ASSR technique. However, in terms of efficiency defined as more thresholds estimated in less time and even with smaller amplitudes, the multiple-ASSR technique outpaces the single-ASSR method.[85,86] Nevertheless, efficiency will vary with the ASSR-stimulus type; the broader the stimulus spectra, the less efficient the stimulus is due to interactions,[84,87] perhaps even more so in infants than in adults. One strategy to optimize testing time is to use multiple simultaneous stimuli at lower-to-mid stimulus levels then switch to single frequencies when greater presentation levels are needed.

What about **recording AC- and BC-ASSRs at the same time**, taking further advantage of coding of the carrier frequency and/or test mode (such as two ears at the same time, as previously discussed)? Results of a recent study recording ASSRs in two ears simultaneously to AC and BC stimuli demonstrated that this novel approach could potentially shorten testing time for infants.[88] ASSR amplitudes were compared when AC and BC stimuli were presented at 2000 Hz and 500 Hz, respectively, in young infants; AC and BC were either presented simultaneously or for one mode only. No significant reductions in amplitude were reported when the simultaneous AC/BC conditions were compared to either mode alone. These preliminary findings support that assessing AC and BC thresholds simultaneously may be clinically feasible.

In summary, what is the state of the science for BC threshold estimation in infants today? Currently, accurate methods for estimation of BC hearing in infants are in daily use. However, there is room for many improvements of conventional methods for this population. As discussed in this episode, there indeed are some gaps in our understanding of BC hearing in infants which, for the most part, is not the case for adults. The BC-ABR test is currently the most studied and applied method to estimate BC hearing sensitivity in infants. To echo a key comparison of methods in Episode 6.3, the subjectivity of interpreting of ABR waveforms is documented to be difficult for clinicians who do not routinely test infants (either for AC or/more so BC threshold estimations). This has certainly been the experience in the provincial EHDI program. BC-ASSRs still have potential as a more objective, straightforward clinical tool. Yet, more data are needed, particularly for BC testing, to embrace fully this method as a replacement for the more established BC-ABR technique.

Episode 3: Testing Patients Under Natural Sleep or Medically Induced Sedation/Unconsciousness

This episode further explores the combination of factors of the test environment and subject state as well as patient management when it comes to evaluations of ABRs/ASSRs in uncooperative patients, particularly the very young. Audiology clinics often are well appointed and have the necessary tranquility and controlled environments to conduct testing in near-ideal patient states. However, this is just a part of the real world of AEP evaluations that derive from a diverse clinical population. The emphasis here primarily will be on testing infants and young children, but in general principles that also are more broadly applicable. Overall then, this episode pertains to those patients who intellectually and/or behaviorally cannot be expected to participate effectively in conventional audiological assessments that require at least "trainable" voluntary response—as in visual reinforcement audiometry—or even to remain adequately sedate for objective tests—as in clinical electrophysiology. Relaxation and remaining adequately quiet are also voluntary issues, and the subject's willingness or ability to do so will naturally impact one of the major factors for AEP recordings of adequate quality (recall Figures 4–2 and 4–3). In those patients who cannot "cooperate" at least in this respect, whatever the reasons, they are considered "difficult-to-test" and present particular challenges as to how best to evaluate them. They frequently present the double jeopardy of being incapable both of cooperation and understanding what is happening, starting indeed with the young child.

This nominal level of cooperation, as touched upon in the last episode in the context of working in newborn nurseries, suggested frequently taking advantage of **natural sleep**. In the broader scheme of patient management, the difficult-to-test patient may require **sedation/anesthesia**. This again is the importance of the ABR/80-Hz ASSR not being sensitive to the patient's state of arousal. The largest percentage of patients who undergo ABR/80-Hz ASSR evaluations are infants and young children for this very reason, perhaps begging the question, is not insensitivity to state of arousal enough? Actually, no. Muscle contraction by the patient is typically the largest source of artifacts encountered during evoked response testing. EMG "noise" (recall Figure 4–14) often involves large potentials interfering with the desired response by degrading or obliterating the averaged signal of the response itself, especially when testing at the lower stimulus levels. Filtering and artifact rejection helps, but constant adjustment can make the acquisition inefficient, if not flatly unsuccessful for any reliable measure, and can bring the examination to a hasty halt. Young children do not and cannot understand the concept of relaxation. Even older children who are cooperative often hear "relax" and try not to move during the test, yet end up seemingly contracting every muscle in their body. While they then may not move, they still are creating even larger sources of noise than before being asked to relax. Nevertheless, for the more cooperative children, having them watch a favored video can be useful. (Note: The sound typically is turned off; video, especially if captioned, needs to be projected/played on a relatively small screen to minimize eye-movement artifact.) This approach was mentioned in the last chapter for testing AEPs requiring the patient to be alert during testing of longer-latency AEPs. It thus is possible for the patient to sufficiently focus on the video as to remain adequately sedate for successful completion of the test. Technology also has developed further that is useful for patients who are awake and have some involuntary muscular noise. Nevertheless, for the youngest children, sleep remains the easiest way to complete tests of the brainstem responses.

Newborns are one of the first and most demanding groups overall for consummating complete assessments, sometimes requiring more than one visit to the clinic, and initial testing (hearing screening, as presented in the first episode of this

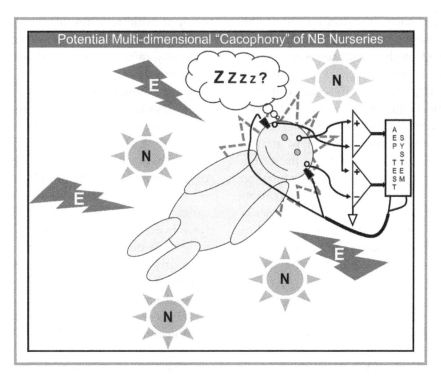

Figure 9–10. The challenges for recording good auditory evoked responses in the environment of well-baby and neonatal intensive care nurseries, another world from acoustically and electrically isolated test booths often used in audiology clinics (see text).

chapter), will not even be conducted in the audiology clinic. Furthermore, newborns, older children, and other difficult-to-test patients often are evaluated in nurseries or outpatient clinical settings, including same-day surgical units, should the need to know and case be difficult enough to warrant testing under a general anesthesia. Alternatively, in cases having to be operated, it is possible that they might best be served by scheduling testing in the operating (OR) or recovery room before waking the patient up. Testing in these environments will demand that the examiner have not only competent knowledge and well-honed skills of good practices of evoked response measurement but also knowledge beyond regarding orchestration of the necessary support service(s) and knowledge of related medical practices. This is to ensure due consideration for the patient's safety.

The newborn also is featured in such discussion as they are special because of demands to meet follow-up milestones, as presented in Episode 9.1. Expediency of initiation of intervention is of paramount importance. Figure 9–10 is a cartoon to remind the reader of some of the challenges to quality of AEP recordings with further emphasis on factors more prevalent in environments like newborn nurseries. Between the patient's own state and essential personnel working in the environment, there will be multiple sources of potential acoustic noise (N) bouncing off strongly reflective surfaces and/or electro-magnetic/electro-static noise (E) from various electrical instruments/sources, perhaps the AEP test system itself. Both the environments of well-baby and NICU nurseries place effective AEP testing at additional risk for interference (in comparison to acoustically and electrically shielded test booths, often available in audiology clinics). As discussed earlier, subject state indeed is an important variable, such as whether or not the baby is sleeping (Z) and/or substantially moving, especially the head (represented by the zig-zag pattern about Baby Doe's head).

Ways were presented earlier by which some of these issues are addressable, up-front and/or in posttest processing, such as artifact rejection, filtering, and weighted averaging. In general, the signal-processing tools of modern AEP test systems do a fairly good job at limiting adverse effects of noise. For instance, 60 Hz/50 Hz interference from powerlines/mains and neighboring equipment can be effectively treated with a notch filter. Alternatively, electrical interference from equipment may be reduced adequately simply by moving the offending equipment as far away as possible or turning it off for the test duration. Finally, filtering recordings can be accomplished digitally by the test system's computer in endeavoring to reduce offending/interfering signals (whatever the source), especially if only partially overlapping the spectrum of the targeted response.

Earplug and earcap types of couplers of the transducer to the ear can help to reduce environmental, acoustical noise to minimize masking effects (Figure 9–11). Tubal insert earphones, as broadly popular for a wide range of AEP measurements and their audiological applications, can be used, given tips "miniaturized" for baby ears (panel A, insert) or an ear-cap type of coupler (panel B). At face value, the earcap type appears to be applicable with the least agitation of the baby, but the infant tubal inserts also can be used without difficulty, with practice and patience. The tubing and insert are supple, so as to be easily inserted and to not cause discomfort. Noise levels of nurseries always have been of concern for the well-being of newborns. Results of studies have documented the high levels of noise exposure to infants in these environments as well as the adverse effects of noise on behavioral and physiological responses of infants.[89,90] Noise reduction techniques such as quiet times and specialized earmuffs (panel C) also have been tried with positive outcomes.[91,92]

While electrical noise certainly can play havoc with any AEP tests, being some of the smallest-amplitude potentials, the transient-ABR/80-Hz ASSR are particularly susceptible to false identification of waves and/or misinterpretation of recordings, as demonstrated by Figure 9–12. Welcome once more to the "Game of Waves"—final edition. The objective this time is not about finding the VDL, rather a game of judging a response component wave and/or its apparent consistency for a given trial, even with knowledge of exactly what the true response looks like—same models employed throughout

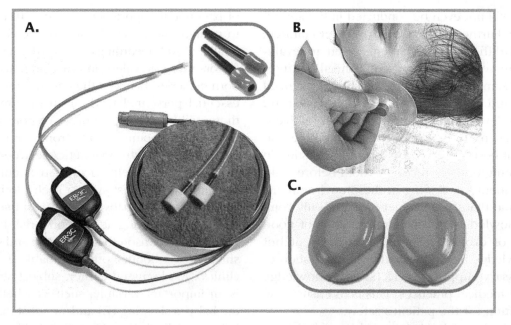

Figure 9–11. A. Tubal-insert type earphones and (inset) ear tips for newborns/young infants. **B.** Earcap type coupler (adaptation of circumaural, rather than supra-aural earphone cushions). **C.** Earmuff type ear defenders for newborns, for more "peace and quiet" in the nursery.

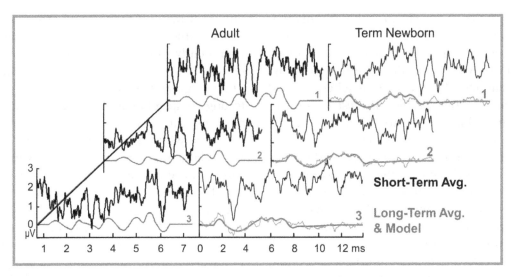

Figure 9–12. Brainstem response in noise simulations in examples of relatively shorter- versus longer-term averages and comparing term-newborn-like (immature) responses with adultlike (mature) responses (see text). For the term-newborn simulation, several test–retest trials also are simulated for relatively longer-term (higher-N) averages, directly overlaid on the model signal for closer scrutiny.

the simulation and simply reseeding the random-numbers generator of the background noise for each trial—statistically the same but fine structure randomized. "Piece of cake?" Look closely. For instance, in the adult sequence, trial 1—how convincing is the presumptive ABR-wave complex, even given the noise-free waveform for reference? If judged to be reasonably good, what about the other peaks of the undulating, residual noise floor of the average? Render judgments similarly for trial 2 in the term-newborn sequence, pending the judgement for the "bumps" in the recording. Feel free to play comparable rounds for all three trials. Lastly, supposing the short-term averages were as good recordings as permitted by time and/or state of the patient, how much and/or for which waves do test–retest comparisons give adequate confidence to render a verdict of a valid response?

Bottom line: One of the greatest dangers of residual noise in the recording is that it can look like a response, even having the right polarity and latencies as a (potentially) real response. This is especially true when a purely subjective analysis is applied. However, this also can trip up results for computer algorithms applied, but at least rule-based decisions have just that for consistent reference—just what rules actually were applied in the interpretation, whether or not the examiner concurs (for whatever reasons and/or extenuating circumstances prevailing in a given trial/test). Reasons that noise can look like a response may be that there was insufficient number of sweeps collected and/or the noise in the recording had prominent peak(s) that serendipitously (unfortunately) fell within the time window of the recording and that mimicked the actual response features. The latter can occur by way of substantially overlapping spectra of the interference and a real response. The spectrum of the background noise (as recorded and regardless of its own spectrum) naturally has a bias toward that of the response, due to front-end band-pass filtering. Any nonstationarity in the noise (recall Episode 4.1) will make the appearance of false responses more likely, such as EMG interference inherent to incidental swallowing. EMG-based artifacts, indeed, are notorious interference and often have wavelike characteristics in their fine structure (rather than truly random noise). Subsequently, there rarely is enough time for such artifacts to be "averaged out" over the number of sweeps available for computing the average response, in practice.

The responses again were models, such as in Figure 6–8 for the adult, in turn adapted per trends of changes in waveform with early maturation, as illustrated in Figure 6–9. The adult model reasonably approximates the 3-year-old's model. As noted in previous episodes, maturation of the ABR (per latency of wave V) is reached around 2 years of age.[93] However, the ABR test in younger children—including newborns at term or earlier (premature being <42 months gestational age)—adds different response morphology to the challenge,[94] hence including in the demonstration a model resembling more that of the full-term newborn versus the now-familiar adult response. Why not actual recordings for this demonstration? The computer-modeled responses make the overall outcome perfectly predictable in principle, permitting demonstration of the effects of noise alone for both shorter-term—such as what pops up on the monitor soon after acquisition has started—versus longer-term averages, as might be accepted finally as a truly reliable ABR recording (recall Figures 4–11 and 6–1). How realistic is the demonstration? While the virtual recordings can be repeated over and over, this certainly is not a "luxury" of real-world testing. Still, the underlying approach to the noise—random-number generation being reseeded per trial—is something (in effect) that is inevitable in test–retests of human subjects. At the same time, demonstrated were responses that, with enough averaging, illustrated that reasonably good approximations to the known/model responses can be realized. The perfectly repeated signal, naturally, is not realistic, although generally consistent with the notion that the AEP signal is stationary and/or noise free enough as to not compromise SNR improvement from increased numbers of repetitions/trials (recall Figures 4–5 and 4–13B). Yet, life on the frontline of service can and likely will present cases of just too much noise and/or not enough time. Experience then helps the clinician not to be "taken in" readily by spurious bumps in the recording.

For example, the examiner must consider that if a certain "bump" at X ms is to be believed, what does that say about one or more bumps of similar magnitude and morphology before and/or after the presumed response? This likely will include peaks of potentials with apparent latencies at which true-response components are likely not even possible, pending both test parameters and known effects of maturation/age and other nonpathological variables. Working with very young children over a fairly short and dynamically changing period of life clearly demands of the examiner detailed knowledge and plenty of experience to carry out testing competently and to interpret the data of the recordings accurately.

Even with replication of responses, noise that is fundamentally random for a given epoch has some chance to seem repeatable. This theoretically could be worse in some patients who, in fact, have hearing loss. This especially is possible if the test stimulus is effectively low-level for the response, recalling that low-level ABRs (for example) tend to have waveforms appearing as merely a singular "lump" above the noise floor (recall Figures 6–5A and 9–5B). Here is where age-specific confidence limits of latencies become particularly important for recognizing true responses, as a cross-check that the assumed response's latency and changes thereof (across stimulus level) make sense as a true response. Another possible mitigating issue may be (as implied earlier) the inexperience of the examiner. Fortunately, many EP test instruments on the market now provide estimates of SNR to aid the examiner in appraising the quality of the overall recording and the presumptive response.

ASSR test instruments provide statistically based scoring of responses (recall Episodes 4.1 and 6.3). As a reminder, these methods may substantially reduce issues of subjectivity of the examiner and bias of inexperience. However, a machine is a machine. It is only as good as the algorithms in the software of the test program as well as the examiner having met conditions delimiting reliability of the test(s) applied (appropriate subject preparation and test protocol). In any event, the human operator is the responsible party and must be prepared to troubleshoot any results that seem incoherent, noisier, or bespeaking other conditions that may seem unusual or event(s) raising suspicion that the instrument may not be working normally.

However, the "big picture" is framed well beyond these technical matters of the electrophysiological test itself, hence dedication of the remainder of this episode to still broader issues particular to such testing. In the test population and environment under consideration, not only examiner competency but also efficiency is extremely important. Unnecessary retesting may be costly in time—or worse, cost more time and create circumstances still leading to unreliable results. If testing during a period of **natural sleep**, for example, it is difficult to count on a set amount of time. If sleep has to be induced medically—through the use of sedation (at narcotic/sleep-inducing doses) or anesthetics—there is both limits of time for the drug used to "wear off" as well as the anesthesiologist's concern for keeping any patient "under" for any longer than absolutely necessary.

The typical minimal age in most clinics for the use of sedation is around 6 months. There may be circumstances when an infant younger than 6 months is given sedation or is tested under anesthesia. This typically occurs when there have been unsuccessful attempts at testing during natural sleep, yet with only partial results suggestive of the presence of elevated response levels, in turn indicating further testing needed with the patient in a more controlled state. Sometimes sedation will be used, but there again may be times that the child is scheduled for a procedure in the OR. It is advantageous for the patient and their family to examine ABRs/other evoked responses during other procedures scheduled in the OR, as it lessens the number of times the child will need anesthesia or sedation. This is true not only for the young child but also for older children who have complex medical needs and/or cognitive and physical problems that prevent getting reliable information from them through behavioral testing. Examples of other procedures that require patients to be sedated or anesthetized are endoscopies, bilateral myringotomy with ventilation tubes, other medical examinations (like MRI), and even dental procedures. It behooves the audiologist to make contact and stay in good standing with other departments and physicians to accomplish the coordination of services. As an aside, what needs to be remembered by those performing the testing is that when evoked response tests are carried out in the OR/another inpatient service, it takes away from the other services' time. Therefore, sensitivity to this and efficiency while conducting the ABR test is again of the utmost importance.

At one time, sedation for children more than 6 months of age was routinely done in outpatient clinic settings, doctor's offices, or within hospitals, yet with little medical oversight. There was almost a lackadaisical approach for the use of sedation. The physician wrote a prescription (typically for **chloral hydrate**), the family/caregiver or medical personnel administered the drug, and the audiologist conducted the test alone in the room with the patient and caregiver. Even if administered by medical personnel, there was no **monitoring** of the patient's status throughout the test. The level of patient monitoring changed dramatically by way of guidelines of the American Academy of Pediatrics emphasizing strict protocols for the use of sedation.[95,96] Furthermore, chloral hydrate was removed from the commercial market.[95]

The guidelines call for medical personnel to be involved to constantly monitor the child's vital statistics including pulse oximetry, thus ensuring greater safety for the patient. The particular sedations used also have changed over time and with anesthesiologists or nurse anesthetists often administering the drugs used intravenously. These procedures are mostly conducted in the "procedure" room/centers of the hospitals—thus not the OR—yet in an environment wherein the health and safety of the patient is ensured. Other details and choice/use of drugs deemed both safe and useful of evoked response testing are beyond the scope here, but further information is readily available in the literature.[97–99]

The indications for the **need for sedation** also must be defined with insight and rigor. When there is a strong suspicion of impairment, timely diagnosis is critical. To remind, the last JCIH position statement[4] continued to adhere to the 1-3-6 milestones for audiological management initiated via UNHS (in effect, minimally; recall Episode 9.1). While the guideline does not put forth strict protocols, the rationale is dictated by results of much research having shown (indeed) that early diagnosis and treatment are core to optimizing language development to age-appropriate or near age-appropriate skills. Here again, partnering with the family throughout the scheduling of follow-up evaluations can lead to best outcomes for both the family and the audiologist.

When testing patients who are sedated or are to be tested under natural sleep, the importance of good scheduling and instructions cannot be emphasized enough. It is not always intuitive to families/caregivers why they need to strictly follow the instructions. Furthermore, it is not always clear to the scheduler how important it is to be clear with such explanations so that families/caregivers know exactly what to expect on the day of the appointment. The appointment schedulers need to be well educated themselves about what is going to happen on the day of the appointment. Having them well abreast of the importance of the instructions is critical. The schedulers should be familiar with the test environment and what is going to happen during the appointment so they too can help/reinforce information requiring complete understanding by the families/caregivers. Having scheduling personnel observe a test can be very helpful to their understanding of the goals of the appointment and the information that they are to convey to caregivers. Schedulers should understand, as well, the frustration families have when the appointment does not go as planned, especially when the family needs a return visit. As most evoked response testing is on very young babies who have not passed the newborn hearing screening, this often brings much stress to the family, as many such infants are found subsequently to have hearing loss. These children often have no evident risk factors for hearing loss, the caregiver may have little to go on at the young age of the infant, so the potential hearing loss comes as a surprise. When testing cannot be completed, it thus adds another layer of stress and anxiety, as the caregiver does not have all of the answers that were presumed to be revealed by test results obtained during their child's appointment.

For testing infants during natural sleep, instructions are often given to caregivers to keep their infant awake on the way to the appointment and withhold the last feeding so that the patient arrives both hungry and sleepy. This is not an easy task for caregivers to accomplish, especially to keep an infant hungry and awake in a car and at the risk of the child being very agitated/crying upon arrival. Often, the caregivers are not told why this is important and what the rationale is. The caregivers may have received "blanket" instructions instead and without inquiry about the infant's sleep habits and feeding times. It is neither always intuitive nor obvious to caregivers what the goals of the appointment are, nor that the appointment will likely require the child to remain asleep for an hour or longer in the clinic. The assumption is that most infants readily fall asleep after feeding, hence the rationale for having the child come in hungry, then nurse/eat and fall asleep for the test. Lastly, one set of instructions likely will not fit all cases.

Questions also may not have been asked about the mode of transportation to get to the appointment: will it be public or private; will the caregiver be coming alone; will they be accompanied? To request a caregiver who is coming by car to keep an infant awake during the car ride assumes that (minimally) two people will accompany the patient to the appointment. Also at issue is how long does it take the infant to feed? Does the infant indeed fall asleep typically right after feeding? What time of day does the infant sleep the most? Families may not also understand why siblings should not come to the appointment, as is the clinical preference. Yet, there may not be options for them (like babysitting of the children remaining at home), so the caregiver may show up with (for instance) both a newborn and a toddler. The time spent initially in the scheduling process thus can save time by way of planning and making for a more pleasant experience for the entire family.

Sending written instructions to the family is common practice but not necessarily with knowledge of the caregiver's literacy. Making assumptions is easy, getting such information may not be as easy, but this is one area where gathering good information is really important. Therefore, it is necessary for the clinic to have both verbal and written instructions to get to all the facts (including possible need of a translator) and, in general, to ensure conveyance of ancillary information. This includes where caregivers should park (if driving), what entrance to use at the facility, and where to register the patient as well as in which department, unit, or clinic the patient will be seen. Thereafter, the caregiver needs to be informed of the amount of time needed for the appointment overall (not only test time itself), what they need to bring with them, who they will be seeing that day, and whether results will be given at the end of the appointment and/or to what other professional/facility results should be sent a copy of the report (such as to a referral source).

Even the most experienced clinicians can often find that they cannot test the child under natural sleep if the child is not a good sleeper. Consequently, insufficient evidence may be obtained to confirm the type and degree of hearing loss that the patient may experience. Efficiency entails not only working fast but also working smart. The evaluation must be goal oriented. The evaluation is to answer the question of why the patient is really there. Did the infant simply fail the newborn hearing screen as a false positive, or does the child truly have a clinically significant, congenital hearing loss. Either way, the patient is there now and in the clinician's care for thorough follow-up, which includes a comprehensive history. Hence the question, might that child be at risk for later onset hearing loss, such as from the effects of cytomegalovirus[100] or other medical and/or familial history? Given suggestion from the screen of possible hearing loss, this appointment also is not just another screening, thus not only more evidence that a hearing loss may exists, but actually estimating hearing thresholds across a significant frequency range of hearing (including those critical to speech detection/recognition and ultimately speech-language development).

The choice of test protocol (ABR vs. ASSR and among possible stimulus paradigms) with which to start also may vary depending on the information obtained upfront. Narrowband chirps again—low-, mid-, and/or high-frequency range stimuli—can enhance efficiency for assessing whether a hearing loss exists and roughly the configuration that it may follow. In addition as noted in the last episode, a couple of selected mid-frequency tone bursts presented at low, borderline-normal levels can help with quick decisions about next steps in the evaluation. There are still other protocols (including ASSR-based) that can lend comparable/other efficiencies. Regardless, babies only sleep for a limited time under natural sleep and there again are practical time limits for drug-based sedation, hence the "pressure" to optimize success during the test session. In general, whatever the circumstances, test times per session need to be scheduled for longer time slots than routinely required to accommodate the general patient population. The principal point is that of having a well-conceived strategy toward utmost efficiency and, if having to prematurely terminate testing, still likely yielding some useful results.

Evaluation of the young pediatric or other difficult-to-test patients while sedated presents additional challenges, namely beyond routine clinical electrophysiology. If likely efficacious to carry out the evaluation with the patient in natural sleep, it must be appreciated that sleep-on-demand (in effect) is not a given. While drug-induced sedation effectively addresses this issue, there are some risks and expenses associated with its use and more so with anesthesia. Not every clinic is equipped and/or situated for the use of sedation and the need for constant monitoring. The objective here was to give a perspective on the general scope and nature of considerations that must be made in order to attain the goals of the testing itself. The audiologist's role clearly exceeds performance/interpretation of the AEP test alone, rather at the same time being a team player in a game of "need to know." Success only can be gained with utmost cooperation of ancillary services and most critically that of the patient's caregiver(s).

HEADS UP

Testing Patients Who "Exaggerate" Their Hearing Thresholds

Much emphasis throughout the preceding chapters was on the general importance of undertaking—to the extent possible—clinical electrophysiology in persons in relatively sedate states, even if they need to be attentive to the stimulus, as may be the case for the long-/late-latency responses. Although transient-ABR and 80-Hz ASSR permit testing patients who are asleep or under drug-based sedation or anesthesia (to optimize SNR of the recorded potentials), it could be alluring to conclude that in any case for which results of conventional audiological assessment seem unreliable, when in doubt, "do an ABR" (in common clinical parlance). In many cases, testing the brainstem's response is the best choice. In this feature story, the contention will be to pause and consider other options in certain cases at both ends of the auditory pathway. It is also the opportunity to highlight another aspect of the clinical utility of tests of both otoacoustic emissions and long-latency responses—inhabitants of opposite ends of the auditory pathway. A clinical subgroup particularly in need of such open mindedness is cases of **nonorganic hearing losses**.

As fundamentally objective measures of auditory function, OAE and/or AEP measures are wholesome choices for the clinician to consider including in management of the patient whose conventional audiometric findings are suspicious of not reflecting an organic disorder. There are two broad categories of such cases, although both present the same practical problem for the clinician—the paramount need to discern the true hearing status. These cases are malingering (willfully misleading the clinician, particularly for some gain) and hysterical hearing losses (a psychologic/psychiatric issue). Individual patients may have their own reasons. One patient confessed, "I was having so much trouble with this ear, I wanted to make sure you noticed." He was found to have an acoustic neuroma. Another tried to fake normal hearing—he wanted to get into the police academy. Still another feigned substantial hearing losses; she was motivated by the desire to be perhaps more accepted by the deaf community. The why of such behavior is naturally an important part of the patient's history. The history itself may give the clinician some suspicion of nonorganic involvement from the get-go. These issues are well-known in clinical audiology. Indications of the need for supplemental testing often are present within the basic audiological evaluation— conflicting pure-tone and speech threshold estimates being a classical hallmark. Thereafter are more specialized/elaborate tests designed to demonstrate (in principle) a discordance of results, largely based on the patient's perception of loudness. It is beyond the scope here to delve into technical details, rather considering basic scenarios and underlying principles that will set the stage for another important application of objective tests.

To feign a loss of hearing by way of the conventional audiogram requires the "suspect" to play the audiometry game; yes, a game as it really is between examiner and examinee. The latter is instructed to listen and respond (like raise a hand) upon hearing a beep, even if it is very soft. Malingerers simply set their criterion to respond, not to just barely detect sounds, but rather to respond to a certain loudness of the beep. This actually makes the game more challenging for the malinger. To apply and maintain their criteria (as extreme variability would certainly raise suspicions of the audiologist), examinees must remain alert and attentive. The most basic results by which the nonorganic case may be uncovered is that of the discordance between the **average of pure-tone thresholds** at 500 Hz, 1000 Hz, and 2000 Hz (**PTA**) and the **speech reception threshold** (**SRT**). Malingering individuals are not likely to realize that the relatively broadband speech and pure tones at the same hearing levels will not have the same loudness; the speech tokens will sound louder, but attempts to equate their loudness to the pure tones are likely to fail. Consequently, the malingerer will have a lower SRT than PTA. (Note: Poor word recognition ability may increase the SRT; thus, SRT > PTA is not indicative of nonorganic involvement.)

Even after obtaining fairly convincing conventional test results, the audiologist may still have some lingering doubts. The additional support of objective test results may, or may not, provide confirmation of the results obtained; whichever way the answer goes, the audiologist has clues as to what step to take next. The one evoked response test that may help in the shortest amount of time is the **DP-gram** (agan, graph of distortion-product otoacoustic emissions plotted as a function of frequency). Recall from Episode 5.1, that the OAEs, in general, are acutely sensitive to status of the outer hair cells. Setup and running the test adds little time to the patient's visit and can reflect readily the presence of nearly any organic hearing loss or organic component of hearing loss that is clinically significant. The rationale for using OAE measurements for suspected nonorganic hearing loss is much the same as in cases suspected of having a retrocochlear lesion. As noted in other clinical populations, OAE measures are a useful supplement in differential diagnosis.[33] In a way of thinking, what the malingerer is doing is a retrocochlear function, as certainly the cochlea did not decide whether or not to raise the patient's hand when the beep was presented.

The results in Figure 9–13A, audiogram #1 are the sort of findings that would be possible in a case of suspected nonorganic involvement. Actually, two possible scenarios are represented by the two ears. One is relative to the DP-grams 1 and 2 in panel B which suggest a completely feigned loss, exemplified by audiogram #2 in panel C. Here the audiogram is shown for the right ear only (for simplicity), but the left-ear results would appear overlapping that of the right ear, plus/or minus the normal variance of pure-tone audiometry (~5 dB) and/or any actual (yet subclinically significant) asymmetry. In this scenario, the thresholds supposed initially were biased by the patient's criteria of response, maintained roughly uniformly across the audiometric frequency range and bilaterally.

The other scenario is exemplified by DP-gram #3 and audiogram #3 in Figure 9–13 (both left ear only for simplicity). This is a realistic alternative and the sort of outcome that may be encountered especially in cases of malingering for profit (for instance, as in a claim for compensation for hearing loss alleged to derive from the patient's line of work). Just about any degree of organic peripheral hearing loss adversely affects DPOAE output; still, some intact end-organ function may be detectable in such cases (namely, DP SPL significantly above the noise floor). The DP SPL over frequency in this case (panel B #3) is sharply reduced around 4000 Hz and overall mimics the true hearing loss (panel C, audiogram #3). In this case, the scenario is that the malingerer exaggerated sensorineural loss, yet the feigned threshold responses (panel A, audiogram #1) may not be substantially different. Although the configuration of the loss in audiogram #3 is one commonly observed bilaterally in patients with significant histories of noise exposure, acoustic trauma (like noise for a fire-cracker having exploded nearby and to one side of head) can manifest similarly and unilaterally. Were this the case, audiogram #1 was the initial audiogram indeed, and both ear's audiograms (#2 and #3) portrayed the truth in this case, then the slight asymmetry (greater degree) of the feigned loss in the left ear (audiogram #1) would have been an element of truth. Still, the DP-gram gives a better idea of where the whole truth might lie. Therefore, the inclusion of DPOAE testing certainly is warranted in the management of the nonorganic suspect.[101]

Nevertheless, there are substantial limitations to the DP-gram, starting with it not being a tool directly applicable to predicting a patient's complete audiogram. The accurate audiogram naturally is ultimately the goal. Some individuals with the nonorganic loss can be led to participate more honestly just knowing that the objective test might reveal their true hearing status. As noted earlier (recall Episode 8.1), hearing-compensation cases in Canada for decades have been required routinely to undergo evoked response testing, specifically by way of CAEP (cortical auditory evoked response) testing.[102] It then is not surprising that, given a case suspected of nonorganic involvement, to think first of the ABR and 80-Hz ASSR. The trustworthiness accorded SLR-ERA is largely well deserved but also may lead the clinician to be a bit cavalier in taking this direction in follow-up—like, what is there to lose? In fact, three things! The first is time of the clinician and the patient. Second, there are consequences in patient management beyond the primary goal of a reliable evaluation of the patient's hearing status. Neither party wins if mutual respect is

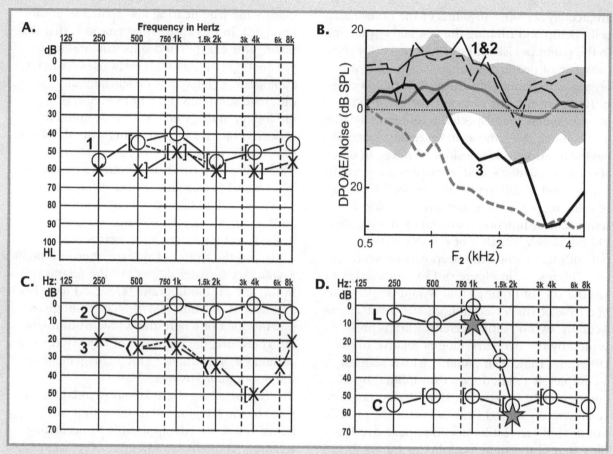

Figure 9–13. A. Audiogram #1: Exemplary results with degree and configuration of apparent hearing loss that can be encountered in nonorganic cases. Note: There is no typical audiogram, as such, although an overall flat configuration is often encountered. **B.** DP-grams #1&2: Data from an actual nonorganic case, suggesting normal sensory function bilaterally, thus portending hearing thresholds well within normal limits (see audiogram #2 in panel C; right ear only, for simplicity). DP-gram #3: Results suggestive of an organic component, consistent with a true audiogram like #3 in panel C (left ear only), typically manifested binaurally but could be a unilateral loss. DPOAE analysis: norms of the clinic—average (*solid gray line*), +/−2 standard deviations (*light-gray-shaded area*); mean noise-floor limit (*dashed gray line*); primaries 65/55 dB SPL. Panel **C.** As indicated previously. Panel **D:** Case of nonorganic hearing loss in a patient with history of partial sudden-onset (organic) hearing loss. C—Audiogram of involved ear the day of the "crisis" of perceiving hearing to have become worse; L—250 Hz to 2000 Hz portion of last/prior audiogram, which had been stable for some time. Stars: Thresholds estimated by ERA, testing the cortical (N_1-P_2) complex (see text).

lost in the process, regardless of the basis of the nonorganic loss/component. The third is the truth and the whole truth (to the extent possible) of the patient's hearing status.

In the discussion of ABR-ERA in particular, various potential limitations were noted. ASSR-ERA had others. In presenting the methods, much attention was given to frequency specificity; yet, there is at least the possibility for some configurations of hearing losses escaping the most accurate picture of the "organic" status. At the same time, there is the pervasive requirement of having the patient be relatively sedate (by volition, natural sleep, or medication). In short, the ideal objective test of the suspected nonorganic hearing loss ought to be

(1) that which can be used most confidently to estimate the audiogram, or at least it should elicit enough frequency-specific responses to determine what the actual hearing status is. At the same time, (2) the test should allow the best results actually to be obtained with the patient alert and attentive to the stimuli. That candidate AEP is the CAEP. Although adequate CAEPs may be recorded with the subject in a passive state of attention, a better outcome is achieved if the subject selectively attends to the stimulated ear.[103] The trick to this trick can be as simple as asking the examinee to count the number of times the stimulus was audible (if audible at all). The examiner will know that number per trial, namely the sum of the numbers of accepted and rejected sweeps of stimulus response from the artifact-rejection algorithm. This will vary a bit from the number of sweeps preset for the average, yet quasi-randomly due to the patient's movements and/or other transient changes in the level of the background noise that likely will trip rejection of some sweeps. Starting at a reasonable level likely to elicit any response—in reference to the suspected "unreasonable" audiogram previously obtained—will give some quantitative basis by which the examiner can be confident (or not) of the initial response. Thereafter, the VDL can be pursued for the test frequencies of interest. The following is a case in point for ALLR-ERA in follow-up testing of the patient suspected of having a nonorganic hearing loss.

An established patient of the otology division of the health center had been treated medically and regularly followed up for his misfortune of a unilateral sudden-onset hearing loss. Sudden hearing losses are typically idiopathic, they may be complete or partial, and they may be temporary or permanent. Some more prevalent configurations include low-frequency, rising configurations or one that is more or less flat. These losses can be associated with or without dizziness and/or tinnitus. When the loss occurs, a medical regimen may be tried, with no guarantee of success. Timing, however, seems to be of the essence—the sooner the treatment begins, the better the outcome is likely to be. The case reviewed here had suffered a partial loss, with the most uncommon presentation audiometrically, as shown in panel D of Figure 9–13, audiogram-L. Not only is the loss predominantly high-frequency, the configuration is that of a "ski-slope" (like "expert" trails on the slopes). This configuration is particularly worrisome as results of testing are vulnerable to adverse effects of frequency splatter, possibly causing the degree of high-frequency loss to be substantially underestimated. The clinic's past audiograms for this patient had demonstrated stability of the degree and configuration of this loss. This middle-aged gentleman had a negative history for other otoneurological involvement and denied a significant history of acoustic trauma or noise exposure (whether events and/or occupationally related). He returned to the clinic as an emergency case, believing that he had lost more hearing in the same ear, as is sadly but entirely possible. That day, the audiogram obtained, labeled "C", showed an essentially flat configuration, but his otologist was not entirely convinced of its validity. The patient was sent to the audiology clinic, asking for "an ABR." The audiologist inheriting the case was concerned that the ABR might not be successful if the previous audiogram was accurate (especially with regard to configuration) and if the patient was rather agitated (indeed, he was). Expressing these concerns to the otologist, the audiologist offered instead "a CAEP" and explained the rationale. With the recommendation accepted, the test was administered. The patient was compliant and awake throughout the test. The estimated thresholds are indicated by stars in the figure. Only two frequencies were tested or needed—just above and below the ski-slope (regarding the last audiogram on file—L). If the slope proved "skiable,, then the new, low-frequency component was likely not organic. Upon counselling by the otologist, armed with assurance of the patient by way of the objective measures—explained to him as suggestive of no significant change in his hearing status— retest of his low-frequency thresholds reconfirmed his previous audiogram (L).

The particular configuration featured in this account might not permit a reliable DP-gram where it was most needed, given the inherent, rising noise level with decreasing frequencies below 1000 Hz or so. Other nonorganic cases, however, are good candidates; even in this case, the results would corroborate the organic component (1000 Hz and above). In a study of nonorganic hearing losses, results from a cohort of 35 patients (early teens to nearly 70 years of age) were analyzed. These cases were from the referring professional or audiologist who raised the concern of nonorganic involvement. These patients were largely characterized by another working diagnosis as well—everything from ear and/or head trauma to a variety of types of sensorineural hearing losses (even retrocochlear suspects). Only a small minority were presumed only to be feigning hearing loss, a subset of which were cases of failure on a hearing screening in a secondary school. Despite the heterogeneity of the patient sample, nearly half ($N = 17$) of the patients suspected of nonorganic involvement were confirmed, even if they had an organic component of their initial audiogram.[101] The DPOAE was proven to be useful in the management of the patient with nonorganic hearing loss. It should always be remembered though, identification of the nonorganic hearing loss is only the first step. In order to develop a treatment plan (if indicated), the referring professional needs to know the true status of the hearing in any given patient.

In the broad population of patients whom clinicians must see, the audiologist must be prepared to explore one end of the auditory pathways or the other, both, and/or the middle—wherever/whenever the facts of the case present themselves and however they evolve. Any case in which there is hearing loss/other dysfunction in the presence of OAEs certainly must be followed up with AEP testing. Evoked response test systems of today readily provide the capability to do all the tests presented in this textbook, often with little increase in time to complete, as another AEP is only a mouse click away. With a solid foundation of information and experience, travel in the time-space continuum of AEPdom should not be scary but, in fact, embraced.

■ Episode 4: Testing Patients With Cochlear or Brainstem Implants

The text to this point has presented AEPs largely in the context of applications in which energy of the stimulus—even in the face of possible outer-/middle-ear impairment—is delivered by electroacoustic devices, as in conventional AC (via an earphone or loudspeaker) and BC (via a bone vibrator) stimuli. Suppose a case having a workable outer/middle ear, yet the hearing organ and/or auditory nerve is so profoundly impaired that acoustically elicited AEPs are minimal to none. This dilemma plagued treatment of some hearing-loss patients using implantable electronic devices until the latter part of the last century. **Cochlear (CI)** and **auditory brainstem (ABI) implants** were developed to process sounds effectively to activate the CANS through remaining nerve fibers or directly at the brainstem. Direct **electrical stimulation** was innovated so as to encode sound in a manner at least roughly emulating the defective organ and in such a way to restore the best quality of hearing possible. For the moment, the focus will be dedicated to the CI, as by far the more successful device and (relatively) more straightforward to be understood, used, and evaluated. The additional tools needed have emerged efficaciously, nearly on the heels of that of AEP-related technology, especially toward the application of CI treatment with confidence in the restoration of hearing. Indeed, the two together have made implants feasible in children as young as 6 months of age.

The general goal of clinicians is to obtain specific information about auditory processing at different levels of the CANS based on measures of **electric-evoked auditory potentials (EEAPs)** in implant recipients. Dependent on the underlying question, this involves auditory processing at the level of signal detection (presence/absence of sound), auditory discrimination (perceiving differences), and/or identification and linguistic interpretation.

As sound-evoked AEPs have been used for decades in clinical audiology in order to estimate auditory thresholds in children, it is this population of CI "users" that has strongly driven interest of the CI clinician in clinical electrophysiology. Application of objective electrophysiological assessment is of utmost importance for very young children who receive a CI, even before the age of 1 year, but also for older pediatric patients who might be unable to respond adequately well behaviorally. In such cases, EEAP recordings are indispensable for programing the *speech processor*, thereby supplying the CI clinician information important to "fitting" the processor of each patient optimally, in the sense of a proper hearing-aid fitting.

Besides determining detection levels of electrical responses, it is absolutely necessary to avoid any chance of intracochlear electrical overstimulation by the CI postoperatively, since this may lead to trauma or nonuse of the implant. Intra- and postoperative EEAP tests can help to predict behavioral thresholds per electrode or to obtain a rough profile of how to "map" the CI frequency allocation of the implanted electrode array. At least, the test results give the clinician information of minimal current levels needed to evoke an auditory neural response.

Since the late 1980s, many CI research studies have been performed at all levels of the CANS. Even until recently, the search has continued for variables that might lead to optimal postoperative performance, especially in terms of speech perception. Tests of some of these EAPs have already found their way into clinical practice; others are still under development for clinical application.

Testing of patients with a CI—hence using electrical stimulation, as characterized by the promontory test (recalling the Heads Up of Episode 8.2)—is in a sense electrocochleography in reverse, yet rather more complicated in detail. Still, the fundamental notion is (again) that the electrical path for recording the sound-evoked, whole-nerve action potential (AP) from scala tympani (recall Figure 5–9) also must provide a path for injecting electrical current to reach the 8th nerve. This was confirmed empirically wherein single-unit discharges from auditory nerve fibers were shown to be manifested in recordings from the round window.[104] The implication is that the modiolus (core) of the cochlea does not fully insulate the nerve in the IAC from the perilymphatic fluid space. As ECochG can be performed from more distal sites than basal-turn scala tympani, it follows that even more distal sites like the round window membrane and again the promontory also permit electrically stimulating the 8th nerve. Historically, all have been tried. However, an electrode/electrode array placed directly in scala tympani has proven to be the most efficacious approach overall, including for use in early intervention and in deference to the need of long-term reliability of the indwelling devices involved.

Performing AEP measurements in users of CIs is very similar to those obtained in nonimplanted patients. When the clinician has sufficient basic knowledge and practical experience in measuring acoustically evoked potentials, EEAP recordings are relatively easy to perform, taking into account only a few differences in the practical setup of the AEP test system. However, this does not mean that the best mode of stimulation would be to place an earphone over the microphone of the patient's ear-level, hearing-aid-like component. Even if seemingly workable in theory, in practice, the story is far more complicated. In any event, first things first; it still is important to consider what the CI's workings do with sound. This starts with an understanding of the main difference between acoustical and electrical stimuli; they are not merely different forms of energy. What mainly makes EEAP stimuli different is that they are typically a biphasic pulse or pulse train (somewhat like square waves) generated by the CI-programming software. The electrical (output) signal is intended to directly stimulate auditory neurons rather than drive an electroacoustic/electromechanical transducer (like an earphone or loudspeaker). The inherent nuances of each mode of stimulation—acoustic (A) and electric (B) are contrasted in Figure 9–14.

The potential interference of extraneous electrical signals is enough of a concern in conventional AEP testing, but it truly is "sobering" in CI

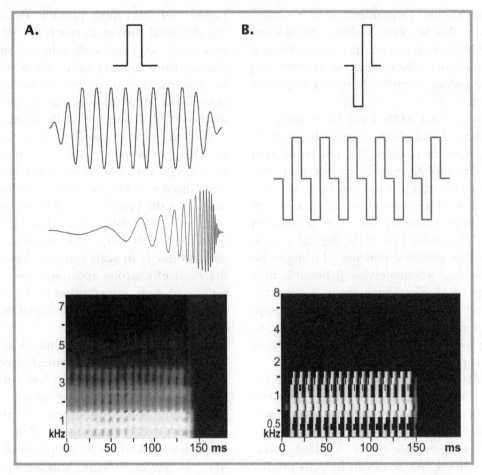

Figure 9–14. A. Examples of electric signals transduced to produce acoustic stimuli of common audiological interests (*from top to bottom*): click, tone burst, chirp (time histories), and speech (spectrograph—frequency by time domains). **B.** Examples of electric stimuli used in operating cochlear implants (*from top to bottom*): biphasic pulse, pulse train (time histories), and CI processor-streamed speech (spectrograph).

testing, hence the next important thing to know. Measurement of EEAPs is at extreme risk for contamination of the recording by **stimulus artifacts**. A few more technical details are then in order, regarding getting the electrical stimulus to the electrode array implanted in the cochlea. The input signal is effectively communicated internally by a hearing-aid-like electronics "package," but with an antenna rather than an acoustic delivery system. The external processor encodes sound as a modulated radio signal that readily passes through the scalp/skin overlying the indwelling receiving antenna/coil to be further processed internally. AEPs have energy falling entirely within the audio frequency range, not overlapping with that of **radio-frequency (RF)** signals. Yet (recalling Episode 4.1), electronic devices (such as amplifiers and digital circuits) involve nonlinear circuit elements that can pick up RF signals and rectify them, thereby demodulating the RF signal. This is akin to the effects of the nonlinear transfer function of hair cells and the eliciting of ASSRs. A modulated high-frequency carrier that when rectified yields an envelope following response (recall Episodes 6.2 and 6.3 as well as Figure 6–21 in particular). The result is the creation of strong **electrical artifacts** that can overlap substantially with the time history of the targeted AEP, whether impulse responses

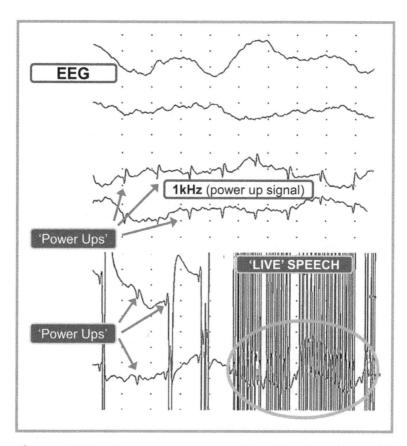

Figure 9–15. Top two traces: ongoing EEG, CI turned "off"; middle two traces: CI "on," but no stimulation, only "power up" spikes visible in EEG; bottom two traces: CI "on," stimulation initiated (speech) with high processor sensitivity.

(to be demonstrated shortly) or quasi-steady-state signals (shown in Figure 9–14). Their shear signal strength and broad spectra are difficult to suppress adequately by routine means of filtering or artifact rejection of conventional AEP-test instruments (for technical reasons beyond the scope here). Suffice it to say that there have been developed approaches to extensively deal with stimulus artifact, as will be presented briefly and noting possible limitations thereof. The principles therein need to be familiar to any examiner seeking to apply AEP testing to CI-related evaluations.

Illustrated in Figure 9–15 are electrical artifacts deriving from *transcutaneous electro-magnetic induction*; two types need to be distinguished: (1) the "power-up" artifact and (2) the actual electrical stimulus artifact. The first is caused by small "packages" of energy (analogous to packets in digital telecommunications), typically presented subthreshold. These are continuously sent to the implant literally to power up the implanted stimulator. It is this energy that is needed to keep the implant working and to deliver sufficient electrical charge to stimulate the auditory nerve. The power-ups are usually recognized as low-amplitude periodic "spikes" in the recording of the free-running EEG and can be temporarily switched off in some CI systems during times of recording to avoid interference—a "RF free period." Generally, they will not significantly influence AEP morphology. The second and much larger stimulus artifact is the actual demodulated electrical signal of the RF transmission that is responsible for communication between the external sender and the internal receiver of the CI. Hence, it usually has exactly the same duration as the electrical stimulus that is

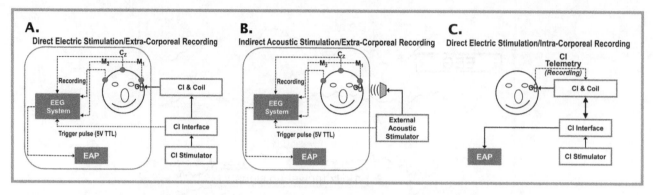

Figure 9–16. Stimulating and recording hardware setup: **A.** Extracorporeal direct stimulation via CI processor. **B.** Extracorporeal indirect stimulation in the sound field. **C.** Intracorporeal recording via the CI test system using telemetric transmission of signals recording from the indwelling electrode array.

delivered by the electrode array, thus the length of the biphasic pulse train streamed in and representing the sounds encoded. However, it is this "ringing" of the artifact that can interfere significantly with the AEP, making interpretation of waveform peaks sometimes difficult (see Figure 9–15, 'live' speech). Both types of artifacts are captured by the surface recording electrodes, picking up RF activity around the area of the external coil (the transmitter antenna) and the subcutaneously implanted device (the receiver).

Nevertheless, it is possible to manage these interferences. In real-time for instance, this can be accomplished simply by using shorter stimuli than the latency of the AEP peak of interest or by filtering. Alternatively, statistical/other computational techniques can be applied off-line. An example of the latter approach is the use of independent component analysis to discern artifacts from the real morphology of the auditory response but also requiring multichannel recordings.[105,106]

Also remarkably different than conventional AEP testing is the extra hardware requirements, which are several, as seen in Figure 9–16. First, there is the **CI stimulator** (CI system-dependent soft- and hardware); stimulation can be direct or indirect. Second, recordings can be made either using external recording electrodes with an AEP test system—*extracorporeal*—or using the CI itself to acquire the signals—*intracorporeal*. In the case of an extracorporeal setup, usually the CI stimulator is sending an external trigger pulse to the test system. This typically is a 5V-TTL (transistor-transistor logic) signal to enable time locking between stimulator and signal averaging system.

Depending on the aim of the measurement, AEPs can be tested using a variety of clinical setups, whether by **direct** or **indirect (electrical) stimulation** and extra- or intracorporeal acquisition. With direct stimulation, the CI itself generates biphasic stimuli, directly activating one or more intracochlear electrodes, thus bypassing all preprocessing functionalities of the speech processor (for example, filtering and automatic gain control). The advantage of direct stimulation is that the clinician is 100% in command of all stimulation parameters, such as stimulation rates, pulse widths, amplitudes, or interphase gaps. Therefore, the examiner exactly knows what, how, and when the predefined stimuli are presented to the cochlear nerve.

In contrast, indirect stimulation makes use of the individual settings of the speech processor. One variant is presentation of stimuli in the sound field using the patient's individual daily-life presettings, thus involving all preprocessing. Another variant of indirect stimulation is to use the audio input of the speech processor, whether or not bypassing all preprocessing options. In contrast to direct stimulation, the advantage of indirect stimulation is that it is relatively easy to apply speech stimuli as input signals and that reflect the patient's daily-life use. EEAPs can be acquired in different modes: electrical bi-phasic pulses (eBP) or pulse trains (eBP-Trains) are typically presented in direct stimulation mode via the CI, while acoustic tone bursts (aTB) or speech stimuli are typically presented in an indirect mode, such as a loudspeaker for testing in the sound field.

To recap AEP acquisition, the distinction between extra- and intracorporeal setups is as follows: extracorporeal recordings require the use of an external AEP test system; intracorporeal recordings use the CI itself via signal averaging incorporated in *telemetry* of the CI system. Telemetry is the back-and-forth communication of the implant, enabling feedback from the CI hardware, such as the *intracochlear electrode impedance measurements (IM)* or *voltage measurements (VM)* and/or neural responses, such as electrocochleography or *intracochlear spread of excitation (SOE)* recordings (see Figure 9–16C). The advantage of an extracorporeal setup is that the clinician is able to test most AEPs along the complete auditory pathway—cochlea to cortex—using their clinical AEP test system (otherwise, analyses/tools familiar to them). The advantage of an intracorporeal approach is that a conventional AEP test system is not needed. Another is that the recordings are less sensitive to a variety of external environmental noises—physiological, powerline/mains, electromagnetic field, and so forth.—particularly in noisy operating theaters.[107] Unfortunately for the intracorporeal approach using CI devices presently in clinical use, it is only possible to capture the EEAPs from the peripheral nerve, namely via a method known commercially as Neural Response Telemetry (NRT), Auditory Response Telemetry (ART), or Neural Response Imaging (NRI)—depending on CI manufacturer.

The applications and possible value of other AEP tests in CI recipients largely parallel those of conventional recordings of AC-/BC-elicited AEPs (extracorporeal approach). This topic is expansive, and a comprehensive overview is beyond the scope here. Still, it will be useful to summarize some of the underlying objectives and highlight interest for the respective AEPs per classical latency classifications. The preceding chapters detailed these evoked responses and have presented numerous applications of AEPs along the auditory pathway. These all are, at least in principle, fundamentally applicable to CI patient management, when paired with technically appropriate modes of electrical stimulation. Choices of tests and approaches, as should be true of any conventional AEP-related test, depend on the clinical question. As one of the hottest areas in AEPdom today, the range of aims and/or foci of such protocols are quite impressive: (1) test results that might inform *preoperative counseling* for realistic expectations and/or choice of the better ear (if unilateral implant planned), such as by assessing behavioral responses to extra-tympanic or trans-tympanic (TT) electrical stimulation[108,109]; (2) findings *predictive of chance of success* in specific populations, like children who are suspected of ANSD[110]; (3) evaluation of the value in patients with some residual hearing of *bimodal* use of a hearing aid with the CI postoperatively[111]; (4) *intraoperative assessment* of possible cochlear damage during electrode array insertion[112]; (5) assessment of *neural and/or hardware integrity* and even predicting electrical thresholds[113]; and (6) objective evaluation of *auditory discrimination*.[114,115]

Preoperative promontory or *round window stimulation (RWS)* in general is an approach of varied history and response modality. Initially (as noted earlier, but to recap some specifics for comparison), the promontory stimulation test was used fairly routinely to evaluate CI candidates, using a transtympanic electrode and promontory placement (recall Figure 5–13A). The test required behavioral responses to electrical stimulation. The RWS approach requires a tympanotomy for access. A noninvasive variant is to present electrical stimulus by way of *ear canal stimulation (ECS)*. Instead of transtympanic electrode placement, the electrode tip is placed in the ear canal in a saline-soaked cotton ball to aid conductivity (essentially a tymptrode, recall Figure 5–13B). Though coming to less broad/routine use, the promontory stimulation test and variants still merit consideration, for instance, in completely deaf candidates. These are patients who do not demonstrate auditory responses by conventional audiometry but whose outcomes of preoperative imaging studies do not permit ruling out neural dysfunction, as occurs in cases of no or inconclusive visibility of auditory nerves. These candidates presumably have hypoplasia of the 8th nerve.[116] An objective variant of this approach is to obtain eABR in the same setup. A clinical AEP test system is used to obtain ABRs using surface recording electrodes. "Preop-eABR" also may be used to predict auditory nerve function in young children who are suspected of ANSD. Preoperative TT-eABRs preferably are performed only to predict possible success of CI and for parent counseling purposes to create realistic expectations.

The electrically evoked compound action potential (*eCAP*) was discussed previously preliminarily with regard to CI telemetry (again Figure 9–16C). Since the introduction of cochlear implants, researchers strived to find objective pre- and intraoperative predictors that can be used for speech processor fitting. Initially, eABRs were examined (extracorporeal setup) to predict electrical thresholds. The disadvantage was that this measurement took relatively long recording times, especially since external noise levels in the operating room are significantly higher than in the clinical laboratory. Thus, more signal averaging is required to obtain good quality eABRs. As a result, a significant prolongation of surgical time was needed, in turn keeping the patient under anesthesia longer than required for the surgery itself.

There nevertheless are several reasons to obtain eCAPs: (1) verify successful insertion without damaging any/all implant electrodes (hardware testing); (2) test the electro-neural interface (neural integrity testing); (3) use as a predictor for postoperative *threshold/comfort (T/C)* stimulus levels; and (4) use such information for (future) automatic fitting paradigms. The acquisition of eCAPs is much easier today than with earlier test hardware and programs. Responses are captured completely intracorporeally, and intracochlear electrodes are used for electrical stimulation (biphasic pulses), while another (usually neighboring) electrode functions as a recording electrode. This then permits measuring the neural response from the spiral ganglion cells in relation to that electrode. To avoid any disturbance from electrical artifacts, a smart but simple paradigm is applied to minimize this artifact—the *subtraction-paradigm*. By consecutive stimulation of two biphasic stimuli (such as one masker and one probe stimulus) presented within the refractory period of the auditory nerve, both stimuli evoke an electrical signal. However, the second stimulus should not evoke a neural response, due to the recovery time required.[117] Recording of the eCAP in CI patients has found its way into clinical practice; most CI systems offer telemetry to estimate fitting parameters for postoperative thresholds, although eCAP thresholds show wide variances between threshold (T) and comfort (C) levels. Multicenter studies have shown that eCAP-thresholds may be used to inform the clinician about the *fitting profile* of the electrode mapping, instead of defining exactly the individual electrode thresholds.[113]

To obtain eABRs, most CI devices provide the capability to deliver a single biphasic pulse in all three modes—positive, negative, and alternating polarities—thus an electrical variant of the acoustic click stimulus. A conventional extracorporeal test system is used to capture, average, and analyze these brainstem responses, examples of which are shown in Figure 9–17. Electrically evoked brainstem responses are similar to those obtained acoustically with the only differences as follows: (1) due to the high-level electrical stimulus artifact, the first peak of the eABR is obscured; (2) all peak latencies are earlier, typically around 1.0 ms to 1.5 ms because the outer and middle ear are skipped, such that wave V (for example) typically shows latencies between 3.5 ms to 4.5 ms; and (3) wave V especially grows rather more dramatically as the stimulus intensity is increased and without latency shifts observed in acoustic ABRs, since the sound transducer's transfer function, the cochlear macro- and micromechanical systems, and the hair cell-to-axon synapse no longer contribute to generation of the response.

For many years, tests of eABRs were performed to predict electrical thresholds in CI patients but with disappointing success. Alternatively, the results were sought to confirm a functioning implant and neural stimulation during surgery. Since the introduction of intracorporeal eCAP recordings (NRT/ART/NRI), the clinical application of eABR has been reduced. This is because (again) eABR testing requires more equipment and is more time consuming, thus perceived as being impractical. Nevertheless, in specific circumstances, eABR evaluations are still applicable, such as in children who are suspected of ANSD (preoperatively). The presentation of the electrical stimulus is similar to that of transtympanic RWS. The main difference is that no behavioral responses are obtained but that electrophysiological brainstem responses are now recorded using a conventional EP instrumentation, thus measuring the *W-eABR*.

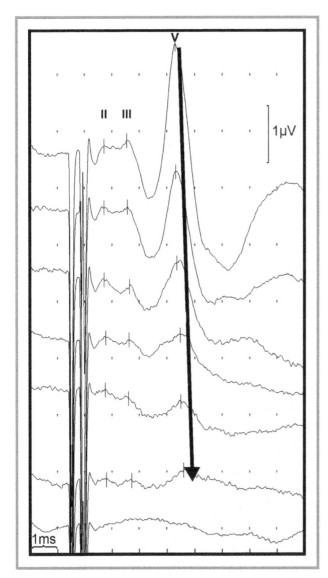

Figure 9–17. Typical example of eABR in response to single biphasic electrical pulse: electrical stimulus artifact is bigger than from that of earphones and even bone vibrators (recall Figures 6–7 and 9–9), and both the peak latencies are 1.0 ms to 1.5 ms shorter and the slope of the latency- intensity function is far steeper (recall, for example, Figures 6–3 and 6–5).

Recipients of ABIs are yet another clinical group that has helped to maintain interest in the eABR, including tests conducted intraoperatively. It is essential to confirm auditory responses for specific electrodes, thus inactivating any electrodes that are not stimulating uniquely auditory neurons. Testing the eABR also is important for redefinition of the frequency allocation of each active electrode. Although working on much the same soft- and hardware platform and the device functioning much on the same system in concept as the CI, moving the electrode array out of the cochlea is a real "game changer," so its nuances require additional discussion.

The ABI's use is considered specifically in the face of deformities or other problems precluding development or any likelihood of development of a functional 8th nerve in the candidate's auditory system. To be clear, the CI relies upon the 8th nerve, even if only a remnant that is functional and/or functioning abnormally for electrically encoded acoustic stimulation. Therefore, anything less precludes efficacious stimulation of the CANS from the cochlea. Figure 9–18 shows conceptually bypassing the defective cochlea and 8th nerve entirely by implanting a specialized multichannel array effectively onto the surface of the brainstem overlying the DVCN. Consequently, tonotopy is not straightforwardly accessible from an electrode array applied to the brainstem's surface (the only practical approach), as it is along the basilar membrane via scala tympani.[118]

To explain, unlike the CI electrode array, that of the ABI has far fewer electrodes (~1/2 in number) and without the advantage of a site of implantation that readily ensures a straightforward frequency allocation to the electrodes. Although coiled a bit inside the cochlea, the CI electrode array is one dimensional. The number of electrodes inserted thus scales the distance along the basilar membrane. In principle, that array gives access to the cochlea's place frequency map (although limited by additional parameters determined by the cochlear electroanatomy and distribution of surviving neurons). The ABI electrode hedges a bet on *tonotopy* with an oblong two-dimensional array, but still without quite the same level of certainty of correct insertion (see Figure 9–18). Despite the problem of less direct access to tonotopy of the central pathways, the approach permits a test protocol to define somewhat of a ***place-frequency (tonal) axis***, as expected from the systematic wiring of the cochlea to this nucleus complex (recall Figure 3–13). As a reminder, the CI effectively initiates stimulation as if at the distal end of the 8th nerve, effectively jumping ahead more than a

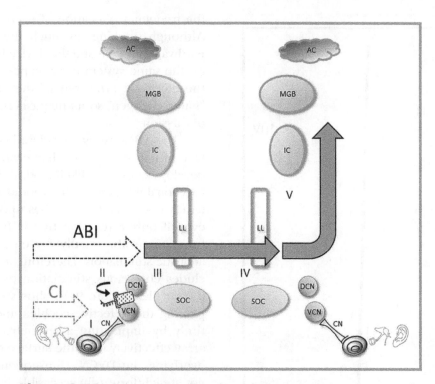

Figure 9–18. Time-space recap focusing on central auditory pathways involved with brainstem versus cochlear implants and their dominant pathway of activation in the CANS. Note the site of implantation, semi-circular arrow symbolizing insertion of the electrode array of the ABI. Brainstem responses thus show different response morphologies, effectively skipping not only the outer and middle ear and hydromechanical part of the inner ear but also the 8th nerve, resulting in still shorter eABR peak latencies—typically 0.5 ms to 1.0 ms compared to CI-eABRs and 1.0 ms to 1.5 ms compared to normal/acoustic ABRs, furthmore often consisting of only waves IV and V. Pop Quiz: Define abbreviations of the auditory pathways; check answers by reviewing Episode 3.2. (As with learning the multiplication table, practice makes perfect, and perfect in this "game" is recall of neuroanatomy that becomes second nature.)

millisecond relative to the acoustically elicited ABR in the normal ear. However, the eABR elicited via an ABI typically only shows one or two peaks, thus losing all earlier brainstem peaks compared to the acoustic response.

Another reason to apply eABR assessments in general is to discern whether sounds are processed normally at the level of the brainstem. If not and/or for still other reasons, an investigation of sound processing at other levels of the CANS is warranted, even up to the cortex. The motivation is to diagnose possible central processing disorders, as might cause (for instance) stagnation of speech-language development. It is known that the relation between eABR and postoperative speech recognition is rather poor.[119,120] It should also be kept in mind that, similar to the eCAPs, there is a discrepancy between the relatively low rate of stimulation applied in the promontory test or eABR and the higher rate of electrode stimulation in patients' daily lives (via the implant),[121,122] although the literature is not consistent on this issue.[123]

Given that the eABR, especially in the ABI cases, is technically challenging to have more than just parts of the response that clearly are distinguishable, it simply is limited in the turf of its generators in the CANS. There thus is plenty of motivation to look beyond the pontine brainstem. All other potentials along the central auditory pathway potentially offer the bases for metrics by which to assess neural processing in children showing no speech and language development, after it has been confirmed that CI/ABI hardware is functioning properly. Yet, evaluations of auditory middle latency responses in CI/ABI patients hardly have been described for the last two decades. Until now, besides the feasibility to evoke *eAMLRs* in CI patients, their evaluation appears not to have come to be employed in practice in CI treatment, such as for prediction of electrical thresholds or otherwise. It is tempting to conclude that, like other AEPs, longer-latency and/or higher-amplitude responses seem to correlate better with both postoperative CI performance and neural plasticity.[124–126]

Clinical applications of cortical responses usually have similar rationales to be of interest when it comes to acoustically evoked AEPs.[127] For signal detection, the targeted potentials of cortical responses (typically) are the P_1 component in children and the N_1-P_2-complex in adults. Auditory long latency responses, including cortical obligatory responses and beyond, are excellent for testing CI/ABI users. Determining auditory thresholds with *e-ALLR* is much the same as with acoustic stimulation in the overall approach, with far less risk of contamination by electrical artifacts, especially when the length of the electrical stimulus is chosen in such a way that the electrical artifact (that has the same duration of the stimulus) will not interfere with the AEP of interest. Examples of typical settings for direct-stimulation testing to evoke the slow vertex potential or N_1-P_2-complex in adults are as follows: biphasic pulse train of 60 ms duration (thus not interfering with the N_1/P_2 detection component); repetition rate of 1.1 Hz; HP-filter cutoff at 0.1 Hz; and LP-filter cutoff at 30 Hz. As shown in Figure 9–19, these responses can be quite robust, in this case, the P_1-N_1-P_2 complex. (Recall, for instance, Figures 4–12 and 8–3 for comparison to similar sets of tracings of acoustically elicited responses in a hearing-impaired and normal-hearing subject, respectively.) Since long latency responses reflect signal processing along nearly the complete auditory pathway, it is assumed

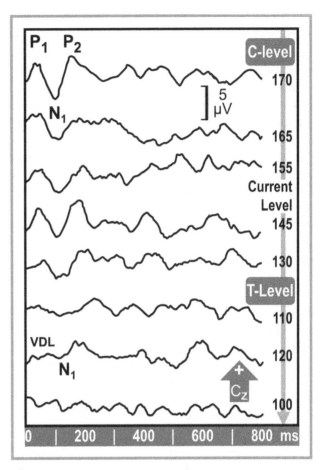

Figure 9–19. Auditory-cortical-response threshold estimation (see VDL) in a CI recipient: peak morphologies (latencies and amplitudes) are much like those obtained in acoustically evoked responses of subjects with normal hearing.

that these responses better predict the individual behavioral thresholds and might be used for speech processor fitting, similar to the application of cortical responses to evaluate acoustic hearing aid fitting in young children,[128] as touched upon in the last chapter.

Many studies have been performed to assess eALLRs in CI patients for the last decade or so. Main goals of measuring eALLRs are determining the relation of their VDLs to subjective auditory thresholds,[129] tracking longitudinally auditory maturation or cross-modal reorganization in children,[130–131] and obtaining measures predictive of postoperative speech recognition ability, namely toward optimizing speech processor fitting.[132]

An example of measuring discrimination is the use of the ***acoustic change complex (ACC)*** (recall Heads Up, Episode 8.3). The ACC has been tested acoustically to detect perception of differences within the presented stimuli, as can be effected in CI users by a sudden change of the stimulating electrode, stimulus amplitude, or other parameters.[114,133] Other auditory potentials focused on cortical discrimination that have been considered are the ***mismatch negativity (MMN)*** or the classical P_{300} ***(P3b)*** or ***cognitive potential***. The latter is relatively easier to recognize and interpret, since P_{300} amplitudes generally are substantially larger than those of the MMN, thus offering significantly higher SNRs and fostering more reliable results, case by case. However, P_3s are more difficult to obtain in young children (especially less than 6 years old), since a relatively long session is required to complete the test and wherein the patient must actively attend to the stimuli, yet remain otherwise sedate. Nevertheless, P_3 measurement is a useful electrophysiological tool to assess auditory discrimination of tone and/or speech contrasts in different populations (such as CI vs. non-CI users or good vs. poor performers) and overall to evaluate cortical endogenous processing.[115] An overview of the main AEPs and their application is presented in Table 9–6.

CIs/ABIs are all about providing the patient renewed input to the CANS, given a wonderfully designed "replacement" (in effect) for the peripheral hearing apparatus. These are patients in whom their native "model" failed to work or work good enough for optimal speech, language, and learning development (in children) or for a level of hearing restoration not realizable via conventional hearing-aid fitting and/or medical treatment (in adults). By progression of latency of AEPs considered, all the way to "the late-late show" of AEPdom, it certainly would be reasonable to close out the episode at this juncture. However, it also is timely to reset the time-space coordinates, for the upcoming episode. Coincidentally, it is interesting to see ECochG playing as much of a role in the CI clinical arena, as appears the trend. Might CI/ABI advances also be a harbinger of an ECochG revival? Overall, the research and development of the CI and ABI has been one of the most highly acclaimed success stories of implantable bioelectric devices. At the same time and as suggested at the outset of this episode, no small role has been played in CI/ABI research and develoment by neurophysiological methods on both pre-and postsides of implant management of the candidate/patient. While no replacement for reliable tests of behavioral responses (if efficacious), the objective measures have compelling value already evident for very young and other difficult-to-test patients as well as for cross-checks and/or assisting troubleshooting. The latter includes issues of hearing preservation, evaluation of surgical insertion techniques, and assessment of invasiveness of electrode arrays (for instance, straight vs. modiolus-hugging designs). For this reason, ECochG has been introduced to evaluate possible cochlear damage pre-, intra- and postoperatively to assess structural preservation in patients with residual hearing.[134] In CI candidates having potentially useful residual low frequency hearing, it can be tested intraoperatively using acoustic stimulation via TT-ECochG with surface or one of the intracochlear electrodes or evaluated postoperatively.[135] Aside from the previously introduced eCAP, recordings that were focused mainly on electrical auditory threshold prediction, intracorporeal ECochG applications of today focus on inner-ear structure preservation "post-op"—the outer hair cells. Other applications of ECochG are optimization of CI clinical programming of patients with hybrid electric-acoustic devices[136,137] or to evaluate preservation of inner ear structures apropos different electrode designs.[138] In general, further research and development of ECochG is anticipated to boost not only the development of new electrophysiological applications to benefit CI patients but also refinement of site-of-lesion studies, perhaps by greater/more innovative use of measurement of the cochlear microphonics and summating potentials.[112,135]

Whatever the course of history brings, it is clear, overall in the research and development of AEP test methods, few things have remained on the back shelf of the "stock of tools" for very long. Some would say "reinventing wheels," but that seems harsh in the face of ultimate progress that has been both great and, on numerous fronts, often dependent on or (at least) facilitated by the considerable leaps of technological progress coming into and continuing in the new century. At the

Table 9–6. Overview of the Main AEPs and Their Application

	Stimulation				Clinical Aim							
	Freq specific	Speech	Direct/ Sound Field	Thr-predict	MAP Profile	Discrim	Intraop Int	Other apps	Pediatric appl	Invasive	Attention needed
ECS/RWS	(behavioral)	eBP	—	Direct	—	—	—	—	Ear choice	—	(ET) / (TT) Yes	Yes
RW-eABR	CM/peak V	eBP	—	Direct	(—)	—	—	Yes	Ear choice/ Pred	Yes	(TT) Yes	—
ECochG	eCAP (NRT/ ART/NRI)	eBP	—	Direct	(—)	Yes	—	Yes	IM/VM	Yes	—	—
	CM (ANN/ SP/AP)	aTB	—	Insert/Sound Field	—	—	—	Yes	SOE/ StructPres	Yes	—	—
eABR	CM/peak V	eBP / aTB	—	Direct	(-)	Yes	—	Yes	(maturation)	Yes	—	—
eMLR	N0P0/ NaPa/NbPb	eBP (Train) / aTB	(Yes)	Direct/Sound field	(?)	Yes	—	(Yes)		Yes	—	—
eACR	SVP: P1 (Pb)	eBP (Train) / aTB	Yes	Direct/Sound field	Yes	Yes	—	—	(maturation)	Yes	—	Yes
eACR	SVP: N1P2	eBP (Train) / aTB	Yes	Direct/Sound field	Yes	Yes	—	—		(Yes)	—	Yes
eACC		eBP (Train) / aTB	Yes	Direct/Sound field	—	—	Yes	—		(Yes)	—	Yes
eMMN		eBP (Train) / aTB	Yes	Direct/Sound field	—	—	Yes	—	(Pre-attent proc)	Yes	—	—
eP300	P3b	eBP (Train) / aTB	Yes	Direct/Sound field	—	—	Yes	—	(Cogn proc)	(Yes)	—	Yes

411

same time, the story of the interface of electronic implantable hearing devices and AEP technology certainly has made for much excitement. This includes still other arenas mentioned along the way but now will be considered more broadly in the upcoming chapter dedicated to applications essentially of clinical electrophysiology in the operating room and beyond.

Take Home Messages

Episode 1

1. The objectives of newborn screening are substantially different from ERA.
2. UNHS embraces various other considerations for implementation according to rigorous milestones in the progression from detection, to diagnosis, to (early) intervention.
3. Family history, prenatal history, and neonatal intensive care are long-recognized risk factors and justifications for NHS in NICUs, ultimately extended to well-baby nurseries.
4. Auditory evoked response tools are matters of approach in UNHS, including otoacoustic emission and/or brainstem response measurement.
5. Fundamentally more than one technology potentially is applicable, including computer automated technology.
6. As important for any test, pass/fail criteria must be set with an understanding of statistical decision making, relevant probability functions, and cost/benefits.
7. This cannot be emphasized enough: NHS must be applied in a systematic manner to ensure effectiveness/benefit.
8. ERA is broadly of interest for any difficult-to-test patient (via conventional audiometry), so it is an essential tool for follow-up to UNHS/other NHS.
9. Consideration of effects of early maturation is critical for proper interpretation of ABRs.
10. Sooner or later, if failing to obtain reliable results via conventional audiologic testing, will likely need to consider more ERAudiometry using ABRs and/or longer-latency AEPs.

Episode 2

1. Reliable AC threshold estimation is essential to ERA as in conventional audiometry but may require correction factors for infants for best estimates.
2. BC test results are substantially different between infants and adults and that differs across audiometric test frequency, and this challenges accurate air-bone gap estimations.
3. BC in infants reveals a curious, yet quite useful, asymmetry of crossover stimulation.
4. Multiple factors contribute to the BC-asymmetry effect and must be well understood.
5. Stimulus artifact in BC testing is a substantial concern, especially when using brief tone bursts, yet manageable for ERA when understood.
6. Effective masking as in BC-pure-tone audiometry is a particular challenge in infants.
7. There remains insufficient data in infants for such effects as interaural attenuation to apply (as in conventional audiometry) to ERA for the most accurate threshold estimations.

Episode 3

1. Although the brainstem responses are robust for ERA, the pervasive requirement is a kind of cooperation—voluntarily or otherwise—in the interest of a low noise floor for reliability.
2. Involuntary relaxation can be achieved by way of natural or drug-induced sedation, introducing a number of additional aspects to patient management for competent testing.
3. The environment of newborn and more so NICU nurseries is a world apart from audiology clinics with more risks of both significant acoustic and electrical interference.
4. Fortunately, there are specialized eartips/earcaps to use with newborns to present sounds with some acoustic noise isolation.
5. Familiarity/experience with young infants and their less-than-mature ABRs is important for proper interpretation of recordings.

6. Beyond experience on the frontline of nurseries is that required in follow-up testing of what still are immature patients—requiring appropriate methods and still dealing with patient state.
7. Beyond natural sleep, if unavoidable but clear need to know, testing patients under sedation/anesthesia will require considerations/organization beyond the actual clinic.
8. Whether natural or induced sleep, proper scheduling and instruction of the caregiver is critical for success to have ample time for thorough and reliable testing.
9. Scheduling is not about what is convenient for clinic and caregiver, rather symbiotic with the infant's daily routine; for example, feeding/nap times if testing under natural sleep.
10. The audiologist must be prepared and use a well-planned protocol (per type of test and stimuli used) as well as make possible adaptations for whatever reasons.

Heads Up

11. In conventional audiometry, patients inevitably have criteria for responding, a nonsensory variable that can bias results unacceptably if exaggerated (whether purposefully or otherwise).
12. Objective measures can help get to the truth but need to meet the special circumstances of the individual and (again) have the full auditory pathway in mind.

Episode 4

1. The electric signal through the cochlear implant differs remarkably from the acoustic input.
2. Testing via the CI naturally requires additional technology; today, testing the patient with their device is possible given an interface and computational "tools" for the audiologist to use.
3. Relative to conventional AEP testing, the signals transmitted to the indwelling device to power and command it create an extraordinarily large electrical-stimulus artifact.
4. There are several configurations of instrumentation that permit testing of the CI patient, either essentially using a conventional AEP test system or telemetry from the implant.
5. Clinicians desire readily accessible and straightforward measures of performance, comparable to input-output measurements, hence the development of telemetry in CIs.
6. The telemetry option is dedicated to a test of the (residual) 8th nerve, but via the other configurations, the EABR (and later Rs) can be tested as well.
7. In the face of deformities/other problems precluding development of a functional nerve, an alternative to the CI is to stimulate centrally, hence the development of the ABI.
8. ALLRs—cortical obligatory potentials and beyond—are excellent for testing CI/ABI users.

References

1. Harrison, M., & Roush, J. (1996). Age of suspicion, identification and intervention for infants and young children with hearing loss: A national study. *Ear and Hearing, 17*(1), 55–62.
2. Watkin, P. M., Baldwin, M., & McEnery, G. (1991). Neonatal at risk screening and the identification of deafness. *Archives of Disease in Childhood, 66*(10), 1130–1135.
3. Yoshinaga-Itano, C., Sedey, A. L., Coulter, D. K., & Mehl, A. L. (1998). Language of early- and later-identified children with hearing loss. *Pediatrics, 102*(5), 1161–1171.
4. Joint Committee on Infant Hearing. (2019). Year 2019 position statement: Principles and guidelines for early hearing detection and intervention programs. *Journal of Early Hearing Detection and Intervention, 4*(2), 1–44.
5. National Institutes of Health. (1993). Early identification of hearing impairment in infants and young children. *NIH Consensus Statement, 11*(1), 1–24. https://consensus.nih.gov/1993/1993hearinginfantschildren092pdf.pdf
6. Joint Committee on Infant Hearing. (1994). Joint committee on infant hearing 1994 position statement. *Pediatrics, 95*(1), 152–156. http://www.jcih.org/JCIH1994.pdf

7. Joint Committee on Infant Hearing. (2000). Position statement: Principles and guidelines for early hearing detection and intervention programs. *Pediatrics, 120*, 898–921.
8. Joint Committee on Infant Hearing. (2007). Year 2007 position statement: Principles and guidelines for early hearing detection and intervention programs. *Pediatrics, 120*(4), 898–921.
9. European Consensus Statement on Neonatal Hearing Screening. Finalized at the European Consensus Development Conference on Neonatal Hearing Screening. Milan, 15–16 May 1998. (1999). *Acta Paediatrica, 88*(1), 107–108.
10. Erenberg, A., Lemons, J., Sia, C., Trunkel, D., & Ziring, P. (1999). Newborn and infant hearing loss: Detection and intervention. American Academy of Pediatrics. Task Force on Newborn and Infant Hearing, 1998–1999. *Pediatrics, 103*(2), 527–530.
11. Newborn Hearing Screening Programmes Clinical Group. (2013, July). Guidelines for the early audiological assessment and management of babies referred from the Newborn Hearing Screening Programme. British Society of Audiology (Version 3.1, p. 44). *British Society of Audiology.* https://www.thebsa.org.uk/wp-content/uploads/2014/08/NHSP_NeonateAssess_2014.pdf
12. Norton, S. J., Gorga, M. P., Widen, J. E., Folsom, R. C., Sininger, Y., Cone-Wesson, B., . . . Fletcher, K. (2000). Identification of neonatal hearing impairment: Evaluation of transient evoked otoacoustic emission, distortion product otoacoustic emission, and auditory brain stem response test performance. *Ear and Hearing, 21*(5), 508–528.
13. Kanji, A., Khoza-Shangase, K., & Moroe, N. (2018). Newborn hearing screening protocols and their outcomes: A systematic review. *International Journal of Pediatric Otorhinolaryngology, 115*, 104–109.
14. Watkin, P. M. (2001). Neonatal screening for hearing impairment. *Seminars in Neonatology, 6*, 501–509.
15. Watkin, P. M., & Baldwin, M. (1999). Confirmation of deafness in infancy. *Archives of Disease in Childhood, 81*(5), 380–389.
16. Kemp, D. T., Ryan, S., & Bray, P. (1990). A guide to the effective use of otoacoustic emissions. *Ear and Hearing, 11*(2), 93–105.
17. Hyde, M. L. (2005). Newborn hearing screening programmes: Overview. *Journal of Otolaryngology, 34*(Suppl. 2), S70–S78.
18. Herrmann, B. S., Thornton, A. R., & Joseph, J. M. (1995). Automated infant hearing screening using the ABR: Development and validation. *American Journal of Audiology, 4*(2), 6–14.
19. Vohr, B., Carty, L. M., Moore, P. E., & Letourneau, K. (1998). The Rhode Island hearing assessment program: Experience with statewide hearing screening (1993–1996). *Journal of Pediatrics, 133*(3), 353–357.
20. Lin, H. C., Shu, M. T., Lee, K. S., Ho, G. M., Fu, T. Y., Bruna, S., & Lin, G. (2005). Comparison of hearing screening programs between one step with transient evoked otoacoustic emissions (TEOAE) and two steps with TEOAE and automated auditory brainstem response. *Laryngoscope, 115*(11), 1957–1962.
21. Lin, H. C., Shu, M. T., Lee, K. S., Lin, H. Y., & Lin, G. (2007). Reducing false positives in newborn hearing screening program: How and why. *Otology & Neurotology, 28*(6), 788–792.
22. Chapchap, M. J., & Segre, C. M. (2001). Universal newborn hearing screening and transient evoked otoacoustic emission: New concepts in Brazil. *Scandinavian Audiology, 30*(2), 33–36.
23. Hayes, D. (June, 2008). *Auditory neuropathy guidelines development conference.* Presented at the International Newborn Hearing Screening Conference, Como, Italy. http://www.infanthearing.org/meeting/ehdi2009/EHDI%202009%20Presentations/36n.pdf
24. Hyde, M. L., Riko, K., Corbin, H., Moroso, M., & Alberti, P. W. (1984). A neonatal hearing screening research program using brainstem electric response audiometry. *Journal of Otolaryngology, 13*(1), 49.
25. Hyde, M. L., Riko, K., & Malizia, K. (1990). Audiometric accuracy of the click ABR in infants at risk for hearing loss. *Journal of the American Academy of Audiology, 1*(2), 59–66.
26. Olusanya, B. O., Wirz, S. L., & Luxon, L. M. (2008). Hospital-based universal newborn hearing screening for early detection of permanent congenital hearing loss in Lagos, Nigeria. *International Journal of Pediatric Otorhinolaryngology, 72*(7), 991–1001.
27. Wood, S. A., Sutton, G. J., & Davis, A. C. (2015). Performance and characteristics of the Newborn Hearing Screening Programme in England: The first seven years. *International Journal of Audiology, 54*(6), 353–358.
28. U.S. Preventive Services Task Force. (2008). Universal screening for hearing loss in newborns: U.S. Preventive Services Task Force recommendation statement. *Pediatrics, 122*(1), 143–148.
29. Berruecos, P. (2008). National newborn hearing screening program in Mexico. *Community Ear and Hearing Health, 5*(7), 8–10.
30. Smith, A. (2003). Preventing deafness—An achievable challenge. The WHO perspective. *International Congress Series, 1240*, 183–191.

31. Zakzouk, S. (2002). Consanguinity and hearing impairment in developing countries: A custom to be discouraged. *The Journal of Laryngology & Otology, 116*(10), 811–816.
32. Gorga, M. P., Reiland, J. K., Beauchaine, K. A., Worthington, D. W., & Jesteadt, W. (1987). Auditory brainstem responses from graduates of an intensive care nursery: Normal patterns of response. *Journal of Speech, Language, and Hearing Research, 30*(3), 311–318.
33. Durrant, J. D., & Collet, L. (2007). Integrating otoacoustic emissions and electrophysiologic measures as the basis for differential diagnostic applications. In M. S. Robinette & T. J. Glattke (Eds.), *Otoacoustic emissions: Clinical applications* (3rd ed., pp. 273–295). Thieme.
34. John, M. S., & Picton, T. W. (2000). MASTER: A Windows program for recording multiple auditory steady-state responses. *Computer Methods and Programs in Biomedicine, 61*(2), 125–150.
35. Cone, B., & Whitaker, R. (2013). Dynamics of infant cortical auditory evoked potentials (CAEPs) for tone and speech tokens. *International Journal of Pediatric Otorhinolaryngology, 77*(7), 1162–1173.
36. Tlumak, A. I., Durrant, J. D., Delgado, R. E., & Boston, J. R. (2012). Steady-state analysis of auditory evoked potentials over a wide range of stimulus repetition rates: Profile in children vs. adults. *International Journal of Audiology, 51*(6), 480–490.
37. Small, S. A., & Stapells, D. R. (2003). Normal brief-tone bone-conduction behavioural thresholds using the B-71 transducer: Three occlusion conditions. *Journal of the American Academy of Audiology, 14*(10), 556–562.
38. Stapells, D. R., & Ruben, R. J. (1989). Auditory brain stem responses to bone-conducted tones in infants. *Annals of Otology, Rhinology and Laryngology, 98*(12), 941–949.
39. Cone-Wesson, B., & Ramirez, G. M. (1997). Hearing sensitivity in newborns estimated from ABRs to bone-conducted sounds. *Journal of the American Academy of Audiology, 8*, 299–307.
40. Vander Werff, K. R., Prieve, B. A., & Georgantas, L. M. (2009). Infant air and bone conduction tone burst auditory brain stem responses for classification of hearing loss and the relationship to behavioral thresholds. *Ear and Hearing, 30*(3), 350–368.
41. Ferm, I., Lightfoot, G., & Stevens, J. (2014). Provisional stimulus level corrections for low frequency bone-conduction ABR in babies under three months corrected age. *International Journal of Audiology, 53*(2), 132–137.
42. Small, S. A., & Stapells, D. R. (2017). Frequency-specific threshold assessment in infants using frequency-specific auditory brainstem response and the auditory steady-state response. In A. M. Tharpe & R. C. Seewald (Eds.), *Comprehensive handbook of pediatric audiology* (2nd ed., pp. 505–549). Plural Publishing.
43. Small, S. A., & Stapells, D. R. (2008b). Maturation of bone conduction multiple auditory steady-state responses. *International Journal of Audiology, 47*(8), 476–488.
44. Small, S. A., & Stapells, D. R. (2006). Multiple auditory steady-state response thresholds to bone-conduction stimuli in young infants with normal hearing. *Ear and Hearing, 27*(3), 219–228.
45. Small, S. A., Hatton, J. L., & Stapells, D. R. (2007). Effects of bone vibrator coupling method, placement location, and occlusion on bone-conduction auditory steady-state responses in infants. *Ear and Hearing, 28*(1), 83–98.
46. Valeriote, H., & Small, S. A. (2015, May). *Comparison of air- and bone-conduction auditory brainstem and multiple 80-Hz auditory steady-state responses in infants with normal hearing and conductive hearing loss.* Presented at the XXIV Biennial Symposium of the International Evoked Response Audiometry Study Group, Busan, Korea.
47. Small, S. A., Smyth, A., & Leon, G. (2014). Effective masking levels for 500 and 2000 Hz bone conduction auditory steady-state responses in infants and adults with normal hearing. *Ear and Hearing, 35*(1), 63–71.
48. Nagashima, H., Udaka, J., Chida, I., Shimada, A., Kondo, E., & Takeda, N. (2013). Air-bone gap estimated with multiple auditory steady-state response in young children with otitis media with effusion. *Auris Nasus Larynx, 40*(6), 534–538.
49. Ferm, I., & Lightfoot, G. (2015). Further comparisons of ABR response amplitudes, test time, and estimation of hearing threshold using frequency-specific chirp and tone pip stimuli in newborns: Findings at 0.5 and 2 kHz. *International Journal of Audiology, 54*(10), 745–750.
50. Cobb, K. M., & Stuart, A. (2016). Neonate auditory brainstem responses to CE-chirp and CE-chirp octave band stimuli I: Versus click and tone burst stimuli. *Ear and Hearing, 37*(6), 710–723.
51. Rodrigues, G. R., & Lewis, D. R. (2014). Establishing auditory steady-state response thresholds to narrow band CE-chirps(®) in full-term neonates. *International Journal of Pediatric Otorhinolaryngology, 78*(2), 238–243.

52. Elberling, C., Callø, J., & Don, M. (2010). Evaluating auditory brainstem responses to different chirp stimuli at three levels of stimulation. *Journal of the Acoustical Society of America, 128*(1), 215–223.
53. Elberling, C., & Don, M. (2010). A direct approach for the design of chirp stimuli used for the recording of auditory brainstem responses. *Journal of the Acoustical Society of America, 128*(5), 2955–2964.
54. Jeng, F. C., Brown, C. J., Johnson, T. A., & Vander Werff, K. R. (2004). Estimating air-bone gaps using auditory steady-state responses. *Journal of the American Academy of Audiology, 15*(1), 67–78.
55. Small, S. A., & Stapells, D. R. (2004). Artifactual responses when recording auditory steady-state responses. *Ear and Hearing, 25*(6), 611–623.
56. British Columbia Early Hearing Program. (2012). *Diagnostic audiology protocol*. http://www.phsa.ca/Documents/bcehpaudiologyassessmentprotocol.pdf
57. Small, S. A., & Hu, N. (2011). Maturation of the occlusion effect: A bone conduction auditory steady state response study in infants and adults with normal hearing. *Ear and Hearing, 32*(6), 708–719.
58. Studebaker, G. A. (1967). Clinical masking of the non-test ear. *Journal of Speech and Hearing Disorders, 32*(4), 360–371.
59. Stenfelt, S. (2012). Transcranial attenuation of bone-conducted sound when stimulation is at the mastoid and at the bone conduction hearing aid position. *Otology and Neurotology, 33*(2), 105–114.
60. Reinfeldt, S., Stenfelt, S., & Håkansson, B. (2013). Estimation of bone conduction skull transmission by hearing thresholds and ear-canal sound pressure. *Hearing Research, 299*, 19–28.
61. Edwards, C. G., Durieux-Smith, A., & Picton, T. W. (1985). Neonatal auditory brainstem responses from ipsilateral and contralateral recording montages. *Ear and Hearing, 6*(4), 175–178.
62. Stapells, D. R., & Mosseri, M. (1991). Maturation of the contralaterally recorded auditory brain stem response. *Ear and Hearing, 12*(3), 167–173.
63. Sininger, Y. S., & Hyde, M. L. (2009). Auditory brainstem response in audiometric threshold prediction. In J. Katz, L. Medwetsky, R. Burkard, & L. Hood (Eds.), *Handbook of clinical audiology* (6th ed., pp. 293–321). Lippincott Williams & Wilkins.
64. Stapells, D. R. (1989). Auditory brainstem response assessment of infants and children. *Seminars in Hearing, 10*, 229–251.
65. Hatton, J. L., Janssen, R. M., & Stapells, D. R. (2012). Auditory brainstem responses to bone-conducted brief tones in young children with conductive or sensorineural hearing loss. *International Journal of Otolaryngology, 2012*, 1–12.
66. Small, S. A., & Love, A. (2014). An investigation into the clinical utility of ipsilateral/contralateral asymmetries in bone-conduction auditory steady-state responses. *International Journal of Audiology, 53*(9), 604–612.
67. Steele, D. G., & Bramblett, C. A. (1988). *The anatomy and biology of the human skeleton*. Texas A&M University Press.
68. Carlson, B. M. (1999). *Human embryology and developmental biology* (2nd ed., pp. 166–170). Mosby.
69. Stuart, A., Yang, E. Y., & Stenstrom, R. (1990). Effect of temporal area bone vibrator placement on auditory brain stem response in newborn infants. *Ear and Hearing, 11*(5), 363–369.
70. Foxe, J. J., & Stapells, D. R. (1993). Normal infant and adult auditory brainstem responses to bone conducted tones. *Audiology, 32*(2), 95–109.
71. Stuart, A., Yang, E. Y., & Botea, M. (1996). Neonatal auditory brainstem responses recorded from four electrode montages. *Journal of Communication Disorders, 29*(2), 125–139.
72. Small, S. A., & Stapells, D. R. (2008a). Normal ipsilateral/contralateral asymmetries in infant multiple auditory steady-state responses to air-and bone-conduction stimuli. *Ear and Hearing, 29*(2), 185–198.
73. Stamatas, G. N., Nikolovski, J., Mack, M. C., & Kollias, N. (2011). Infant skin physiology and development during the first years of life: A review of recent findings based on in vivo studies. *International Journal of Cosmetic Sciences, 33*(1), 17–24.
74. Mackey, A. R., Hodgetts, W. E., & Small, S.A. (2018). Maturation of bone-conduction transcranial attenuation using a measure of sound pressure in the ear canal. *International Journal of Audiology, 57*(4), 283–290.
75. Yang, E. Y., Rupert, A. L., & Moushegian, G. (1987). A developmental study of bone conduction auditory brain stem response in infants. *Ear and Hearing, 8*(4), 244–251.
76. Sohmer, H., Freeman, S., Geal-Dor, M., Adelman, C., & Savion, I. (2000). Bone conduction experiments in humans—A fluid pathway from bone to ear. *Hearing Research, 146*(1–2), 81–88.
77. Moore, J. K., Ponton, C. W., Eggermont, J. J., Wu, B. C., & Huang, J. Q. (1996). Perinatal maturation of the auditory brain stem response: changes in path length and conduction velocity. *Ear and Hearing, 17*(5), 411–418.
78. Ponton, C. W., Moore, J. K., & Eggermont, J. J. (1996). Auditory brain stem response generation by parallel pathways: differential maturation of axonal conduction time and synaptic transmission. *Ear and Hearing, 17*(5), 402–410.

79. Hood, J. D. (1960). The principles and practice of bone conduction audiometry: A review of the present position. *Laryngoscope, 70*(9), 1211–1228.
80. Hansen, E., & Small, S. A. (2012). Effective masking levels for bone conduction auditory steady-state responses in infants and adults with normal hearing. *Ear and Hearing, 32*(2), 257–266.
81. Lau, R., & Small, S. A. (2020). Effective masking levels for bone conduction auditory brainstem response stimuli in infants and adults with normal hearing. *Ear and Hearing*. Advance online publication. https://doi.org/10.1097/AUD.0000000000000947
82. Herdman, A. T., & Stapells, D. R. (2001). Thresholds determined using the monotic and dichotic multiple auditory steady-state response technique in normal-hearing subjects. *Scandinavian Audiology, 30*(1), 41–49.
83. John, M. S., Lins, O. G., Boucher, B. L., & Picton, T. W. (1998). Multiple auditory steady-state responses (MASTER): Stimulus and recording parameters. *Audiology, 37*(2), 59–82.
84. Ishida, I. M., & Stapells, D. R. (2012). Multiple-ASSR interactions in adults with sensorineural hearing loss. *International Journal of Otolaryngology, 2012*, 1–9.
85. Hatton, J. L., & Stapells, D. R. (2011). Efficiency of single- vs. multiple-stimulus auditory steady-state responses in infants. *Ear and Hearing, 32*(3), 349–357.
86. Hatton, J. L., & Stapells, D. R. (2013). Monotic versus dichotic multiple-stimulus auditory steady state responses in young children. *Ear and Hearing, 34*(5), 680–682.
87. Mo, L., & Stapells, D. R. (2008). The effect of brief-tone stimulus duration on the brain stem auditory steady-state response. *Ear and Hearing, 29*(1), 121–133.
88. Torres-Fortuny, A., Hernández-Pérez, H., Ramírez, B., Alonso, I., Eimil, E., Guerrero-Aranda, A., & Mijares, E. (2016) Comparing auditory steady-state responses amplitude evoked by simultaneous air- and bone-conducted stimulation in newborns. *International Journal of Audiology, 55*(6), 375–379.
89. Wachman, E. M., & Lahav, A. (2011). The effects of noise on preterm infants in the NICU. *Archives of Disease in Childhood-Fetal and Neonatal Edition, 96*(4), F305–F309.
90. Berg, A. L., Chavez, C. T., & Serpanos, Y. C. (2010). Monitoring noise levels in a tertiary neonatal intensive care unit. *Contemporary Issues in Communication Science and Disorders, 37*, 69–72.
91. Zahr, L. K., & de Traversay, J. (1995). Premature infant responses to noise reduction by earmuffs: Effects on behavioral and physiologic measures. *Journal of Perinatology, 15*(6), 448–455.
92. Abdeyazdan, Z., Ghassemi, S., & Marofi, M. (2014). The effects of earmuff on physiologic and motor responses in premature infants admitted in neonatal intensive care unit. *Iranian Journal of Nursing and Midwifery Research, 19*(2), 107–112.
93. Ponton, C. W., & Eggermont, J. J. (2007). Electrophysiological measures of human auditory system maturation. In R. E. Burkard, M. Don, & J. J. Eggermont (Eds.), *Auditory evoked potentials: Basic principles and clinical application* (pp.358–402). Lippincott Williams & Wilkins.
94. Salamy, A., Mc Kean, C. M., & Buda, F. B. (1975). Maturational changes in auditory transmission as reflected in human brain stem potentials. *Brain Research, 96*, 361–366.
95. Coté, C. J., & Wilson, S. (2006). Guidelines for monitoring and management of pediatric patients during and after sedation for diagnostic and therapeutic procedures: An update. *Pediatrics, 118*(6), 2587–2602.
96. Coté, C. J., & Wilson, S. (2016). Guidelines for monitoring and management of pediatric patients before, during, and after sedation for diagnostic and therapeutic procedures: Update 2016. *Pediatric Dentistry, 38*(4), E13–E39.
97. Schmidt, C. M., Knief, A., Deuster, D., Matulat, P., & am Zehnhoff-Dinnesen, A. G. (2007). Melatonin is a useful alternative to sedation in children undergoing brainstem audiometry with an age dependent success rate-a field report of 250 investigations. *Neuropediatrics, 38*(1), 2–4.
98. Casteil, L., Viquesnel, A., Favier, V., Guignard, N., Blanchet, C., & Mondain, M. (2017). Study of the efficacy of melatonin for auditory brainstem response (ABR) testing in children. *European Annals of Otorhinolaryngology, Head and Neck Diseases, 134*(6), 373–375.
99. Behrman, D. B., Bishop, J. L., Godsell, J., Shirley, B., Storey, S., Carroll, W. W., & Prosser, J. D. (2020). Efficacy of melatonin for auditory brainstem response testing in children: A systematic review. *International Journal of Pediatric Otorhinolaryngology, 131*, 109861.
100. Fowler, K. B., McCollister, F. P., Sabo, D. L., Shoup, A. G., Owen, K. E., Woodruff, J. L., . . . Boppana, S. B. (2017). A targeted approach for congenital cytomegalovirus screening within newborn hearing screening. *Pediatrics, 139*(2), e20162128.
101. Durrant, J. D., Kesterson, R. K., & Kamerer, D. B. (1997). Evaluation of the nonorganic hearing loss suspect. *American Journal of Otology, 18*(3), 361–367.
102. Hyde, M., Matsumoto, N., Alberti, P., & Li, Y. L. (1986). Auditory evoked potentials in audiometric

assessment of compensation and medicolegal patients. *Annals of Otology, Rhinology & Laryngology, 95*(5), 514–519.
103. Picton, T. W., & Hillyard, S. A. (1974). Human auditory evoked potentials. II: Effects of attention. *Electroencephalography and Clinical Neurophysiology, 36*, 191–200.
104. Kiang, N. Y. S., Moxon, E. C., & Kahn, A. R. (1976). The relationship of gross potentials recorded from the cochlea to single unit activity in the auditory nerve. In R. J. Ruben, C. Elberling, & G. Salomon (Eds.), *Electrocochleography* (pp. 95–115). University Park Press.
105. Gilley, P. M., Sharma, A., Dorman, M., Finley, C. C., Panch, A. S., & Martin, K. (2006). Minimization of cochlear implant stimulus artifact in cortical auditory evoked potentials. *Clinical Neurophysiology, 117*(8), 1772–1782.
106. Viola, F. C., Thorne, J. D., Bleeck, S., Eyles, J., & Debener, S. (2011). Uncovering auditory evoked potentials from cochlear implant users with independent component analysis. *Psychophysiology, 48*(11), 1470–1480.
107. Kileny, P. (2019). *The audiologist's handbook of intraoperative neurophysiological monitoring.* Plural Publishing.
108. Kuo, S. C., & Gibson, W. P. (2002). The role of the promontory stimulation test in cochlear implantation. *Cochlear Implants International, 3*(1), 19–28.
109. Polterauer, D., Neuling, M., Müller, J., Hempel, J. M., Mandruzzato, G., & Polak, M. (2018). PromBERA: A preoperative eABR: An update. *Current Directions in Biomedical Engineering, 4*(1), 563–565.
110. McMahon, C. M., Patuzzi, R. B., Gibson, W. P., & Sanli, H. (2008). Frequency-specific electrocochleography indicates that presynaptic and postsynaptic mechanisms of auditory neuropathy exist. *Ear and Hearing, 29*(3), 314–325.
111. Van Yper, L. N., Dhooge, I. J., Vermeire, K., De Vel, E. F., & Beynon, A. J. (2020). The P300 auditory event-related potential as a method to assess the benefit of contralateral hearing aid use in bimodal listeners: A proof-of-concept. *International Journal of Audiology, 59*(1), 73–80.
112. O'Leary, S., Briggs, R., Gerard, J. M., Iseli, C., Wei, B. P., Tari, S., . . . Bester, C. (2020). Intraoperative observational real-time electrocochleography as a predictor of hearing loss after cochlear implantation: 3 and 12 month outcomes. *Otology & Neurotology, 41*(9), 1222–1229.
113. Cafarelli Dees, D., Dillier, N., Lai, W. K., von Wallenberg, E., van Dijk, B., Akdas, F., . . . Smoorenburg, G. F. (2005). Normative findings of electrically evoked compound action potential measurements using the neural response telemetry of the Nucleus CI24M cochlear implant system. *Audiology & Neuro-Otology, 10*(2), 105–116.
114. He, S., McFayden, T. C., Shahsavarani, B. S., Teagle, H. F., Ewend, M., Henderson, L., & Buchman, C. A. (2017). The electrically evoked auditory change complex evoked by temporal gaps using cochlear implants or auditory brainstem implants in children with cochlear nerve deficiency. *Ear and Hearing, 39*(3), 482–494.
115. Jacquemin, L., Mertens, G., Schlee, W., Van de Heyning, P., & Gilles, A. (2019). Literature overview on P3 measurement as an objective measure of auditory performance in post-lingually deaf adults with a cochlear implant. *International Journal of Audiology, 58*(12), 816–823.
116. Sennaroğlu, L., Colletti, V., Lenarz, T., Manrique, M., Laszig, R., Rask-Andersen, H., . . . Bayazıt, Y. (2016). Consensus statement: Long-term results of ABI in children with complex inner ear malformations and decision making between CI and ABI. *Cochlear Implants International, 17*(4), 163–171.
117. Abbas, P. J., & Brown, C. J. (1991). Electrically evoked auditory brainstem response: Refractory properties and strength-duration functions. *Hearing Research, 51*(1), 139–147.
118. Deep, N. L., Choudhury, B., & Roland, J. T., Jr. (2019). Auditory brainstem implantation: An overview. *Journal of Neurological Surgery: Part B, 80*(2), 203–208.
119. Hirschfelder, A., Gräbel, S., & Olze, H. (2012). Electrically evoked amplitude modulation following response in cochlear implant candidates: Comparison with auditory nerve response telemetry, subjective electrical stimulation, and speech perception. *Otology & Neurotology, 33*(6), 968–975.
120. Lundin, K., Stillesjö, F., & Rask-Andersen, H. (2015). Prognostic value of electrically evoked auditory brainstem responses in cochlear implantation. *Cochlear Implants International, 16*(5), 254–261.
121. Dees, D. C., Dillier, N., Lai, W. K., Von Wallenberg, E., Van Dijk, B., Akdas, F., . . . Chanal, J. M. (2005). Normative findings of electrically evoked compound action potential measurements using the neural response telemetry of the Nucleus CI24M cochlear implant system. *Audiology and Neurotology, 10*(2), 105–116.
122. McKay, C. M., & Smale, N. (2017). The relation between ECAP measurements and the effect of rate on behavioral thresholds in cochlear implant users. *Hearing Research, 346*, 62–70.

123. Davids, T., Valero, J., Papsin, B. C., Harrison, R. V., & Gordon, K. A. (2008). Effects of stimulus manipulation on electrophysiological responses of pediatric cochlear implant users. Part II: Rate effects. *Hearing Research, 244*(1–2), 15–24.
124. Firszt, J. B., Chambers, R. D., Kraus, N., & Reeder, R. M. (2002). Neurophysiology of cochlear implant users I: Effects of stimulus current level and electrode site on the electrical ABR, MLR, and N1-P2 response. *Ear and Hearing, 23*(6), 502–515.
125. Kurnaz, M., Satar, B., & Yetiser, S. (2009). Evaluation of cochlear implant users' performance using middle and late latency responses. *European Archives of Oto-Rhino-Laryngology, 266*(3), 343–350.
126. Deshpande, S. B., Lu, Z., Pan, T., & Ma, F. (2017). The relationship between electrical auditory middle-latency response components and measures of auditory performance and speech intelligibility in pediatric cochlear implant recipients. *Journal of the Acoustical Society of America, 141*(5), 3815.
127. Kileny, P. R. (2007). Evoked potentials in the management of patients with cochlear implants: Research and clinical applications. *Ear and Hearing, 28*(2), 124S–127S.
128. Visram, A. S., Innes-Brown, H., El-Deredy, W., & McKay, C. M. (2015). Cortical auditory evoked potentials as an objective measure of behavioral thresholds in cochlear implant users. *Hearing Research, 327*, 35–42.
129. Liebscher, T., Alberter, K., & Hoppe, U. (2018) Cortical auditory evoked potentials in cochlear implant listeners via single electrode stimulation in relation to speech perception. *International Journal of Audiology, 57*(12), 933–940.
130. Cardon, G., & Sharma, A. (2019). Somatosensory cross-modal reorganization in children with cochlear implants. *Frontiers in Neuroscience, 13*, 1–14.
131. Silva, L. A. F., Couto, M. I. V., Magliaro, F. C., Tsuji, R. K., Bento, R. F., de Carvalho, A. C. M., & Matas, C. G. (2017). Cortical maturation in children with cochlear implants: Correlation between electrophysiological and behavioral measurement. *PLoS One, 12*(2), e0171177.
132. Távora-Vieira, D., Wedekind, A., Marino, R., Purdy, S. C., & Rajan, G. P. (2018). Using aided cortical assessment as an objective tool to evaluate cochlear implant fitting in users with single-sided deafness. *PLoS one, 13*(2), e0193081.
133. Brown, C. J., Etler, C., He, S., O'Brien, S., Erenberg, S., Kim, J. R., . . . Abbas, P. J. (2008). The electrically evoked auditory change complex: Preliminary results from nucleus cochlear implant users. *Ear and Hearing, 29*(5), 704–714.
134. Haumann, S., Imsiecke, M., Bauernfeind, G., Büchner, A., Helmstaedter, V., Lenarz, T., & Salcher, R. B. (2019). Monitoring of the inner ear function during and after cochlear implant insertion using electrocochleography. *Trends in Hearing, 23*, 1–18.
135. Dalbert, A., Pfiffner, F., Hoesli, M., Koka, K., Veraguth, D., Roosli, C., & Huber, A. (2018). Assessment of cochlear function during cochlear implantation by extra-and intracochlear electrocochleography. *Frontiers in Neuroscience, 12*, 1–9.
136. Koka, K., Saoji, A. A., & Litvak, L. M. (2017). Electrocochleography in cochlear implant recipients with residual hearing: Comparison with audiometric thresholds. *Ear and Hearing, 38*(3), e161–e167.
137. He, S., Teagle, H. F., & Buchman, C. A. (2017). The electrically evoked compound action potential: From laboratory to clinic. *Frontiers in Neuroscience, 11*, 339.
138. Ramos-Macias, A., O'Leary, S., Ramos-de Miguel, A., Bester, C., & Falcon-González, J. C. (2019). Intraoperative intracochlear electrocochleography and residual hearing preservation outcomes when using two types of slim electrode arrays in cochlear implantation. *Otology & Neurotology, 40*(5S), S29–S37.

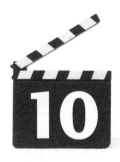

10

Testing Potentially Beyond Hearing-Related Yet of Interest in Audiology the Profession

> **The Writers**
>
> Heads Up: John D. Durrant,
>   David L. McPherson, and
>   Lionel Collet
> Episode 1: Abreena I. Tlumak and
>   John D. Durrant
> Heads Up: John D. Durrant and
>   Abreena I. Tlumak
> Episode 2: Suzanne C. Purdy

HEADS UP

Not Only Electric Fields, Magnetic Fields Too—Confirming Origins

In first discussing basic principles of measurement and generation of signals to record electrically from the auditory system and (next step) tapping into such signals on the scalp of humans, the concern was to have an appropriate interface so that bioelectricity can be optimally measured using instruments that operate on physical electricity. It was sufficient to consider Ohm's law for direct current (DC) circuits and note just a few concepts that extend it to alternating current (AC) circuits: auditory evoked potentials are largely AC signals. The law expresses the most fundamental concept of the relation among voltage (electrical pressure), current (electrical flow), and resistance (electrical friction), readily exemplified by the simple DC circuit of the common flash light. All three of these physical quantities are readily measureable in principle and are equally expressed in bioelectric systems. However, the measure used in conventional/clinical electrophysiology is that of voltage, as it is the most accessible metric of bioelectricity, noninvasively. Just put electrodes on the scalp (with due diligence, of course) and watch those little electroencephalographically recorded voltages go up and down.

Dipole estimation to predict actual locations of the neural generators of signals is

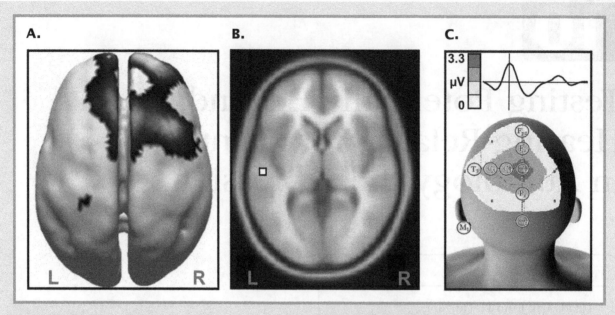

Figure 10–1. Looking into the brain by way of "imaging" its electrophysiological activity or other signs of neural activation: **A.** sLORETA; **B.** fMRI; **C.** basic topographical mapping. (See text.)

a considerably longer story than has been pursued thus far or shall be within the scope of this foundational textbook. Not that it is less than an intriguing enough story to tell, rather one of epic proportion. Indeed, the method of dipole estimation is a seductive statistical tool for producing curious and fascinating "imaging" by which to display auditory and other sensory responses of the brain from high-density recordings across the scalp (recall Figure 3–2B). The hope always has been that such quantitative techniques can localize and characterize the spread of the brain's electrical activity, if not discern loci of lesions. For generator dipole localization, the approach does and it does not; mostly, it does not from electroencephalography data. Figure 10–1A shows an example of results of multielectrode recordings and analysis using sLORETA (standardized low resolution brain electromagnetic tomography, here applied to EEG data). They are plotted as contours (colorized in practice, rendered in gray tone here) overlaid on a brain model. The results are from grand averages of data from this feature's second author laboratory, wherein the oddball paradigm was used to elicit the mismatch negativity (recall Figures 8–13 and 8–17). The stimulus paradigm was binaural stimulation with the standard-deviant contrast being diphthongs in English versus Khmer. Responses were recorded in a Native Khmer group of young adult listeners. It is notable how the sLORETA figure clearly shows various areas of activation from a 64-channel recording—left frontal and right midfrontal lobes (the "hottest areas" translated here to lighter-gray tones). In the same study, fMRI (functional magnetic resonance imaging) was used, having the ability to yield more precise localization data, as seen in panel B. Here, the statistical analysis applied was to find, in effect, the area of singularly most significant difference of MMN response. In other words, the fMRI permitted virtually pinpointing a structural location of activity—the left midtemporal lobe.[1]

The principal objective of dipole estimation is to give coordinates and orientation of the generator. So what's wrong with voltage/EEG-based methods to do so? Whatever may be lacking cannot be any fault of voltage, and it is going to be there regardless! Well, there is one thing; its measurement requires "touching" the subject, even if a bit indirectly with the metal electrode (somewhat floating on a cushion of electrolyte paste; recall Figure 3–1A). There also was nothing wrong in how well voltage can be sampled across the scalp, even if the interest was to record from sometimes 100 sites at a time, again using an electrode cap. The basic idea is exemplified (more modestly) in Figure 10–1C. This can be considered as a follow-up to the virtual demonstrations of Figure 3–4A and B, taking that next step and then some. It portrays the relative spread at the peak of P_2 of a cortical auditory evoked potential, thus a replot of the response recorded at C_Z from Figure 3–4B. This record is one of several that were used regarding front-to-back changes in the CAEP across the scalp, but actually comes from a subset of recordings from some 20 electrodes over the scalp. The data were processed with a program to produce a "brain map"—more formally, topographic map of the auditory/other evoked potentials, essentially the first-generation method of high-density recordings and analyses.[2] In Episode 4.1, the "trick" for extracting stimulus-elicited responses from the EEG and extraneous interference was that of tapping into the coherence of a true response's signal versus the incoherence of the virtually random background. The trick here can be thought of as tapping into the coherence of the signal across the scalp's surface. Such surface-mapping provided pretty pictures by which to visualize spread of activity recorded (far easier on the user's brain than looking at numerous tracings of responses, recalling Figures 3–4 and 7–6A). Nevertheless, the method proved insufficient for "zeroing-in" on loci of AEP generators. Since this debut, continued research and development, advances in computer technology, employment of more and more channels of recording, and further advances in mathematical modeling have led to continued refinements and interests. Indeed, that level of fruition has come to be realized by technological advances in recordings of EEG/evoked responses permitting routine use of 64 or many more electrodes and software development for relatively broad (research or clinical) use, thus providing powerful tools for certain applications. Yet, less than ideal for dipole estimation, as such. So, if there is a better "mouse trap," then what can be its basis? What else is there than voltage as a signal source in the domain of noninvasive electrophysiology? Back to the flashlight circuit.

Pulling out the light bulb and battery and substituting a couple lengths of insulated wire to complete the circuit would readily demonstrate another consequence of the flow of electrical current. Rather than trashing a perfectly good portable light source, this demonstration (as before) can be a mind game, but can be explained with the aid of Figure 10–2A. Grasping the wire from the positive pole of the battery with the right hand, as illustrated, and extending the thumb toward the light bulb or other resistive load indicates the direction of current flow away from the positive pole of the battery (by convention). The fingers curled around the lead demonstrate another effect. Direction of *lines of flux* of an *electromagnetic field* circling the wire counterclockwise; this is the *right-hand rule*.[3] Bottom line: the flow of electricity through a conductor generates a magnetic field. That is, current flow is a moving electrical charge in the wire, which in turn causes an electromagnetic field surrounding the wire to develop. Therefore, sensing this field is not about contacting the bare wire, and although often a matter of electrical safety, the insulation of wire is largely inconsequential. Common insulations include the likes of rubber, plastics, some lacquers, and (in biology) myelin. In this example, the electromagnetic field is minuscule, although its presence is confirmable using a compass. There also are means of concentrating electromagnetic fields, as done

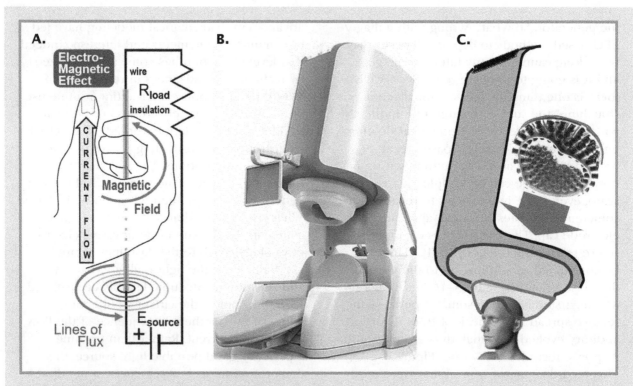

Figure 10–2. A. Right-hand rule of direction of rotation lines of magnetic flux around a wire conducting electricity. E_{source}—battery/source of direct current in this example; R_{load}—resistive load "drawing" current, like a flashlight's bulb. **B.** Magnetoelectroencephalography (MEG) system, as used to measure auditory evoked fields (AEFs), courtesy of CTF MEG Neuro Innovations, Incorporated. **C.** Sketch of subject head positioning and the dewar—helmetlike device that supports the sensors (see text). Note: inset image of the dewar virtually enlarged ~2× for illustration purposes.

in appliances, similar to electromagnetic transducers in earphones and loudspeakers, and when superconcentrated in design of electromagnets that can pick up whole automobiles in the junk yard. In earphones/loudspeakers, AC is applied to coils of wire to push and pull alternatingly a permanent magnet attached to the diaphragm or a speaker cone, thus generating alternating pressures (namely, sound pressure) following the reversals of the magnetic field. Although bioelectricity is somewhat different and neurons' body types vary along the auditory and other pathways to form complex groupings, these electrical devices still must obey the laws of physics. They too must and do give off measureable electromagnetic fields. The measurement of the ongoing electromagnetic fields of the brain is termed ***magnetoelectroencephalography (MEG)***. Consequently, in parallel to the concept and phenomena of the AEP is the ***auditory evoked field (AEF)***, thus another basis by which to explore auditory event-related responses.

Seems simple enough in principle, yet technically far more difficult practically. If measurement of micro- or even picovolts is a sobering challenge in measuring AEPs, they are nothing compared to sampling the incredibly minute magnetic fields in question. The latter was a substantial problem in the earliest years of practical exploration of AEFs, but long since addressed by solid-state electronics and a combination of the equivalent of high-quality audio recording instruments and computing. The **biomagnetic fields** of interest here are for brain waves, more than 10^7 times weaker and for AEFs, more than 10^9 times weaker than earth's magnetic field. The sensing of diminishingly small magnetic fields is the epitome of the expression, "a whole new ballgame," requiring extremely low-noise amplifiers of ultracooled circuit components (just for starters). For instance, resistances distributed in any circuit must be minimalized, as they are substantial sources of voltage (signal) loss and/or internal/thermal noise. The good news is that sensors and other electronics have been developed to do the job and to do so by noninvasive methods—no touching—just sort of hoovering nearby. Interestingly, some of the more fundamental technology underlying the ultimate practical demonstrations of MEG, including sensory evoked fields, was seeded at about the same time (late-1960s to early 1970s) as AEP technology was coming to the fore in hearing science and clinical electrophysiology in audiology. It took a bit longer for MEG to be brought to human research laboratories and medical facilities, but vigorous research and development ensued along with work in MEG/AEF, generating the voluminous literature of today.

The modern evoked (voltage) response test system can serve both clinical and bedside or cribside uses wherein a cart to transport the instrumentation needed is generally larger than the instrumentation itself, computer included. Interface to the patient employs several wires or an electrode cap. A modern MEG system is shown in Figure 10–2B and an accompanying sketch in panel C further characterizes the overall dimensions involved. A more sobering detail of what it takes to accommodate such a system is that the adjustable semireclining couch supporting the patient (as seen in panel B) is indeed an integral part of the apparatus. This is due to the need for highly stable and safe support of the front end of the system—a good part of which is looming over the head of the subject. For advanced imaging techniques, forget bedside testing. This paraphernalia and other supporting hardware, computer, and other electronics consume a lab space of equal to or greater dimensions than the typical single-patient hospital room. For purposes here, the part of the system parallel to an electrode cap for high-density EEG/AEP recordings is the **dewar** (see insert, panel C). This is a helmetlike support for the numerous sensors—**SQUID (superconducting quantum interference devices) gradiometers**—and which circulates liquid helium around them. Situated above the dewar, but not shown in the figure, is a tank of liquid helium. The price tag is also substantial, on the order of cost of instrumentation like that a MRI system. Given a substantial need for funds, space, and additional personnel with the necessary expertise, the immediate reaction may be, "This better be good, really good!" It is.

If not off the starting blocks of MEG/AEF research and development quite as quickly as that of AEP technology, it was quick to catch up and come to command essentially parallel and complementary AEP-related interests. Like EEG, MEG has both research and clinical interests (as in neurology and psychiatry). AEFs proved to provide better precision of specifying dipole generator location and orientation, more approximating capabilities of fMRI. AEFs essentially have been used to examine most of the same effects of stimulus parameters and nonpathological variables including maturation, effects of aging, effects of hearing loss, pursuit of objective indications of tinnitus, and (more recently) even research relevant to cochlear implantation. The MEG counterpart of the LLR N_1 component, $N_{100}m$ (or simply N_1m), has received and continues to receive much attention. At the same time, the method has been applied to AEFs from brainstem and beyond for both transient and steady-state paradigms, also those necessary for testing discrimination responses, like MMN and the cognitive potentials. For instance, in one of the most recent works, AEFs have

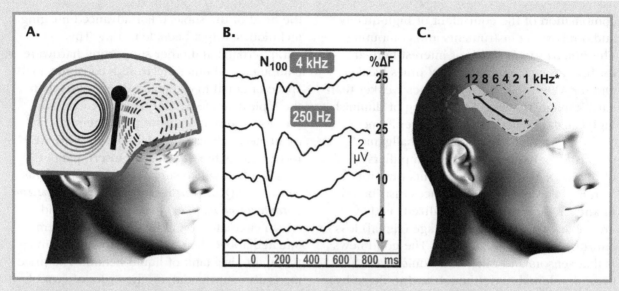

Figure 10–3. A. Outline of the dewar and cartoon illustrating nature of lines of flux and symbol of a dipole representing both magnitude and orientation in place of view. **B.** $N_{100}m$ (or N_1m) corresponding to N_1 of the auditory evoked potential, P_1-N_1-P_2 complex, in this case elicited by brief frequency modulations—upward changes of frequency for 100 ms every 1.4 s of a steady carrier—carrier frequencies and percent changes as indicated (based on data of Dimitrijevic and associates [2008][7]). **C.** Illustrated summary of results of a MEG study exploring AEFs over a range of upper frequencies (1 kHz–12 kHz); see text. Size of quasigraphical "projections" on the manikin's head exaggerated for purposes of illustration; overall length of the black-line function (for example) is only about 0.5 cm in situ (based on data of Gabriel and coworkers [2004][14]).

been examined using modulation of interaural timing.[4] The nature of the electromagnetic dipole is illustrated in Figure 10–3A (compare to voltage dipoles in Figure 3–5, bearing in mind that the orientation of the magnetic field is perpendicular to that of the voltage field). The literature is so expansive that it would be impractical to do it justice by an overview within the scope and space of a Heads Up. Hence, the rest of the story highlights a couple of specific interests exemplary of both the progressive evolution of the technology and its capabilities.

Even in earlier exploration of cortical AEPs, more than clicks and tone bursts were tried. In the mid-1970s, ramps of frequency modulation to an otherwise steady tone were demonstrated to be effective stimuli as well.[5] Given the advent of the capability to search for AEFs in humans, the same investigator in the early 1980s demonstrated AEFs to such stimuli.[6] More recently (using current technology, mid-2000s), this general idea was investigated further. Brief changes of frequency of a steady carrier served as the stimulus for the desired event-related response and were examined for effects of carrier frequency and limits of detection of percent change, as illustrated in Figure 10–3B. The $N_{100}m$ was shown to be robust for a broad range of carrier frequencies, although a bit more so for the lower frequencies, and present down to small percentages of change.[7] How the auditory system processes frequency has been and is one of the most pervasive issues of hearing science. Therein lies pursuit of evidence of tonotopy in the organization the CANS, if not mechanistically the underpinning of the place theory of frequency encoding (recall Episode 3.2).

Not surprisingly, AEF technology came to be applied to the question of tonotopical organization of the human auditory cortex.[8] The implication was presented earlier in reference to the maintenance of tonotopical organization originating from the bottom-up wiring of the auditory pathways. Historically, strong functional evidence appeared in the 20th century from results of animal research.[9] Around the mid-1960s, compelling data compiled from single-unit records in the animal cortex seriously challenged the extent (and thus importance) of tonotopical organization of the auditory cortex.[10] In a decade, however, the tide of opinion would turn more favorably again, wherein the researcher had refined the technique of recording single-unit neuronal responses in the cortex.[11] The folds in the cerebral tissue (with its gyri and sulci) demand special care to maintain proper orientation at the surface for penetration into the depths of the cortex with an electrode. By the turn of the century, AEF researchers began to take on the challenge in humans.[12] Early in the 2000s, an AEF-research team in Japan mounted a study with an interest to extend the frequency range of inquiry to substantially above that of 8000 Hz (per the conventional audiogram), including ultrasounds (nominally, 20000 Hz and above).[13] However, they were unable to detect responses (N_{100m}) above 14 kHz; responses at 8 kHz and above also were found to be smaller, likely from the roll-off of the frequency response of the middle-ear "filter" (recall Episode 2.3).

Soon after, an "AEP-research team" from Lyon headed to Paris to collaborate with an MEG-research team to explore further the frequency range of evident totopicity, from midaudiometric to 12 kHz (although also testing 14 kHz, but with less reliable results).[14] Portions of their findings are illustrated in Figure 10–3C. In this figure, the data emphasized are right hemisphere results with left-ear stimulation from 1 kHz to 12 kHz. The mean coordinates derived from the recordings are represented approximately by the thick black line, portraying the most straightforwardly appearing trend observed. The area of the light-gray shadow expresses approximately standard errors of these measures, yet supporting the trends of the means.

However, other results reflected a somewhat different orientation of the overall scatter of data, both in terms of a substantially more variant and complex pattern. The dashed line in panel 10–3C approximates the area of the standard errors of the mean for the left hemisphere, as if viewed through the head. The coordinates fell on average pretty much along a more horizontal orientation overall with means (not shown for simplicity) forming a zigzag pattern across test frequencies (like a flattened, backward "Z"). There was also the complication overall of significant variance looking down from above the head at the level of the superior temporal gyrus. Meanwhile, as the artwork is not anatomically scaled in dimensions of actual areas of the data, all is "happening" in a volume of roughly 1 × ½ × ¼ centimeter at the same time demonstrating how good MEG technology really is. Consequently, as hinted earlier (Episode 3.2), tonotopical organization at the cortical level appears more complicated than a virtual "rainbow" of tonal frequencies laid out neatly along the superior plane of the superior temporal gyrus, as often had been portrayed at one time in colorful anatomical illustrations of the functional anatomy of the CANS.

Numerous auditory researchers now have pursued and carried out successful and enlightening work in the area of AEFs. The method remains prohibitive for routine use in clinical electrophysiology in audiology. Still, the "good work" goes on. Nothing says success technologically as well as continued refinement of the this tool and thus continued investment in research and development and marketing for decades after the seminal work. In reference to the predominantly pediatric interest pursued in Chapter 9, another benchmark also has been achieved—MEGs in the young infant and even the fetus. Whether instrumentation and cost-benefit can bring MEG/AEF testing into more routine accessibility in the clinic in due course remains to be seen. In any event, progressively more applications can be anticipated and results generated with increasingly direct clinical relevance, especially for site-of-lesion testing of the auditory primary and association cortical areas. Meanwhile, they can be expected to continue to provide bases of validation of the more conventional and/or basic AEP tests, even screening tests, to further support their clinical applications and the mandate of evidence-based practices. Collaborations between research and development efforts in AEP and AEF science and technologies thus can be expected to help build an ever-stronger foundation for understanding and interpretation of AEPs.

Episode 1: Quick Look at Intraoperative Neuromonitoring and Other Evoked Potentials

This episode overviews, firstly, the concept of conducting the assessment of evoked potentials. In principle, some of the methods of clinical electrophysiology surveyed throughout this book readily lend themselves to intraoperative uses, as well as other—yet technologically related—circumstances that certain surgeries can present, such as recording from an electrode directly on exposed nerves. Secondly discussed are other evoked potentials in general, either as natural spinoffs of intraoperative monitoring interest, but also of possible clinical interest to audiologists. Both include *sensory* and *motor evoked potentials*. The most fundamental definition of *intraoperative monitoring (IOM)* is the use of real-time electrophysiological information to *continuously monitor* (assess and track) the functional integrity of the central and peripheral nervous systems during high-risk surgeries. However, the development of the concept of IOM, in the broadest sense, is found outside of audiology and clinical electrophysiology, initially in the field of anesthesiology.

The history of IOM commences at the turn of the last century, in the hands of medical student Harvey Cushing.[15] He and a fellow medical student created what is known today as the *anesthesia record*, depicting the *intraoperative course* of anesthesia administered and the patient's corresponding vital signs during surgery. Several decades later, Dr. Cushing's student Wilder Penfield would begin a practice of what is known today as *intraoperative neurophysiological monitoring (IONM)*, deriving from the motivation to monitor brain function intraoperatively.[16] Table 10–1 shows the historical framework and summarizes the breadth of electrophysiological and other measures used in IONM. These metrics were adapted to or developed apropos a broadening scope of cranial and spinal surgeries that inevitably put the integrity of not only more of the brain but also the spine and (ultimately) peripheral nerves in the hands of surgeons. Although comprehensive, the focus of this episode is the EPs that audiologists—upon development of the necessary knowledge base and specialized expertise—typically monitor, especially working in services in/or affiliated with departments of head and neck surgeries. The history of the particular areas and applications is relatively more recent, in part thanks to technological developments and advancements in neurosurgical and related treatments (see Table 10–1, 1970s and on). Before pursuing specific examples, it will be useful to consider various basics that separate IONM from clinical neurophysiology and/ or related audiological interests.

The approach in IONM differs considerably from the practice of electrophysiology in audiology and related clinical areas. Neuromonitoring, more often than not, employs *multimodal* electrophysiology—recording simultaneously more than one type of neurogenic and/or myogenic potentials. IONM is practiced routinely today during surgical procedures in neurosurgery of the brain and spine,

Table 10-1. Historical Backdrop to Intraoperative Neuromonitoring

	Methods	Innovators and Academia	Surgical Apps
1930–1940s	Direct cortical stimulation on exposed cortex of conscious patients during neurosurgery	Penfield and Boldrey[17] (neurology)	Neurosurgery of the brain
	Intracranial electroencephalogram (iECG); Electrocorticography (ECoG)	Foester and Alternburger[18] (neurology); Jasper[19] (neurology)	Neurosurgery of the brain
1960s	Electrocochleography (ECochG) used in otolaryngology surgery	Rubin et al.[20] (otolaryngology)	Otology/neurology
	Electrical stimulation to identify recurrent laryngeal nerve (CN 10) in thyroid/radical neck dissection	Shedd and Burget[21] (surgery)	Neurosurgery of the brain, otolaryngology
	Phase reversal for cortical localization	Goldring[22]; Goldring and Gregorie[23] (neurology)	Neurosurgery of the brain
	Raw/analog EEG (rEEG)	Harris et al.[24] (neurology)	Neurosurgery of the brain and spine, vascular/cardiovascular
1970s–1980s	Visual evoked potentials (VEP)	Feinsod et al.[25] (neurosurgery)	Neurosurgery of the brain
	Somatosensory evoked potential (SSEP)	Nash et al.[26] (orthopaedics)	Neurosurgery of the brain and spine, vascular/cardiovascular
	Language mapping	Whitaker and Ojemann[27]; Ojemann[28] (neurological surgery)	Neurosurgery of the brain
	Transcranial magnetic stimulation of the motor cortex	Merton and Morton[29] (neurology)	Neurosurgery of the spine
	Quantitative/digital EEG (qEEG)	Levy et al.[30] (Anesthesiology and neurosurgery)	Neurosurgery of the brain and spine, vascular/cardiovascular
	ABR from surface electrodes and directly from CN VIII	Grundy et al.[31] (anesthesiology and neurosurgery); Moller et al.[32] (otolaryngology and neural surgery)	Neurosurgery of the brain, otology/neurotology

continues

Table 10-1. *continued*

	Methods	Innovators and Academia	Surgical Apps
	MLR as an adjunct for anesthetic monitoring	Thornton et al.[33] (anesthesiology)	Still under research and development
	Spontaneous/triggered electromyography (EMG)	Sekhar and Moller[34] (neurological surgery); Niparko et al.[35] (otolaryngology-head and neck Surgery); Mishler and Smith[36] (audiology and otorhinolaryngology-head and neck surgery)	Neurosurgery of the brain and spine, otology/neurotology/laryngology
	D-wave to monitor motor pathways from the spinal chord	Boyd et al.[37] (orthopaedics)	Neurosurgery of the spine
	ECochG to supplement ABR	Lambert and Ruth[38] (otolaryngology-head and neck surgery)	Neurosurgery of the brain, otology/neurotology
1990s	Transcranial motor evoked potential (tcMEP)	Burke et al.[39] (orthopaedics and anestheisa)	Neurosurgery of the brain and spine
	Direct cortical motor evoked potential (tcMEP)	Taniguchi et al.[40] (neurological surgery)	Neurosurgery of the brain
	Electrically evoked ABR (EABR)	Kileny et al.[41] (otolaryngology-head and neck surgery)	Otology/neurotology
	Pedicle screw testing via triggered EMG	Maguire et al.[42] (orthopaedics)	Neurosurgery of the spine
	Deep brain stimulations (DBS) for treatment of Parkinson's disease	Benabid et al.[43] (neurosurgery and neurology); Limousin et al.[44] (clinical and biological neurosciences)	Neurosurgery of the brain
	Distortion product otoacoustic emissions (DPOAE)	Filipo et al.[45] (neurology and otolaryngology)	Otology/neurotology
2000s	Auditory steady-state response (ASSR)	Oghalai et al.[46] (otolaryngology-head and neck surgery, audiology); Verhaegen et al.[47] (otorhinolaryngology)	Otology/neurotology
	Intracochlear ECochG during CIElectro insertion	Koka et al.[48] (reseach and technology, otolaryngology)	Otology/neurotology

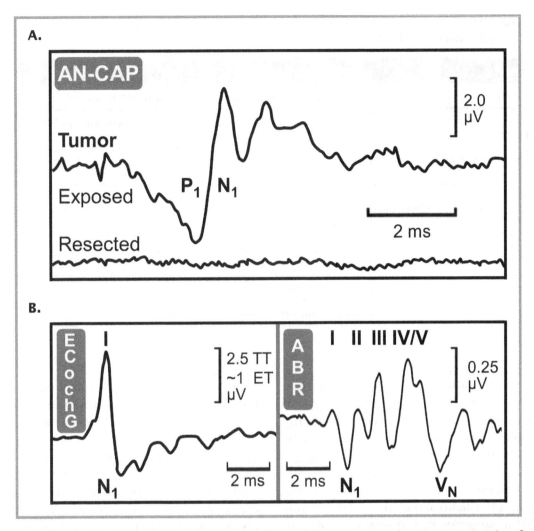

Figure 10–4. A. Example of the sort of near-field, compound action potentials of the auditory nerve that can be recorded during surgery, such as in the resection of an acoustic tumor or other procedures wherein the proximal auditory nerve is exposed (including pathologies of the neighboring vestibular and facial nerves). Decreases in the magnitude/morphology of the response may indicate compromised integrity of the 8th nerve. Complete resection of such tumors unfortunately may not leave an intact nerve (*bottom trace*). **B.** Recap of clinically familiar AEPs that also are useful in IONM: ECochG (both trans- [TT] and extratypmpanic [ET]) and ABR, essentially as conventionally stimulated and recorded. Panels A and B together portray approximate relative magnitudes among these potentials. (Figure concept from an AN-CAP model based on data of Martin and Shi [2009].[51])

otology/neurotology, and in vascular/cardiovascular surgeries. This allows ongoing evaluation of the functional integrity of neural pathways to identify surgically related changes, as (in effect) in the abbreviated record in Figure 10–4A.

The objectives of IONM include reducing surgical risks by providing guidance to the surgeon to localize and identify important neural structures in the operative field that are congenitally abnormal, severely damaged, or obscured by disease or previous surgery. The next objective is that of improving outcomes by identifying potential neurological insults, permitting immediate intervention to avoid, and/or limit significant postoperative impairment.

Table 10–2. Utility of Auditory Evoked Potentials in IntraOperative Neurophysiological Monitoring.

AEP	Surgical Procedure
ABR	Acoustic neuroma/vestibular schwannoma resection
	Microvascular decompression of CN V, VI, VII, VIII, and IX
	Posterior fossa aneurysm and arteriovenous malformation
	Skull-base surgery
	Suboccipital decompression surgeries
	Vestibular neurectomy
ECochG	Intracanalicular acoustic neuroma surgery Vestibular neurectomy
	Superior semicircular canal dehiscence surgery
	Middle and other inner ear surgeries

The ultimate objective is to reduce postoperative morbidity and mortality by providing the surgeon with information regarding the functional integrity of neural pathways/structures that would not be available otherwise.

The conventionally recorded AEPs commonly monitored (Figure 10–4B) are the auditory brainstem response (far field) and electrocochleography (near field) in surgeries that involve the posterior and middle fossa as well as the brainstem to improve the probability of preservation of hearing, restoration of hearing, and/or preservation of brainstem-dependent functions. However, the choice of AEP modality(ies) to be monitored is dependent on the type of surgery and the neural structures within the auditory pathway that are inherently at risk. The ABR and ECochG can be used independently of each other or concomitantly in cases when the ABR via surface electrodes are not recordable or reliable. In addition, the ABR and ECochG can also be utilized to identify anatomical landmarks as well as predict postoperative outcomes. Monitoring other AEPs have been investigated as potentially useful tools; for instance, the auditory middle latency response (AMLR) has been considered for the objective assessment of anesthetic depth.[49] Given that cortical auditory evoked potential is well-known to be acutely affected by level of consciousness (recall Episode 8.1), it has not been pursued for use in IONM. Table 10–2 summarizes examples of surgical procedures in which the AEPs are used as an index of auditory function.[50]

In cases where surface electrodes are not enough to record a clear ABR wave I and/or the *compound action potential (CAP; a.k.a., AP)* of the 8th nerve, there are several options.[51] The least invasive are extratympanic (ET) electrocochleography or transtympanic (TT) with a needle electrode on the promontory (recall Episode 5.3 and the accompanying Heads Up). Recording also can be made from an electrode in the round window niche with a myringotomy or a posterior tympanotomy to gain access (recall Episode 5.4). Recall that *ECochG-CAP* (and thus ABR wave I) is generated and recorded distal to most lesions of the 8th nerve, like an acoustic tumor. However, *AN-CAP* can be recorded proximal to lesions via a specialized electrode positioned by the surgeon directly on the 8th nerve (again Figure 10–4A). Such intracranial recordings are made possible only after some degree of dissection is performed by the surgical team, and there is appropriate exposure of the auditory nerve. Responses evoked via direct contact with the nerve can be acquired with fewer epochs of signal averaging than required clinically for an adequately stable ABR, facilitating virtually continuous real-time monitoring of the status of the peripheral nerve. To avoid false-negative results, the AN-CAP must be recorded proximal to the lesion to be resected. The ECochG-CAP and/or AN-CAP are particularly advantageous during microvascular decompression for cranial nerve dysfunction (7th, 8th, and 9th) and vestibular nerve resection (situated within the 8th nerve) as well as mapping cochlear nerve fibers during acoustic tumor resection. ECochG is also relevant to IONM for its sensory side (not just neural) side; recall Figure 5–21 and its associated Heads Up, demonstrating use of monitoring the summating potential in surgical treatment of semicircular canal dehiscence. Changes in AEP responses are considered to be related to surgical maneuvers if they cannot be accounted for by the effects of hypotensive episodes (drops in blood pressure), significant hypothermia, acoustical masking from drill-generated noise, electrical noise (including interference from electrocautery used to reduce bleeding at the site of dissection), or other technical factors that could compromise or prevent recording an evoked response when one is actually present. Technical factors to consider include incorrect stimulus and/or acquisition parameters, dislodged foam eartip or kinked/blocked tubing from the tubal insert earphone, and suboptimal SNR. Potentially injurious surgical maneuvers include drilling bone (for access to tumors and the like), debulking or total tumor resection/excision, and cerebellar retraction—which can stretch cranial nerves, put pressure on the brainstem, or put traction on parts of the cerebrum (which also can put pressure on brainstem by pushing it against the foreman magnum). Direct mechanical injury, arterial vasospasm, vascular compromise, and/or thermal injury are concomitant to these maneuvers. All such causes of dysfunction, as well as improper closure of the dura, can affect both latency and amplitude of the targeted AEP(s), including a specific wave component, combination of components, or all waves. Although an exhaustive compilation of these effects is beyond the scope of this book, more comprehensive and detailed discussion of vulnerabilities and nuances of changes of SLRs is available in the literature.[52] An example of some such changes in the ABR, based on an actual surgical case,[53] is illustrated in Figure 10–5.

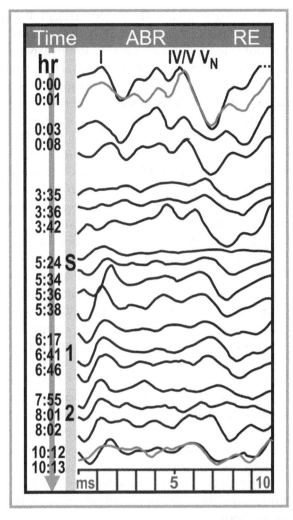

Figure 10–5. "Waterfall display" (excerpts) of recorded ABRs during course of neurosurgery involving exposure of the frontal poles of the cerebrum and their retraction, applied for exposure of a tumor. This can cause significant compression of the brainstem, as believed to have occurred in this case. Also exemplified is a midcourse change in the test paradigm and (in effect) reference for judging a significant change that had to be adjusted, namely no longer the baseline responses at the beginning of surgery, as follows: baseline, test/retest during preparation postanesthetic induction, at nominally zero hours (hr, in hours:minutes, for purposes of illustration); S, sudden/unexplained change in sensitivity, thus increased stimulus by 10 dB; 1 and 2—changes after brainstem compression suspected—retraction removed (1), replaced, then removed for good (2); finally, a reasonably stabilized ABR observed, including IV/V/V_N headed back to the patient's normal latencies (based on data of Durrant and Sclabassi [1993][53]).

The particular case illustrated brings out several other inherent differences between clinical electrophysiology and minimally/noninvasive applications of the same tools in IONM. However, it suffices for the purposes of this episode to summarize only those differences that are the most salient. The interested reader can refer to a guideline of the American Society of Neurophysiologic Monitoring (ASNM) for recommended stimulus and recording parameters for IONM of AEPs.[54] Reporting of findings in some clinical settings may be right after the patient's consultation. The report, which may reach the referral source several days later, likely will include not only necessary measurements but also deviations from normative values (if applicable) and further (post hoc) analyses and recommendations. Reporting of findings in the operating room (OR) is "on the fly," instantly when needed. "Needed" is when there is a significant change in the response that constitutes warning the surgeon. Changes must be conveyed immediately to the surgical team and/or anesthesiologist or upon demand by the surgeon for a status report. Most technicians support an arbitrary warning criterion of a 50% decrease in amplitude and/or a 10% increase in latency for most evoked potentials. However, for the auditory system, a prolongation of latency more than 1 ms and/or decrease in amplitude more than 50% pragmatically is used as an alarm criterion.

Measurement in IONM is about expediency, as well, and involves far more test–retests than are typical of clinical evaluations. Seemingly countless repetitions of stimulus presentations are launched once a baseline response is established. Neuromonitoring is continuous throughout most of the procedure and often for nearly as long as the patient is "on the table." Emphasis in the clinic is upon a set/subset of high-quality recordings from relatively few test/retests via averages over high numbers of stimulus repetitions, hence somewhat lengthy response-acquisition times. Quality of recording certainly is not to be discounted in IONM. Yet, the "game" is to have relatively expedient averages and counting on the frequently repeated trials to help judge the response(s) by way of observing a "waterfall" display of the responses collected and generated automatically as surgery progresses. Then an "on-the-spot" decision must be made of what, indeed, is a significant change versus just a momentary fluctuation in morphology due to an inherently electrically noisy recording environment. If a seemingly salient change in the response emerges in the "waterfall," another decision must be made—is it due to the overall status of the patient (depth of anesthesia, core body temperature, etc.) or related to the surgery itself? The example in Figure 10–5 demonstrates that the monitoring and judgment call may have to be tempered at times by a "reality check." If the surgical and anesthesia teams have decided that nothing needs to/can be done about an observed change, the paradigm may have to be revised (such as increased stimulus level, as in this case) and either way, the baseline must be redefined—the new reality.

Surgical experience, thorough anatomical knowledge, and good surgical technique are the most important tools for protecting against neural injury. However, use of IONM as an adjunct to lowering the risk of postoperative permanent neurological deficits is also an economic matter, requiring critical assessment and justification of its cost-benefit. The National Institute of Health's Consensus Conference on Acoustic Neuroma[55] acknowledged the benefits of 8th nerve monitoring in the surgical management of acoustic tumors in minimizing the risk of *iatrogenic injury* (injury secondary to treatment). Also acknowledged is the possibility of improved hearing preservation by the use of IONM in such cases. Some acoustic tumors (recall Episode 6.5) develop substantially within the internal auditory canal—intracanalicular tumors. The surgery required is particularly delicate to debulk such tumors, placing at risk injury to the nerve itself (it may be stretched or otherwise damaged), if not also to the vestibular-nerve branch and the 7th nerve (recall Figure 3–13A, inset) and/or the cochlear artery. Furthermore, large acoustic and other types of tumors can be situated in the cerebellopontine angle and may come to compress the adjacent brainstem. Such tumors may additionally affect still other cranial nerves (5th, 9th, 10th, or 12th). Consequently, the consensus was that intraoperative monitoring should be included in surgical management to minimize risk of cranial nerve injury. In addition, the American Society of Neurophysiologic Monitoring (ASNM) developed a position statement,[56] recommending the monitoring of AEPs in cases of acoustic tumor, vestibular nerve resection, microvascular decompression, other cerebellopontine angle and fourth-ventricle tumors, arteriovenous malformations of the brain, and suboccipital decompression surgeries for preservation of the 8th nerve.

Results of studies of skull-based surgery, especially involving large tumors where there is intricate involvement of lower cranial nerves (9th and/or 12th), show that IONM has been shown to reduce cranial nerve morbidity while facilitating total tumor resection.[57,58] Furthermore, skull-based tumors that invade the cavernous sinus can involve the 3rd, 4th, and 6th cranial nerves. Since tumors of the skull base tend to be relatively large (relative to the confined spaces of the skull), mapping cranial nerves for intraoperative localization and identification of extraocular muscles reduces their incidence of injury.[59]

The utility of IONM during middle ear and mastoid surgery may not be immediately obvious but, at the same time, should not be underestimated. The facial nerve is at risk during these surgeries as the surgeon is working near the internal auditory meatus where the 7th nerve runs a tortuous course through the facial canal to fan out and innervate muscles serving facial expression and taste sensation. The tympanic segment of the 7th nerve is especially vulnerable in the presence of chronic otitis media and cholesteatoma, while the descending portion of the nerve is at risk for iatrogenic injury during mastoidectomy and posterior tympanotomy. Research findings in such cases have shown that facial nerve **electrical stimulation** and monitoring, during both primary and revision surgeries, enables more reliable identification of dehiscence (thinning) of the overlying bone and/or aberrant facial nerve anatomy than simply visual inspection of the nerve. IONM leads to reduction of the incidence of facial paralysis and has been advocated as a useful adjunct to middle ear and mastoid surgery.[60,61] The American Academy of Otolaryngology-Head and Neck Surgery recently developed a position statement, *Intraoperative Nerve Monitoring in Otologic Surgery*,[62] that attests to **facial nerve monitoring** as not only cost-effective but also beneficial for both otoneurologic and mastoid surgeries.

Investigations of the use of IONM in other head and neck cases, specifically involving the parotid and thyroid glands, have provided less compelling evidence of reduction of iatrogenic nerve injury. Facial nerve monitoring during parotidectomy has been observed to reduce the incidence of transient postoperative facial paresis. However, there was no statistical difference in incidence of permanent facial nerve injury with versus without IONM, given the use of nerve visualization alone.[63] Although the use of IONM during parotid surgery is still controversial, monitoring is considered useful in surgery where there is a higher risk of injury to the facial nerve, such as total parotidectomy or reinterventions, or in cases with histories of chronic inflammation.

Meta-analyses likewise have not shown IONM to provide greater protection of the 10th cranial nerve, that is against nerve paresis or paralysis after either routine or high-risk thyroid surgeries.[64,65] However, despite the lack of evidence in the literature, the American Academy of Otolaryngology-Head and Neck Surgery in a practice guideline[66] recommends that surgeons consider IONM in bilateral thyroid surgery, revision thyroid surgery, and surgery wherein an existing recurrent laryngeal nerve paralysis exists.

The nature of the environment of IONM and technical knowledge base beyond routine clinical testing of AEPs[67] begs the question of who should perform AEP monitoring intraoperatively. The American Speech-Language-Hearing Association (ASHA) and the American Academy of Audiology (AAA), for example, acknowledge IONM as within the scope of practice of audiologists. However, having a doctor of audiology (AuD) or other professional or master's degree with clinical certification does not automatically qualify someone to practice IONM. Competency in IONM requires comprehensive knowledge beyond that of clinical audiology and is thusly not ensured by a knowledge base and clinical competency in audiological applications of electrophysiology alone. Extensive training overall and for each type and modality of intraoperative monitoring (again, see Table 10–1) is expected of the IONM practitioner and essential for the patient's welfare. Academic audiology programs simply do not provide all the necessary knowledge base and skill sets essential to competency in IONM. In some academic audiology programs, especially in or with close affiliation with medical centers, there have been opportunities for students to get some technical background and observational experience in IONM. To the writers' knowledge, there are only three academically accredited IONM training programs in the United States.[68] In any event, audiologists with competency in clinical electrophysiology in audiology are good candidates for being educated and mentored subsequently in IONM. Their knowledge base, abilities, and experience are very useful foundations for success.

Although few standardized training programs for **IONM technologists**, there nevertheless are paths to becoming certified by the American Board of Registration of Electroencephalographic and Evoked Potential Technologists (ABRET), after passing the certification examination in neurophysiologic intraoperative monitoring (CNIM).[69] Outside of accredited IONM training programs, readers can seek guidance on requisite education and supervised practice from organizations such as the ABRET and ASNM (mentioned earlier), ASET (American Society of Electroneurodiagnostic Technologists), ABNM (American Board of Neurophysiologic Monitoring), and AABIOM (American Audiology Board of Intraoperative Monitoring).

Practically (as hinted earlier), as inherently involving other neural pathways than auditory, IONM in a given surgical case likely will involve tracking more than one potential simultaneously. Furthermore, for procedures within the purview of otolaryngology/neurology, this may or may not include AEP(s). A primary example is the **somatosensory evoked potential (SSEP)**. On the one hand, the underlying principles for eliciting the SSEP and the processing of the transient event-related response are readily familiar from earlier episodes, as demonstrated by Figure 10–6A (as indicated). A largely brainstem-level SSEP component is highlighted therein, being reminiscent of the AMLR. There are also longer-latency, cortical SSEPs, but they are beyond the scope of interest here. In any event, it will be the earlier components that will be featured in the virtual demonstrations of IONM of the SSEP, although often concomitant changes will be seen in the later components. Incidentally, Cz is a reasonably good site for recording the SSEPs, but others, particularly toward the Ps, are preferable, at least in this line of work. Also as learned well from the AEPs, it is a matter of preferences which polarity points up, hence "ups and downs" across examiners of these evoked potentials as well.

On the other hand, SSEPs are elicited using electrical stimulation via **surface electrodes** or **subcutaneous needles**. The time course of the amplitude and latency in SSEPs can serve as a practical indicator of cerebral blood flow, hence there is a major attraction for their use in IONM (see Table 10–1). Eliciting the SSEPs also evokes robust motoric responses, whether using (for instance) stimulus sites in the upper or lower extremities. A thumb twitch can be seen during stimulation when electrodes are applied on the undersurface of the wrist (see Figure 10–6B, XX with "MS" denoting direction of neural activation of the motor system). Likewise, a foot twitch can be seen during stimulation of the tibial nerve when electrodes are applied around the ankle. Generally, both sides will be prepared, just as it is most convenient and prudent in AEP evaluations to have bilateral stimulation and recordings sites prepared—from the "get-go." In clinical tests, the same sites are used, but the electrical stimulus is applied by surface contact with electrodes at significantly less intensity (this mode will shortly be considered further, for other purposes.) Electrical stimuli actually can be used to elicit robust transient responses from all along the somatosensory pathway (again panel B) and providing overall a powerful tool of IONM (see panel C).

Descending/motor pathways from the brainstem and cortex also are very important to monitor in many cases.[67] A spontaneous/free-running **electromyograph (EMG)** is the first "available" signal to monitor and is an inherently prevalent signal. Any "events" (response-like signals) or other signals (noise/interference of possible concern) generally are readily oberved in the free-running signal analysis (much like the time history of EEG recordings from the scalp). EMG monitoring thus allows for continuous feedback on the functional status of selected cranial nerves or spinal roots throughout the surgical procedure. Changes that occur in activity suggest manipulation in the vicinity of the innervating nerve/root. At rest, a healthy nerve should cause little or no activation of muscles, especially given that the patient is rendered immobile by the anesthesia. Electrically triggered EMG potentials

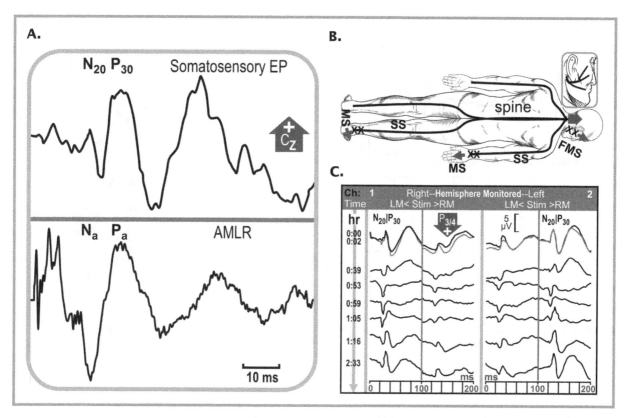

Figure 10–6. A. The somatosensory evoked potential compared to the AMLR. **B.** Somatosensory pathways that can be stimulated electrically for SSEP testing and common sites of stimulation (XX, using pairs of electrodes) with direction of motor response activated (MS). Inset: Schematic to represent fan-out of major branches of the facial nerve (to be discussed subsequently). (Illustration courtesy of Mr. M. A. Durrant). **C.** Partial display of SSEPs tracked during a skull-base surgical case. Recordings are two-channel while stimulating both the right (RM) and left (LM) median nerves, but interleafing R-L stimuli, at 25 volts and rate of 3.3/s. As the somatosensory pathway crosses over, the RM-elicited SSEP is registered primarily in the left hemisphere and the right hemisphere for LM. Events and time lines were as follows: 0:00 to 0:02—test/retest baseline responses; 0:39 and 0:53 still opening/approaching site of lesion; 0:59—advised anesthesiology of observed SSEP reduction and EEG suppression overall; 1:05—anesthesia reported decreased level of iso-flurane (anesthetic gas employed); 1:16—SSEPs/EEG recovering; anesthesia reported no longer using iso-flurane, only narcotics; 2:33—last recording before starting to head patient to recovery room (based on data of Durrant and Sclabassi [1993][53]).

(Figure 10–7, top panel) are useful for directly testing the integrity of the nerve/roots; a consistently elicited response can ensure the integrity distally to the possible site of injury. On the EMG side of the "test," recordings are made from subcutaneous needle electrodes on the face, for example to monitor the 7th nerve. Spontaneous trains of such potentials (bottom panel) also are stimulated readily during incidental surgical manipulation or acute thermal changes in the vicinity of the nerve. Mechanical irritation of the nerve roots/nerve due to traction or thermal injury elicit such neurotonic, unit-muscle discharges (spikes or bursts of activity) associated with a risk of permanent injury to the corresponding nerve, either immediately or upon repetitive trauma. The degree of irritation to the nerve/nerve roots roughly correlates with the magnitude and duration of the EMG activity. EMG activity due to nonmechanical causes may be benign, such as from temperature changes caused by below-body-temperature water in flushing the surgically exposed area, use of electrocautery devices,

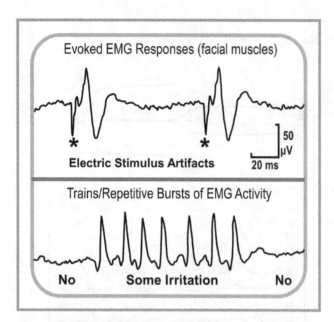

Figure 10–7. Electromyographic signals common to motor nerve monitoring, 7th nerve in the examples shown.

and low depth of anesthesia. Cutting of the nerve, intentionally or otherwise, produces a final burst of activity—like at the end of the train of pulses in Figure 10–7, so thereafter nothing but noise floor. In order for EMG activity to be correctly interpreted, the IONM technologist must have in-depth knowledge regarding EMG waveform as well as surgical orientation and awareness of ongoing surgical events. Monitoring instrumentation can provide a response detector that generates an audible alert (with adjustable threshold), thus "beeps" that the surgeon can hear as well. The technologist is not "out of the picture" here, rather critical to helping rule out false alarms. This includes a dialogue with the surgeon, namely toward valid interpretation of activity observed/heard.

In IONM, electrical stimulation/triggered EMG potentials are an extension of the clinical *electroneuronography (ENoG)*, arguably more technically correctly referred to as *facial evoked electromyography*.[70] This test permits objective evaluation of the integrity of the facial nerve.[71,72] Consequently, modern test systems for measuring AEPs and other EPs are packaged or can be upgraded to provide the stimulator (Figure 10–8A) and additional software for performing ENoG. The

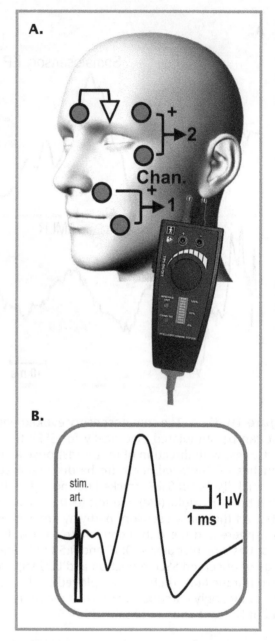

Figure 10–8. Overview of electroneuronography. **A.** Recording montage and mode of stimulation. (Images courtesy of Dr. R. E. Delgado.) **B.** Example of facial evoked electromyographic response (stim. art.—electrical stimulus artifact).

examiner familiar with AEP testing should be "at home" with the operation of the test system, having to master only the specific additional parameters of the test and thereafter benefiting from the tools typical of systems for AEP recording and analysis (panel B). These tools include signal conditioning, storage, further processing digitally, and plotting/report generation. The required basic knowledge for competency in ENoG may have derived from degree/certification programs in clinical audiology. However, full mastery of the skill set needed for competency likely will require additional training. This is a procedure that can lead to substantial discomfort to the patient and misleading/misinterpreted results without a thorough understanding.

The essence of ENoG is provided in Figure 10–8. Unlike IONM, evaluating the integrity of the facial nerve noninvasively provides only information relevant to the status the distal facial nerve trunk—the portion outside of the temporal bone. This is because the stimulus is generally applied on the skin overlying the temporomandibular joint (TMJ) or just under the zygomatic arch (cheek bone) posteriorly (apropos a large area of facial muscle involvement). Stimulation generally is applied with a handheld device for fine positioning toward optimal stimulation and convenience in adjusting stimulus strength. The response is recorded generally to sample two main fields of muscle activity, using pairs of electrodes that are placed both along nasolabial folds and above and below the eye laterally (ground electrode on the forehead; panel A). This montage thus permits measuring compound motoric potentials of main branches of the facial nerve.

One of the most typical cases for use of (clinical) ENoG is that of Bell's palsy (a 7th nerve disorder); this commonly is a unilateral, peripheral paralysis which can arise (for example) from unknown causes or postoperative trauma. The test thus is applicable for both diagnostic purposes and postoperative monitoring of recovery.[72,73] Somewhat like differential-diagnostic ABR testing (involving relatively high-level stimulation at times; recall Episode 6.5), the ENoG examiner must find the voltage needed to achieve maximal ("saturated") stimulation of the 7th nerve—in principle, all neurons activated within the nerve, if possible. Comparison of the affected versus the nonaffected side can help to determine the amount of denervation that might have occurred on the affected side, which is critical in predicting the grade of facial nerve recovery.[74] Appling electricity to the skin is not pleasant at the voltage that often is necessary to drive enough current to adequately stimulate the nerve, situated some millimeters below the skin's surface. However, with skill, along with good patient orientation and with compassion, ENoG can be performed relatively quickly and with minimal/brief discomfort.

Naturally, the cochlea's equally close neighbor (by way of their respective nerves) and even more intimate relation (sharing fluid systems in their peripheral systems) is the ***vestibular peripheral system***. Balance-sensory, neurogenic evoked responses have yet to be demonstrated that quite parallel auditory evoked neurogenic responses. However, great success in clinical electrophysiology applicable to the vestibular system has been realized, based on evoked motor responses, yet has been elicited by sensory stimulation. But surprise, the stimulus in question is acoustic! These clinically evaluated responses are the ***vestibular evoked myogenic potentials (VEMPs)*** (Figure 10–9). The generators are subsets of muscles that control movement of the eyes and neck, reminiscent of the postauricular muscle response (recall the second Heads Up of Episode 6.5 dedicated to the subject). The balance system overall is inherently a multimodal system with well-known interactions among the visual, vestibular, and motor systems.[75] Processing of balance-related signals input to the CNS results in interactive control of eye movements, especially as the head turns and (ideally) whatever the position of the rest of the body. The VEMPs are relatively short-latency potentials in response to sounds of high hearing levels (≥ 90 dB).[76] This in part explains how the cochlea's neighbor also can be affected by sound, bearing in mind that the oval window opens directly into the vestibule and the fluids of the inner ear course throughout both peripheral systems (recall the first Heads Up, Episode 6.5, Case 3). Interestingly, bone-conducted sounds are effective too and at much lower hearing levels (by some 35 dB–50 dB). Although clicks work here too, particularly effective stimuli are tone bursts of mid-low frequencies, like 500 Hz.

The VEMPs, nevertheless, are motor responses. They can be recorded with surface electrodes over the ipsilateral sternocleidomastoid (neck) muscle—the cervical, ***cVEMP***. They also arise from ocular muscles—the ocular, ***oVEMP***—but are recorded contralaterally. Both scenarios are covered using the recording montage summarized in Figure 10–9.

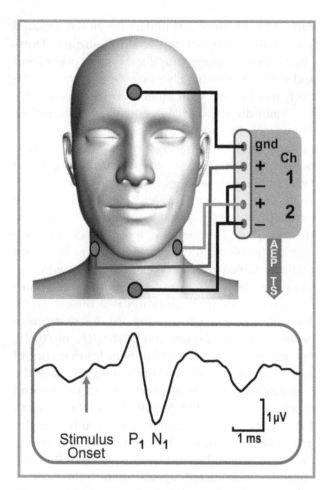

Figure 10–9. Overview of recording of a vestibular evoked myogenic potential. The recording montage permits cervical (recorded ipsilaterally) and/or ocular (recorded contralaterally) VEMP assessment. Sample recording of a response (*bottom figure*). AEP TS— indication of electrode cable connection to an AEP test system (yes "auditory"), as indeed an earphone or bone vibrator is needed to provide the effective stimulus. (Concept and data courtesy of Dr. K. Barin.)

Short latency in this area of clinical electrophysiology in "AEP-time" is more akin to that of early AMLR components or (perhaps not surprisingly) the latency of the PAMR. The VEMPs are relatively easy to measure by way of a protocol that is "patient friendly" to administer. The VEMP test is an emergent clinical tool to complement classical vestibular diagnostic tests (like the caloric, rotary chair, and optokinetic tests using electronystagmography [ENG] or video nystagmography [VNG]). Reduced VEMPS can indicate involvement of the otoliths or inferior portion of the vestibular nerve.

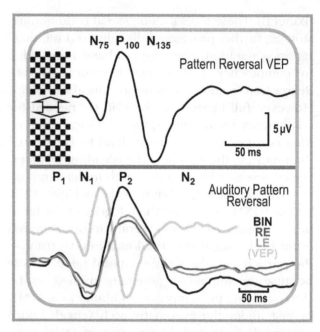

Figure 10–10. Visual evoked potential recorded at Oz (overlying the occipital cortex, top figure) versus a conceptually related approach to the corresponding cortical evoked auditory potential (recorded at Cz). VEP stimulated by alternating checkerboard pattern (see inset) at 2 reversals/s. (Courtesy of Dr. R. E. Delgado.) The "auditory pattern reversal" was that of an alternating 8-tone complex in which the component tones were spaced at (on average) two critical bands of frequency resolution by the auditory system, alternately shifted by one critical bandwidth (fundamentally, by equal intervals on the basilar membrane), at the rate of 1.1/s at 55 dB SPL. This paradigm was designed to approximate reversal of light-dark stripes which also is efficacious for eliciting a VEP, showing substantial enhancement of binaural over monaural responses (the latter in turn shown to be essentially the same as a 500-Hz tone burst of the same peak-equivalent SPLs, namely transient versus the steady-state pattern stimulus).

Other nuances of findings can point to possible central-system involvement. Cases of possible interest include differential diagnosis including Meniere's disease and semicircular canal dehiscence (recall Heads Up of Episode 5.3).

This tour of other evoked potentials could not be wrapped up without a "tip of the hat" to one other neighbor, the visual system, specifically the ***visual evoked potential (VEP)*** (Figure 10–10)— another sensory-neurogenic evoked response and that also can be evaluated clinically with instrumentation that only differs in terms to the stimulator and particular software.[77] Indeed, commercially available EP test systems can be outfitted to support AEP, VEMP, SSEP, ENoG, and VEP measurement—one to all on the same test system. Not only being in physical proximity to the auditory system, the visual system is a close sensory neighbor in many ways functionally, even in the face of remarkably different neural "wiring" of both their respective peripheral and central pathways. The click-evoked cortical AEP and flash-evoked VEP are analogous fundamentally, thus assessable by way of a comparable transient stimulus-response paradigm and yielding comparably robust responses. However, just as tones, speech, and other signals have been seen to work well or better for testing some longer-latency AEPs, a substantially more robust VEP is obtained by none other than a mere on-off stimulus paradigm. However, a particularly effective stimulus is an alternating checkerboard pattern—*pattern reversal*—presented to the viewer (see inset to left of top subpanel). As such, the stimulus is not just being turned on and off to elicit an event-related potential; there is continuous (steady-state) stimulation but with coherent signal averaging being synchronized to the reversal of the pattern. Yet, the response is quite robust in neurologically intact subjects (again, upper subpanel). This is because this paradigm taps well into the way that the eye is exquisitely wired for up-front, peripheral-system processing to enhance contrast of the visual image. It then is not about the overall intensity of the "light" from the light squares (that is constant!), rather the flip-flopping of the pattern-reversal about the edges among them. Pattern-reversal of light and dark stripes also works, just not eliciting quite as robust a pattern-reversal VEP (given thereby greatly reducing the number of edges about which the flip-flopping is occurring). While the checkerboard pattern is conceptually a difficult paradigm to match in hearing science, an analogous paradigm for pattern-reversal of stripes (in effect) is possibly using alternating frequency patterns of a multitone complex—an FM steady-state paradigm. Such pattern reversal for binaural (diotic) stimulation yields comparable enhancement of CAEPs, particularly in reference to that elicited by simpler-pattern (effectively broader "stripes") or tone-bursts presented monaurally (bottom subpanel).[78,79]

The science, technology, and practical experience underlying the clearly broad areas of clinical neurophysiology has not occurred like a "horse race" among them, wherein blinders are put on the horses to keep them focused straight ahead, and less attentive to other horses on either side. Applications have emerged and evolved in parallel and with lessons learned among them. This permits considerable transference of innovations from one to the other, such as paradigms to optimize EPs whatever the sensory and/or motor system, and their novel applications.

Acknowledgment:

The writers are indebted to Dr. William H. Martin, professor of otolaryngology and director of the audiology MSc programme, Centre for Hearing, Speech and Balance, National University of Singapore, for his sage counsel at the inception of this episode as a former worker in IONM and, in general, as a long-time contributor to AEP research and development and the field of audiology.

HEADS UP

Heads Up: A Case of Elective Surgery That Could Have Gone Badly Were It Not for IONM

Although the OR is one of the most complex work environments, this case shows the level of teamwork and communication that is necessary amongst different disciplines. This case, which takes place in the early 1990s when innovations and use of IONM was growing dramatically,[80] could have ended tragically. However, all persons involved innately understood the importance of patient safety, and everyone collaboratively accepted their role in minimizing the patient's risk of neurological, iatrogenic injury.

The grave importance of anesthesiology is never as well appreciated as in such a case as this one. The surgical team does the work, but it is the anesthesiologist who is responsible for patient care throughout the surgical experience: before, during, and after the surgery itself. A thorough preoperative medical history, physical examination, and review of laboratory results—as well as continuous monitoring of the patient's vital signs—contribute to the successful perioperative monitoring and management of the patient. In this case, while performing the preoperative assessment, the anesthesiologist noted a history of carotid artery stenosis. Although at the time the patient's laboratory tests and vital signs were unremarkable, this was of concern to the anesthesiologist, knowing the way in which the surgeon likely would have to position the patient's head during surgery. Thus, prior to intubation, the patient's head was turned to one side whereupon the patient reported tingling sensation in the fingers and toes. The anesthesiologist relayed his observations and concerns to the surgeon. Surgical considerations/risks were then addressed so the patient could make a well-informed decision to consent.

Since the patient decided to proceed with the surgery to be performed in the otolaryngology and head and neck surgical block of the medical center, anesthesiology placed an urgent call to the director of audiology, section of otology (the first author) to discuss the possible need for intraoperative monitoring. The director, also a member of the IONM team, conveyed the particulars of the case to the head of the IONM team in the neurosurgery department.[80] Although the surgery itself posed no risk of neurological deficit, a carotid artery stenosis potentially posed a significant neurological risk overall for this patient, namely from possible compromise of cerebral blood flow during the course of the procedure. It readily was agreed that IONM was indicated, specifically monitoring SSEPs to reduce the risk of a stroke during the procedure. In the OR, timeliness is paramount, which this case clearly demonstrates. The test modality to be used was discussed with the surgical team and the surgery commenced.

The best outcome would be to see no change of SSEPs throughout the surgery, other than minor changes attributable to core temperature and/or anesthetic, as long as the patient's vitals were being well maintained by the anesthesiology team. In Figure 10–11 is a condensed representation of the tracked waterfall display of the SSEP responses recorded in this case. Initially, responses bilaterally are seen to be robust and reproducible. However, within approximately half an hour, a progressive decline in the amplitude of the response became evident. This trend was reported to the surgeon, although at this time, the change was not yet suggestive of eminent danger. However, the SSEPs continued to decrease in amplitude, and the surgeon was alerted; it was becoming depressed rapidly and indeed nearly extinguished on one side. Surgery was temporarily suspended (demarked by the star in the figure). The patient's head was then turned so that the neck was in a neutral position and vital signs were analyzed. To lessen the chances of permanent neurological injury, the surgical procedure was then modified—the patient's head was repositioned so as to cause minimal torque to the neck. Surgery was resumed. Although, the patient's vital signs remained unremarkable, the SSEP display did not change appreciably immediately. However, after about one hour, the SSEPs slowly started to show recovery. By the time the patient was awakened, responses were reproducible and nearly back to baseline.

Anesthesiologist vindicated? IONM "proved" its value? Yes, yes, and more. That patient on that day was, in all likelihood, spared a stroke during surgery. In fact, not long afterward the same patient returned for

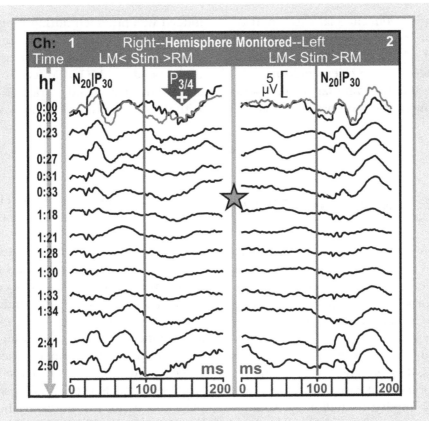

Figure 10–11. Representation of highlights of tracked/waterfall display of SSEPs recorded during a head and neck surgery procedure in a patient at risk per a preexisting medical condition. As in the case presented in Figure 10–6C, SSEPs were recorded using a two channel-system and bilateral electrode pairs nominally at F3-P3 and F4-P4. The "parietal (P)" electrodes actually were placed 2 cm anterior (regarding the international 10-20 system). Right (RM) and left median (LM) nerves were stimulated alternately at 3.3/s. Again, time-lapse following establishment of baseline responses (approximately start of the surgical procedure itself) is indicated per trial. The "game changing" event is demarked by the star (see text). By the end of surgery, the patient's responses had fully recovered (based on data of Durrant and Sclabassi [1993][53]).

a second procedure contralaterally, which required the surgeon to turn the head to the opposite side. Learning from the first procedure, as a precaution, the approach for the next surgery was planned accordingly, including IONM, to reduce the patient's potential risk. The SSEPs were observed to be stable throughout, thus without significant departure from baseline recordings.

This case was unique in that the head/neck positioning for this procedure had not been perceived as a risk factor. As so often in the evolution of medical science, it is that one case that is needed to raise the issue,

> even if challenging conventional wisdom. It is uncommon, but cases may arise now and again wherein a brief ad hoc tutorial for the surgical team may be necessary to orient and/or educate them about the importance and usefulness of IONM modalities and protocols, as indeed was provided during preparation of this patient for the first procedure. In any event, these circumstances also serve as a reminder of the need for the IONM technologist to be on cooperative terms and work as a team player with the entire surgical team.

■ Episode 2: Whose Land Is This?

Audiologists with expertise in auditory electrophysiology can combine this knowledge with their unique understanding of the auditory pathway, hearing disorders, audiometry, and auditory science to greatly advance their understanding of auditory function and better serve their patients.

Although audiologists do not "own" auditory evoked potentials, they do have a unique and important contribution to make in the area of clinical electrophysiology applied to audiology. Audiologists have knowledge that spans many clinical and hearing science domains, bringing an advanced ability to understand well-established evoked potential approaches, such as ABR measurement (for purposes of ERA and differential diagnosis), and contributing to the development of novel clinical applications that will advance electrophysiological approaches in clinical audiology (such as being a team player in the treatment of deafness with a cochlear implant).

Audiologists work alongside otolaryngologists, pediatricians, neurosurgeons, neurologists, cognitive neuroscientists, and many others who also have expertise in clinical electrophysiology, namely across other sensory/motor domains, including the evaluation of somatosensory, visual, and other evoked potentials as well as overlapping interests in EPs, including AEPs. Clinical audiologists and hearing scientists thus have the unique ability to encourage and enhance the use of AEP technologies in these other fields, if opportunities arise and should they choose to actively participate in multidisciplinary collaborations. Indeed, it is multidisciplinary collaborations that have greatly contributed to advancements via the research and development of clinical electrophysiology in audiology to bring this specialty to where it is today.

Audiologists have tools to test hearing sensitivity and discrimination abilities in order to determine if these abilities should be considered or will be impacted by neurological conditions or medical/surgical procedures. To recap, evoked potentials are routinely used for monitoring multiple sclerosis, for example. Sensorineural hearing loss affects a significant proportion of patients with multiple sclerosis[81] and hence audiologists have a role to play. This is not just in testing hearing sensitivity but also in understanding how hearing sensitivity and configuration of the hearing loss interact audiometrically/audiologically—thus evaluating the virtual transfer function through the peripheral system (recalling Episode 6.5). Might this affect the results of evoked-potential monitoring of disease status?[82] Patients with cerebellopontine angle tumors typically present with a hearing loss, and the surgical procedure to remove the tumor can then worsen hearing. Because of this situation, audiologists can also contribute uniquely to the care of these patients, for example, through use of intraoperative monitoring to support hearing preservation[83]—one of the several overlapping interests of clinical audiology and intraoperative monitoring, as just learned (Episode 10.1). Furthermore, the audiologist can provide postsurgery rehabilitation as needed for the patient, and in some patients, may beg supplementary AEP testing. Then, as the past attests, the future can be expected to further intertwine the technologies of hearing assessment/diagnosis with treatment monitoring by way of both behavioral and objective measures. Figure 1–1, at the outset of this book, broadly illustrated the range of auditory EPs in time and brain space that are in the clinical domain. In wrapping up this foundational textbook, it will be worthwhile to reflect, in parting, upon the several key interests clinically in the use of the audiologist's electrophysiological toolbox.

Extracting signals from noise: Peak latencies and amplitudes and spectral composition of the peaks can be extracted from the waveform using simple methods such as visual peak-picking or from more sophisticated or even automated algorithms.[84] The fundamental problem, however, remains: AEP measurement techniques rely on the extraction of small electrical auditory signals out of noise. It was learned that this extraction is especially challenging when the signal of interest is very small and buried in myogenic/other noise on top of the background EEG, such as might occur during the recording of the ABR in a fidgety, awake adult rather than a sleeping baby. Elsewhere in this text, techniques for reducing noise and amplifying the signal of interest are described. Automated techniques for identifying responses are also defined, thus providing audiologists with an opportunity to develop a fundamental understanding that can enable them to go beyond blindly following test protocols, or indeed perhaps even help to see possible improvements or even propose innovations.

Measuring perception–detection versus discrimination: The original suite of objective, auditory electrophysiological measures (the electroencephalogram, auditory brainstem response, and cortical auditory evoked potentials) was used to address fundamental questions, starting with, "Is there neural evidence in scalp recordings for the detection of sound?" It took more than three decades of research and development to get there beyond the Davis' first "plunge" into brainwaves.[85] Now there is a range of evoked potentials that can be measured at threshold levels that correlate well with a behavioral audiogram. The choice of optimal stimulus and recording paradigm to achieve frequency-specific estimates of hearing depends on whether the patient is an infant or an adult, asleep or awake. Further, tests of AEPs can address the origin of any hearing deficits, helping answer the question: "Is the problem affecting hearing thresholds in the peripheral auditory system, the auditory nerve, the brainstem, or at higher levels in the auditory pathway?" Audiologists are very familiar with these considerations; tests of AEPs gives them more tools with which to pursue them.

Auditory neuropathy/spectrum disorder, as was discussed frequently in this book, is both an intriguing and challenging disorder. It also is an example of a complex audiological condition for which the electrophysiological measures traditionally used for objective audiometry in infants, such as the transient or steady-state ABR, proved not to correlate well with behavior.[86,87] So, it is important to have a means to identify an AN, but then what? Audiologists are able to use their clinical judgment in cases where ANSD is suspected/confirmed and do more. This was the all-important point of the audiologist being able to call/rely upon cortical evoked potentials to get a broader assessment of functional hearing.[88,89]

A range of EP-testing techniques can be used to measure discrimination of complex sounds in people with hearing difficulties, such as sensorineural hearing loss and auditory processing disorders (APD). Advances in the use of complex stimuli, recording paradigms, and evoked response analysis in both time and frequency domains with sophisticated automated analysis are pushing the boundaries of clinical audiology; for example, in the understanding of the effects of sensorineural hearing loss on speech perception in noise.[90] This is the common problem affecting people with sensorineural hearing loss as well as synaptic-level APD from the distal 8th nerve and beyond. These developments are important—after years of hearing research and clinical practice, significant advances in related technologies, and debates over levels of the auditory system where APDs can occur—have brought audiologist/other professionals to face the reality of differences across individuals with the same audiometric thresholds/configurations in the perception of speech, especially in ever-challenging, everyday listening environments. Therein still remains audiological challenges for the efficacious detection, diagnosis, and clinical management of hearing losses/APDs.

Ultimately, functional use of hearing/behavioral measures can provide this information for many patients, but it is very helpful to have EEG-based/other objective indicators that can be relied upon to indicate whether a patient can both detect and discriminate sounds. These measures are needed especially for the very young and perhaps those who are older and have cognitive impairment and cannot express what they are hearing.[91] There has been clear progress toward this goal. For decades indeed, it had been known that the cortical, N_1 potential is a reliable indicator of hearing sensitivity,[92] yet it is only recently that the measurement of this component's latencies and amplitudes has been shown to inform the clinician about speech perception in noise.[93]

Understanding auditory stimuli: Having a nuanced understanding of auditory signals is helpful in knowing which stimuli are optimal for EP testing. Both temporal and spectral features of stimuli matter. Clicks, brief tone bursts, and chirps were touted for testing the auditory brainstem. It seems clicks still have certain advantages/attractions.[94] Yet, there are more advanced EP measures that can address speech processing, such as the frequency and/or envelope following response(s), and thereby facilitate a more comprehensive understanding of how the brain processes speech stimuli.[95] Results of recent studies suggest that, indeed, novel test paradigms are being used to measure speech-evoked envelope following responses, with great promise to provide useful outcome measures for people with hearing loss and wearing hearing aids.[96]

Transducers, stimulus levels, and standards: Considerations such as which transducer is used (insert earphone versus loudspeaker versus direct electrical stimulation) impacts the "view" of auditory functions in general and in measures of AEPs in particular as well as what measures are used for stimulus intensity—logarithmic "levels" per calibration approach (dB SPL, peSPL, dBA/dBC/dBZ, dB nHL, etc.)—or relative/sensation level (hearing-threshold-referenced). Thereafter is the decisive issue of where within the dynamic range of hearing to work (such as "soft" versus conversational versus loud speech level), which also includes frequency range. The conventional audiogram happens not to be comprehensive in covering the latter; frequencies above 8 kHz are only lightly embraced in conventional audiometry and largely neglected in ERA. These, indeed all, are issues within the realm of communication science and disorders and are points of departure for endeavors to detect and interpret findings of both behavioral and objective measures of auditory function and which continue to be refined in practice. With advances in sound level meter technology, it is possible to record fast and slow time-weighted sound levels, including both impulse and peak measures,[97] making it easier to calibrate a wide range of auditory stimuli. Advances in AEP and related test equipment (otoacoustic emissions and wideband middle-ear absorbance) have made stimulus calibration more accessible. More fundamentally, accurate auditory electrophysiology requires of audiologists understanding of sounds/acoustics for competent practice. Fundamental considerations also include attention to the (potential) effects of ambient noise levels on measurements of thresholds or even suprathreshold measures (pending test environment, like hearing clinic versus cribside)—equally for behavioral and electrophysiological tests. These are areas where audiological expertise can ensure the correct approach is used and accuracy is ensured when delivering auditory stimuli. Still, herein are needs begging further advances than reflected in methods used currently, such as real-ear calibration. This is integral to the measurement of otoacoustic emissions, yet not in "prime time" for auditory clinical electrophysiology, or even in conventional audiological evaluations.

The most commonly used transducer today, the tubal insert earphone, when used with clicks and tones, comes with at least a long-established calibration procedure,[98] based on standardization directly cross-referenced to the previously predominate transducer (supraaural type) but strongly dedicated to pure tones. Increasingly however, clinicians and hearing researchers are moving away from using simple stimuli in favor of more complex sounds, such as chirps, speech, and speech-like stimuli that can be used (again) to measure both limits of detection and/or discrimination.[99-101] Thus, there is a need to understand transducer and other stimulus and calibration effects on the evoking stimulus, and communication science is more important than ever for ensuring the reliability and validity of auditory-electrophysiological test results.

Amplification: As hearing loss is often diagnosed at very young ages today, interest in the use of electrophysiological measures to ensure that amplification is optimized has grown. Audiologists want the benefits of early detection and treatment of hearing loss to be realized to the extent possible and are aware that stimulus audibility is key to amplification success.[102] Auditory evoked potentials can support decisions about choices of amplification, amplification benefits, or whether it is time to move from hearing aids to cochlear implants.[103] Evoked potential amplitudes and detectability are linked to stimulus audibility.[104,105] Cortical evoked potentials can help speed up habilitation decisions in children with ANSD, for example,[106] and show in general the effects of hearing aid processing on audibility of speech sounds especially in children.[107] They can also demonstrate central auditory maturation (including intactness of binaural processing) in children, including with bilateral cochlear implants.[108]

Evoked responses and auditory processing: Cortical responses were shown in Chapter 8 to be quite suitable and, in fact, in Episode 9.4 robust for measurement in CI recipients, which has also been this writer's experience in both pediatric and adult users.[109] The value of tests of the acoustic change potential, featured in the last Heads Up of Chapter 8, demonstrated taking the classical CAEP to the next level, from serving as a metric of response detection to one sensitive to a stimulus difference. Multiple metrics otherwise were extensively overviewed in the same episode, suggesting a broad range of tests (P_3 and all) with progressively more ability to reflect hearing in its broadest sense. However, with CIs being implanted now in cases with various hearing impairments and over the life span, this area is not just a "replay" of issues confronted historically and today—with conventional amplification and its technology—although with parallels. One especially is the issue of maturity (in effect) of the metric itself in a given patient. Use of the CAEP and/or other indicators (early versus late onset of deafness) is complicated by such matters for defining the most efficacious utilities of AEP measurement. Meanwhile, this all is prime turf for the audiologist who is on the front line of programming the habilitative/rehabilitative device and ensuring optimal performance of device and patient alike.

In general, immature cortical responses are seen in children with APD.[110] In this area, audiologists work alongside a range of professionals including speech pathologists, teachers, and psychologists. There can be confusion regarding the auditory basis for listening difficulties that co-occur, for example, alongside reading, language, learning, or attention difficulties.[111] AEPs "help" to provide the evidence bases for listening and learning difficulties.[110,112,113] Equally importantly, AEP tests can show the benefits of treatment, such as that of using remote-microphone hearing aids in cases of APD.[114,115]

In conclusion, if the question of, "Whose land is this?" is merely about the technology and who "owns" it, the answer (hopefully resoundingly from Episode 10.1) is no one profession. While audiological applications of evoked responses in the early days were mainly in threshold measures and diagnostic audiology, interest in using evoked-response technology for guiding habilitation/rehabilitation decisions and monitoring progress has been growing nonstop. As the field of audiology moves toward increasingly complex applications of evoked responses, it becomes more critical that basic steps are followed to ensure the capture of a response optimal for addressing the problem of interest, and with an informed and open mind. For example, most responses covered in this text were neurogenic, and key culprits lurking in the background often were myogenic. However, the oft-belittled PAMR was demonstrated potentially to prove useful for some purposes (recall the second Heads Up of Episode 6.5). Is artifact then a matter of "the eye of the beholder?" Audiologists who understand hearing instruments and transducers appreciate that stimulus artifact indeed can mimic or obliterate a neural response, leading to false results and/or rendering the evoked response test a waste of time. It may be impossible to eliminate all artifacts, but errors of interpretation can be avoided through comprehensive knowledge of them and careful attention to the timing and morphology of the targeted response. Audiologists have played a major role in the development of the expanding suite of applications of auditory and other evoked responses that can solve clinical audiologic problems. While a whole range of people are experts in clinical electrophysiology, there are key challenges that audiologists are substantially qualified to address. Clinically competent audiologists bring with them an understanding of conductive and sensorineural hearing loss and disorders of neural dyssynchrony and of the central auditory system. They also know about the temporal and spectral features of auditory stimuli and how these stimuli are transduced by hearing instruments. And audiologists, like psychologists, also bring behavioral science, as well as biomedical science "to the table" of the patient's management. If this knowledge is coupled with that of physiological bases of evoked responses and technical aspects of their recording and processing, as presented in this text, audiologists then are clearly well placed to help advance this field and should be confident that this is their land. Audiologists will have the keys to the castle!

Take Home Messages

Heads-Up Special

1. From classical EEG on, the desire to peer into the brain has lured technological advances leading to computational processing of high-density recordings to estimate EP-generator loci.
2. Several methods have been more or less successful, yet not like functional MRI/other modern high-tech imaging methods.
3. Voltage measurement is not all there is; the synchronous activation of neurons in the brain gives rise to minute magnetic fields that permit eliciting and recording measurable AEFs.
4. MEG technology provides better estimation of generator dipoles, also helping to confirm AEP components' origins and to test auditory phenomena more directly in humans.

Episode 1

1. IONM of A/OtherEPs serves different objectives than in clinical electrophysiology.
2. IONM must be well justified; success depends on timely and systematic observations.
3. Differences in approach for IONM (in reference to clinical testing) are the needs for sampling of responses often and recurrently and for interpreting results pretty much "on the spot."
4. Working in IONM requires additional training and experience toward competency with the different skill sets involved.
5. Knowledge base of IONM spans still broader areas of neuroanatomy/neurophysiology than that of the auditory system, such as knowledge of pathways and methods of monitoring SSEPs.
6. It often is not enough to monitor responses only evoked via ascending pathways, rather descending/motor pathways, if not the primary purpose—like "protection" of the 7th nerve.
7. Returning to clinical neurophysiology, appropriately trained audiologists may become involved with tests of evoked muscle responses, like ENOG and testing VEMPs.
8. In general, it is useful at times to look across areas of neurophysiology for what may be learned/shared from one field to the other, like the impressively robust pattern-reversal VEP.

Heads Up

9. IONM is a part of a team effort; monitoring the SSEP is often (in some cases more) about protecting the well-being of the patient, as the case in point dramatically demonstrated.

References

1. McPherson, D., Harris, R., Sorensen, D. (2020). Functional neuorimaging of the central auditory system. In S. Hatzopoulos (Ed.), *Advances in audiology, speech pathology, and hearing science*. Apple Academic Press.
2. Tonnquist-Uhlén, I. (1996). Topography of auditory evoked long-latency potentials in children with severe language impairment: The P2 and N2 components. *Ear and Hearing, 17*(4), 314–326.

3. Amateur Radio Relay League. (2018). *The ARRL handbook for radio communications, volume 1: Introduction and fundamental theory* [Kindle edition]. ARRL.
4. Van Yper, L. N., Undurraga, J. A., Johnson, B., Monaghan, J., & McAlpine, D. (2019). Neural representations of interaural time differences in the human cortex—An MEG study. *IERAG (International Evoked Response Study Group).* http://www.ierasg.ifps.org.pl/index.php?s=meetings
5. Arlinger, S. D., Jerlvall, L. B., Aren, T., & Holmgren, E. C. I. (1976). Slow evoked cortical responses to linear frequency ramps of a continuous pure tone. *Acta Physiologica Scandinavica, 98*, 412–424.
6. Arlinger, S., Elberling, C., Bak, C., Kofoed, B., Lebech, J., & Saermark, K. (1982). Cortical magnetic fields evoked by frequency glides of a continuous tone. *Electroencephalography and Clinical Neurophysiology, 54*, 642–653.
7. Dimitrijevic, A., Michalewski, H. J., Zeng, F-G., Pratt, P., & Starr, S. (2008). Frequency changes in a continuous tone: Auditory cortical potentials. *Clinical Neurophysiology, 119*, 2111–2124.
8. Pantev, C., Bertrand, O., Eulitz, C., Verkindt, C., Hampson, S., Schuierer, G., & Elbert, T. (1995). Specific tonotopic organizations of different areas of the human auditory cortex revealed by simultaneous magnetic and electric recordings. *Electroencephalography and Clinical Neurophysiology, 94*, 26–40.
9. Walzl, E. M. (1947). Representation of the cochlea in the cerebral cortex. *Laryngoscope, 57*, 778–787.
10. Whitfield, I. C. (1967). *The auditory pathway.* Williams & Wilkins.
11. Merzenich, M. M., Knight, P. L., & Roth, G. L. (1975). Representation of cochlea within primary auditory cortex in the cat. *Journal of Neurophysiology, 38*, 231–249.
12. Verkindt, C., Bertrand, O., Perrin, F., Echallier, J. F., & Pernier, J. (1995). Tonotopic organization of the human auditory cortex: N100 topography and multiple dipole model analysis. *Electroencephalography and Clinical Neurophysiology, 96*, 143–156.
13. Fujioka, T., Kakigi, R., Gunji, A., & Takeshima, Y. (2002). The auditory evoked magnetic fields to very high frequency tones. *Neuroscience, 112*, 367–381.
14. Gabriel, D., Veuillet, E., Ragot, R., Schwartz, D., Ducorps, A., Norena, A., . . . Collet, L. (2004). Effect of stimulus frequency and stimulation site on the N1m response of the human auditory cortex. *Hearing Research, 197*, 55–64.
15. Sundararaman, L. V., & Desai, S. P. (2017). The anesthesia records of Harvey Cushing and Ernest Codman. *Anesthesia & Analgesia, 126*(1), 322–329.
16. Preul, M. C., & Feindel, W. C. (1991). Origins of Wilder Penfield's surgical technique. The role of the "Cushing ritual" and influences from the European experience. *Journal of Neurosurgy, 75*(5), 82–120.
17. Penfield, W., & Boldrey, E. (1937). Somatic motor and sensory representation in the cerebral cortex in man as studied by electrical stimulation. *Brain, 37*, 389–443.
18. Reif, P. S., Strzelczyk, A., & Rosenow, F. (2016). The history of invasive EEG evaluation in epilepsy patients. *Seizure, 41*, 191–195.
19. Jasper, H. (1949). Electrocorticograms in man. *Electroencephalography and Clinical Neurophysiology, 1* (Suppl. 2), 16–29.
20. Ruben, R. J., Bordley, J. E., & Lieberman, A. T. (1961). Cochlear potentials in man. *Laryngoscope, 71*, 1141–1164.
21. Shedd, D. P., & Burget, G. C. (1966). Identification of the recurrent laryngeal nerve. *Archives of Surgery, 92*(6), 861–864.
22. Goldring, S. (1978). A method for surgical management of focal epilepsy, especially as it relates to children. *Journal of Neurosurgery, 49*(3), 344–356.
23. Goldring, S., & Gregorie, E. M. (1984). Surgical management of epilepsy using epidural recordings to localize the seizure focus. Review of 100 cases. *Journal of Neurosurgery, 60*(3), 457–466.
24. Harris, E. J., Brown, W. H., Pavy, R. N., Anderson. W. W., & Stone, D. W. (1967). Continuous electroencephalographic monitoring during carotid artery endarterectomy. *Surgery, 62*(3), 441–447.
25. Feinsod, M., Madey, J. M., & Susal, A. L. (1975). A new photostimulator for continuous recording of the visual evoked potential. *Electroencephalography and Clinical Neurophysiology, 38*(6), 641–642.
26. Nash, C. L., Jr., Lorig, R. A., Schatzinger, L. A., & Brown, R. H. (1977). Spinal cord monitoring during operative treatment of the spine. *Clinical Orthopaedics and Related Research, 126*, 100–105.
27. Whitaker, H. A., & Ojemann, G. A. (1977). Graded localization of naming from electrical stimulation mapping of left cerebral cortex. *Nature, 270*(5632), 50–51.
28. Ojemann, G. A. (1979). Individual variability in language. *Journal of Neurosurgery, 50*, 164–169.
29. Merton, P. A., & Morton, H. B. (1980). Stimulation of the cerebral cortex in the intact human subject. *Nature, 285*, 227.
30. Levy, W. J., Shapiro, J. M., Maruchak, G., & Meathe, E. (1980). Automated EEG processing for intraoperative monitoring: A comparison of techniques. *Anesthesiology, 53*(3), 223–236.
31. Grundy, B. L., Lina, A., Procopio, P. T., & Jannetta, P. J. (1981). Reversible evoked potential changes with

retraction of the eighth cranial nerve. *Anesthesia & Analgesia, 60*(11), 835–838.

32. Moller, A. R., Jannetta, P. J., & Moller, M. B. (1981). Neural generators of brainstem evoked potentials. Results from human intracranial recordings. *Annals of Otology, Rhinology & Laryngology, 90,* 591–596.

33. Thornton, C., Cately, D. M., Jordan, C., Lehane, J. R., Royston, D., & Jones, J. C. (1983). Enflurane anaesthesia causes graded changes in the brainstem and early cortical auditory evoked response in man. *British Journal of Anaesthesia, 55,* 479–486.

34. Sekhar, L. N., & Moller, A. R. (1986). Operative management of tumors involving the cavernous sinus. *Journal of Neurosurgy, 64*(6), 879–889.

35. Niparko, J. K., Kileny, P. R., Kemink, J. L., Lee, H. M., & Graham, M. D. (1989). Neurophysiologic intraoperative monitoring: II. Facial nerve function. *American Journal of Otolaryngology, 10*(1), 55–61.

36. Mishler, E. T., & Smith, P. G. (1995). Technical aspects of intraoperative monitoring of lower cranial nerve function. *Skull Base Surgery, 5*(4), 245–250.

37. Boyd, S. G., Rothwell, J. C., Cowan, J. M. A., Webb, J. P., Morley, T., Asselman, P., & Marsden C. D. (1986). A method of monitoring function in corticospinal pathways during scoliosis surgery with a note on motor conduction velocities. *Journal of Neurology, Neurosurgery and Psychiatry, 49,* 251–257.

38. Lambert, P. R., & Ruth, R. A. (1988). Simultaneous ABR for use in recording of noninvasive ECoG intraoperative monitoring. *Otolaryngology-Head and Neck Surgery, 98*(6), 575–580.

39. Burke, D., Hicks, R., Stephen, J., Woodforth, I., & Crawford, M. (1992). Assessment of corticospinal and somatosensory conduction simultaneously during scoliosis surgery. *Electroencephalography and Clinical Neurophysiology, 85,* 388–396.

40. Taniguchi, M., Cedzich, C., & Schramm J. (1993). Modification of cortical stimulation for motor evoked potentials under general anesthesia: Technical description. *Neurosurgery, 32*(2) 219–226.

41. Kileny, P. R., Zwolan, T. A., Zimmerman-Phillips, S., & Telian, S. A. (1994). Electrically evoked auditory brain-stem response in pediatric patients with cochlear implants. *Archives of Otolaryngology-Head and Neck Surgery, 120,* 1083–1090.

42. Maguire, J., Wallace, S., Madiga, R., Leppanen, R., & Draper, V. (1995). Evaluation of intrapedicular screw position using intraoperative evoked electromyography. *Spine, 20*(9), 1068–1074.

43. Benabid, A. L. Pollak, P., Hoffmann, D., Benazzouz, A., Gao, D. M., Laurent, A., ... Parret, J. (1994). Acute and long-term effects of subthalamic nucleus stimulation in Parkinson's disease. *Stereotactic and Functional Neurosurgery, 62,* 76–84.

44. Limousin, P., Pollak, P., Benazzouz, A., Hoffmann, D., Le Bas, J. F., Broussolle, E., ... Benabid, A. L. (1995). Effect of parkinsonian signs and symptoms of bilateral subthalamic nucleus stimulation. *Lancet, 345*(8942), 91–95.

45. Filipo, R., Attanasio, G., Barbaro, M., Viccaro, M., Musacchio, A., Cappelli, G., & De Seta, E. (2007). Distortion product otoacoustic emissions in otosclerosis: Intraoperative findings. *Advances oto-rhino-laryngology* (Vol. 65, pp. 133–136).

46. Oghalai, J. S., Tonini, R., Rasmus, J., Emery, C., Manolidis, S., Vrabec, J. T., & Haymond, J. (2009). Intra-operative monitoring of cochlear function during cochlear implantation. *Cochlear Implants International, 10*(1), 1–18.

47. Verhaegen, V. J., Mulder, J. J., Noten, J. F., Luijten, B. M., Cremers, C. W., & Snik, A. F. (2010). Intraoperative auditory steady state response measurements during Vibrant Soundbridge middle ear implantation in patients with mixed hearing loss: Preliminary results. *Otology & Neurotology, 31*(9), 1365–1368.

48. Koka, K., Riggs, W. J., Dwyer, R., Holder, J. T., Noble, J. H., Dawant, B. M., ... Labadie, R. F. (2018). Intracochlear electrocochleography during cochlear implant electrode insertion is predictive of inal scalar location. *Otology & Neurotology, 39*(8), e654–e659.

49. Bell, S. L., Smith, D. L., Allen, R., & Lutman, M. E. (2006). The auditory middle latency response, evoked using maximum length sequences and chirps, as an indicator of adequacy of anesthesia. *Anesthesia & Analgesia, 10*(2), 495–498.

50. Simon, M. V. (2011). Neurophysiologic intraoperative monitoring of the vestibulocochlear nerve. *Journal of Clinical Neurophysiology, 28*(6), 566–581.

51. Martin, W. H., & Shi, Y-B. (2009). Intraoperative neurophysiology: Monitoring auditory evoked potentials. In J. Katz, L. Medvetsky, R. Burkard, & L. Hood (Eds.), *Handbook of clinical audiology* (6th ed., pp. 351–372). Lippincott-WW.

52. Legatt, A. D. (2002). Mechanisms of intraoperative brainstem auditory evoked potential changes. *Journal of Clinical Neurophysiology, 19*(5), 396–408.

53. Durrant, J. D., and & Sclabassi, R. J. (1993). Neurophysiologic monitoring in cranial base surgery. In Principles in Cranial Base Surgery, I. P. Janecka, Vol. Ed.; *Problems in Plastic and Reconstructive Surgery, 3*(1), 91–101.

54. American Clinical Neurophysiology Society. (2009, October). *Guideline 11 C: Recommended standards for intraoperative monitoring of auditory evoked*

potentials. https://www.acns.org/pdf/guidelines/Guideline-11C.pdf

55. National Institutes of Health. (1991). Acoustic neuroma. *NIH Consensus Statement, 9*(4), 1–24. https://consensus.nih.gov/1991/1991AcousticNeuroma087html.htm

56. Martin, W. H., & Stecker, M. M. (2008). ASNM position statement: Intraoperative monitoring of auditory evoked potentials. *The Journal of Clinical Monitoring and Computing, 22*, 75–85.

57. Schlake, H.-P., Goldbrunner, R. H., Milewski, C., Krauss, J., Trautner, H., Behr, R., ... Roosen, K. (2001). Intra-operative electromyographic monitoring of the lower cranial motor nerves (LCN IX–XII) in skull base surgery. *Clinical Neurology and Neurosurgery, 103*(2), 72–82.

58. Topsakal, C., Al-Mefty, O., Bulsara, K. R., & Williford, V. S. (2008). Intraoperative monitoring of lower cranial nerves in skull base surgery: Technical report and review of 123 monitored cases. *Neurosurgical Review, 31*, 45–53.

59. Schlake, H.-P., Goldbrunner, R. H., Siebert, M., Behr, R., & Roosen, K. (2001). Intra-operative electromyographic monitoring of extra-ocular motor nerves (Nn. III, VI) in skull base surgery. *Acta Neurochirurgica, 143*, 251–261.

60. Noss, R. S., Lalwani, A. K., & Yingling, C. D. (2001). Facial nerve monitoring in middle ear and mastoid surgery. *Laryngoscope, 111*, 831–836.

61. Wilson, L., Lin, E., & Lalwani, A. (2003). Cost-effectiveness of intraoperative facial nerve monitoring in middle ear or mastoid surgery. *Laryngoscope, 113*, 1736–1745.

62. American Academy of Otolaryngology-Head and Neck Surgery Foundation. (2017). *Position statement: Intraoperative nerve monitoring in otologic surgery*. https://www.entnet.org/intraoperative-nerve-monitoring

63. Sood, A. J., Houlton, J. J., Nguyen, S. A., & Gillespie, M. B. (2015). Facial nerve monitoring during parotidectomy: A systematic review and meta-analysis. *Otolaryngology-Head and Neck Surgery, 152*(4), 631–637.

64. Higgins, T. S., Gupta, R., Ketcham, A. S., Sataloff, R. T., Wadworth, J. T., & Sinacori, J. T. (2011). Recurrent laryngeal nerve monitoring versus identification alone on post-thyroidectomy true vocal fold palsy: A meta-analysis. *Laryngoscope, 121*, 1009–1017.

65. Sanabria, A., Ramirez, A., Kowalski, L. P., Silver, C. E., Shaha, A. R., Owen, R. P., ... Ferlito, A. (2013). Neuromonitoring in thyroidectomy: A meta-analysis of effectiveness for randomized controlled trials. *European Archives of Oto-Rhino-Laryngology, 270*, 2175–2189.

66. Chandrasekha, S. S., Randolph, G. W., Seidman, M. D., Rosenfeld, R. M., Angelos, P., Barkmeier-Kraemer, J., ... Robertson, P. J. (2013). Clinical practice guideline: Improving voice outcomes after thyroid surgery. *Otolaryngology-Head and Neck Surgery, 148*(6S), S1–S37.

67. Kileny, P. R. (2019). *The audiologist's handbook of intraoperative neurophysiological monitoring*. Plural Publishing.

68. Commission on Accreditation of Allied Health Education Programs. https://www.caahep.org/Students/Find-a-Program.aspx

69. American Board of Registration of Electroencephalographic and Evoked Potential Technologists. https://www.abret.org/candidates/credentials/cnim/

70. May, M., Blumenthal, F., & Klein, S. R. (1983). Acute Bell's palsy: Prognostic value of evoked electromyography, maximal stimulation, and other electrical tests. *American Journal of Otolaryngology, 5*, 1–7.

71. Esslen, E. (1973). Electrodiagnosis of facial palsy. In A. Miehelke (Ed.), *Surgery of the facial nerve* (pp. 45–51). W.B. Sanders Company.

72. Mannarekki, G., Griffin, G. R., Kileny, P., & Edwards, B. (2012). Electrophysiological measures in facial paresis and paralysis. *Operative Techniques in Otolaryngology-Head and Neck Surgery, 23*(4), 236–247.

73. Zhao, Y., Feng, F., Wu, H., Aodeng, S., Tian, X., Volk, G. F., ... Gao, Z. (2020). Prognostic value of a three-dimensional dynamic quantitative analysis system to measure facial motion in acute facial paralysis patients. *Head & Face Medicine, 16*, 15. https://doi.org/10.1186/s13005-020-00230-6

74. House, J. W., & Brackmann, D. E. (1985). Facial nerve grading system. *Otolaryngology-Head and Neck Surgery, 93*, 146–147.

75. Barin, K., & Durrant, J. D. (2000). Applied physiology of the vestibular system. In R. F. Canalis & P. R. Lambert (Eds.), *The ear: Comprehensive otology* (pp. 113–140). Lippincott W&W.

76. McCaslin, D. L., & Jacobson, G. P. (2021). Vestibular-evoked myogenic potentials (VEMPs). In G. P. Jacobson, N. T. Shepard, K. Barin, R. F. Burkard, & K. Janky (Eds.), Balance function assessment and management (3rd ed., pp. 399–438). Plural Publishing.

77. Odom, J. V., Bach, M., Brigell, M., Holder, G. E., McCulloch, D. L., Mizota, A., & Tormene, A. P. (2016). ISCEV standard for clinical visual evoked potentials: (2016 update). *Documenta Ophthalmologica, 133*, 1–9. 10.1007/s10633-016-9553-y

78. Durrant, J. D. (1987). Auditory evoked potential to pattern reversal stimulation. *Audiology, 26*, 123–132.
79. Durrant, J. D. (1987). Pattern reversal auditory evoked potential. *Electroencephalography and Clinical Neurophysiology, 68*, 157–160.
80. Sclabassi, R. J., Krieger, D. N., Weisz, D., & Durrant, J. (1993). Methods of neurophysiological monitoring during cranial base tumor resection. In L. N. Sekhar & I. P. Janecka (Eds.), *Surgery of cranial base tumors* (pp. 83–98). Raven Press.
81. Di Stadio, A., Dipietro, L., Ralli, M., Meneghello, F., Minni, A., Greco, A., . . . Bernitsass, E. (2018). Sudden hearing loss as an early detector of multiple sclerosis: A systematic review. *European Review for Medical and Pharmacological Sciences, 22*, 4611–4624.
82. Pokryszko-Dragan, A., Bilinska, M., Gruszka, E., Kusinska, E., & Podemski, R. (2015). Assessment of visual and auditory evoked potentials in multiple sclerosis patients with and without fatigue. *Neurological Sciences, 36*(2), 235–242. 10.1007/s10072-014-1953-8
83. Morawski, K. F., Niemczyk, K., Bohorquez, J., Marchel, A., Delgado, R. E., Ozdamar, O., & Telischi, F. F. (2007). Intraoperative monitoring of hearing during cerebellopontine angle tumor surgery using transtympanic electrocochleography. *Otology & Neurotology, 28*(4), 541–545. 10.1097/mao.0b013e3180577919
84. Bardy, F., Van Dun, B., Seeto, M., & Dillon, H. (2020). Automated cortical auditory response detection strategy. *International Journal of Audiology, 59*(11), 835–842.
85. Davis, P. A. (1939). Effects of acoustic stimuli on the waking human brain. *Journal of Neurophysiology, 2*(6), 494–499.
86. De Siati, R. D., Rosenzweig, F., Gersdorff, G., Gregoire, A., Rombaux, P., & Deggouj, N. (2020). Auditory neuropathy spectrum disorders: From diagnosis to treatment: Literature review and case reports. *Journal of Clinical Medicine, 9*(4), 1074. 10.3390/jcm9041074
87. Rance, G., & Starr, A. (2015). Pathophysiological mechanisms and functional hearing consequences of auditory neuropathy. *Brain, 138*(Pt. 11), 3141–3158. 10.1093/brain/awv270
88. Cardon, G., & Sharma, A. (2011). Cortical auditory evoked potentials in auditory neuropathy spectrum disorder: Clinical implications. *Perspectives on Hearing and Hearing Disorders in Childhood, 21*(1), 31–37.
89. Gardner-Berry, K., Chang, H., Ching, T. Y., & Hou, S. (2016). Detection rates of cortical auditory evoked potentials at different sensation levels in infants with sensory/neural hearing loss and auditory neuropathy spectrum disorder. *Seminars in Hearing, 37*(1), 53–61. 10.1055/s-0035-1570330
90. Fuglsang, S. A., Marcher-Rorsted, J., Dau, T., & Hjortkjaer, J. (2020). Effects of sensorineural hearing loss on cortical synchronization to competing speech during selective attention. *Journal of Neuroscience, 40*(12), 2562–2572. 10.1523/JNEUROSCI.1936-19.2020
91. Bott, A., Hickson, L., Meyer, C., Bardy, F., Van Dun, B., & Pachana, N. A. (2020). Is cortical automatic threshold estimation a feasible alternative for hearing threshold estimation with adults with dementia living in aged care? *International Journal of Audiology, 59*(10), 745–752. https://doi.org/10.1080/14992027.2020.1746976
92. Davis, H. (1965). Slow cortical responses evoked by acoustic stimuli. *Acta Oto-Laryngologica, 59*(2–4), 179–185. https://doi.org/10.3109/00016486509124551
93. Billings, C. J., McMillan, G. P., Penman, T. M., & Gille, S. M. (2013). Predicting perception in noise using cortical auditory evoked potentials. *Journal of the Association for Research in Otolaryngology, 14*(6), 891–903. 10.1007/s10162-013-0415-y
94. Keesling, D. A., Parker, J. P., & Sanchez, J. T. (2017). A comparison of commercially available auditory brainstem response stimuli at a neurodiagnostic intensity level. *Audiology Research, 7*(1), 161. 10.4081/audiores.2017.161
95. Coffey, E. B. J., Nicol, T., White-Schwoch, T., Chandrasekaran, B., Krizman, J., Skoe, E., . . . Kraus, N. (2019). Evolving perspectives on the sources of the frequency-following response. *Nature Communications, 10*(1), 5036. https://doi.org/10.1038/s41467-019-13003-w
96. Easwar, V., Birstler, J., Harrison, A., Scollie, S., & Purcell, D. (2020). The accuracy of envelope following responses in predicting speech audibility. *Ear and Hearing, 41*(6), 1732–1746. https://doi.org/10.1097/AUD.0000000000000892
97. Laukli, E., & Burkard, R. (2015). Calibration/standardization of short-duration stimuli. *Seminars in Hearing, 36*(1), 3–10. 10.1055/s-0034-1396923
98. Elberling, C., Don, M., & Kristensen, S. G. (2012). Auditory brainstem responses to chirps delivered by an insert earphone with equalized frequency response. *The Journal of the Acoustical Society of America, 132*(2), EL149–154. 10.1121/1.4737915
99. Cho, S. W., Han, K. H., Jang, H. K., Chang, S. O., Jung, H., & Lee, J. H. (2015). Auditory brainstem responses to CE-Chirp(R) stimuli for normal ears and those with sensorineural hearing loss. *International*

Journal of Audiology, 54(10), 700–704. 10.3109/1499 2027.2015.1043148

100. Easwar, V., Purcell, D. W., & Scollie, S. D. (2012). Electroacoustic comparison of hearing aid output of phonemes in running speech versus isolation: Implications for aided cortical auditory evoked potentials testing. *International Journal of Otolaryngology, 2012*. https://doi.org/10.1155/2012/518202

101. Stone, M. A., Visram, A., Harte, J. M., & Munro, K. J. (2019). A set of time-and-frequency-localized short-duration speech-like stimuli for assessing hearing-aid performance via cortical auditory-evoked potentials. *Trends in Hearing, 23*. https://doi.org10.1177/2331216519885568

102. McCreery, R. W., Walker, E. A., Spratford, M., Bentler, R., Holte, L., Roush, P., . . . Moeller, M. P. (2015). Longitudinal predictors of aided speech audibility in infants and children. *Ear and Hearing, 36*(Suppl. 1), 24S–37S. 10.1097/AUD.0000000000000211

103. Purdy, S. C., Katsch, R., Dillon, H., Storey, L., Sharma, M., & Agung, K. (2004). Aided cortical auditory evoked potentials for hearing instrument evaluation in infants. In R. C. Seewald (Ed.), *A sound foundation through early amplification* (pp. 115–127). Phonak AG.

104. Chang, H. W., Dillon, H., Carter, L., van Dun, B., & Young, S. T. (2012). The relationship between cortical auditory evoked potential (CAEP) detection and estimated audibility in infants with sensorineural hearing loss. *International Journal of Audiology, 51*(9), 663–670. 10.3109/14992027.2012.690076

105. Van Dun, B., Kania, A., & Dillon, H. (2016). Cortical auditory evoked potentials in (un)aided normal-hearing and hearing-impaired adults. *Seminars in Hearing, 37*(1), 9–24. 10.1055/s-0035-1570333

106. Gardner-Berry, K., Purdy, S. C., Ching, T. Y., & Dillon, H. (2015). The audiological journey and early outcomes of twelve infants with auditory neuropathy spectrum disorder from birth to two years of age. *International Journal of Audiology, 54*(8), 524–535. 10.3109/14992027.2015.1007214

107. Ching, T. Y., Zhang, V. W., Hou, S., & Van Buynder, P. (2016). Cortical auditory evoked potentials reveal changes in audibility with nonlinear frequency compression in hearing aids for children: Clinical implications. *Seminars in Hearing, 37*(1), 25–35. 10.1055/s-0035-1570332

108. Easwar, V., Yamazaki, H., Deighton, M., Papsin, B., & Gordon, K. (2017). Cortical representation of interaural time difference is impaired by deafness in development: Evidence from children with early long-term access to sound through bilateral cochlear implants provided simultaneously. *Journal of Neuroscience, 37*(9), 2349–2361. 10.1523/JNEUROSCI.2538-16.2017

109. Purdy, S. C., Lin, R. Y.-C., Welch, D., Giles, E., Kelly, A. S., & van Dun, B. (2009, June). *Speech-evoked cortical auditory evoked potentials in children and adults with cochlear implants: Stimulus effects, test-retest stability, and characterization of the cochlear implant artifact.* Paper presented at the International Evoked Response Study Group (IEARSG) XXII Biennial Symposium, Moscow, Russia

110. Tomlin, D., & Rance, G. (2016). Maturation of the central auditory nervous system in children with auditory processing disorder. *Seminars in Hearing, 37*(1), 74–83. 10.1055/s-0035-1570328

111. Sharma, M., Purdy, S. C., & Kelly, A. S. (2009). Comorbidity of auditory processing, language, and reading disorders. *Journal of Speech, Language, and Hearing Research, 52*(3), 706–722. 10.1044/1092-4388(2008/07-0226)

112. Barker, M. D., Kuruvilla-Mathew, A., & Purdy, S. C. (2017). Cortical auditory-evoked potential and behavioral evidence for differences in auditory processing between good and poor readers. *Journal of the American Academy of Audiology, 28*(6), 534–545. 10.3766/jaaa.16054

113. Cunningham, J., Nicol, T., Zecker, S., & Kraus, N. (2000). Speech-evoked neurophysiologic responses in children with learning problems: Development and behavioral correlates of perception. *Ear and Hearing, 21*(6), 554–568. 10.1097/00003446-200012000-00003

114. Purdy, S. C., Smart, J. L., Baily, M., & Sharma, M. (2009). Do children with reading delay benefit from the use of personal FM systems in the classroom? *International Journal of Audiology, 48*(12), 843–852. 10.3109/14992020903140910

115. Sharma, M., Purdy, S. C., & Kelly, A. S. (2014). The contribution of speech-evoked cortical auditory evoked potentials to the diagnosis and measurement of intervention outcomes in children with auditory processing disorder. *Seminars in Hearing, 35*(1), 51–64.

116. Choi, S. M. S., Wong, E. C. M., & McPherson, B. (2019). Aided cortical auditory evoked measures with cochlear implantees: the challenge of stimulus artefacts. *Hearing, Balance and Communication, 17*(3), 229–238.

Index

Note: Page numbers in **bold** reference non-text material.

NUMBERS

1-3-6 milestones, for audiological management, 393
3CLTs (Three-channel Lissajous trajectories), 59–61
40-Hz ASSR, 210
80-Hz ASSR, 209, 230

A

AABR (Automated ABR), 369
ABI (Auditory brainstem implants). *See* Auditory brainstem (ABI) implants
ABR (Auditory brainstem response), 58, 150, 177
    AC elicited, 187
    AEPs (Auditory evoked potentials/responses) recording and, 83
    air conduction frequency-specific, 224
    automated, 369
    BC, infant, **384**
    bone-conduction, 378
    click-elicited, **236**
    differential diagnosis, **247–254**
    ECochG (Electrocochleography) and, **171**
    ERA
        ALLR-ERA, 324
        AMLR-ERA alternative/supplement, 284
        AMLR, 284
        applying bone conduction to, 316
    evaluation findings of lesions, **242**
    frequency-specific, bone conduction, 224
    hearing
        loss, **233**
        threshold estimation and, 326
    ideal/modeled, **191**
    interpretation of, 178
        findings, 240–241
    latencies of, 238
    main positive peaks, **112**
    NHS, 367
    normal, **179**
    norms for, 239
    older children/young adults, **110**
    to rarefaction, **183**
    recordings, **182**
        examples, **85**
        parameters for, **181**
    simultaneous recording of, 180
    stacked, 246–247
    stimulus rate and, **183**
    tests, vestibular responses, 379
    transducer and, 186
    VDL relationship with, 326
    wave amplitudes, 246
    waveforms, 233–234
Absorbance
    1-ER, 44
    measurement, **44–45**
AC (Air conduction). *See* Air conduction
AC (Alternating current). *See* Alternative current (AC)
ACC (Acoustic change complex), 352–353, 410
Acoustic
    broadband click, 144
    calibration, **219**
        equipment, **42**
    change complex (ACC), 352–353, 410
    click, 34
        AMLR, **274**
    coupler, defined, 35
    evoked motor response, PAMR and, 255
    filtering, 16
    intensity (I), 38
    nerve tumors, 241
    output, measured, 38
    stimulus, 34
    transients, standards, **42**
    tumors, 241, 434
Action potentials, 65
    adaptation, 147
Active transducer, 122
A–D (Analog to digital), conversion, 17
Adaptation, 147, 184, 201, 214, 218, 257, 277, 284, 346
ADHD (Attention deficit hyperactivity disorder), 343

Advanced age, AMLR and, 280–281, 297
AEF (Auditory evoked field), **424**
AEPs. *See* Auditory evoked potentials/responses (AEPs)
　derived, example *See* binaural interaction component (BIC)
Afferents, IHCs (Inner hair cells) and, 65
Ag-AgCl (Silver-silver-chloride), 51
　electrodes, 52
Age
　advanced, AMLR and, 297
　related hearing loss, 297
Aging
　dementia, 343
　effects, maturation and, 341–342
Air/bone conduction brief-tone ABRs, summary of, **221**
Air-bone gap, amplitudes/latencies and, 234
Air conduction (AC), 187–188
　ABR testing and, 381
　artifactual responses, 229
　ASSRs
　　infants and, 379
　　predict behavioral thresholds, 226–228
　　thresholds, 379
　BC, recording ASSRs at same time, 387
　ear specific thresholds, 222
　EMLs, 225
　frequency-specific
　　ABR (Auditory brainstem response), 224
　　stimuli, 219
　narrowband level-specific CE-chirp, 379
　stimulus, 377
　　parameters, **220**
　thresholds
　　electrophysiological assessment of, 380
　　estimates, 228
　　searches, at audiometric frequencies, 222
Algorithms, **32**
Aliasing, 18
　low-pass filter and, 94
ALLR (Auditory long latency response), 285, 302, 313
　determining auditory thresholds with, 409
　ERA, 377
　　vs. ABR-ERA, 324
　　CAEP measurement approaches and, 332
　　in workman's compensation, 314
Alternating
　current (AC), 50, **421**
　polarity/phase, stimuli, 92
Alzheimer's disease, 297, 343
　late-late AEPs and, 347

AM (Amplitude). *See* Amplitude (AM)
American Academy of Otolaryngology-Head and Neck Surgery, *Intraoperative Nerve Monitoring in Otologic Surgery*, 435
American Academy of Pediatrics, sedation guidelines, 393
American National Standards Institute (ANSI), 41
AMLR (Auditory middle latency response), 271–284, 409, 432
　40-Hz ASSR, **279**, 280
　acoustic click, **274**
　advancing age effect on, 280–281
　amplitude-intensity functions of, **299**
　differential diagnostic applications of, 292–302
　electrically elicited, 301
　ERA and, 284–292
　example of, **272**
　generators, 273, 293
　limitations, P_{50}, 297
　illustrated, **301**
　latencies
　　amplitudes values of, **272**
　　responses recorded, **285**
　measures, during sleep, 287
　obtained
　　at various stimulus rates, **278**
　　using 4000 clicks, **275**
　P_b of, 314
　recorded at C_Z, **276**
　salient features of, **294**
　simulation, **279**
　　diotic versus monotic, 274
　somatosensory evoked potential compared to, **437**
　stimulus/recording parameters, **273**
Amplification, 16, 446–447
Amplifier, differential, 95–96
　inverted versus noninverted inputs, 96
Amplitude (AM), 10–11, 26
　air-bone gap and, 234
　AMLR and, 271–284
　ASSRs, 83
　CAEP, 316–317
　LLR, 83
　nonlinearity of, 15
　of P_a and P_b components, **282**
　of potentials, recorded via TT-ECochG, 165
　ratio, (V/I) of ABR, 183
AN-CAP, 432–433
Analog
　electrophysiological signals, 17
　filter, high-pass (HP) setting of, 152

filters, 95
signal, 17
   signal conditioning, 111
   to digital (A–D) conversion, 17
Analysis, 8
Ancillary circuits, computer interface and, **30**
Anesthesia record, 428
ANSD (Auditory neuropathy spectrum disorder), 165
ANSI (American National Standards Institute), 41
   S3.1, **42**, 43
   S3.6, 41, **42**, 43
AP, latency-intensity shifts of, **170**
Apex (of cochlea), 63
Aphasia, injury, 347
AP(N_1)/ABR, **169**
A_{p-p} (Peak-to-peak amplitude), 10–11
   nonlinearity of, 15
A_{RMS}, 11
Arousal
   defined, 341
   effects, 341
Artifact rejection
   principle of, **91**
   reducing noise and, 86, 90–92
Artifactual responses, 229
Ascending pathway/nerve fibers, 65
ASSRs (Auditory steady-state responses), 75, 83, 197, 209–219
   80-Hz ASSR, 209
   80-Hz/brainstem ASSR-ERA, 230
   40-Hz ASSR, 279–280
   air-bone gap and, 379
   AC-ASSR thresholds, 379
   amplitude of, 83
   bone-conduction, 378
      vestibular response, 379–380
   CAEP measurement of, 329–330
   ERA, threshold estimates, 326
   M-ASSR (multiple stimuli), 216–**217**
   measurement of, 326
   multiple, 387
      BC stimuli, 378
   NHS/UNHS, 370
   polar plot, 215
Asymmetry, 15
Attention
   effects, 338, 341
   responses and, 338
Attention deficit hyperactivity disorder (ADHD), 343
Attenuation, 16
   filters and, 16
Audiogram, ripple effect, 122

Audiological management, 1-3-6 milestones for, 393
Audiology, 7
   computers and, **29–33**
Audiometry
   objective, 210
   pure-tone, 26
   pure-tone average (PTA), 396
   speech reception threshold (SRT), **251**, **351**, 396
   testing, standards, **42**
Auditory brainstem
   implants, 400
   response (ABR), 58, 83, 150, 177, 367
      AC elicited, 187
      AEPs (Auditory evoked potentials/responses) recording and, 83
      air conduction frequency-specific, 224
      amplitude ratio, (V/I) of ABR, 183
      BC, infant, **384**
      bone-conduction, 378
      British Society of Audiology (guideline), 91
      click-elicited, **236**
      differential diagnosis, 244, **247–254**
      ECochG (Electrocochleography) and, **171**
      electrode hedges, 407
      evaluation findings of lesions, **242**
      hearing loss, **233**
      hearing-threshold estimation and, 326
      ideal/modeled, **191**
      interpretation of, 178, 240–241
      latencies of, 238
      main positive peaks, **112**
      normal, **179**
      norms for, 239
      older children/young adults, **110**
      to rarefaction, **183**
      recording parameters for, **181**
      recordings, **182**
      simultaneous recording of, 180
      stacked ABR, 246–247
      transducer and, 186–187
      wave amplitudes, 246
   waveforms, 233–234
   microstructure, 122
   nerve
      near-field, compound action potentials, **431**
      fibers, IHCs (Inner hair cells) and, 64–65
   pathways
      central, 63
      lesions in, 245
   processing
      disorders, 344
      processing, evoked responses and, 447–448

Auditory brainstem (*continued*)
  steady-state responses (ASSRs), 75, 197, 209–219, 370
  system
    peripheral, **4**, 62
      stimulating, signal-issues particular to, 34–43
  training, 344–345
Auditory evoked potentials/responses (AEPs), **2**, 7, 22, 50, 83
  amplitude, interpolation method, 324
  bioelectrical systems and, 50
  block diagram of, **29**
  dependent variables of, 37
  derived from recordings, **283**
  extracting, from noise background, 84
  eye-related potential artifacts of, **109**
  field (AEF), **424**
  grammar/meaning and, 347
  in IONM, **432**
  late-late, 347
  LLR (long latency responses) and, 58
  long-latency and, **332**
  measurement applications, steady-state stimuli, 41
  obligatory, 313, 336
  online test assessment, 280
  overview of, **3**
  peak latency, 170
  recording, 83, 165
    examples, **85**
    infants, **389**
  review of, **411**
  sound, 401
  specifying sounds and, 28
  stimulus repetition
    effects on, 328
    rate function, **290**
  time continuum, 347
Auditory long latency response (ALLR), 285
  AMLR recording and, 285
  determining auditory thresholds with, 409
  ERA, 377
    vs. ABR-ERA, 324
      CAEP measurement approaches and, 332
      in workman's compensation, 314
Auditory meatus
  external, 63
  internal, 66
    nerve exits, 70
Auditory microstructure (ripple effect), 122
Auditory middle latency response (AMLR), 271–284, **274**, 409, 432
  acoustic click, **275**
  advancing age effect on, 280–281

artifacts, 277
  eyeblink/eye movement, 278
  power line, 277–278
  stimulus, 278
binaural interaction, 300, 302
deconvolution, 277
  developmental changes, 280
differential diagnostic applications of, 292–302
electrically elicited, 301
ERA and, 284–292
example of, **272**
generators, 293
illustrated, **301**
latencies/amplitudes values of, **272**
latency responses recorded, **285**
measures, during sleep, 287
obtained at various stimulus rates, **278**
obtained using 4000 clicks, **275**
P_b of, 314
recorded at C_z, **276**
salient features of, **294**
sex (of examinee), 283–284
simulation, **279**
stimulus/recording parameters, **273**
Auditory nerve fibers
  type I and II, 64–65
Auditory processing disorders, 343
  auditory training, 343
Auditory Response Telemetry (ART), 405
Auricle, 63
Autism, 343–344
Automated
  ABR (AABR), 369
    auditory brainstem response (AABR), 369
Automatic gain control, 66
Averaging, weighted, 90
Axons, demyelination of, 241

B

Background
  activity, random, 86
  noise, time history of, **107**
Backward TWs, 122
Band-pass filters, 16, 94
Basalward shift, 189
Base (of cochlea), 63
Basilar membrane (BM), 63–64, 123, **161**
  appearance of, 169
  displacement, **127**
Batteries
  DC (Direct-current) and, 50
  rotating, 61–62

in-vivo, 123
Bayesian weighting, 90
BC (Bone-conduction). *See* Bone conduction (BC)
BC-CAEP-ERA, 316
Beating, tones, 195
Bekesy's theory, of linear cochlea, 122
Bell-shaped curve, 372
Binaural
  difference potential, 194
  hearing, 193
  interaction component, **194–195**, 246, 296, 300, 302–306
  interaural timing differences, 320
  masking level differences, 320
Bioelectric signals
  hearing and, 62
  neurophysiology and, 49
  recording, 50
  systems, auditory evoked potentials/responses (AEPs) and, 50
Biomagnetic fields, **425**
Bipolar neurons
  myelinated, 66
  unmyelinated, 66
Blackman window, 23, 190
  tone bursts and, 274, 286
Block-mode averaging, 103
Bluetooth, **31**
BM (Basilar-membrane), 63–64, 123, **161**
  appearance of, 169
  displacement, **127**
Bone conduction (BC), 187
  ABR (Auditory brainstem response), **382**, 378
    applying to ERA, 316
    infant, **384**
  AC, recording ASSRs at same time, 387
  ASSRs, 378
    infants and, 379
    predict behavior, 226–228
    thresholds, adult, 379
  frequency-specific stimuli, 219, 224
  friendly adaptations for, infants, 381
  head positioning and, 381
  hearing
    maturational difference, 378
    sensitivity, 378
  infant sensitivity, applied in clinic, 380
  indirect measures, 385
  interaural attenuation (IA), 382
  narrowband level-specific CE-chirp, 379
  stimulus, 377
    for infants, **385**
    parameters, **220**
  testing, 377–388
    evoked response in infants, 377–378
    protocol, recommended, 380–381
  thresholds, electrophysiological assessment of, 380
  vibrator, 187
Box-whisker plot, **133**
Brain
  injury, late-late AEPs and, 347
  responses, illustration of spectrum, **197**
  waves, **3**
    AEPs (Auditory evoked potentials/responses) and, 28
    electroencephalogram (EEG) and, 49
Brainstem
  ASSR, 230
  implants, testing patients with, 400–412
  montage of, recording vertical component, **60**
  response. *See* Auditory brainstem response
  testing, **332–336**
Brainwaves, 3
British Society of Audiology, 91
  ABR testing and, 91
Broadband acoustic click, 144
Burst, tone, 9, 22
Bytes, 17

C

C (Condensation), electrical input/acoustical output signals, 37
CA (Cochlear amplifier), 123
CAEP (Cortical auditory evoked potential), 313
  amplitude of, 316–317, 318
    stimulus levels and, 324
  ASSR measured by, 329–330
  detection
    limits of sound, 327
    testing, 329
  developmental latency data for click-evoked, 319
  ERA and, 322–332
  evaluating visual limit of, 314
  latency of, 318
    stimulus levels and, 316, 324
  listener-related variables, 318
  measurements of, 328
  N_1 component, 314
  P_1, versus P_b (*See* AMLR), 314
  P_2 component, 314
  neuromaturation and, 328
  P_1-N_1-P_2 complex, **315**
  partial replots of, **325**
  recording, **317**
    young adults and elders, **320**

CAEP (Cortical auditory evoked potential) (*continued*)
   stimulus/recording parameters, **322**
   Stimulus-response dependencies, 315
   test system, 329
Calibration
   acoustic, **219**
   defined, 37
CANS (Central auditory nervous system), **4**, 63, 71–72, 169
   input signal to, 169
   schematic representation of, **71**
CAPDs (Central auditory processing disorders), 295–296
Capacitance, 52
Carhart-Jerger, Hughson-Westlake method modified, 324
Carrier
   gating of, 9
   sinusoidal pulse and, 22
CE-chirps, vs. clicks, 220–221
Central
   auditory
      input signal to, 169
      nervous system (CANS), **4**, 63, 71–72
         central auditory pathways, 63
         schematic representation of, **71**
      auditory pathway, lesions in, 245
Central processing unit (CPU), **31**
CEOAE (Clicked-evoked otoacoustic emission), 122, 130, 369
   comparison results, **370**
   example of, **132**
Cerebellopontine angle, 70
Cerebral spinal fluid (CSF), 63
Cerebrum
   international 10-20 system definitions, **55**
   photographs of, **76**
Certification in neurophysiologic intraoperative monitoring (CNIM), 436
Chewing, LLR (Long latency responses) and, 108
Chirps, 379
   stimulus, 190
      narrowband, 220
CI (Cochlear implants). *See* Cochlear implants (CI)
Circuits, ancillary, computer interface and, **30**
Claudius' cells, 64
Clicks
   acoustic
      AMLR, 34
      broadband, 144
   alternating polarity of, 92
   CE-chirps vs., 220–221

elicited ABR, **236**
evoked
   cochlear potentials, **145**
   otoacoustic emissions (CEOAE), 122, 130, 132, 369, **370**
Clinical
   evaluation, 293
   masking
      for infants, 386
      protocol, 222
   measures of interest, 293
   neurophysiology, 63
   protocols, with testing sequencing, 222
Clock, for computing, 18
CM (Cochlear microphonic), 142
CMR (Common mode rejection), 96–97
CN (Cochlear nucleus), 70
CNIM (Certification neurophysiologic intraoperative monitoring), 436
CNS (Central nervous system), 63
Cochlea, 17, 63
   active, 122
   electroanatomy of, **140**
   electrophysiological and, 138
   essential nonlinearity of, 143
   linear, Bekesy's theory of, 122
   potentials
      action, 141
      stimulus-related, 141
   promontory, 141
   properties of
      linear, 121
      passive, 121
   round-window recording, 141
   traveling wave and, 125
Cochlear
   amplifier (CA) 123
   filter, 232
   hearing loss, 232
   implants (CI), 164, 301, **332, 408**
      stimulator, 404
      telemetry incorporated in, 405
      testing patients with, 400–412
   microphonic, 65, 142
      recording, **167**
   nonlinearity, 122
   nucleus (CN), 70
   potentials, 139, 142
      click evoked, **145**
   sensorineural hearing loss, 235
Cognitive response, 313
Coherent averaging, reducing noise and, 86–90, **88**
Commissure of Probst, 70

Common mode rejection (CMR), 96–97
Communication systems, neurophysiology and, 49
Compensation-related utilization of neural circuits hypothesis (CRUNCH), 342
Complex, function/waveform, 9
Compound action potentials, 68, **69**, 142, 178, 432
Computers, importance of, **29–33**
   general-purpose, 29
   hard-, firm-, and software, 29
   CT scan/Computerized tomography, imaging, 248
Condensation (C), electrical input/acoustical output signals, 37
Conductive hearing loss, 234
   audiometric results, **234**
   recording sample case, **223**
Conductivity, 51
Consonant vowel (CV), 318
Continuous
   monitor, 428
   spectra, 21
   spectrum, 13
Conservation of energy, law of, 10
Copus callosum, 75
Cortical auditory evoked potential (CAEP), 313
   amplitude of, 316–317, 318
      stimulus levels and, 324
   ASSR measured by, 329–330
   detection
      limits of sound, 327
      testing, 329
   developmental latency data for click-evoked, 319
   ERA and, 322–332
   evaluating visual limit of, 314
   latency of, 318
      stimulus levels and, 316, 324
   measurements of, 328
   N1-P2 components of, 324
   neuromaturation and, 328
   P_1-N_1-P_2 complex, **315**
   partial replots of, **325**
   recordings, **317**
      young adults and elders, **320**
   stimulus/recording parameters, **322**
   test system, 329
   testing AEP, **332–336**
Cortical responses, obligatory, 338
Cortilymph, 64
Cost/benefit, NHS, 367
Counseling, preoperative, 405
Coupler, acoustic, defined, 35
CPU (Central processing unit), **31**
Crest factor, 39
Crossover stimulation, asymmetry of, 382

CRUNCH (Compensation-related utilization of neural circuits hypothesis), 342
CSF (Cerebral spinal fluid), 63
Cutoff frequencies, 15, 16
CV (Consonant vowel), 318
cVEMP, 439
C_Z
   ABR measurement and, 179
   AMLR recorded at, **276**
   CAEP recordings and, 317
   electrode
      montage and, 178
      placed at, 56, 61, 168
   hairline strategy, 55
   PAMR recorded at, **257**
   referent of, 54

D

D (Duration), pulse, 21
D-A (Digital to analog), conversion, 17
Dallos, Peter, **161**
Data, response to, 98–100
Davis, Hallowell, 123, 313
   ERA and, 323
Davis, Pauline, 323
dB (Decibel), 38
DC (Direct-current), **421**
   batteries and, 50
   pulse, 21
      time-domain representations of, **27**
   resting potentials, 139
Decibel (dB), 38
Deconvolution (of signals), 33, 201, 277, 284
Degenerative diseases, neural, 241
Dementia
   aging, 343
   Alzheimer's, 297, 343
Dendrites, 66
Descending (nerve fibers/pathways)
   efferent nerve fibers (auditory), 65
   motor pathways, 436
Detectability index, 213
Detection
   testing, CAEP, 329
   vs. discrimination, 445
Deterministic, effect, 180, 211
Deviant
   stimuli, 336
   target/nontarget, 338
Dewar, **425**
   outline of, **426**
Dieters' cells, 64

Difference tones, 15
Differential
    amplification, 95
        reducing noise and, 86
    amplifier, 95–96
    diagnostic
        applications, 231–247
        defined, 231
    neurodiagnosis, AMLR and, 294–295
Digital
    filtering, 95, 111
    sampling, 18
        of analog (input signal), **19**
    signal processors (DSP), **30**, **31–32**
    to analog (D–A), conversion, 17
Diotic presentation, AMLR and, 274
Dipole estimation, **421–422**
Direct
    current (DC), **421**
        batteries and, 50
        pulse, 21
        resting potentials, 139
    electrical synapses, 49
Discrete spectra, 13
Discrimination potentials, 336
Diseases, degenerative neural, 241
Distortion, 15
    harmonic, 35
    intermodulation, 35–36
    of output signal, 16
    product OAEs (DPOAEs), 126–134, 370
        BM displacement, **127**
        secondary source, 127
        system distortion, 128
Domain, 7
Dorsal-ventral cochlear nucleus (DVCN), **64**
    AEP peak latency, 170
    compression of the proximal 8th nerve, 243
    lesions beyond, 244–245
DP-gram, 128, **129**
    ABR and, 243
    of OAEs, 142
DPOAEs (Distortion product OAEs). See Distortion
        product OAEs (DPOAEs)
DSP (Digital signal processors), **30**, **31–32**
Duration (D), pulse, 21
DVCN (Dorsal-ventral cochlear nucleus). See Dorsal-
        ventral cochlear nucleus (DVCN)

E

Ear
    canal

pipe, 17
static pressure, on middle ear absorbance, **45**
stimulation (ECS), 405
middle, 17
outer, schematic representation of, **148**
ringing in, 134
Earcap, noise reduction, 390
Eardrum, 63
Early
    left anterior negativity (ELAN), 347
    maturation, AMLR and, 297
Earphone, 34
    frequency response of, **188**
    tubal insert, 390
Earplug, noise reduction, 390
ECG (Electrocardiogram), 10, 50, 106–107
ECochG (Electrocochleography), 147–159, 163
    ABR testing and, **171**
    CAP, 432
    chi-squared results, **156**
    examples of, **152**
    transtympanic, **164**
ECochGm, 154
    SP/AP measures, **155**
Ecologically valid stimuli, 284
EEAPS. See Electric-evoked auditory potentials
EEG (Electroencephalogram). See
        Electroencephalogram (EEG)
Effective
    duration, window, 23–24
    masking levels (EMLs), 225, 386–387
        bone conduction, auditory brainstem response,
        226
Efferent/descending nerve fibers, 65
Efficiency
    described, 395
    of multiple stimuli, 228
EFRs (Envelope-following responses), 197, 198
    amplitude, FFRs and, 198
    scalp recorded, 199
eHL (Estimated Hearing Level) correction factors, 380
ELAN (Early left anterior negativity), 347
Elastic headband, bone vibrator and, 381
Elective surgery, **442–444**
Electric
    evoked auditory potentials (EEAPs), 400
        stimulus artifacts and, 402
    shock, avoiding, 96
Electrical
    artifacts, 402
    current flow, 50
    isolation, 96
    shock, 96

Electrically
    elicited AMRLs, 301, 408
    evoked compound action potential (*eCAP*), 405
Electroacoustics, 34
Electrocardiogram (ECG), 10, 50, 106–107
Electrocochleography (ECochG), 147–159, 163
    chi-squared results, **156**
    examples of, **152**
    transtympanic, **164**
Electrocochleogram (ECochGm), 150
Electroculogram, 108
Electrode, 50
    clinically popular, **53**
    ground, 96
    impedance, 53
    metal, **51**
    montage, **53**, 56
    placement of, 54, 165
    surface, electric stimulation via, 436
    TM, 149
        recording parameters, **151**
Electroencephalogram (EEG), **3**, 50, 83
    analyses via advanced signal processing, 349–352
    brain waves and, 49
    data, **87**
    as extraneous signals, 83
    typical magnitudes of, **84**
Electrolyte paste, 52
Electromagnetic
    field, lines of flux, **423**
    induction, 96
    radiation, stimulus artifacts and, 188
Electro-motility, OHCs (Outer hair cells), 123
Electromyographic (EMG)
    interference, controlling, 86
    signals, common to motor nerve monitoring, **438**
Electromyography, facial evoked, 438
Electroneuronography (ENoG), 438
Electrophysiological
    cochlea and, 138
    imaging of brain, **422**
    objective measures, goals of, 219
    recordings, reducing noise in, 86
    signals, 17
    tools, **2**
Electrostatic interference, 97
ELH (Endolymphatic hydrops), 147–148
    ECochG (Electrocochleography), 164
    idiopathic, 153
EMG (Electromyographic) interference, controlling, 86

EMLs (Effective masking levels), 225, 386–387
    bone conduction, auditory brainstem response, **226**
    clinical masking procedures in infants, 387
Endocochlear potential (EP), 139
    test system, filters and, 95
Endogenous
    ERP, 313
    response, 336
Endolymph, 63
Endolymphatic hydrops (ELH), 147–148
    ECochG (Electrocochleography), 164
    idiopathic, 153
Energy reflectance (ER), **44**
Engineering, 7
ENoG (Electroneuronography), 438
Envelope
    following responses (EFRs), 197, 198
    local rate, 202
    periodicity of, **205**
    spectral, 13
    temporal, 22
EP (Endocochlear potential). *See* Endocochlear potential
Ephaptic coupling, 49
ER (Energy reflectance), **44**
ERA (Evoked response audiometry), 114, 134, 209, 365
    ASSRs, threshold estimates, 326
    CAEP and, 322–332
    Hallowell Davis and, 323
    hearing threshold estimates, 326
    using AMLR, 284–292
ERD (Event-related desynchronization), 351–352
ERP (Event-related potential), 313
    endogenous, 313
ERS (Event-related synchronization), 351
ERSP (Event-related spectral perturbation), 351
Estimation, hearing thresholds, 116
Estimated Hearing Level (eHL) correction factors, 380
ET (Extratympanic), 148
    recording, 146
ET-ECOCHG, applications of, **158**
Event-related
    desynchronization (ERD), 351–352
    potential (ERP), 313
    spectral perturbation (ERSP), 351
    synchronization (ERS), 351
Evoked
    potentials, 63
        audiometry, using auditory brainstem response/auditory steady-state response measurements, 219–231

Evoked (*continued*)
   response audiometry (ERA), 114, 134, 209, 284, 365
      ASSRs, threshold estimates, 326
      CAEP and, 322–332
      Hallowell Davis and, 323
      hearing threshold estimates, 326
      using AMLR, 284–292
   responses
      auditory processing and, 447–448
      recording, statistical detection methods, **99**
      test systems, 97
      testing, stimuli used in, **227**
Exogenous ERP/response, 313, 338
Expectation, effects, 338
Experiments, N-of-1, 1–2
External
   auditory meatus, 63
   ear, 63
Extratympanic (ET), 148
   recording, **146**
Eye/eyeblink movement
   ABR testing and, 278
   LLR (Long latency responses) and, 108

F

F test, **99**
Facial
   evoked electromyography, 438
   nerve
      monitoring, 435
      stimulation of, 435
False
   negatives, 371
      rate, 99
   positives, 371
      rate, 98–99
   signals, 18
Far field, 58
Faraday cage, 97
Fasciculus, superior longitudinal, 75
Fast function, 38
Fast-Fourier transform (FFT), 11, 126
FFRs (Frequency following responses), 197, 198
   amplitude, EFR and, 198
   line spectrum for, **208**
FFT (Fast-Fourier transform), 11, 126
Filtering
   concepts of, 93
   digital, 95, 111
   preamplifier stage, 111
   reducing noise and, 86

Filters, 16
   analog, 95
   anti-aliasing, 20
   attenuation and, 16
   band-pass, 16, 94
   high-pass, 16, 93
   low-pass, 16, 93
      aliasing and, 94
   notch, 94–95
   settings, high-pass (HP), 325–326
Fine-structure, 7, 195
   following responses, 198
   temporal (TFS), 205
   temporal varying feature (slowly vs. rapidly), 205
Firmware, **29**
First-order neurons, 139
Flowchart, 372, **373**
FM (Frequency modulation), 26
F_{mp} method, **99**
Force fields, three-dimensional, illustrations of, **58**
Formants, 13
Forward TWs, 122
Fourier, analysis/transform, 11, 126, 195
Frequency, 27, 170
   components, 10
   cutoff, **15**, 16
   domain representations, **35**
   following responses (FFRs), 197, 198
   fundamental, 196
      sample of, **12**
   line spectrum for, **208**
   "get rid of," 94–95
   makeup, 7
   missing fundamental, 196
   modulation (FM), 26
   Nyquist, 18, 20
   per latency, 170
   place coding of, 66
   of reciprocal, 8
   response, 16
      earphone, **188**
      of a notch, **94**
      SPL (Sound pressure level) and, 41
      ABRs, bone conduction, 224
   specificity, 22
   spectral nulls, 21–22
   stimuli, 336
      specific, 219
   time-domain-based metrics and, **205**
Fronto-vertex (F_Z) positions, recordings, 318
Frowning, LLR (Long latency responses) and, 108
F_{sp} method, 98, **99**

Fundamental frequency, 196
    sample of, **12**
F_Z (Fronto-vertex)
    CAEP recordings and, 317
    MMN and, 345
    positions, 318
    referent of, 54

G

Gain, output signal, 16
Galambos, Robert, 209
"Game of Waves," 104, **105**, 113
Ganglia, spiral, 66
Gated, sinusoidal pulse and, 22
Gating, of carrier, 9
Gaussian
    noise, 13, **14**
    window, frequency specificity, 286
Gd-DTPA MRI, tumor detection and, 245–246
Generation, 8
"Get rid of" frequencies, 94–95
Glutamate, hair cells, 66
Gold, Thomas, 121–122
Grammar, 347–**348**
Graphical user interface (GUI), **31**
Ground electrode, 96
GUI (Graphical user interface), **31**

H

Hair cells
    receptor potentials, 139
    transduction, **160**
Halfwave rectification, 214
Hansen's cells, 64
Hardware, **29**
    setup, **404**
Harmonic distortion, 35
Head, positioning of, audiometry and, 381
Headband, bone vibrator and, 381
Hearing, perception, 116
    aids/amplification, 301, 447
    binaural, **193**
    bioelectrical signals and, 62
    screening, 365
        newborn, 365, 367
            UNHS. see UNHS (Universal newborn hearing screening)
        universal newborn, 367
    sensitivity, bone-conduction, 378
    threshold,
        estimates, **166**, 326
    testing patients who exaggerate, 395–400
Hearing loss
    age-related, 297
    conductive, 234
    nonorganic, 396
        malingering, 396
    postlingual, 344
    sensorineural
        CAEP and, 321
        trend analysis of, **237**
Heisenberg uncertainty principle, 25
Heschl's gyrus, 75, 314
High-frequency controlled oscillator, 18
High-pass (HP) filters, 16, 93
    filter setting, 325–326
Hookup, flip-flop of, 169
Hormones, neurophysiology and, 49
Hotelling T^2, 98, 329
HP (High-pass)
    filters, 16, 93
    setting, 325–326
HT^2 method, **99**
Hubs, 13
Hughson-Westlake method, Carhart-Jerger modified, 324

I

I (Intensity), acoustic, 38
IA (Interaural attenuation), 224–225
    BC, 382
    values, 222
Iatrogenic injury, 434
IC (Inferior colliculus), 70
    midbrain and, 70
Idiopathic endolymphatic hydrops (ELH), 153
IEC (International Electrotechnical Commission), 41
    60645-3, **42**, 43
IHCs (Inner hair cells), 64–65
    Auditory nerve fibers and, 64–65
IID (Interaural intensity differences), 74
IL (Intensity level), 38
IM (intermodulation distortion), 126
Impedance, 53
    measurement, intracochlear electrode, 405
Impulses, signals, 26
Incus, 63
Induction, electromagnetic, 96
Infants
    BC testing, friendly adaptations for, 381
    bone-conduction, evoked response, 377–378
    CAEP and, 319
    clinical masking for, 386

Infants (*continued*)
  recording, auditory evoked responses, **389**
  REM sleep and, 287
Inferior colliculus (IC), 70
Infrequent stimuli, 336
Inner
  ear, 63
  hair cells (IHCs), 64–65
    auditory nerve fibers and, 64–65
Input-output (I-O) function, of CEOAE, 122
Input signal, gain, 16
Integrated circuit, 29
Insula, 75
Intensity (I)
  acoustic, 38
  functions, latency, comparison of, **375**
  level (IL), 38
Interaural
  attenuation (IA), 222, 224–225
  BC, 382
  indirect measures of, **385**
  latency difference, 239
  time differences (ITD), 74, 320
  values, 222
Interference, 30
  electrostatic, 97
  EMG (Electromyographic), controlling, 86
  reducing, 96, **97**
Intermodulation distortion (IM), 35–36, 126
Internal
  auditory meatus, 66
    nerve exits, 70
  capsule, 70
    MGB neurons, 75
International 10-20 system, **55**
International Electrotechnical Commission (IEC), 41
International Organization of Standards (ISO), 41
Interpeak (latency) intervals (IPLs), 184
Interpolate, 18
Interstimulus interval (ISI), ABR and, 184
Intertrial phase coherence (ITPC), 352
Intracochlear
  electrode, impedance measurement, 405
    recordings, signals of, **143**
    spread of excitation (SOE), 405
Intracranial, matter/fluid volume, **159**
Intraoperative
  course, 428
  monitoring (IOM), 428
  neuromonitoring, 428–441
    historical backdrop to, **429–430**

neurophysiological monitoring (IONM), **159**, 428, 431
IOM (Intraoperative monitoring), 428
IONM (Intraoperative neurophysiological monitoring), **159**, 428, 431
  historical backdrop to, **429–430**
  facial nerve monitoring, 435
  multimodal electrophysiology, 428
  position statement, 435
  technologists, 436
Ions, currents and, 50
IPLs (Interpeak (latency) intervals), 184
Ipsi- versus contralateral differences, **180**
Irritability, defined, 50
ISI (Interstimulus interval), ABR and, 184
ISO (International Organization of Standards), 41
  389-6, **42**, 43
Isolation, electrical, 96
ITD (Interaural time differences), 74
ITPC (Intertrial phase coherence), 352
  discrimination, **352**

J

JCIH (Joint Commission on Infant Hearing), 366, **368**
  1-3-6 milestones, 393
Jitter, 185
Judgment (of reliability), 104

K

KEMAR, 186
  time histories of clicks, **187**
Kemp, David, 122

L

Large-scale integration, of logic circuits, **30**
Late-late AEPs, 347
Latency
  ABR, 238
  action potentials and, **67**
  air-bone gap and, 234
  AMLR and, 271–284
  artificial shifts, 111
  defined, **4**
  functions, 181–182
    comparison of, **375**
  intensity (L-I), 170
    effects, **185**
    functions, 170

hypothetical, **171**
shifts of AP, **170**
interaural difference, 239
latency-shift, artificial, 111
measurement of, 68
of P_a and P_b components, **282**
per frequency, 170
response, 101
auditory middle, 271–284
stimulus level and, 316
variation trends of, **342**
Late-novelty P_3 or nP_3, 339
Lateral lemniscus (LL), 70
peri-olivary nuclei of, 70
Law, of conservation of energy, 10
Lesion, pure conductive, 232
Lesions
beyond DVCN, 244
in central auditory pathway, 245
evaluation of, **242**
peripheral nerve, 243
in pontine brainstem, **245**
space-occupying, 241
studies of, 340
L-I (Latency-intensity). *See* Latency
Line spectra, 13
Linear
coherent, OAEs (Otoacoustic emissions), 126
passive properties, cochlea, 121
protocol, CEOAE (Clicked-evoked otoacoustic emission), 130
Lissajous pattern/segments, 60
Listener-related variables, 318
LL (Lateral lemniscus), 70
peri-olivary nuclei of, 70
LLASSR (Long latency auditory steady-state response), 330
LLR (Long latency responses), **4**, 313
AEPs (Auditory evoked potentials/responses) and, 58
eyeblink and, 108
slow part of, 104
Lobes, spectral, 22
Local envelope rate, 202
Logic circuits, large-scale integration of, **30**
Long-latency
AEP, measurement, **332**
auditory steady-state response (LLASSR), 330
response (LLR), **4**, 313
AEP (Auditory evoked potentials/response) and, 58
amplitude of, 83
eyeblink and, 108

slow part of, 104
Loop-back adaptor, 111
Loudness, 10
Low-pass (LP) filters, 16, 93
aliasing and, 94
settings, 326
LP (Low-pass filters), 16, 93, 94
settings, 326

M

Magnetic resonance imaging (MRI), 250
Magnetoelectroencephalography (MEG), **424**
Magnitude
perceived, 10
resolution, 18
Malleus, 63
Masking
clinical, for infants, 386
level differences, binaural, 320
protocol, clinical, 222
M-ASSR, 216–217
Maturation, 318
ABR (Auditory brainstem response) and, 192
aging effects and, 341–342
early, AMLR and, 297
effects of, on N_a and P_a components, **282**
maturational difference in BC, 378
Maximum length sequences (MLS), 201
MCI (Mild cognitive impairment), 297
MD (Meniere's disease), 147–148
ECochG (Electrocochleography) and, 163
SP/AP complex and, 156
Meaning, responses and, 338
Media, scala, 63
Medial geniculate body (MGB), 70
MEG (Magnetoelectroencephalography), **424**
Memory, working, 339
Meniere's disease (MD), 147–148
ECochG (Electrocochleography) and, 163
SP/AP complex and, 156
Metal electrode, **51**
MGB (Medial geniculate body), 70
brachium, 70
Microphone, 34
probe, **44**
Midbrain, IC (Inferior colliculus) and, 70
Middle
ear, 17
absorbance, ear-canal static pressure, **45**
cavity, 63
latency response (MLR), **4**, 210
audiological applications, 284

Mild cognitive impairment (MCI), 297, 343
Mismatch negativity (MMN), 410
Missing fundamental, 196
MLR (Middle latency response), 4, 210
   audiological applications, 284
MLS (Maximum length sequences), 201
MMN (Mismatch negativity), 345–347
Modiolus, 64
Modulation, **9**
Monaural response, AMLR and, 274
Monotic response, AMLR and, 274
Montage, electrode, 56
Motility (of outer hair cells), 66
   motile response, 123–124
Motor
     acoustic-evoked motor response, 255
     evoked potentials, 428
     nerve monitoring, compared to
       electromyographic signals, **438**
Multiple sclerosis (MS), 241–244
   AMLR and, 295
Myelin, nerve conduction velocity and, 68
Myelinated bipolar neurons, 66
Myogenic responses, 108

N

N_1 component, 65, 314
   tracked to limit of visual detection, **316**
Narrowband
   chirp, 379
     stimuli, 220
   level-specific CE-chirp (NB CE-Chirp LS), 222
Natural sleep, 388
   testing during, 393
NB CE-Chirp LS (Narrowband level-specific CE-chirp), 222
Near field, 58
Negative damping, 122
Negativity that peaks at 400 ms, 347
Nerve
   conduction velocity, 68
   facial
     monitoring, 435
     stimulation of, 435
   fiber firing, spontaneous rate, 67
Neural
   arborization, 70
   degenerative diseases, 241
   generators, 273
     P_1-N_1-P_2 and, 314
   lesions, 240
   periodicity, strength of, **206**

Neural Response Imaging (NRI), 405
Neural Response Telemetry (NRT), 405
Neuroanatomy, of AEP space, 62–77
Neurodegenerative disorders, AMLR and, 295
Neurodiagnosis, differential, 294–295
Neurogenic responses, 108
Neuromaturation, 328
Neuromonitoring, Intraoperative, 428–441
Neuronal potentials, 67
Neurons, first-order, 139
Neurophysiology
   clinical, 63
   communication systems, 49
Nerve conduction velocity, 68
Newborn hearing screening (NHS), 365, 367
Newborn intensive care unit (NICU), 365
   AABR screening in, 369
   recording, auditory evoked responses, **389**
NHS (Newborn hearing screening), 365, 367
NICU (Newborn intensive care unit), 365
   AABR screening in, 369
   recording, auditory evoked responses, **389**
NLL (nuclei of the LL), 70
Nodes of Ranvier, 68
N-of-1 experiments, 1–2
Noise
   artifact rejection of, 90–92
     principle of, **91**
   background
     extracting response signal from, 83–100
     random, 86
     time history of, **107**
   coherent averaging of, 86–90
   extracting signals from, 445
   Gaussian, 13, **14**
   methods of reducing, 86
   nonphysiological, 84
     controlling, 86
   nursery levels of, 390
   physiological, 84
     controlling, 86
   as a quasi-steady-state phenomenon, 28
   random, 13, 88
   reducing, on electrophysiological recordings, 86
   reduction, 390
   residual, 106
   simulators, brainstem response, **391**
   stationary, 88
   white, 13
     stationary, effect of averaging, **89**

Nonlinear protocol, CEOAE (Clicked-evoked otoacoustic emission), 131
Nonlinearity, 15
  cochlea and, 122
  essential nonlinearity, 143
  nonlinear effect pf cochlear hearing loss, 232
Nonorganic hearing loss, 396
  malingering, 396
Nonphysiological noise, 84
  controlling, 86
Nonsensory variable, 213
Notch
  filter, 94–95
  frequency response of, **94**
Nuclei of the LL (NLL), 70
Nulls, spectral, 21
Nurseries, noise levels of, 390
Nyquist frequency, 18, 20

O

OAEs (Otoacoustic emissions). *See* Otoacoustic emissions (OAEs)
Objective
  audiometry, 210
  auditory tests, 138
  electrophysiological measures, goals of, 219
  objective measure of acoustic discrimination (*See* ACC)
  tests (statistical), for response detection, 280
  online assessment, 280
Obligatory
  AEP, 336
  cortical responses, 338
  response, 313, 354
OCB (Olivo-cochlear bundle), 165
Occlusion effect, 381
OHCs (Outer hair cells), 64
  depolarization of, 123
  electro-motility of, 123, **124**
Ohm's law, 38, **421**
Olivo-cochlear bundle (OCB), 165
On-effect, 74
Online, test assessment, AEP, 280
Onset response, 313
Operating system, 32
Organ of Corti, 63
  BM (basilar membrane) and, 64
  drawing of, **65**
  electrical properties of, 139
  endolymph production and, 154–155
  quasischematic representation, **67**
  receptor potentials, 138

Oscillographic display, voltage on, 39
Ossicular chain, 63
Otoacoustic emissions (OAEs), 122, 134–137
  absence of, 244
  click-evoked, 130, 369
  distortion product, **370**
  DP-gram, 142
  measurement of, 125–126
  NHS, 367
  stimulus frequency, 126
  suppression, **137**
Outer
  ear, 63
    schematic representation of, **148**
  hair cells (OHCs), 64
    depolarization of, 123
    electro-motility of, 123, **124**
Output signal
  asymmetry in, 15
  distortion of, 16
  gain, 16
oVEMP, 439

P

P1 component, 314
P_1-N_1-P_2 complex, 313, 314, 320–321
  CAEP, **315**
P_2 complex, 314
P_3 recording
  response to speech-token, standard and deviant, **341**
  settings for, **340**
P_{600} (Positivity that peaks at 600 ms), 347
PAC (Primary auditory cortex), 70
PAMR (Postauricular muscle response), **254–260**, 440
Parkinson's disease, late-late AEPs and, 347
Pass-fail criteria
  NHS, 371
  probability functions, 371
  statistical decision making, 371
  UNHS, 366
Passive-linear properties, cochlea, 121
Pathology, categories of, 241
Pathways, descending/motor, 436
Patients
  asleep, testing, 388–395
  testing, who exaggerate thresholds, 395–400
Pattern reversal, 441
Peak
  amplitude, sinusoid, 11
  equivalent SPL (peSPL), 38
    acoustic click, **40**

Peak (*continued*)
   process, 39
      using ppV, 39
   magnitudes, 10
   SPL (pSPL), 38
Peak-to-peak
   amplitude (A_{p-p}), 10–11
   voltage, peSPL (peak equivalent SPL) and, 39
Percept, measured, 37
Perception, measuring, 445–446
Perilymph, 63
Period, 8
   periodicity, envelope, 195, 205
   periodicity, neural, strength of, **206**
Peri-olivary nuclei, 70
   of LL (Lateral lemniscus), 70
Peripheral
   auditory system, **4**, 62
      illustrations of, **64**
   devices, **30**
   vestibular system, **159**
Peri-Sylvian area, 75
peSPL (Peak equivalent SPL), 38
   acoustic click, **40**
   process, 39
   using ppV, 39
Petrous portion, 70
Phase, 8
   coherence, **99**
   dispersion, 189
   locking, **205**
   shifts, 13
   of sine wave, 8
Phasor, 10
Phasor summation, 181
Physiological noise
   controlling, 86
   typical magnitudes of, 84
Pinna, 63
Pitch, voice, 202
Place-coding of frequency, 66
Placed-fixed reflection, OAEs (Otoacoustic emissions), 126
Place-frequency (tonal) axis, 407
Planum
   polare, 75
   temporale, 75
Plaques, MS and, 241
Plateau, window and, 24
Polar plot (ASSR), 215
Polarity, 36
Pons (of brainstem), 70
   pons-medulla junction, 70, 178

Porus acousticus, 70
Positivity that peaks at 600 ms (P_{600}), 347
Post
   stimulus-time histograms (PSTHs), 74
   synaptic potentials, 66–67
Postauricular muscle response (PAMR), **254–260**, 440
Postlingual hearing loss, 344
Post-stimulus-time histogram (PSTH), 73, 74
Potential
   action/spike-action, 141
   difference, 194
   myogenic, 93, 108
   neural/neurogenic, 141
   receptor/sensory, 67
   resting, 50
ppV (peak-to-peak voltage), peSPL (peak equivalent SPL) and, 39
Prestin, 123
Primary auditory cortex (PAC), 70
Principal component analysis, 339
Prism, **351**
Probability density function, 372
Probe microphone, **44**
Promontory, 141
Protocols, clinical, with testing sequencing, 222
pSPL (peak SPL), 38
PSTH (Post-stimulus-time histogram), 73, 74
Psychiatry, sensory gating and, 296–297
Psycho-physical method, hearing testing, 116
   Hughson-Westlake method, Carhart-Jerger modified, 324
   subjective, tests, 116
Pulse
   direct-current (DC), 21
   sinusoidal, 22
      time domain and, **23**
Pure
   conductive lesion, 232
   tone, 8
      audiometry, 26
      threshold comparisons, 324
P-values, 98
Pyramid, 70
P_z, referent of, 54

Q

Q samples test, 98, **99**

R

Radio-frequency (RF) signals, AEPs, 402
Random

magnitude, 10
noise, 13, 88
period, 10
random background activity, 86
Rapidly varying temporal feature, **205**
Rare stimuli, 336
Reactance, 53
Receiving operator characteristics/curves (ROCs), 213
Receptor potentials, hair cells, 139
Recording, 50
   AEPs (Auditory evoked potentials/responses), 83
   montage, clinical evaluation, 293
   sites, 56
   time history, 101, **102**
Rectification, halfwave, 214
Rectilinear window, 22–23
Reference sound level, 38
Refractory periods, 73
Reissner's membrane, 63, **161**
   distention of, **154**
Reliability, 133
REM sleep, 287
Repetition rate, 27
Reproducibility, 131
Residual noise, 106
Resistance, 50
Resistors, 50
Resolution, magnitude, 18
Response
   signal, extracting, from noise background, 83–100
   spectrum, 198
Responses
   adaptation, 184
   artifactual, 229
   cortical obligatory, 338
   detection of, objective (statistical) tests, 280
   endogenous, 336
   myogenic, 108
   neurogenic, 108
Resting DC potentials, 139
Retrocochlear pathology, 240
Retrograde traveling wave, 125
Ribbons, synaptic, 66
Right-hand rule, of direction of rotation of lines of flux, **423**, **424**
Ringing
   acoustic signal, 35
   in ear, 134, 300
Ripple effect, audiogram, 122
Rise-fall times, window and, 24
RMS (Root-mean-square) amplitude, 11
   split-buffer's difference, 106
   value, 13

ROCs (Receiving operator characteristics/curves), 213
Roll-off, cutoff frequencies and, 16
Root-mean-square (RMS) amplitude, 11
   split-buffer's difference, 106
   value, 13
Round-window
   stimulation (RWS), 405
   recording, cochlea, 141

S

Saltatory conduction, 68
SAM (Single-modulation frequency), 210
SAM (Sinusoidally amplitude modulated), 199
Sampling
   digital, 18
   rate, 18
   theorem, 18
   rate effects, demonstration of, **20**
Scala tympani, 63
   intracochlear recordings, signals of, **143**
Scales, time-weighted, 38
Schizophrenia, 342–343
Schwann cells, 241
Screening hearing responses, vs. threshold estimation/estimating audiometric configuration, 365–377
Secondary DPOAE source, 127
Sedation
   American Academy of Pediatrics on, 393
   need for, 393
Sensitivity
   microphone, 41
   test performance and, 371
Sensorineural hearing loss
   CAEP and, 321
   cochlear, 235
   trend analysis of, **237**
Sensory
   evoked potentials, 428
   gating, 296–297
Sensory psychology, 1
Sex effects, 342
SFOAE (Stimulus frequency OAE), 126, 130
Shock, electric, avoiding, 96
Short latency response (SLR), **4**, **138**, 177
Signal-to-noise ratio (SNR), 13–14, 88, 198
Signal detection theory, 213
   detectability index, 213
   receiver operating characteristics (ROC), 213
Signals
   analog, 17

Signals (*continued*)
   analyses of, 10
   conditioning, 93
   detection theory, 213
   extracting from noise, 445
   false, 18
   generation/analysis/conditioning, analog vs. digital, 7–20
   impulses, 26
   sample of, **9**
   steady-state, 26
   transients, 26
Silver-silver-chloride (Ag-AgCl), 51
   electrodes, 52
Sine wave, phase of, 8
Single-unit discharge/potential, 67
Sinusoid/sinusoidal, 8
   combining two, 10, **11**
   generation of, 8, **8**
   harmonically related, 10
   peak amplitude, 11
   pulses, 9
Sinusoidal pulse, 9, 22
   time domain and, **23**
Sinusoidally amplitude
   Modulated (SAM), 199, **281**
      carrier, **215**
      noises-broadband vs. narrowband, 201
Sleep, 287–288
   natural, 388
      testing during, 393
   REM, 287
   testing patients, 388–395
SLM (Sound level meter), 38, 41
sLOETA (standardized low resolution brain electromagnetic tomography), **422**
Slow
   negative wave (SN_{10}), 111
   wave, 339
Slowly varying temporal feature, **205**
SLR (Short latency responses), **4**, **138**, 177
SN_{10} (slow-negative wave), 111
SNR (Signal-to-noise ratio), 13–14, 88, 198
   higher amplitude responses and, 327
SOAEs (Spontaneous otoacoustic emissions), 134, **134–137**
SOC (Superior olivary complex), 70
Software, **29**
Somatosensory evoked potential (SSEP) 436, compared to AMLR, **437**
Sound
   defined, 34

   level meter (SLM), 38, 41
   pressure, 38
SP (Summating potential), 65, 144
Space-occupying lesions, 241
SP/AP
   amplitude ratio, 150
   complex, duration of, **155**
   measurement of, **157**
   ratio, computation of, 156
Spectra
   discrete, 13
   line, 13
Spectral
   analyses, 7, 13
   envelope, 13
   lobes, 22
   nulls, 21
   ripple noise, spectrogram of, **353**
   views, temporary vs., 20–33
Spectrum, continuous, 13
Speech-evoked, EFR/FFR, **205–209**
Spike-action potentials, 67
Spiral
   ganglia, 66
   ligament, 64
   limbus, 66
SPL (Sound pressure level), 38
   frequency response, 41
   microphone sensitivity, SLM, 41
Splatter
   Blackman window and, 23
   sinusoidal pulse and, 22
Split-buffer averaging, 92, 105
Spontaneous
   otoacoustic emissions (SOAEs), 134
   rate, nerve-fiber firing, 67
SP-to-AP ratio, 167
SQUID (superconducting quantum interference devices) gradiometers, **425**
SSC (Superior semicircular canal), **159**
SSCD (Superior semicircular canal dehiscence), **159**
SSEP (Somatosensory evoked potential), 436
   recording and, 436
Stacked-ABR, 246
Standard deviation, 11
Standard, national/international, 38
   calibration and, 39
   current, 42
   organizations, 41
Standing waves, 16
   generating, on a string, **17**

Stapes, 63
Stationarity of response, noise and, 90
Stationary
  noise, 88
  signal, 90
Steady state, 9
  responses, 98
  signals, 26
  stimuli, AEP measurement applications and, 41
Stereocilia, 139
  tip links and, 66
Stimulating hardware setup, **404**
Stimulation, electrical, CI-related
  direct/indirect, 404
  ear canal, 405
  electrical, facial nerve (IONM), 435
  round window, 405
Stimuli, auditory, understanding, 446
Stimulus
  artifacts, 92, 188, 278, 402
  ecologically valid, 284
  efficiency of multiple, 228
  frequency OAE (SFOAE), 126, 130
  frequent, 336
  level, AMLR and, 274
  level dependence, 232
    CAEP latency and, 316
  parameters, **220**
  rate, 144
    ABR and, **183**, 184
  response dependencies, CAEP and, 315
  speech, 14, 203
Stimulus-related potentials, 141
Stria vascularis, 64
Stroke, AMLR and, 295
Subcutaneous/needle electrodes, 436
Subjective judgment, 220
Summating potential (SP), 65, 144
Superconducting quantum interference devices
    (SQUID) gradiometers, **425**
Superior
  longitudinal fasciculus, 75
  olivary complex (SOC), 70
  semicircular canal (SSC), **159**
    dehiscence (SSCD), **159**
  temporal gyrus, 56, 75
Supporting cells, 64
Surface electrodes, electric stimulation via, 436
Swallowing, interference and, 108
Synapses, operating time, 167
Synaptic
  cleft, 66
  delays, 68
  ribbons, 66
  transmission, 49
Synchronously (coherently) averaged, 198
System distortion, 128
  sweeps (epochs taken for average), 88
Synchronized, 87
Synthesis, 8

T

Target population, of AMLR, 292–293
TB (Trapezoid body), 70
TBI (Traumatic brain injury), AMLR and, 295
T-complex, 314
TEABR (Telehealth-enabled ABR), 230
Technologists, IONM, 436
Tectorial membrane, 66
Telehealth-enabled ABR (TEABR), 230
Telemetry, incorporated in cochlear implants, 405
Template cross-correlation, **99**
Temporal
  analyses, 7
  bone, peripheral auditory system and, 63
  envelope, 22
  fine structure (TFS), **205**
  time history and, 8
  views, vs. spectral, 20–33
Testing sequencing, clinical protocols with, 222
Test-retest
  recordings, 100
  repeatability, 98
TFS (Temporal fine structure), **205**
Thalamocortical
  pathway, 75
    potentials, 293
    response, 314
Thalamus, 70
Theorem, sampling, 18
Three-channel Lissajous trajectories (3CLTs), 59–61
Thresholds
  comparing, 324
  estimation/estimating audiometric configuration, vs.
      screening hearing responses, 365–377
  hearing, testing patients who exaggerate, 395–400
Time
  history
    recording, 101, **102**
    temporal analyses and, 8
  resolution, adequate, 18

Time (*continued*)
  space
    continuum, 4
    time-space recap, **408**
  weighted scales, 38
Time domain
  pulses, 21
  representations, **26, 36**
    DC (Direct-current) pulse, **27**
    of two tones, **196**
    sinusoidal pulse and, **23**
Time-frequency
  analysis, 350
    normalizing, 350–351
    realities, **202**
Tinnitus, 134, 300
TM electrodes, 149
  recording parameters, **151**
TOAE (Transient-evoked otoacoustic emission), **136**
Tones
  adjust level of, 40
  bursts, 9, 22, 141
    alternating polarity of, 92
    Blackman-windowed, 274, 286
    detection limits of sound, 327
  difference, 15
  envelope for, 195
  original, 195
  spectrum of pair, **197**
Tonotopical organization, 72
  tonotopicity, 72, **73**
  tonotopy, ABI electrode array and, 407–408
Tonotopical organization/tonotopicity, 72
Tract (definition of, versus nerve), 70
Transcutaneous electro-magnetic induction, 403
Transducers,
  ABR and, 186–187
  active, 122
  stimulus levels and standards, 446
Transduction
  acoustic stimulus measuring and, 34
  processes, 63
  of signal, 8
Transfer functions, 34, 232
Transformative transduction processes, 63
Transient, 9
  evoked response, 122
  otoacoustic emission (TOAE), 136
  signals, 9, 26
Translational research, 345–347
Transmission, wideband, **43–45**

Transtympanic
  ECochG, **164**
  (TT) recordings, 148, **150**
Trapezoid body (TB), 70
Traumatic brain injury (TBI), AMLR and, 295
Traveling wave, 64, 121
  backward, 122
  cochlea and, 125
  development of, **125**
  forward, 122
  retrograde, 125
  reverse, energy and, 122
Triggered, 87
True
  negatives, 371
  positives, 371
TT (Transtympanic)
  ECochG, 165
  electrode, 146
  recordings, 148, **150**
    vs. Extratympanic (ET) ECochG, **150**
Tubal insert earphones, 390
Tumors
  ABR testing and, 241
  acoustic, 241, 434
    nerve, 241
  detection of, 245–246
Tunnel of Corti, 64
TW (Traveling wave), 64, 121
  forward/backward, 122
  reverse, energy and, 122
Tympani, scala, 63
Tympanic membrane, 63
Tympanometry, conventional, **43**
Tymptrodes, 149
  placing a, **151**

U

UART (Universal asynchronous receiver/transmitter), **31**
Uncertainty principle, Heisenberg, 25
UNHS (Universal newborn hearing screening), 365–368
  1-3-6 milestones, 393
    identification, diagnosis, intervention, 365–366
    pass-fail criteria, 366
  justifications, **367**
  most common tests
    OAEs and ABR, 367
  recommendations, **373**
Universal asynchronous receiver/transmitter (UART), **31**

Universal newborn hearing screening (UNHS), 365–368
   1-3-6 milestones, 393
   justifications, **367**
   recommendations, **373**
Universal serial bus (USB), **31**
Unmyelinated bipolar neurons, 66
USB (Universal serial bus), **31**

V

VDLs (Visual detection limit), 182, 375
   ABR relationship with, 326
   estimating, **212**
   replot of data, **214**
   virtual demonstration of, 291
VEMPs (Vestibular evoked myogenic potentials), 439
   reduced, 440
Vertex-positive peaks, of ABR, 178
Vestibular
   apparatus, **159**
   evoked myogenic potentials (VEMPs), 439
   overview of, c- versus oVEMPS, 439, **440**
      responses, 379
   peripheral system, 439
   reduced, 440
Vestibuli, 63
Visual detection limit (VDL), 182, 375
   ABR relationship with, 326
   estimating, **212**
   replot of data, **214**
   stimulus levels and, 324
   virtual demonstration of, 291
Visual evoked potential (VEP), 440–441
Voice pitch, 202

Voltage, 50
   measurements, 405
   on oscillographic display, 39
   three-dimensional, illustrations of, **58**

W

WAI (Wideband acoustic immittance), **44**
Wave
   amplitudes, ABR (Auditory brainstem response), 246
   fixed, OAEs (Otoacoustic emissions), 126
   V component, determining presence or absence of, 222
Waveform, 7
   ABR, 233–234
   visual inspection of, 98
WBNs (Well-baby nurseries), **368**, 369
Weber's law, 38
Weighted averaging, 90
Well-baby nurseries (WBNs), **367**, 369
Wever, Glen, 139
White noise, 13
Whole-nerve
   action potential, 65, 178
   response, 142
Wideband
   acoustic immittance (WAI), **44**
   transmission, **43–45**
Window
   Blackman, 23
   effective duration, 23
   rectilinear, 22–23
   sinusoidal pulse and, **24**
   spectra for two different, **24**
Windowing, of carrier, 9
Working memory, 339